Photodynamic Therapy in Dermatology

Xiuli Wang • Bo Wang
Editors

Photodynamic Therapy in Dermatology

Springer

同济大学出版社
TONGJI UNIVERSITY PRESS

Editors
Xiuli Wang
Institute of Photomedicine
Shanghai Skin Disease Hospital, School of Medicine, Tongji University
Shanghai, China

Bo Wang
Avera Medical Group Dermatology
Aberdeen, SD, USA

ISBN 978-981-96-8914-9 ISBN 978-981-96-8915-6 (eBook)
https://doi.org/10.1007/978-981-96-8915-6

Jointly published with Tongji University Press Co., Ltd.

The print edition is not for sale in China (Mainland). Customers from China (Mainland) please order the print book from: Tongji University Press Co., Ltd..

This Springer imprint is published by the registered company Springer Nature Singapore Pte Ltd.
The registered company address is: 152 Beach Road, #21-01/04 Gateway East, Singapore 189721, Singapore

Contents

Editors and Contributors

About the Editors

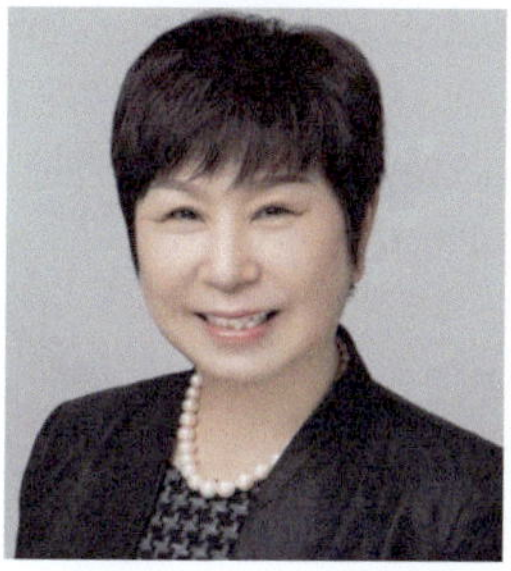

Xiuli Wang the chief physician at Shanghai Skin Disease Hospital, has been leading basic photodynamic therapy (PDT) and clinical research on skin diseases since 1996. In China, Dr. Wang pioneered the use of ALA-PDT for treating urethral genital warts and subsequently expanded its indications to include acne, skin cancer, and other HPV-related diseases. Her work on PDT for HPV-related diseases has influenced the guidelines for managing genital warts and female lower reproductive tract diseases. Dr. Wang serves as a Board Member of the International Photodynamic Association (IPA), Chair of the Chinese Association of Rehabilitation Dermatology, Deputy Editor-in-chief of *Photodiagnosis and Photodynamic Therapy*, and Chief Expert at the Chinese Medical Association's PDT Research Collaboration Group, promoting PDT through training and advocacy in more than 1000 hospitals. She has authored 350 scientific papers, including 220 in English, and contributed to eight critical guidelines, such as "Chinese Guidelines on the Clinical Application of 5-Aminolevulinic Acid Photodynamic Therapy in Dermatology" and "Clinical Practice Guidelines for 5-Aminolevulinic Acid Photodynamic Therapy for Acne Vulgaris in China (2022)." She was honored with the "Clinical PDT Research Excellence Award" from the IPA in 2022. As a frequent speaker at major dermatology societies, she has led 16 national PDT projects, organized 7 Shanghai PDT Summits, and hosted 9 international conferences. Dr. Wang has secured 25 research grants and 6 NSFC programs and has coauthored 19 books, including *Photodynamic Therapy for Skin Diseases*

(2023), *Technical Specifications for Photodynamic Therapy* (2020), and *Practical Applications of Photodynamic Therapy in Dermatology: Pocket Book* (2016). Dr. Wang and her research team hold nine Chinese national patents. Her impact on PDT and dermatology is transformative and globally recognized.

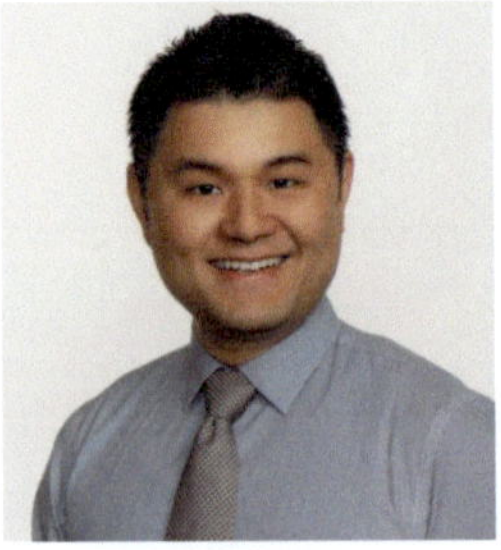

Bo Wang is a dermatologist at Avera Medical Group Dermatology and a Clinical Assistant Professor at the University of South Dakota, Medical School. He earned his M.D. from Shanghai Jiao Tong University, Medical School, and his PhD in neuroscience from the University of Michigan, Ann Arbor. He completed his internship at Lincoln Medical Center, Weill Cornell Medicine, followed by dermatology residency training at the University of Michigan. He is double board-certified in Dermatology and Mohs Micrographic Dermatologic Surgery by the American Board of Dermatology. He also serves as a reviewer for multiple international journals, including JAAD, BJD and JAMA Dermatology.

Dr. Wang has studied and worked on photodynamic therapy (PDT) for skin diseases for more than 10 years. Dr. Wang proposed the threshold theory of photodynamic pain, published in the *British Journal of Dermatology* in 2014, and then promoted research on painless photodynamic therapy. Dr. Wang has published 56 peer-reviewed English articles on dermatology and PDT, including "Clinical Practice Guidelines for 5-Aminolaevulinic Acid Photodynamic (2022)."

Dr. Wang participated in Photodynamic Therapy for Skin Diseases (2023), Practical Applications of Photodynamic Therapy in Dermatology: Pocket Book (2016).

Contributors

Yajing Cao Institute of Photomedicine, Shanghai Skin Disease Hospital, School of Medicine, Tongji University, Shanghai, China

Zhi Cao Institute of Photomedicine, Shanghai Skin Disease Hospital, School of Medicine, Tongji University, Shanghai, China

Qihang Chang Institute of Photomedicine, Shanghai Skin Disease Hospital, School of Medicine, Tongji University, Shanghai, China

Chengqian Chen Institute of Photomedicine, Shanghai Skin Disease Hospital, School of Medicine, Tongji University, Shanghai, China

Jiawen Gao Institute of Photomedicine, Shanghai Skin Disease Hospital, School of Medicine, Tongji University, Shanghai, China

Jianhua Huang Department of Dermatology, Huadong Hospital, Fudan University, Shanghai, People's Republic of China

Caihe Liao Institute of Photomedicine, Shanghai Skin Disease Hospital, School of Medicine, Tongji University, Shanghai, China

Chunxiao Li Institute of Photomedicine, Shanghai Skin Disease Hospital, School of Medicine, Tongji University, Shanghai, China

Jiandan Li Institute of Photomedicine, Shanghai Skin Disease Hospital, School of Medicine, Tongji University, Shanghai, China

Xiaojing Liu Institute of Photomedicine, Shanghai Skin Disease Hospital, School of Medicine, Tongji University, Shanghai, China

Zhijie Ruan Institute of Photomedicine, Shanghai Skin Disease Hospital, School of Medicine, Tongji University, Shanghai, China

Shuzhan Shen Institute of Photomedicine, Shanghai Skin Disease Hospital, School of Medicine, Tongji University, Shanghai, China

Jingjuan Shi Institute of Photomedicine, Shanghai Skin Disease Hospital, School of Medicine, Tongji University, Shanghai, People's Republic of China

Lei Shi Department of Dermatology, Huadong Hospital, Fudan University, Shanghai, People's Republic of China

Dixin Wang Institute of Photomedicine, Shanghai Skin Disease Hospital, School of Medicine, Tongji University, Shanghai, China

Hongwei Wang Department of Dermatology, Huadong Hospital, Fudan University, Shanghai, People's Republic of China

Peiru Wang Institute of Photomedicine, Shanghai Skin Disease Hospital, School of Medicine, Tongji University, Shanghai, China

Long Wen Institute of Photomedicine, Shanghai Skin Disease Hospital, School of Medicine, Tongji University, Shanghai, China

Jin Yang Institute of Photomedicine, Shanghai Skin Disease Hospital, School of Medicine, Tongji University, Shanghai, China

Yuling Yang Institute of Photomedicine, Shanghai Skin Disease Hospital, School of Medicine, Tongji University, Shanghai, China

Yutong Yang Institute of Photomedicine, Shanghai Skin Disease Hospital, School of Medicine, Tongji University, Shanghai, China

Jia Yan Institute of Photomedicine, Shanghai Skin Disease Hospital, School of Medicine, Tongji University, Shanghai, China

Yu Yan Institute of Photomedicine, Shanghai Skin Disease Hospital, School of Medicine, Tongji University, Shanghai, China

Qingyu Zeng Institute of Photomedicine, Shanghai Skin Disease Hospital, School of Medicine, Tongji University, Shanghai, China

Guolong Zhang Institute of Photomedicine, Shanghai Skin Disease Hospital, School of Medicine, Tongji University, Shanghai, China

Haiyan Zhang Institute of Photomedicine, Shanghai Skin Disease Hospital, School of Medicine, Tongji University, Shanghai, China

Linglin Zhang Institute of Photomedicine, Shanghai Skin Disease Hospital, School of Medicine, Tongji University, Shanghai, China

Yunfeng Zhang Institute of Photomedicine, Shanghai Skin Disease Hospital, School of Medicine, Tongji University, Shanghai, China

Zijun Zhao Institute of Photomedicine, Shanghai Skin Disease Hospital, School of Medicine, Tongji University, Shanghai, China

History of Photodynamic Therapy

1

Zhi Cao, Hongwei Wang, Bo Wang, and Xiuli Wang

1.1 The Discovery of Photosensitivity

One of the earliest records of photosensitivity can be traced back to the sixteenth century when sunlight exposure followed by buckwheat intake induced a skin response in animals. In the eighteenth century, people in Sicily and Naples reported that white sheep developed severe skin reactions after consuming hypericum, such effects were not observed in black sheep [1].

1.2 Discovery of the Photodynamic Effect

Photodynamic therapy (PDT) traces its origin to Germany in 1900. The first significant observation was made by Oscar Raab, a medical student at the University of Munich, who did not notice that paramecium thrived in culture medium containing acridine and similar dyes in the dark but died when exposed to light. Further investigation indicated that this phenomenon was influenced not only by the concentration of acridine but also by the illumination intensity. This marked the first PDT research that verified the cytotoxic effect of the combined application of light and chemical substances, laying the groundwork for photodynamic research [2].

Raab's supervisor, Professor von Tappeiner, expanded on this research and conducted a series of experiments on the interaction between light and the photosensitization of dyes. His work demonstrated the potential of photosensitizers in photochemotherapy. In 1903, together with Professor Jesionek, Professor von Tappeiner explored the application of eosin combined with light for treating patients with basal cell carcinoma (BCC). The lesions were treated with 1% eosin solution and then exposed to sunlight or a mercury lamp. The results were promising as four of the six patients achieved complete clearance without relapse after 1 year. This study, published in 1907, was the first clinical investigation of photosensitizers combined with visible light for the treatment of skin cancers.

To differentiate this photosensitized response from the photosensitization of photoplate to light, Professor von Tappeiner introduced the term

Z. Cao · X. Wang
Institute of Photomedicine, Shanghai Skin Disease Hospital, School of Medicine, Tongji University, Shanghai, China
e-mail: wangxiuli_1400023@tongji.edu.cn

H. Wang (✉)
Department of Dermatology, Huadong Hospital, Fudan University, Shanghai, People's Republic of China

B. Wang
Avera Medical Group Dermatology, Aberdeen, SD, USA

University of South Dakota, Vermillion, SD, USA
e-mail: makiwang@med.umich.edu

X. Wang, B. Wang (eds.), *Photodynamic Therapy in Dermatology*, https://doi.org/10.1007/978-981-96-8915-6_1

"photodynamic" in *Clinics in Dermatology* in 1904 [3]. He also identified the oxygen-dependent nature of the process, emphasizing that both dyes and light could not induce cell death without the presence of oxygen. This recognition of oxygen as a key element in the photodynamic effect was a crucial advancement [3]. In 1912, Dr. Meyer-Betz conducted a self-experiment with hematoporphyrin (Hp), where he reported that Hp could induce a photosensitive reaction under sunlight. After intravenous injection of 200 mg of Hp, the patient experienced significant edema and pain in his forearms the following day. Subsequent outdoor exposure induced severe acute phototoxic reactions on the patient's face and hands, followed by months of photosensitive response. His findings confirmed that both Hp and light illumination were essential elements for inducing photosensitive reactions in the skin [4].

Later, in 1924, Albert Policard reported more intense red fluorescence from tumors than from surrounding tissue in animal models. This observation laid the foundation for the concept of fluorescence localization in tumors. Unfortunately, this research did not draw immediate attention, and subsequent research progressed slowly over the following two decades [5, 6].

1.3 Mechanistic Study of the Photodynamic Effect

After nearly two decades of stagnation, the application of the photodynamic effect in the diagnosis and treatment of malignancies has gained renewed attention [6]. In 1942, Auler and Figge made a significant breakthrough by reporting the damaging effect of Hp combined with light on tumor tissue. They reported that when Hp was injected into rats, it accumulated in tumor tissue and emitted orange fluorescence when it was excited by ultraviolet light. Upon exposure to sunlight, the tumor tissue is injured, suggesting that Hp combined with light could be a promising new antitumor therapy [7]. In the same year, Auler and Banzer conducted a similar study in which sunlight illumination was replaced with a quartz lamp and reported that Hp combined with this light source promoted tumor necrosis. They initiated clinical experiments using Hp and quartz lamps for tumor patients, but their research was interrupted by World War II.

As research has progressed, more porphyrins, including coprophyrins, uroporphyrins, protoporphyrins, and hematoporphyrin-zinc complexes, have been discovered and purified. In 1948, Figge and Weiland reported that various porphyrins accumulate in tumor, embryonic, and wound tissues and that the emitted fluorescence can be used for tumor diagnosis [8]. In 1951, Manganiello reported that porphyrins also accumulate in wound, lymph node, and placenta tissues [9]. In 1953, Peck reported that metallic porphyrin compounds can accumulate in tumor tissue [10]. In 1955, Rassmussen-Taxdal reported three patients with benign tumors and eight patients with malignant tumors who were injected with a high dose of hemoporphyrin (500–1000 mg). Orange fluorescence could be observed in seven malignant tissues at 3–12 h after injection, while only one case of a benign lesion had detectable fluorescence [11]. Research has shown that fluorescence intensity from the tumor is positively correlated with the hematoporphyrin dose, indicating that the tendency of porphyrin to accumulate in tumor tissue could be used for tumor diagnosis and to define the macroscopic surgical resection margin [11]. This is the first report of photodynamic diagnosis, but the high dose of hematoporphyrin required for tumor fluorescence diagnosis causes severe phototoxic reactions, affecting not only tumor tissue but also normal skin, which limits its clinical application. Improving the efficiency of the fluorescence-based diagnosis of hematoporphyrin while reducing adverse effects has become an urgent challenge.

In 1955, Schwartz reported that the hematoporphyrin used in previous studies was a mixture of porphyrin compounds. He subsequently processed the crude hematoporphyrin with glacial acetic acid and sulfuric acid, obtaining a new porphyrin mixture called hematoporphyrin derivative (HpD). Compared with Hp, this derivative exhibited better specificity and photodynamic toxicity to tumor tissue and accumulated significantly less in lymphatic tissue [12]. Owing to these advantages, HpD has been successfully applied in clinical settings and remains one of the most common photosensitizers today. In 1960, Lipson and Baldes demonstrated the superiority of HpD over Hp in not only tumor fluorescence diagnosis and localization but also photodynamic toxicity. They conducted tumor fluorescence diagnosis and localization with HpD in 50 cases of bronchogenic carcinoma and esophageal carcinoma, and the fluorescence was observed by bronchoscopy as well as esophagoscopy. The concept of "fluorescence endoscopic diagnosis" was proposed for the first time [13]. In 1966, Lipson reported the application of HpD combined with white light irradiation for the treatment of metastatic breast cancer on the chest wall, and partial necrosis of tumor tissue was observed in this study [14]. In 1968, Gregorie and his team reported a study on HpD fluorescence diagnosis involving 226 tumor cases, including 173 cases of malignant tumors. Among these malignant tumors, 132 exhibited orange fluorescence, yielding a positive detection rate of 76.3% (132/173) [15].

1.4 Pioneering Studies in Photodynamic Therapy

In 1972, Diamond and colleagues supplemented the culture medium of glioma cells with Hp and irradiated them with white light, resulting in the complete death of the glioma cells. They further injected Hp into a rat model of cutaneous squamous cell carcinoma followed by light exposure 24 h later. The results showed that the growth and volume of the implanted tumors were significantly reduced, which confirmed the therapeutic effect of Hp-PDT on tumors. This study, reported in *The Lancet*, was the first to use the term "photodynamic therapy (PDT)" to describe this treatment [16].

In 1975, Thomas Dougherty advanced this field by injecting HpD into mouse and rat models with transplanted tumors, followed by illumination with red light. The efficacy of this treatment exceeds that in previous reports [17]. Later, this approach was successfully applied in breast cancer patients who were resistant to traditional therapies [18]. In the same year, Kelly and colleagues established a xenograft tumor mouse model via the subcutaneous injection of tumor cells isolated from human bladder cancer. The tumors became ulcerated and necrotic after HpD-PDT, whereas the surrounding normal tissue showed only mild edema. Conversely, when HpD-PDT was used on mouse models injected with epidermal cells or smooth muscle cells, the treatment was weak or even ineffective [19]. In 1976, Kelly applied PDT to a patient with recurrent bladder cancer. He inserted an optical fiber connected with a 200 W mercury vapor light source into the bladder of the patient via the urethra, with 30 min of illumination. Necrosis of the tumor tissue was observed 48 h after illumination in the treated area, whereas no obvious change was observed in the untreated area. These findings indicate that PDT has good selectivity for tumors [20]. In 1978, PDT was performed on 113 primary or metastatic skin cancers in 25 patients. The primary cancers included cutaneous squamous cell carcinoma (cSCC), BCC, and malignant melanoma. Metastatic cancers originate from the breast, colon, and endometrium. All patients had previously failed to respond to traditional treatments. The results revealed that 98 lesions completely regressed and that 13 showed a partial response after HpD-argon arc illumination. Adverse reactions included local erythema and edema and, in severe cases, local skin necrosis. These adverse reactions can be mitigated by photoprotection after therapy [21]. This study, the largest at the time, demonstrated that PDT was effective for patients with cancers unresponsive to traditional therapies. These findings suggest that an ideal photosensitizer should (1) be biologically nontoxic in the dark, (2) selectively accumulate in tumors, and (3) be excited by light sources with wavelengths above 600 nm. These milestones solidified Dr. Dougherty's status as a pioneer in the development of PDT for cancer treatment.

1.5 Advancement of Photodynamic Therapy

In his pioneering work, Dougty further purified HpD to create Photofrin II. In 1993, Photofrin II was approved for the clinical treatment of bladder cancer in Canada [22]. It was subsequently approved by the U.S. Food and Drug Administration (FDA) for the treatment of esophageal cancer in 1995 [23]. Photofrin II subsequently gained approval in several other countries, including the United Kingdom, Germany, Japan, China, and others, for the treatment of various cancers, such as lung cancer, esophageal cancer, gastric cancer, bladder cancer, and head and neck cancer. However, a notable drawback of Photofrin II is its slow metabolism and clearance from the body, necessitating prolonged protection from light exposure to provoke delayed phototoxic reactions.

In 1990, Kennedy and colleagues in Canada made another breakthrough by reporting the use of 5-aminolevulinic acid (ALA) combined with visible light for the local treatment of skin cancers. Remarkably, a single session of ALA-PDT could clear approximately 90% of BCC lesions [24, 25]. The development and clinical application of ALA, a small-molecule drug, are groundbreaking. ALA can be absorbed through topical administration and is rapidly eliminated from the skin, eliminating the need for light protection after treatment. These advantages make it highly convenient for the clinical application of superficial skin cancers and premalignant lesions, marking a new era in dermatological therapy. After more than 30 years of clinical practice and evidence-based medicine, ALA-PDT has been proven to be a noninvasive and efficient treatment for a wide range of skin conditions, including actinic keratosis (AK), Bowen's disease (BD), BCC, cutaneous squamous cell carcinoma (cSCC), human papillomavirus (HPV) infection, acne, fungal infection, photoaging, cutaneous kala-azar, and other benign and malignant skin diseases.

1.6 Development of Photosensitizers

Photosensitizers, the key agents in PDT, have evolved over time and are generally classified into three generations on the basis of their development timeline [26]. First-generation photosensitizers were discovered in the 1970s and early 1980s and include primarily HpD, dihaematoporphyrin ether (DHE), and Photofrin II. Second-generation photosensitizers include porphyrin derivatives and some chemically synthesized photosensitizers developed in the late 1980s, including 5-ALA, mesotetrahydroxyphenyl chlorin (mTHPC), tin etiopurpurin (SnEtz), methylene blue, toluidine blue, zinc phthalocyanines, aluminum phthalocyanines, benzoporphyrin and its derivatives, as well as lutelium texaphyrins (Lu-Tex) and mono-l-aspartyl chlorine e6 (talaporfin sodium, NPe6). The second generation of photosensitizers addresses some of the disadvantages of the previous generation by having shorter photosensitive periods, longer wavelengths of excitation (allowing deeper tissue penetration), and improved target selectivity. For example, Foscan® (temoporfin), a chlorophyll family member approved by the FDA in 2002 and certified by the European CE, is effective in the palliative treatment of head and neck cancers. However, like Photofrin®, it has significant phototoxicity and limited cancer selectivity. The third generation of photosensitizers involves the modification of existing photosensitizers through coupling or encasing within the carrier, which results in increased tumor specificity and activation by long-wavelength light [27]. While this classification is broad and not strictly defined, it emphasized that newer generations do not necessarily surpass the previous generations in all aspects. Each photosensitizer's application must consider its specific properties and clinical context.

In 1999, the FDA approved Levulan® (5-aminolevulinic acid, 5-ALA) for PDT to treat AK [28]. In addition, products such as Metvix® (methyl-aminolevulinate, MAL) [28, 29] and

Hexvix® (hexyl aminolevulinate, HAL) [28] have become available in Europe and Australia, respectively. Visudyne® (verteporfin), a second-generation photosensitizer, was approved in 2000 for treating age-related macular degeneration and other neovascular eye diseases, significantly impacting millions of patients with these diseases [30]. In 2001, Foscan® (temoporfin) was approved for the treatment of head and neck cancer in Europe [31]. In 2007, 5-ALA was approved for the treatment of condyloma acuminata by the China Food and Drug Administration (CFDA)/National Medical Products Administration, marking the first time this indication was formally recognized globally for PDT. In 2016, hemoporfin (HMME) was approved for the treatment of port-wine stains by the CFDA, establishing HMME-PDT as a new treatment option [32].

With the continued development of new photosensitizers, the use of PDT has expanded beyond treating various cancers to address non-malignant conditions. New challenges and requirements have emerged, prompting ongoing research focused on enhancing efficacy, reducing adverse effects, and optimizing new photosensitizers. Innovations such as targeted modified photosensitizers, photosensitizers combined with various nanocarriers, and efficient two-photon photosensitizers are current research hotspots, driving the future of PDT forward.

1.7 Advancements in Light Sources and Devices in PDT

The development of PDT has been significantly influenced not only by breakthroughs in photosensitizers but also by advancements in light sources and guiding devices. The effectiveness and expansion of the clinical applications of PDT are closely tied to the availability of appropriate light sources. Initially, PDT utilized white light and daylight as light sources [14], which are relatively inefficient. The introduction of the ruby laser in 1960 marked a turning point, leading to the widespread clinical application of various lasers in the 1970s. Lasers, with their excellent monochromaticity and high power, have become crucial in PDT, especially when they are used with optical fibers in endoscopy. This innovation allowed for the treatment of internal diseases and sparked significant interest in PDT research, particularly for cancers. During the late 1970s and 1980s, research focused on improving the activation efficiency of photosensitizers by developing new laser devices that match the absorption wavelengths of these agents. Long-wavelength lasers have been created to increase the efficacy of PDT for treating deep-seated and large tumors. Modifications to optical fibers made it possible to target deep tumors more accurately under endoscopy, increasing the precision and flexibility of PDT.

Today, newer light sources, such as semiconductor diode lasers, organic light-emitting diodes (OLEDs), and radiation light-emitting diodes (LEDs), are being developed and implemented in PDT. These advancements continue to improve the efficiency and applicability of PDT across various medical fields. PDT has also been increasingly integrated with other treatment modalities, such as surgery, radiotherapy, chemotherapy, and immunotherapy. Additionally, the combination of PDT with diagnostic imaging technologies such as CT, MRI, and PET has significantly increased its utility. With advancements in light sources and devices, PDT is now widely used in dermatology and has expanded to treat age-related macular degeneration; arterial restenosis after atherosclerotic angioplasty; and various tumors across multiple systems, including the respiratory, digestive, nervous, and urinary systems. As we progress into the twenty-first century, global clinical and basic research on PDT continues to expand, leading to broader applications and more effective treatments.

1.8 The History of PDT in China

Traditional Chinese medicine has long used Fructus Psoraleae and Radix Angelica, which contain compounds such as psoralen and propionin that, when activated by ultraviolet rays, can induce erythema, edema, and hyperpigmentation in sun-exposed areas. Chlorophyll and other plant-based substances in traditional Chinese herbs also serve as photosensitizers for photodynamic therapy (PDT). Silkworm rearing, a traditional practice in China, has contributed to PDT research. Silkworm excreta, known as silkworm sand, is a traditional medicine used to promote blood circulation and has photosensitive properties, with chlorophyll derivative 4 (CPD4) being isolated from it.

PDT research in China began later than in Europe and the United States but has made rapid progress. Between 1980 and 1981, Chinese scholars, including Jin Zou, Xianwen Ha, and Junheng Li, started basic and clinical studies on PDT [33]. In 1981, Chinese researchers successfully isolated hematoporphyrin and its sodium salt (HpD) for the first time. Beijing Tongren Hospital then treated a basal cell carcinoma patient with HpD-PDT, marking the first application of PDT in China [34]. Following this, the Beijing Area PDT Treatment Collaboration Group was formed with eight participating hospitals. From 1982 to 1984, 421 patients with various tumors were treated with PDT, for an effective rate of 86.7%. PDT was then included as a key scientific research project in China's Sixth and Seventh Five-Year Plans, leading to significant national collaboration in the development of photosensitizers and laser devices. Institutions such as the Institute of Maternology of the Chinese Academy of Medical Sciences and the Beijing Institute of Pharmaceutical Industry played key roles [35]. By the mid-1990s, China had treated thousands of patients with various cancers using domestically developed photosensitizers and lasers, achieving notable success.

However, in the late 1990s, the popularity of PDT declined due to limitations such as the restricted range of photosensitizers and the long protection period from light exposure. Nonetheless, in the twenty-first century, Chinese researchers and entrepreneurs revived PDT by developing unique Chinese photosensitizers such as hypocrellin, a fungus growing on fargesia in Yunnan and Sichuan Provinces. Hypocrellin was developed into an ointment by the Yunnan Baiyao Group for treating vulvar white lesions and hypertrophic scars [36]. Professor Deyu Xu from the Second Military Medical University developed second-generation hematoporphyrin monomethyl ether (HMME) in 1994, a significant advancement internationally. HMME, a monomeric porphyrin with high purity, was later used for treating tumors and port-wine stains [37].

The turn of the century also included the introduction of 5-aminolevulinic acid (ALA)-PDT in China. In 1996, Professor Shizheng Xu introduced ALA-PDT, and his student, Professor Xiuli Wang, established the first PDT treatment room at Wuhan University People's Hospital. The first study on the treatment of Bowen's disease with ALA-PDT in China was published in 1999 [38]. ALA-PDT was found to be effective for various skin conditions, including basal cell carcinoma and squamous cell carcinoma [39]. Additionally, ALA-PDT was innovatively applied to treat condyloma acuminatum, particularly urethral warts, and was highly effective. In 2000, the authors conducted a study on fluorescence dynamics and treatment parameters for ALA-PDT in the treatment of condyloma acuminatum, which was later published in the *British Journal of Dermatology*, garnering international attention [40].

The clinical application of ALA-PDT has expanded in China, with the optimization of treatment protocols for various skin diseases. Professor Wang played a significant role in drafting expert consensus and guidelines to standardize ALA-PDT clinical applications. In 2014, the Photodynamic Therapy Research Center of the Chinese Medical Association Dermatovenereology Branch was established, leading to further advancements in ALA-PDT. By 2015, the first Chinese expert consensus on the clinical application of 5-aminoketovalic acid photodynamic therapy in dermatology was published [41], and by 2021, this consensus was revised and published in English in the *Photodiagnosis and Photodynamic Therapy* journal, marking China's progress in PDT research [42].

In 2006, ALA-PDT was applied for acne vulgaris treatment in China for the first time. Further research should explore the optimal treatment parameters and principles for moderate to severe acne. This work was recognized in the *Guidelines of Care for the Management of Acne Vulgaris* (2016) in the United States [43, 44]. The authors' group also established a human sebaceous gland cell line derived from acne patients in China, providing a crucial model for studying the mechanism of ALA-PDT in acne treatment. In skin tumor research, the group introduced UV-induced skin photoaging and cutaneous squamous cell carcinoma mouse models and established a corresponding cell line. These models demonstrated that ALA-PDT could kill tumor cells and induce an antitumor immune effect, suggesting a role for PDT as a tumor vaccine.

Chinese researchers have continued to explore new indications for ALA-PDT, including skin aging, refractory HPV infection, fungal infection, and androgenic alopecia. Efforts to reduce adverse effects and improve accessibility have led to innovations such as painless PDT and daylight PDT. These advancements earned recognition, such as the first prize in the Top Ten Most Transformable Scientific and Technological Achievements of Tongji University in 2020.

In 2017, Professor Xiuli Wang and her team won the honor of hosting the 19th International Photodynamic Academic (IPA) Conference in Shanghai, and she was elected as an executive director of the IPA. This marked a significant achievement for China in the global PDT community.

PDT has grown from a small discovery to a widely applied clinical therapy. Its development has been a long, arduous process built on the dedication and continuous innovation of researchers. Today, PDT is used worldwide for diagnosing and treating diseases across various medical fields, including dermatology, gastroenterology, and oncology. PDT is now a first-line treatment for several conditions, including actinic keratosis, Bowen's disease, and certain types of basal cell carcinoma. It also provides an alternative palliative treatment for patients unable to undergo surgery. The role of PDT in preoperative diagnosis, postoperative treatment, and photodynamic immunotherapy is expanding, offering advantages in terms of diagnosis, treatment, prevention, and rehabilitation.

In summary, PDT has great potential, and the continued development of photosensitizers, lasers, and photoconductive materials, along with deepening clinical and basic research, will lead to more effective and accessible treatments for patients worldwide.

References

1. Allison RR, Mota HC, Sibata CH. Clinical PD/PDT in North America: an historical review. Photodiagn Photodyn Ther. 2004;1(4):263–77. https://doi.org/10.1016/s1572-1000(04)00084-5.
2. Dolmans DE, Fukumura D, Jain RK. Photodynamic therapy for cancer. Nat Rev Cancer. 2003;3(5):380–7. https://doi.org/10.1038/nrc1071.
3. von Tappeiner H, Jodlbauer A. Uber Wirkung der photodynamischen (fluoreszcrenden) Stoffe auf Protozuan und Enzyme. Dtsch Arch Klin Med. 1904;80:427–87.
4. Meyer-Betz F. Untersuchungen uber die Biologische (photodynamische) Wirkung des Hematoporphyrins und anderer Derivative des Blut-und Galenfarbstoffs. Dtsch Arch Klin Med. 1913;112:476–503.
5. Moan J, Peng Q. An outline of the hundred-year history of PDT. Anticancer Res. 2003;23(5):3591–600.
6. With TK. A short history of porphyrins and the porphyrias. Int J Biochem. 1980;11(3–4):189–200. https://doi.org/10.1016/0020-711x(80)90219-0.
7. Auler H, Banzer G. Untersuchungen uber die Rolle der Porphyrine bei geschwulstkranken Menschen und Tieren. Z Krebsforsch. 1942;53:65–8.
8. Figge FHJ, Weiland GS, Manganiello LOJ. The affinioty of neoplastic em-bryonic and traumatized tissue for porphyrins and met alloporphyrins. Proc Soc Exp Biol Med. 1948;68(3):640.
9. Manganiello LO, Figge FH. Cancer detection and therapy. II Methods of preparation and biological effects of metallo-porphyrins. Bull Sch Med Univ. 1951;36(1):3–7.
10. Peck GC, Mack HP, Figge FH. Study of the effect of hematoporphyrin on hypophyseal-adrenal relationships. Proc Soc Exp Biol Med. 1953;83(2):264–6. https://doi.org/10.3181/00379727-83-20328.
11. Rassmussen-Taxdal DS, Ward GE, Figge FH. Fluorescence of human lymphatic and cancer tissues following high doses of intravenous hematoporphyrin. Cancer. 1955;8(1):78–81. https://doi.org/10.1002/1097-0142(1955)8:1<78::aid-cncr2820080109>3.0.co;2-l.
12. Schwartz SK, Vermund H. Some relationships of porphyrins, X-rays and tumors. Univ Minn Med Bull. 1955;27:7–8.
13. Lipson RL, Baldes EJ, Olsen AM. Hematoporphyrin derivative: a new aid for endoscopic detection

of malignant disease. J Thorac Cardiovasc Surg. 1961;42:623–9.
14. Lipson RL, Baldes EJ, Gray MJ. Hematoporphyrin derivative for detection and management of cancer. Cancer. 1967;20(12):2255–7. https://doi.org/10.1002/1097-0142(196712)20:12<2255::aid-cncr2820201229>3.0.co;2-u.
15. Gregorie HB Jr, Horger EO, Ward JL, Green JF, Richards T, Robertson HC, et al. Hematoporphyrin-derivative fluorescence in malignant neoplasms. Ann Surg. 1968;167(6):820–8. https://doi.org/10.1097/00000658-196806000-00002.
16. Diamond I, Granelli SG, McDonagh AF, Nielsen S, Wilson CB, Jaenicke R. Photodynamic therapy of malignant tumors. Lancet. 1972;2(7788):1175–7. https://doi.org/10.1016/s0140-6736(72)92596-2.
17. Diamond I, Granelli SG, McDonagh SF, Crafts D, Wilson CB. Photodynamic therapy of experimental gliomas. Trans Am Neurol Assoc. 1975;100:185–7.
18. Dougherty TJ, Grindey GB, Fiel R, Weishaupt KR, Boyle DG. Photoradiation therapy. II. Cure of animal tumors with hematoporphyrin and light. J Natl Cancer Inst. 1975;55(1):115–21. https://doi.org/10.1093/jnci/55.1.115.
19. Kelly JF, Snell ME, Berenbaum MC. Photodynamic destruction of human bladder carcinoma. Br J Cancer. 1975;31(2):237–44. https://doi.org/10.1038/bjc.1975.30.
20. Kelly JF, Snell ME. Hematoporphyrin derivative: a possible aid in the diagnosis and therapy of carcinoma of the bladder. J Urol. 1976;115(2):150–1. https://doi.org/10.1016/s0022-5347(17)59108-9.
21. Dougherty TJ, Kaufman JE, Goldfarb A, Weishaupt KR, Boyle D, Mittleman A. Photoradiation therapy for the treatment of malignant tumors. Cancer Res. 1978;38(8):2628–35.
22. Dougherty TJ. Photodynamic therapy. Photochem Photobiol. 1993;58(6):895–900. https://doi.org/10.1111/j.1751-1097.1993.tb04990.x.
23. Davila ML. Photodynamic therapy. Gastrointest Endosc Clin N Am. 2011;21(1):67–79. https://doi.org/10.1016/j.giec.2010.09.002.
24. Kennedy JC, Pottier RH, Pross DC. Photodynamic therapy with endogenous protoporphyrin IX: basic principles and present clinical experience. J Photochem Photobiol B. 1990;6(1–2):143–8. https://doi.org/10.1016/1011-1344(90)85083-9.
25. Taub AF. Photodynamic therapy in dermatology: history and horizons. J Drugs Dermatol. 2004;3(1):8–25.
26. Li L, Xiang L, Qin Z, Wang L, Lin J, Ma Y, Luo R, Huang Z. Photodynamic therapy: clinical research and application in China. Chin J Laser Med Surg. 2012;21(5):278–307.
27. Baskaran R, Lee J, Yang SG. Clinical development of photodynamic agents and therapeutic applications. Biomater Res. 2018;22:25. https://doi.org/10.1186/s40824-018-0140-z.
28. Krammer B, Plaetzer K. ALA and its clinical impact, from bench to bedside. Photochem Photobiol Sci. 2008;7(3):283–9. https://doi.org/10.1039/b712847a.
29. Gardlo K, Ruzicka T. Metvix (photocure). Curr Opin Investig Drugs. 2002;3(11):1672–8.
30. Battaglia Parodi M, La Spina C, Berchicci L, Petruzzi G, Bandello F. Photosensitizers and photodynamic therapy: verteporfin. Dev Ophthalmol. 2016;55:330–6. https://doi.org/10.1159/000434704.
31. Darragh TM, Colgan TJ, Cox JT, Heller DS, Henry MR, Luff RD, et al. The lower anogenital squamous terminology standardization project for HPV-associated lesions: background and consensus recommendations from the College of American Pathologists and the American Society for Colposcopy and Cervical Pathology. Arch Pathol Lab Med. 2012;136(10):1266–97. https://doi.org/10.5858/arpa.LGT200570.
32. Zhang M, Wu Q, Lin T, Guo L, Ge Y, Zeng R, et al. Hematoporphyrin monomethyl ether photodynamic therapy for the treatment of facial port-wine stains resistant to pulsed dye laser. Photodiagn Photodyn Ther. 2020;31:101820. https://doi.org/10.1016/j.pdpdt.2020.101820.
33. Li J. Recent progress of photodynamic therapy. Basic Clin Med. 1997;17(3):8–13.
34. Fansong Liu XL. Photodynamic therapy in China. Chin J Laser Med Surg. 2005;14(1):67.
35. Zhenxiang Dong RG, Liu L. Hema. 2006;21:1895–6.
36. Shangjie X, Chen S, Zhang M, Shen T, Wang Z. Hypocrellin derivative as new photosensitizer: studies and progress. Chin Sci Bull. 2003;48(10):1005–15.
37. Ying G, Wang K, Zhu J, Liang J, Pan Y, Li J. Clinical analysis of 1216 cases of port wine stain treated with photodynamic therapy. Chin J Laser Med Surg. 2001;2:21–4.
38. Xiuli Wang SX, Zhang C, Zheng W. Photodynamic therapy of Bowen's disease using 5-aminolevulinic acid. Chin J Laser Med Surg. 1999;1:13–5.
39. Shizheng X, Zhang C. Treatment of cutaneous basal cell carcinoma and squamous cell carcinoma with 5-aminolevulinic acid photodynamic therapy. Chin J Dermatol. 1999;3:39–40.
40. Wang XL, Wang HW, Wang HS, Xu SZ, Liao KH, Hillemanns P. Topical 5-aminolaevulinic acid-photodynamic therapy for the treatment of urethral condylomata acuminata. Br J Dermatol. 2004;151(4):880–5. https://doi.org/10.1111/j.1365-2133.2004.06189.x.
41. Dermatology I. Experts consensus on the clinical application of 5-aminolevulinic acid-based photodynamic therapy in dermatology. Chin J Dermatol. 2015;48(10):675–8.
42. Shi L, Wang H, Chen K, Yan J, Yu B, Wang S, et al. Chinese guidelines on the clinical application of 5-aminolevulinic acid-based photodynamic therapy in dermatology (2021 edition). Photodiagn Photodyn Ther. 2021;35:102340. https://doi.org/10.1016/j.pdpdt.2021.102340.
43. Wang XL, Wang HW, Zhang LL, Guo MX, Huang Z. Topical ALA PDT for the treatment of severe acne vulgaris. Photodiagn Photodyn Ther. 2010;7(1):33–8. https://doi.org/10.1016/j.pdpdt.2010.01.003.
44. Zaenglein AL, Pathy AL, Schlosser BJ, Alikhan A, Baldwin HE, Berson DS, et al. Guidelines of care for the management of acne vulgaris. J Am Acad Dermatol. 2016;74(5):945–73. https://doi.org/10.1016/j.jaad.2015.12.037.

2 Principles of Photodynamic Therapy and Photosensitizers in Dermatology

Haiyan Zhang, Shuzhan Shen, Peiru Wang, Bo Wang, and Xiuli Wang

2.1 Introduction

The core components of PDT are photosensitizers, light, and oxygen. The theoretical foundation of PDT lies in the process of photodynamic reactions, wherein photosensitizers in their ground state absorb photon energy upon exposure to specific wavelengths of light, such as visible light, near-infrared light, or ultraviolet light, transitioning from the ground state to excited state. The singlet excited state of photosensitizers is inherently unstable and rapidly undergoes physical or chemical de-excitation, releasing energy and reverting to the ground state. The physical de-excitation process generates fluorescence, which is utilized for disease diagnosis.

The mechanism of reactive oxygen species (ROS) generation induced by various photosensitizers is fundamentally similar, differing primarily in the cellular organelles where the photosensitizers accumulate. In China, the most widely used photosensitizers are aminolevulinic acid (ALA), hematoporphyrin monomethyl ether (HMME), and hematoporphyrin derivative (HpD).

H. Zhang · S. Shen · P. Wang · X. Wang (✉)
Institute of Photomedicine, Shanghai Skin Disease Hospital, School of Medicine, Tongji University, Shanghai, China
e-mail: wangxiuli_1400023@tongji.edu.cn

B. Wang
Avera Medical Group Dermatology, Aberdeen, SD, USA

University of South Dakota, Vermillion, SD, USA
e-mail: makiwang@med.umich.edu

2.2 ALA-PDT

It has been 26 years since ALA-PDT was first introduced to dermatology in China in 1996. It has been popularized and implemented in more than 3000 hospitals across China, with its safety and efficacy being widely recognized. ALA-mediated photodynamic therapy (ALA-PDT) is used to treat various skin conditions, including actinic keratosis, basal cell carcinoma, acne, psoriasis, viral warts, port wine stains, and several other dermatological disorders.

2.2.1 Photosensitizer

ALA, a naturally occurring nonproteinogenic amino acid, serves as a precursor for the synthesis of hemoglobin in mammals and chlorophyll in plants, ultimately leading to the generation of Protoporphyrin IX (PpIX) upon intracellular metabolism. Under laser excitation at approximately 400 nm, PpIX emits intense red fluorescence. Upon excitation by red or blue light, it undergoes photodynamic reactions, producing singlet oxygen. This property has been harnessed in PDT. ALA is administered topically, and upon

X. Wang, B. Wang (eds.), *Photodynamic Therapy in Dermatology*,
https://doi.org/10.1007/978-981-96-8915-6_2

penetration into cells, it is involved in the biosynthesis of hemoglobin, which is selectively converted to PpIX in cells in high metabolic states, such as virus-infected cells, inflammatory cells, and precancerous or malignant tissues.

2.2.2 Pharmacokinetics of ALA

Current research indicates that ALA can be administered through various methods, and the pharmacokinetics differ depending on the method of administration.

2.2.2.1 Topical Administration to the Skin

As a small-molecule drug, ALA can be absorbed through the skin. Topical administration can reduce the risk of systemic phototoxicity. Normal skin and tumor-covered skin tissues presented different kinetic patterns after the application of the ALA cream. In normal skin, the concentration of porphyrin peaks at 1.5 h after administration, whereas in tumor-covered skin, the peak concentration of PpIX appears at 3 h post-administration [1].

2.2.2.2 Topical Administration to the Mucous Membrane

ALA-PDT is widely used in dermatology for the treatment of diseases of the cervical mucosa and urethral mucosa. In cervical intraepithelial neoplasia (CIN), fluorescence from 3% ALA solution was detectable between 150 and 450 min post-application but peaked at 300 min. Research from the authors' group demonstrated that the optimal ALA concentration for ALA-PDT of urethral condyloma acuminatum is 5% or 10%, with the best application time being 3–5 h [2].

Owing to its simple structure and small molecular weight, ALA is most suitable for local transdermal administration in dermatology. Topical administration to the skin and mucosa produces a maximum amount of PpIX locally, thereby avoiding the risk of systemic phototoxic reactions associated with the systematic administration route.

2.2.3 Light Source Selection

Light is one of the three essential elements of PDT, directly affecting its efficacy. The role of light is to activate the photosensitizer, initiating the photodynamic reaction. The use of red light with a wavelength of approximately 630 nm in ALA-PDT is recommended. Currently, common light sources for ALA-PDT include laser sources (coherent light) and nonlaser sources (incoherent light). Laser sources include semiconductor lasers and high-power helium-neon lasers. Nonlaser sources include light-emitting diode (LED) light sources and intense pulsed light (IPL).

If a laser light source is used, optical fibers are required for light transmission. The proper selection of optical fibers is a crucial factor in determining the efficacy of treatment.

1. Standard bare optical fibers: suitable for general superficial ALA-PDT.
2. Microlens optical fibers: beneficial for improving the efficacy of superficial ALA-PDT.
3. Cylindrical diffusing optical fibers: suitable for intracavitary ALA-PDT.

2.3 HMME-PDT

In 2016, HMME was marketed as a photosensitizer used in the venous system. Currently, port wine stains (PWS) are the sole indication for HMME-PDT, with adverse reactions, including systemic and local effects.

2.3.1 Photosensitizer

Hemoporfin, an innovative development from China, represents a second-generation photosensitizer with the chemical name hematoporphyrin monomethyl ether (HMME), a refined monomeric porphyrin. Unlike its predecessor, HpD, hemoporfin has a unique composition, structural stability, exceptional tissue selectivity, preferential uptake by vascular endothelial cells, rapid photobleaching kinetics, and a shortened post-treatment light avoidance period.

Upon intravenous administration of HMME, it promptly localizes within vascular endothelial cells, which exhibit significantly higher absorption rates than epidermal cells do. Under appropriate illumination, HMME undergoes a photochemical reaction, inducing swelling, degeneration, and necrosis of endothelial cells, culminating in microvascular occlusion and subsequent attenuation of erythema. The adjacent epidermis remains relatively unaffected due to the minimal presence of photosensitizers, whereas the limited penetration of laser light shields deeper dermal tissues from the therapeutic dose. Furthermore, as the photosensitizer is continuously consumed, the ample surface area of endothelial cells near the vessel lumen facilitates rapid replenishment, in contrast to the more challenging replenishment within epidermal cells. This phenomenon enhances the concentration disparity between the two tissues, increasing the selectivity of photodynamic therapy for the target tissue. Consequently, hemoporfin has clinical utility in the treatment of port wine stain, demonstrating particular efficacy in managing extensive lesions (>5 cm) and potentially eliminating lesions without inducing local scarring. Owing to its stable structure, high photoactivity, and low phototoxicity, HMME is widely used in PDT for PWS in China.

2.3.2 The Pharmacokinetics of HMME

A phase I clinical trial of HMME in healthy Chinese subjects revealed that doses ranging from 2.5 mg/kg to 10 mg/kg were safe and well tolerated [3]. After intravenous injection, HMME is rapidly cleared from the blood, with a short half-life, indicating its high degree of safety, short photoprotection period, ease of care, and short interval for repeated treatments. These features enhance compliance among healthcare providers and patients.

2.3.3 Light Source Selection

The selection of a light source requires consideration of various factors, such as matching the wavelength to the absorption spectrum of the photosensitizer, ensuring sufficient penetration and adequate output power, and effectively illuminating diseased blood vessels. The light sources commonly used in HMME-PDT include lasers and LED. The use of green light with a wavelength of 530 nm is recommended for HMME-PDT.

The absorption peak of the HMME photosensitizer is in the green light band, allowing minimal absorption by the epidermis compared with the blue–purple band, ensuring that sufficient light reaches diseased blood vessels. Furthermore, its penetration only reaches the superficial dermis, effectively protecting the deeper layers. Coherent light sources such as lasers and incoherent light sources such as intense pulsed light and LED are the main light sources. Continuous lasers, such as 532 nm semiconductor lasers or all-solid-state lasers, are preferred because of their high efficiency in exciting photosensitive drugs. Additionally, high-frequency pulse lasers and 630 nm semiconductor lasers can also be used, with the latter having a deeper penetration depth but an increased risk of scar formation after penetrating the dermis. Recently, 532 nm LED machines have become the preferred light source for HMME-PDT because of their small size, face mask design, continuous treatment, stable energy, long lifespan, and low cost.

2.4 HpD-PDT

Hematoporphyrin derivative photodynamic therapy (HpD-PDT) has been shown to have therapeutic effects on squamous cell carcinoma, basal cell carcinoma, extramammary Paget's disease (EMPD), port wine stain, and other skin diseases.

2.4.1 Photosensitizer

HpD, a mixture of porphyrin oligomers, belongs to the first generation of photosensitizers used in PDT. Owing to its systematic administration, HpD requires a long interval of administration and illumination, with prolonged tissue retention and slow excretion. Skin tests are necessary before treatment, and patients must avoid light exposure for an extended period posttreatment to prevent phototoxic reactions. These limitations have restricted its application. HpD is approved by the China Food and Drug Administration (CFDA) for diagnosing and treating superficial cancers in the oral cavity, the bladder, bronchus, lung and digestive systems, precancerous lesions, including leukoplakia, and benign conditions, such as port wine stains.

2.4.2 The Pharmacokinetics of HpD

The authors' group treated 20 patients with non-melanoma skin cancers via HpD-PDT, employing fluorescence diagnosis to assess drug accumulation in lesions, margins, and distant skin areas [4]. The results suggest that the optimal illumination time for HpD-PDT is 48–72 h after intravenous injection, and two sessions of irradiation with red light at 48 and 72 h postinjection are recommended. Strict light avoidance is necessary for at least 1 month post-treatment. Although most HpD is cleared from the body after 3 months, patients should continue to avoid strong light exposure, as photosensitivity may persist.

2.4.3 Light Source Selection

The primary light sources used in HpD-PDT are lasers and LEDs. Although no studies have directly compared the effectiveness of different light sources in the treatment of EMPD, red LEDs and semiconductor lasers are the most commonly used. In some cases, combination therapies, including CO_2 lasers or holmium lasers, can be used. In 2022, the authors treated 11 EMPD patients with HpD-PDT via a 630-nm red light semiconductor laser with an output power of 1000–2000 mW, a power density of 80–150 mW/cm^2, and an energy density of 150–200 J/cm^2. Two sessions of red light irradiation were performed at 48 h and 72 h after a single HpD injection, and no serious adverse reactions were observed. For patients with residual lesions after one treatment, a combination of a holmium laser and ALA-PDT effectively cleared the remaining lesions.

References

1. Casas A, Fukuda H, Batlle AM. Tissue distribution and kinetics of endogenous porphyrins synthesized after topical application of ALA in different vehicles. Br J Cancer. 1999;81:13–8. https://doi.org/10.1038/sj.bjc.6690644.
2. Pahernik SA, Botzlar A, Hillemanns P, Dellian M, Kirschstein M, Abels C, Korell M, Mueller-Hoecker J, Untch M, Goetz AE. Pharmacokinetics and selectivity of aminolevulinic acid-induced porphyrin synthesis in patients with cervical intraepithelial neoplasia. Int J Cancer. 1998;78:310–4. https://doi.org/10.1002/(sici)1097-0215(19981029)78:3<310::Aid-ijc9>3.0.Co;2-y.
3. Sun PH, Zhao X, Zhou Y, Liang Y, Zhang HL, Cui YM, Tao JN. Tolerance and pharmacokinetics of single-dose intravenous hemoporfin in healthy volunteers. Acta Pharmacol Sin. 2011;32:1549–54. https://doi.org/10.1038/aps.2011.132.
4. Wang DX, Wang PR, Li CX, Zhou ZX, Zhang LL, Zhang GL, Wang XL. Efficacy and safety of HpD-PDT for Extramammary Paget's disease refractory to conventional therapy: a prospective, open-label and single arm pilot study. Photodiagn Photodyn Ther. 2022;37:102670. https://doi.org/10.1016/j.pdpdt.2021.102670.

3 Mechanisms of Photodynamic Therapy

Qingyu Zeng, Chengqian Chen, Zhi Cao, Bo Wang, and Xiuli Wang

3.1 Introduction

Photodynamic therapy (PDT) is an innovative therapeutic modality that leverages photodynamic reactions for both disease diagnosis and treatment, blending pharmaceutical and technological methodologies. Clinically, PDT typically refers to the therapeutic application of photodynamic reactions, whereas photodynamic diagnosis (PDD) is often referred to as fluorescence diagnosis. This distinction highlights the dual functionality of PDT, encompassing both diagnostic and therapeutic dimensions, thereby enhancing its clinical versatility.

The core components of PDT include photosensitizers, light, and oxygen molecules. The theoretical basis of PDT lies in photodynamic reactions, where photosensitizers, in their ground state, absorb photon energy when exposed to specific wavelengths of light (e.g., visible light, near-infrared light, or ultraviolet light), causing a transition to the singlet excited state. This singlet excited state is unstable and undergoes either physical or chemical de-excitation, releasing energy and returning to the ground state (Fig. 3.1). Physical de-excitation produces brick-red fluorescence, which is employed in diagnostic applications. Chemical de-excitation occurs when the singlet excited state transforms into a more stable triplet excited state. In this state, photosensitizers interact with molecular oxygen (O_2) via two pathways: type I and II photodynamic reactions. In type I reactions, the triplet-state photosensitizer transfers an electron to O_2, generating superoxide anions ($O_2^{\bullet -}$) and forming reactive oxygen species (ROS), such as hydrogen peroxide (H_2O_2) and hydroxyl radicals (·OH). In type II reactions, the triplet-state photosensitizer transfers energy directly to O_2, producing singlet oxygen ($^1O_2$).

The ROS generated during the chemical de-excitation process trigger a cascade of oxidative reactions with surrounding biomolecules, leading to cytotoxic effects. These effects disrupt cellular structure and function, causing cellular damage or death, thus fulfilling the therapeutic objectives of PDT [1].

The mechanistic basis for reactive oxygen species (ROS) generation induced by various photosensitizers is fundamentally similar, with the primary difference being the specific cellular organelles where the photosensitizers accumulate. Given the widespread use of 5-aminolevulinic

Q. Zeng · C. Chen · Z. Cao · X. Wang
Institute of Photomedicine, Shanghai Skin Disease Hospital, School of Medicine, Tongji University, Shanghai, China
e-mail: zengqingyu2011@tongji.edu.cn; 2211517@tongji.edu.cn; wangxiuli_1400023@tongji.edu.cn

B. Wang (✉)
Avera Medical Group Dermatology, Aberdeen, SD, USA

University of South Dakota, Vermillion, SD, USA
e-mail: makiwang@med.umich.edu

X. Wang, B. Wang (eds.), *Photodynamic Therapy in Dermatology*,
https://doi.org/10.1007/978-981-96-8915-6_3

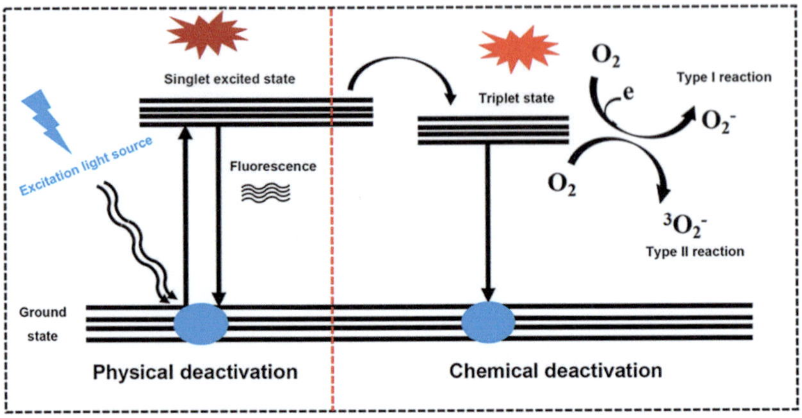

Fig. 3.1 The excitation and de-excitation processes of photosensitizers

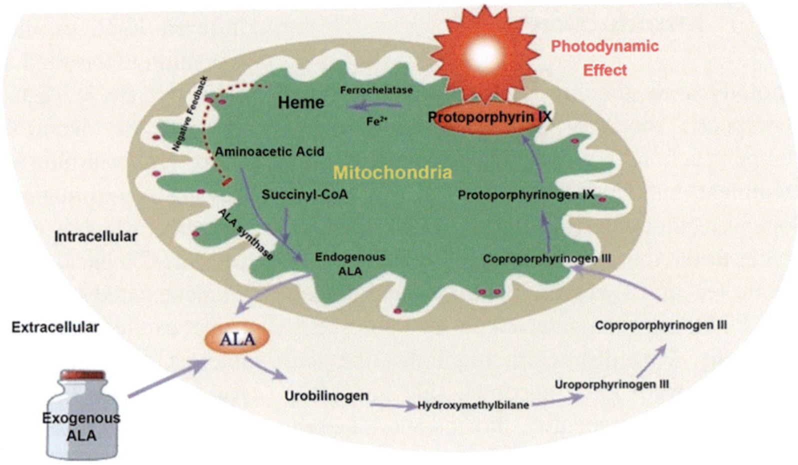

Fig. 3.2 Schematic representation of PpIX generation through ALA metabolism

acid (ALA) in China, this chapter focuses on elucidating the mechanism behind ALA-photodynamic therapy (ALA-PDT).

ALA is a naturally hydrophilic small-molecule compound found abundantly in the mitochondria of both animals and plants. In its native state, ALA lacks photosensitizing properties and acts as an endogenous precursor to the photosensitizer protoporphyrin IX (PpIX). Under normal conditions, endogenous ALA is an intermediate product in the heme synthesis pathway.

Within mitochondria, ALA is synthesized from aminoethyl acetate and succinyl-CoA through the catalytic action of ALA synthase. Once synthesized, ALA enters the cytoplasm, where it undergoes a series of enzymatic reactions, eventually converting into fecal protoporphyrinogen III. This molecule then returns to the mitochondria, where it is catalyzed by protoporphyrin oxidase to form PpIX. Finally, under the action of ferrochelatase, PpIX reacts with Fe^{2+} to produce heme (Fig. 3.2).

Under normal conditions, heme biosynthesis is tightly regulated by negative feedback mechanisms, with ALA synthase and ferrochelatase acting as key rate-limiting enzymes. The end product, heme, exerts negative feedback inhibition on ALA synthase, preventing the excessive accumulation of ALA or PpIX in tissues. However, when a substantial amount of exogenous ALA is introduced into an organism, it is selectively absorbed by tumor cells and other rapidly proliferating cells, bypassing the rate-limiting control of ALA synthase. This leads to significant intracellular buildup of PpIX. Owing to the limitations imposed by ferrochelatase, which converts PpIX into heme, a considerable portion of PpIX remains unconverted, accumulating within the cells. Upon exposure to light at specific wavelengths, PpIX undergoes a photochemical reaction, generating a substantial amount of ROS. This process forms the basis of ALA-PDT.

Currently, the widely accepted mechanisms of PDT are primarily classified into three aspects: (1) direct cytotoxicity to target cells through the generation of ROS during the PDT process. (2) Destruction of the tissue microvascular system by PDT leads to hypoxia or nutrient deprivation in the lesion tissue, resulting in indirect cell death. (3) Induction of an inflammatory response following PDT promotes the aggregation of local immune cells, further activating the body's immune system.

3.2 Direct Cytotoxic Effects of PDT

The direct cytotoxic repercussions of PDT stem from the irreversible damage inflicted on subcellular structures within target cells. This damage is caused by oxidation reactions triggered by the ROS generated during the PDT process, which subsequently interact with neighboring biomolecules. Owing to the short lifespan and limited diffusion range of ROS, the cytotoxic effects remain confined to the localized area surrounding the photosensitizer. When damage surpasses a critical threshold, cellular death occurs.

PDT can induce multiple forms of cell death, including apoptosis, necrosis, and autophagy, as well as more recently recognized pathways such as ferroptosis and pyroptosis [2]. The particular cell death pathway activated by PDT depends on several factors, such as the cell type and metabolic profile, PDT parameters (e.g., photosensitizer concentration, incubation time, and light dose), and the subcellular localization of the photosensitizer. PDT is widely accepted to induce multiple modes of cell death rather than a single pathway. Therefore, further comprehensive research is necessary to fully understand the specific cellular mechanisms by which PDT is activated in different contexts.

3.2.1 Necrosis

Necrosis is an uncontrolled form of cell death induced by intense physical or biological factors. It is characterized by increased membrane permeability, cellular swelling, chromosomal displacement, mitochondrial and nuclear swelling, lysosomal destruction, and eventual rupture of the cell membrane, which triggers a strong local inflammatory response. Traditionally, necrosis is considered an incidental and unregulated process that is primarily observed in pathological conditions. However, recent studies suggest that a variant known as programmed necrosis, or necroptosis, is regulated by intricate signal transduction pathways [3, 4].

PDT-induced cellular necrosis relies on diverse signal transduction pathways, including the RIP3-dependent necrotic pathway, the calcium–calmodulin/calcium–calmodulin kinase II pathway, and the JNK cascade pathway, and is associated with multiple factors, such as tumor necrosis factor (TNF), TRAF2 (TNF receptor-associated factor 2), and lysosomal cathepsins. Upon TNF-α stimulation, the necrosome formed during necrosis contains components such as caspase-8 and Fas associated with death domain protein (FADD). Recent research has shown that PDT can induce the formation of a pronecrotic complex comprising RIP1 and RIP3, excluding caspase-8 and FADD [5]. Additionally, singlet oxygen can introduce lipid hydroperoxides (LOOHs) into the cell membrane or directly cause rapid membrane disruption, culminating in cellular necrosis.

The authors' group has pioneered the application of ALA-PDT for various cutaneous malignancies, including condyloma acuminatum and HPV-related malignancies [6–8]. In 2004, their investigation into the effects of ALA-PDT on condyloma acuminatum, as reported in the *British Journal of Dermatology*, revealed keratinocyte degeneration and necrosis 3 h after ALA-PDT treatment. By 5 h, significant epidermal thinning was observed, with widespread necrotic keratinocytes, which confirmed the effectiveness of ALA-PDT in inducing necrosis in HPV-infected cells [9, 10].

To further understand the mechanisms of ALA-PDT at the animal level, the authors developed a mouse model of ultraviolet (UV)-induced cutaneous squamous cell carcinoma (cSCC) via SKH-1 hairless mice. This model, which simulates human cSCC resulting from UV exposure at the pathological level, was treated with ALA-PDT [11, 12]. Transmission electron microscopy revealed that ALA-PDT induced both necrosis and apoptosis in tumor cells, progressively leading to the destruction of tumor structures [11]. In parallel with in vitro experiments using the PECA cell line (derived from mouse cSCC), ALA-PDT also demonstrated its ability to induce necrosis and apoptosis [13].

3.2.2 Apoptosis

Apoptosis, a controlled and programmed cell death mechanism, plays a crucial role in maintaining internal environmental stability in multicellular organisms by eliminating aberrant or senescent cells. It is characterized by distinct features, such as cell rounding, cytoplasmic condensation, chromatin condensation into crescent-shaped, high-density regions around the nuclear envelope, and subsequent self-segmentation of the cell into membrane-bound apoptotic bodies. Importantly, apoptosis is noninflammatory as it avoids the dissolution of surrounding cells. In the context of PDT, apoptosis can be induced through three interconnected pathways—the mitochondrial pathway, the endoplasmic reticulum signaling pathway, and the death receptor pathway—forming a complex network system.

3.2.2.1 Mitochondrial Pathway

The mitochondrial pathway is the primary route through which ALA-PDT induces apoptosis. This process involves the accumulation of PpIX in the mitochondria, where it leads to the release of cytochrome C (Cyt C) upon light activation. Cyt C triggers the formation of the apoptosome by binding with apoptotic protease activating factor 1 (Apaf-1) and caspase-9. This activates downstream caspases, such as caspase-3, culminating in apoptosis. This pathway is fast and highly efficient. In 1991, Agarwal reported the induction of apoptosis in L5178Y mouse lymphoma cells subsequent to PDT [14]. In 2004, the authors' group demonstrated that ALA-PDT effectively induced mitochondrial disruption in HPV-infected keratinocytes. Following ALA-PDT treatment of genital warts, electron microscopy revealed swelling, fragmentation, and a reduction in mitochondrial structure within 1 h of treatment. Apoptotic changes, such as abnormal chromatin aggregation and the formation of a halo or crescent shape, were observed 3 h after treatment [9]. In animal models of SCC, apoptotic bodies were detected within tumor cells after 3 h and persisted for up to 12 h post-treatment. The degree of apoptosis versus necrosis was dependent on the light fluence used, with lower fluences (0.5 J/cm^2) favoring apoptosis and higher fluences (2 J/cm^2) leading to necrosis [11].

Inoue et al. reported substantial induction of apoptosis in human glioma cells following ALA-PDT, primarily through the mitochondrial pathway [15]. The authors' group established an in vitro model of HPV-infected keratinocytes by transfecting keratinocytes with HPV16E7 (HaCaT/HPV16E7) and demonstrated that ALA-PDT can increase apoptosis and necrosis in a light dose-dependent manner. Low doses predominantly trigger apoptosis, whereas high doses trigger necrosis [16]. Confocal microscopy revealed that mitochondrial depolarization is an early event in apoptosis, followed by phosphatidylserine exposure on the cell surface. These observations suggest a correlation between apoptosis and the structural and functional aspects of mitochondria. The increased expression of cleaved caspase-3 and cleaved caspase-9 supported the conclusion that the mitochondrial pathway plays a central role in ALA-PDT-induced apoptosis [17].

3.2.2.2 Endoplasmic Reticulum (ER) Signaling Pathway

The ER signaling pathway also contributes to PDT-induced apoptosis, primarily through oxidative stress. When photosensitizers localize within the ER, they induce ER stress, increasing intracellular calcium ion (Ca^{2+}) levels. This increase in Ca^{2+} triggers mitochondrial damage and activates calcium-dependent proteases, initiating apoptosis. Additionally, ER stress disrupts protein folding, resulting in the accumulation of unfolded proteins and the unfolded protein response (UPR). Consequently, apoptosis is induced via the activation of the caspase pathway, downregulation of Bcl-2 expression, and activation of MAPK pathways. Although ALA-PDT predominantly targets mitochondria instead of the ER, recent research (2021) has demonstrated that it also induces ER stress in HeLa cells infected with high-risk HPV. This ER stress-activated Caspase-12, promoting apoptosis in HPV-infected cells [18].

3.2.2.3 Death Receptor Pathway

The death receptor pathway operates through apoptosis-related receptors on the cell membrane, such as TNF receptor-1 (TNF-R1) and Fas. Upon binding their respective ligands, these receptors activate the caspase cascade, particularly caspase-8 and caspase-3, leading to apoptosis [3]. While this pathway is a well-established mechanism of extrinsic apoptosis, it is not the predominant pathway involved in PDT-induced cell death.

3.2.3 Autophagy

Autophagy is a vital cellular process responsible for degrading and recycling intracellular components such as damaged organelles and cytoplasmic material. It helps maintain cellular homeostasis by preventing nonprogrammed cell death. The process involves the formation of autophagosomes, which are membrane-bound vesicles that engulf the targeted materials, which are then transported to lysosomes for degradation. The breakdown products are subsequently reused by the cell [3, 19].

Recent research has shown that autophagy can play both protective and destructive roles, depending on the context, especially in PDT. On the one hand, under low-dose PDT conditions, autophagy acts as a cytoprotective mechanism. By isolating and degrading damaged organelles and proteins, autophagy prevents the release of proapoptotic signals, thus inhibiting cell death and supporting survival. This can hinder the therapeutic efficacy of PDT as damaged cells can repair themselves rather than undergo apoptosis or necrosis. In contrast, under high-dose PDT conditions, autophagy can contribute to cell death. Excessive damage to proteins and organelles caused by ROS generation triggers intense oxidative stress that overwhelms the cell's repair mechanisms. When autophagy is excessively activated under these conditions, it fails to maintain the raw materials necessary for repair, leading to the accumulation of defective proteins and organelles, further exacerbating oxidative stress. This ultimately converts autophagy from a survival mechanism into a cell death pathway. High-dose PDT promotes this shift by persistently damaging organelles and proteins such that autophagy-induced degradation becomes counterproductive, leading to autophagic cell death [20]. Consequently, within therapeutic contexts, low-dose PDT demands the suppression of protective autophagy, whereas high-dose PDT necessitates the augmentation of autophagic cell death.

The swift surge in ROS during PDT serves as a key inducer of oxidative stress, triggering autophagy [21]. Moreover, the vascular occlusion that follows PDT leads to nutrient depletion and hypoxia, which are classical stimuli for autophagy induction. These conditions promote the activation of autophagic pathways to remove damaged cellular components in an attempt to restore balance.

In experiments conducted by the authors' group, an increase in the expression of LC3-II, a marker of autophagosome formation, was observed in A431 and SCL-1 cells 24 h after low-dose ALA-PDT treatment, confirming the occurrence of autophagy. By using chloroquine to inhibit autophagy, the study demonstrated enhanced inhibition of cell proliferation, emphasizing the protective role of autophagy under low-dose PDT.

Thus, a more nuanced understanding of how to manipulate autophagy in PDT, on the basis of the light dose and the biological context, is essential for improving treatment strategies. Further studies are needed to explore ways to inhibit protective autophagy during low-dose PDT and enhance autophagic cell death during high-dose PDT, thus optimizing the balance between survival and death pathways for more effective therapeutic outcomes.

3.2.4 Pyroptosis

Pyroptosis, also known as inflammatory necrosis, is a programmed cell death mechanism characterized by cellular swelling and membrane rupture, leading to the release of intracellular contents and a potent inflammatory response. It serves as an essential component of the innate immune system, playing a significant role in the body's defense against infections and promoting antitumor immunity [22].

Pyroptosis is primarily mediated by gasdermin proteins and is uniquely reliant on inflammatory cysteine proteases such as caspase-1, caspase-4, caspase-5, and caspase-11 [23]. Unlike other cell death modalities, such as apoptosis and necrosis, pyroptosis is distinct in terms of morphological features, occurrence, and regulatory mechanisms. Under light microscopy, pyroptotic cells exhibit swelling and numerous bubble-like protrusions. Electron microscopy revealed the emergence of small vesicles, termed pyroptotic bodies, preceding cell membrane rupture. Pores subsequently form on the cell membrane, leading to membrane rupture and the efflux of cellular contents. The activation of a subset of caspase family proteins by inflammasomes, which are multiprotein complexes that detect cellular stress or infection. Once activated, caspases cleave gasdermin proteins, notably gasdermin D (GSDMD), into their active forms. The N-terminal fragment of GSDMD then translocates to the cell membrane, where it forms pores, leading to cell swelling, cytoplasmic efflux, and eventual rupture of the cell membrane. These events trigger a robust local inflammatory response, distinguishing pyroptosis from other forms of cell death, such as apoptosis, which is noninflammatory.

Emerging evidence has demonstrated that PDT can instigate GSDMD-mediated pyroptosis, fostering antitumor immunity [24, 25]. PDT pyrolyzes in human esophageal cancer cells via the PKM2/caspase-8/caspase-3/GSDME axis [26]. Recent investigations by the authors revealed that 4 h after ALA-PDT induction, A431 and SCL-1 human SCC cells undergo pyroptosis. Elevated ALA-PDT intensity is correlated with increased expression of the NLRP3 protein, cleaved caspase 1, and cleaved GSDMD. The increase in IL-1β and IL-18 mRNA expression further confirmed the pyroptotic response. The authors' findings suggest that the JNK signaling pathway is a key regulator of ALA-PDT-induced pyroptosis. When the JNK pathway was inhibited with SP600125, the expression of pyroptosis markers (cleaved caspase-1 and cleaved GSDMD) significantly decreased. These findings suggest that ALA-PDT induces pyroptosis by upregulating the JNK signaling pathway in squamous cell carcinoma cells. Given the novelty of pyroptosis as a mode of cell death, elucidating the mechanisms underlying the PDT-mediated regulation of pyroptosis requires further investigation.

3.2.5 Ferroptosis

Ferroptosis, a distinctive form of programmed cell death, is characterized by its reliance on iron ions and distinct morphological and biochemical features. Unlike apoptosis or necrosis, ferroptosis is driven primarily by lipid peroxidation, particularly involving unsaturated fatty acids in the cell membrane, which is catalyzed by ferrous iron or lipoxygenase enzymes [27]. Notably, the core enzyme of the antioxidant system, glutathione peroxidase 4 (GPX4), is downregulated during ferroptosis. The key manifestations of ferroptosis include the following: (1) morphologically, mitochondrial shrinkage with denser membranes, reduced mitochondrial cristae, and inconspicuous changes in the cell nucleus; and (2) biochemically, elevated lipid peroxidation and increased levels of ROS.

PDT can increase the intracellular levels of reactive oxygen species (ROS), which are crucial for the initiation of ferroptosis. Thus, the link between ferroptosis and PDT is significant. Recent studies have shown that PDT can trigger ferroptosis across various cell types [28, 29]. In research conducted by the authors' group, the Ce6 analog Sontaraporn (STBF)-PDT downregulated the expression of GPX4 and xCT in the sebaceous gland cell line XL-i-20 in a manner that was dependent on both time and concentration. The occurrence of ferroptosis was further validated through intracellular staining for ferrous iron ions. Subsequent pathway analyses indicated that ferroptosis induced by STBF-PDT is associated with the mTOR signaling pathway. Importantly, cells undergoing ferroptosis exhibit high levels of immunogenicity in vivo, suggesting that PDT-induced ferroptosis may play a vital role in mediating the immune response after PDT treatment.

The cytotoxic effects of PDT on target cells are fundamentally linked to oxidative reactions involving the ROS generated during treatment, which interact with nearby biomolecules. This targeted disruption primarily affects subcellular structures that absorb the photosensitizer, leading to irreversible damage and eventual cell death. The types of cell death observed post-PDT are varied and complex. A thorough understanding of the specific mechanisms governing cell death after PDT, identification of the dominant forms of cellular demise, and investigation of potential modifications in cell death pathways under varying PDT conditions for therapeutic enhancement require extensive further study.

3.3 PDT and Vascular Injury

In 1963, Castellani et al. first documented the effects of PDT on tissue microcirculation, highlighting vascular endothelial injury as the key initiating factor behind PDT-induced vascular changes—a crucial mechanism affecting microcirculation in PDT [30]. The PDT process induces immediate hypoxia and generates ROS, leading to endothelial cell damage and triggering a series of events, including vascular constriction, increased permeability, the release of coagulation factors, platelet aggregation, and thrombus formation. These processes culminate in vascular closure, resulting in target cell death due to hypoxia and nutrient deprivation [31]. The endothelial damage caused by PDT, along with subsequent changes in hemorheology, represents a vital mechanistic aspect of the therapeutic effects of PDT. Importantly, the influence of PDT on blood vessels varies on the basis of the specific photosensitizer used.

Under normal physiological conditions, vascular homeostasis is carefully regulated by angiogenic factors such as vascular endothelial growth factor (VEGF) and fibroblast growth factors 1 and 2 (FGF1/2), alongside angiogenic inhibitors such as thrombospondin-1 (TSP-1). TSP-1 is regulated by p53, and its deficiency can lead to abnormal neovascularization. Tumor angiogenesis plays a critical role in tumor initiation, progression, metastasis, and prognosis. In this context, PDT serves as a treatment modality that indirectly targets and damages tumor cells by disrupting the vasculature within the tumor microenvironment. The effectiveness of vascular impairment in PDT is closely related to the selective uptake and accumulation of photosensitizers in tumor tissues. This phenomenon is associated with specific characteristics of the tumor vasculature: (1) irregular morphology and luminal dilation, along with abnormal and discontinuous endothelial structures, which increase the vulnerability of tumor vessels to ROS-induced damage; (2) hypovascular tumors, characterized by inadequate oxygen supply, which enhances glycolysis and acid accumulation, promoting photosensitizer aggregation within tumor vessels; (3) inefficient clearance of accumulated PSs in newly formed tumor vessels; and (4) increased collagen content in the vascular basement membrane, further facilitating photosensitizer aggregation. Collectively, these factors create the basis for the selective effects of PDT on tumor tissues.

In 1986, Star et al. utilized a transparent chamber to directly observe changes in microcirculation within rat-implanted breast cancer and adjacent normal tissues during Hpd-PDT. Their findings revealed an initial constriction of tumor blood vessels, followed by complete stasis of blood flow and instances of bleeding, with platelet aggregation leading to thrombus formation in larger vessels [32]. The authors' group reported a reduction in vascular density within tumors in SKH-1 mice following local ALA-PDT [33]. Researchers have also leveraged the ability of PDT to transiently disrupt microcirculation, employing ALA-PDT to temporarily breach the blood–brain barrier in normal rats, thereby facilitating the efficient delivery of chemotherapy drugs to adjacent tumor tissues. However, damage to the tumor vasculature induced by PDT can lead to adverse effects, such as further hypoxia in tumor tissues, which may reduce the efficacy of PDT. Hypoxic conditions can also trigger the expression and increased activity of hypoxia-inducible factor alpha (HIF-α), increasing the transcription of factors such as vascular endothelial growth factor (VEGF) and erythropoietin. This cascade promotes tumor angiogenesis, and subsequent autophagy may allow residual tumor cells to resist PDT treatment, impacting overall efficacy [34].

The mechanism of vascular damage caused by PDT serves as the conceptual foundation for treating port wine stains, with significant clinical efficacy demonstrated via hematoporphyrin monomethyl ether-mediated PDT (HMME-PDT), particularly with the domestically produced drug hemoporfin (trade name: Fumeida) [35]. As HMME-PDT plays a crucial role in therapeutic interventions, an important question arises regarding the suitability of using the more widely applicable and accessible photosensitizer ALA for treating port wine stains. Preliminary investigations by the authors' group using murine models revealed reduced vascular density in tumor tissues following ALA-PDT. Using a chicken comb model, they compared the effects of ALA-PDT and HMME-PDT. This study revealed that the PpIX fluorescence intensity peaked at 4 h after the local application of ALA, which was localized to the epidermis, whereas intravenous ALA administration resulted in peak fluorescence at 6 h, which was distributed throughout the epidermis and dermal layers. In contrast, intravenous HMME administration elicited an immediate peak fluorescence intensity limited to the superficial vascular tissue surrounding the dermis, with no observable fluorescence in the epidermis. Low-dose local ALA-PDT interventions (80 J/cm^2, 120 J/cm^2) induced minimal comb changes, and histological examination revealed no significant alterations in the epidermis or dermis. High-dose local ALA-PDT (160 J/cm^2, 200 J/cm^2) led to apparent comb necrosis, exudation, and scabbing, with histopathological findings indicating epidermal necrosis, focal cell loss, and marked dermal edema. Systemic ALA-PDT application resulted in immediate purple–black comb changes, with evident black scabbing at 3 days persisting until 14 days; conversely, the HMME-PDT group presented noticeable comb whitening without significant adverse reactions.

In conclusion, HMME-PDT is effective at treating port wine stains, whereas both local and systemic ALA-PDT are ineffective at addressing this condition.

Upon intravenous administration of HMME, rapid uptake occurs within vascular endothelial cells, with absorption rates significantly surpassing those of epidermal cells. The heightened sensitivity of endothelial cells to PDT, driven by substantial HMME absorption, leads to their degeneration and necrosis, resulting in capillary occlusion and subsequent resolution of erythema in the treated area. Moreover, the normal epidermis remains relatively unaffected by lower photosensitizer levels, and deeper dermal tissues are protected by limited penetration of the excitation wavelength. Conversely, intravenous ALA requires conversion to PpIX, necessitating considerable time for adequate accumulation within vascular endothelial cells, during which PpIX also accumulates in the overlying epidermis. This may lead to damage to the dermal capillaries of port wine stains while adversely affecting nontarget treatment areas. Furthermore, preliminary studies indicate that topical ALA application is confined primarily to the epidermis and sebaceous gland units [36], resulting in a limited ability to penetrate the basement membrane and reach the dermis, which is essential for inducing vascular occlusion in port wine stains.

The mechanism of vascular damage induced by PDT has broad implications for various systemic diseases, particularly in ophthalmology for treating age-related macular degeneration (AMD). For example, verteporfin-PDT occludes choroidal neovascularization, effectively alleviating or eliminating exudation and hemorrhage, leading to improved visual outcomes. Careful control of the vascular effects of PDT expands its utility for treating hemorrhagic conditions, such as gastrointestinal mucosal vascular lesions. Moreover, the impact on tumor vascular endothelial cells is intricately connected to inflammatory responses and the initiation of antitumor immunity.

The effectiveness of PDT in tumor treatment faces challenges in hypoxic microenvironments, where ROS generation depends on molecular oxygen. Rapid oxygen consumption during PDT creates a hypoxic environment, which is common in solid tumors and promotes conditions conducive to tumor growth, metastasis, and alterations in gene expression related to metastasis and chemotherapy resistance. Addressing these microenvironment characteristics is critical for enhancing the antitumor efficacy of PDT. Recent advances in nanomedicine, led by the authors' group in 2020, have resulted in biomimetic nanoparticles (MnO_2-ICG@BSA) with significant singlet oxygen generation and photothermal stability. These nanoparticles generate oxygen molecules and Mn^{2+} in response to H_2O_2 under low pH conditions, effectively inhibiting melanoma [37]. Additionally, the research team synthesized HbA@ZIF nanoparticles that encapsulate hemoglobin (Hb) and ALA and were loaded with oxygen molecules to form oxygen-carrying OHbA@ ZIF nanoparticles. These nanoparticles release oxygen molecules stably, alleviating hypoxia in squamous cell carcinoma, enhancing antitumor immunity, and effectively eradicating squamous cell carcinoma cells, thereby inhibiting skin squamous cell carcinoma growth in mice.

In summary, vascular endothelial injury has emerged as a critical mechanism underlying the vascular damage effects of PDT. The rapid action of PDT induces endothelial cell damage, triggering a cascade of reactions that ultimately leads to complete occlusion of target vessels, resulting in the death of target cells due to hypoxia and nutrient deprivation. Vascular damage is a fundamental mechanism in the treatment of tumors and port wine stains through PDT.

3.4 Immunological Mechanisms of PDT

Historically, research on the therapeutic mechanisms of PDT has focused primarily on its direct cytotoxic effects on target cells and its ability to disrupt the vascular system in pathological tissues. However, an increasing body of evidence highlights the role of immunological mechanisms in the damage induced by PDT. While the main objectives of PDT are the direct destruction of target cells and the impairment of vascular structures to treat underlying diseases, the elicitation of adaptive immune responses in the host is emerging as a crucial factor for effective disease control and prevention of disease recurrence.

3.4.1 Immunological Mechanisms of ALA-PDT in the Management of Condyloma Acuminatum

In 1997, the authors' group pioneered the use of ALA-PDT for the treatment of urethral condyloma acuminatum, building on their previous success with ALA-PDT in cutaneous tumors. Their groundbreaking work demonstrated the significant efficacy of ALA-PDT, characterized by low recurrence rates and minimal adverse reactions in managing urethral condyloma acuminatum [10]. Given the immunomodulatory effects of human papillomavirus (HPV) infection, a known inducer of immune evasion, patients with condyloma acuminatum frequently exhibit local immunological dysregulation, which is closely linked to disease onset, recurrence, and prognosis. In a follow-up study in 2001, the authors' group applied ALA-PDT to patients with condyloma acuminatum, revealing noteworthy histological changes. One hour posttreatment, considerable dermal edema accompanied by significant infiltration of neutrophils and eosinophils was observed. Additionally, the epidermis showed a modest influx of neutrophils. By the 3-h mark after treatment, significant neutrophil infiltration in the epidermis was noted, along with pronounced intercellular and intracellular edema. These findings suggest that PDT induces neutrophil infiltration into the treated area [9, 10].

Neutrophils serve as "sentinels" in the immune system and play a critical role in the early treatment response, performing three primary functions: (1) direct phagocytosis and elimination of damaged or tumor cells; (2) recruitment of various immune cells to the tumor site; and (3) secretion of multiple proinflammatory factors, contributing to the inflammatory response following PDT. To comprehensively elucidate the cellular types and immune status involved in the immune response during ALA-PDT treatment of condyloma acuminatum, the authors' group employed immunohistochemical methods to investigate changes in the quantities of CD4+ T cells, CD8+ T cells, and CD68+ macrophages, as well as the CD4+/CD8+ cell ratio in skin lesions before ALA-PDT treatment and at 1, 2, 3, and 48 h post-treatment. The results revealed a significant increase in the number of macrophages in the dermis at 3 h post-ALA-PDT treatment, whereas the number of CD4+ T cells and CD8+ T cells and their ratio increased at 48 h in the dermis. These findings suggest that ALA-PDT enhances cellular immune function, bolsters the antiviral immune response, and predominantly initiates a Th1 response driven by CD4+ T cells in the early stages of treatment for condyloma acuminatum, which is consistent with previously reported findings in the literature [38].

The species specificity of HPV presents challenges for in-depth exploration of the immunological mechanisms of ALA-PDT in treating genital warts owing to the lack of internationally recognized animal models for HPV infection. To address this limitation, the authors developed a model utilizing keratinocytes infected with HPV. They amplified the HPV16E7 gene from CaSki cells via PCR and restriction enzyme techniques and then directionally cloned it into the eukaryotic expression vector pcDNA3.1(+), resulting in the recombinant plasmid pcDNA3.1(+)-HPV16E7. Subsequent transfection of this plasmid into immortalized human epidermal cells (HaCaT cells) and the selection of stable cell lines expressing the HPV16E7 protein via G418 screening led to the establishment of the HaCaT/HPV16E7 cell line [17]. In coculture experiments, HaCaT/HPV16E7 cells treated with ALA-PDT exhibited a notable chemotactic effect on peripheral blood monocytes from patients with genital warts [39]. At the cellular level, this study demonstrated that ALA-PDT not only directly eliminates HPV-infected keratinocytes but also activates the host immune response to further eradicate viral infections. Through its targeted cytotoxic effects on HPV-infected cells and enhancement of cellular immunity, ALA-PDT effectively clears clinical lesions of genital warts and eliminates subclinical and latent infections, providing a significant advantage over traditional treatment methods.

3.4.2 Immunological Mechanisms of ALA-PDT in Acne Treatment

ALA-PDT, a chronic inflammatory disorder affecting the pilosebaceous unit, is recognized as a crucial therapeutic approach, especially for moderate to severe cases [40]. A significant milestone in this area occurred in 2009 when the authors' group first reported the safe and effective use of ALA-PDT for treating severe facial acne in Chinese patients [41]. Following these groundbreaking observations, a series of clinical and foundational studies were conducted, leading to the establishment of standardized treatment principles for acne. These guidelines recommend ALA concentrations between 3% and 5%, a drug incubation period of 3 h, and an initial low-energy dose that can be incrementally adjusted. The efficacy and safety of these principles have been acknowledged and endorsed by various national and international guidelines [42, 43].

The precise mechanisms through which ALA-PDT treats acne remain incompletely understood.

Current hypotheses suggest that ALA-PDT works by targeting various pathogenic factors associated with acne. As noted earlier, ALA-PDT has both direct and indirect biocidal effects on microbes such as *Cutibacterium acnes* as well as on sebaceous gland cells and keratinocytes. This action helps inhibit sebaceous gland hyperactivity, regulate the microbial environment, and normalize abnormal keratinization of follicular epithelial cells. Additionally, ALA-PDT has significant immunomodulatory and anti-inflammatory effects on acne. In cases of severe acne, where nodules and cysts predominate, chronic inflammation presents a major treatment challenge. On the basis of clinical observations, the authors noted a transient inflammatory amplification early in ALA-PDT treatment for severe acne. Interestingly, the extent of acute inflammation correlates with clinical efficacy, suggesting that this immunomodulatory effect, characterized by inflammation amplification, may be a key therapeutic mechanism for severe acne [44].

The research team successfully isolated primary sebaceous gland cells from acne patients' lesions and demonstrated, in both cell cultures and a golden hamster sebaceous gland spotted acne model, that ALA-PDT upregulated CXCL8 expression. This upregulation recruits T cells, B cells, neutrophils, macrophages, and other immune components, amplifying the inflammatory response (Fig. 3.3) [45]. Recent studies by the authors further indicate that ALA-PDT may regulate acne-related inflammation by inducing M1 polarization of macrophages. In an inflammatory microenvironment, macrophages polarize into different states, with M1 being dominant in acute inflammation and M2 playing a role in chronic inflammation [45]. Research by Do et al. revealed that macrophages in acne lesions exhibit M2 characteristics, emphasizing their role in chronic inflammation [46]. However, transcriptomic gene chip analysis performed by the authors revealed that 24 h post-ALA-PDT, several inflammation-related genes, including cyclooxygenase-2 (COX-2) and triggering receptor expressed on myeloid cells 1 (TREM-1), were upregulated. In a *Cutibacterium acnes*-induced mouse ear acne-like inflammation model, ALA-PDT can target keratinocytes, activate the COX-2-TREM-1 axis, and induce M1 macrophage polarization through the NF-κB and p38-MAPK signaling pathways. This promotes the release of proinflammatory cytokines such as IL-1β and IL-6 while inhibiting the anti-inflammatory cytokine IL-10. This inflammatory amplification disrupts the persistent chronic inflammation observed in severe acne, leading to the rapid resolution of inflammation and significant improvements in patients' facial appearance (Figs. 3.4 and 3.5).

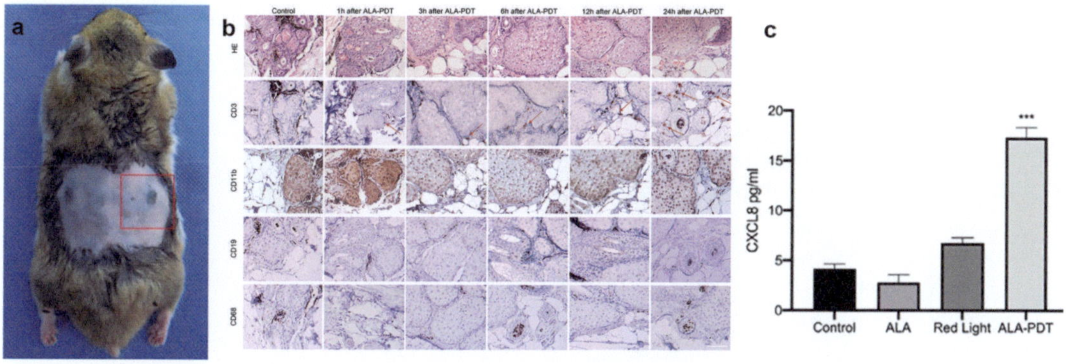

Fig. 3.3 ALA-PDT upregulates CXCL8 expression in the golden hamster sebaceous gland model, recruiting T cells, B cells, neutrophils, and macrophages to amplify the inflammatory response. (**a**) Golden hamster sebaceous gland model; (**b**) many T cells, B cells, neutrophils, and macrophages are recruited in a time-dependent fashion; and (**c**) ALA-PDT upregulates CXCL8 expression in the golden hamster sebaceous gland model

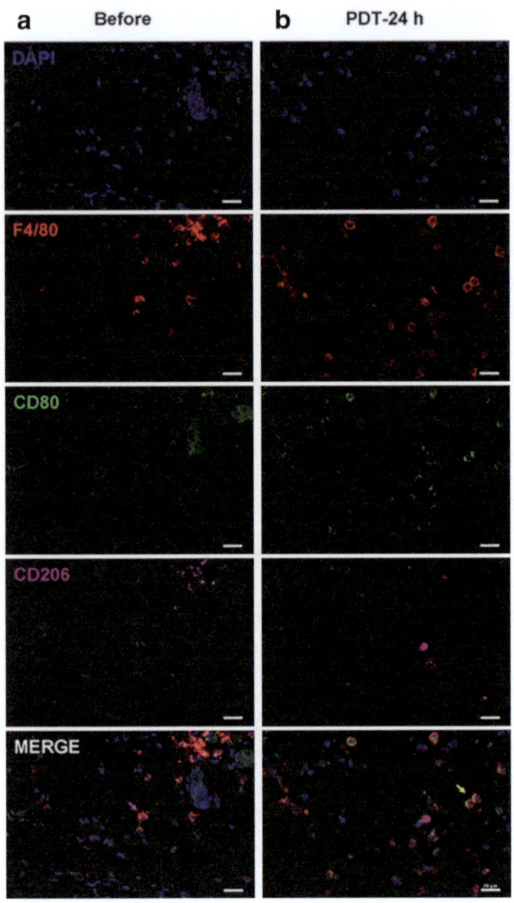

Fig. 3.4 ALA-PDT induces M1 polarization of macrophages. (**a**) Immunofluorescence staining of a mouse acne model. (**b**) 24 h after ALA-PDT, immunofluorescence staining of mouse tissue revealed an increase in the number of M1 macrophages marked by both CD80 and F4/80 and a decrease in the number of M2 macrophages marked by both CD206 and F4/80

3.4.3 PDT-Induced Antitumor Immunity

In the 1990s, the Canadian scientist Korbelik and colleagues pioneered investigations into the immunological effects of PDT, producing a series of pivotal findings. These studies showed that Photofrin-mediated PDT could achieve complete remission of EMT6-related breast cancer in immunocompetent BALB/c mice. However, in immunodeficient BALB/c or nude mice of the same strain, Photofrin-PDT led to only a temporary disappearance of EMT6 breast cancer without full tumor eradication. Notably, transplanting bone marrow or T lymphocytes from immunocompetent BALB/c mice into immunodeficient mice delayed tumor recurrence, indicating a strong link between the immune response and PDT efficacy, with functional lymphocytes playing a crucial role. Further work by Korbelik's group demonstrated that the removal of cytotoxic T lymphocytes (CTLs) from BALB/c mice with EMT6 breast cancer after PDT significantly reduced the tumor cure rate. Similarly, removing CD4+ T cells or blocking IL-2 also lowered the cure rate, although to a lesser extent than CTL removal. These findings highlight that PDT can induce host-specific antitumor immunity, with tumor antigen-specific CTLs acting as key effector cells in the antitumor immune response. As a result, the immune mechanisms triggered by PDT have become a major research focus, drawing significant attention and advancing the field's understanding of the therapeutic effects of PDT.

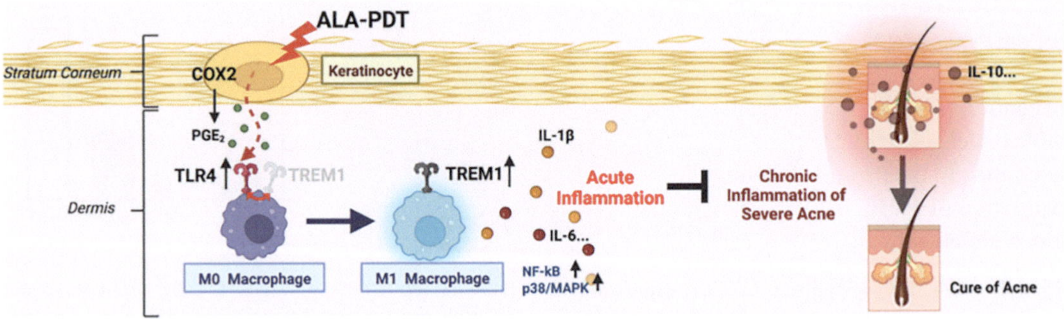

Fig. 3.5 ALA-PDT targets keratinocytes, induces macrophages to polarize toward the proinflammatory M1 type through the COX2-PGE2-TREM1 axis, amplifies the inflammatory response, and disrupts the persistent state of chronic inflammation in severe acne

In 1996, the authors' group initiated pioneering studies on ALA-PDT for skin tumor treatment in China, observing a significant acute inflammatory response post-PDT [6, 7]. This inflammation represents a specific immune response against tumor antigens. Alterations in the tumor vasculature signal PDT-induced inflammation, resulting in hemoglobin leakage and inflammatory cell adhesion. Neutrophils, mast cells, and macrophages rapidly infiltrate the tumor, helping clear damaged tissues and necrotic cells. In a mouse SCC model treated with ALA-PDT, neutrophils accumulated in the tumor vasculature within 3 h and subsequently migrated to the tumor stroma. Electron microscopy at 6 h post-treatment revealed that neutrophils engulfed debris, and by day 7, dendritic cells (DCs), CD4+ T cells, and CD8+ T cells had gathered at the tumor site, with increased TNF-α secretion, indicating a local immune response [11, 12].

To further elucidate the antitumor immune effects of PDT, the authors' group used a UV-induced SKH-1 mouse skin SCC model. They isolated SCC cells from mouse tissue, established an in vitro culture, and developed the XL50 SCC cell line, which they patented. ALA-PDT was applied to treat XL50 cells in vitro, and after subcutaneous injections of ALA-PDT-treated XL50 cells into SKH-1 mice, followed by additional injections of XL50 cells on the opposite side, tumor formation was successfully prevented [46]. This study revealed that the efficacy of ALA-PDT relies on the activation of local tumor-specific immunity. However, questions remain regarding the mechanisms of antitumor immunity post-ALA-PDT and the role of specific immune cells, warranting further investigation.

Dendritic cells (DCs) are specialized antigen-presenting cells that activate naïve T lymphocytes and connect the innate and adaptive immune responses. In their immature state, DCs have low expression of MHC I/II, adhesion, and costimulatory molecules but are still capable of antigen recognition and phagocytosis. Upon exposure to inflammatory stimuli, DCs mature, increasing their antigen-presenting capacity. They process antigen–peptide complexes and present them to T cells, initiating an antitumor immune response. After observing an increase in DCs at tumor sites post-PDT in animal studies, the authors' group performed coculture experiments with DCs and ALA-PDT-treated XL50 cells to sensitize DCs. The results showed that ALA-PDT-treated tumor cells induced DC maturation. These mature DCs exhibited morphological changes (thicker dendritic processes and more lysosomes) and upregulated MHC II, CD80, and CD86 expression, indicating their maturation. Functionally, they secrete relatively high levels of IFN-γ and IL-12, increasing their ability to stimulate T-cell proliferation. Post-PDT treatment of XL50 cells, mature sensitized DCs were then injected into SKH-1 mice, leading to a preventive effect against the development of squamous cell carcinoma [47]. Thus, PDT-induced antitumor immunity relies on the maturation and activation of DCs, which recognize and process immunogenic substances from dying tumor cells post-PDT, along with the processing and presentation of tumor-associated antigens to T cells. Consequently, this instigates acquired immune memory in mice, fostering the proliferation and activation of initial T cells into effector T cells, thereby orchestrating assault on primary tumors and metastatic foci (Figs. 3.6 and 3.7).

CD8+ T lymphocytes play a crucial role in driving specific immune responses after PDT. Studies have shown that the long-term antitumor efficacy of PDT depends on its immunological effects as immunodeficient mice are unable to maintain these effects. However, immunoreconstruction through the administration of bone marrow cells or T cells with intact immune function significantly enhances PDT efficacy. Both murine and human models indicate that reduced CD8+ T-cell activation or decreased tumor infiltration compromises the effectiveness of PDT. After PDT treatment, there was a marked increase in CD4+ and CD8+ T lymphocytes within the tumor tissue. Notably, removing CD8+ T cells from mice via anti-CD8 antibodies greatly reduces the antitumor effects of PDT, highlighting the vital role of CD8+ T lymphocytes in the anticancer response triggered by PDT.

PDT has the ability to induce macrophage infiltration at the tumor site. Studies have shown

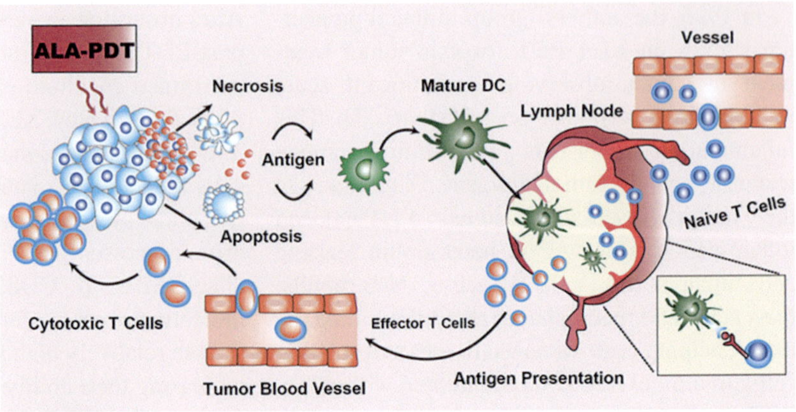

Fig. 3.6 Key role of T cells in the PDT treatment of tumors

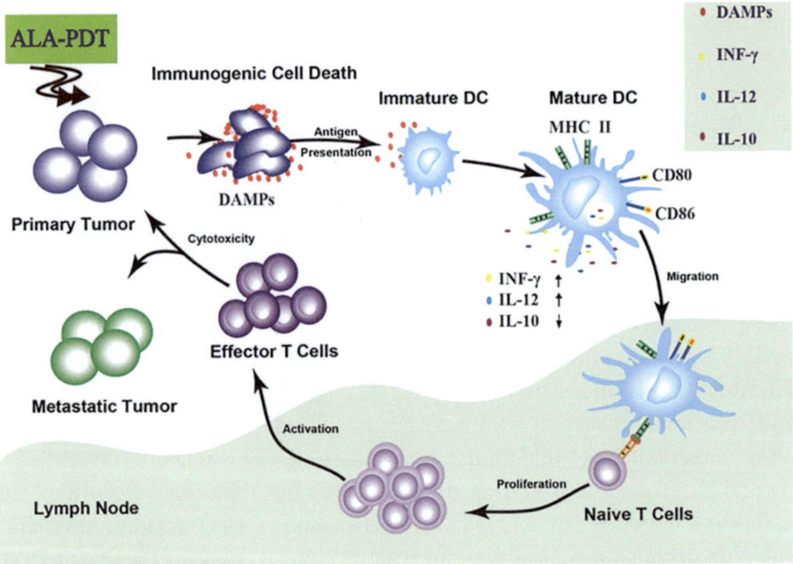

Fig. 3.7 Immunological mechanism of ALA-PDT in tumor treatment

that macrophage infiltration becomes noticeable within 2 h after PDT. Macrophages, key effector cells in the body's immune defense system, play critical roles depending on their activation state. They are generally classified into M1 (classically activated) and M2 (alternatively activated) macrophages, which regulate immune responses in opposing ways. M1 macrophages engage in phagocytosis, process tumor antigens, and present them to T lymphocytes, exerting direct cytotoxic effects on tumor cells, either alone or with antibodies and complement. On the other hand, M2 macrophages promote tumor invasion and metastasis by secreting growth factors such as TGF-β. A study by Demidova et al. demonstrated that selectively eliminating M2 macrophages via a photosensitizer enhanced the efficacy of treating mouse breast cancer [48]. Subsequent investigations suggest that PDT can activate macrophages through the release of various cytokines, including interleukins, TNF, and chemokines.

Immune recognition is crucial for initiating immune responses, particularly in distinguishing between dying tumor cells and normal cell death. In the context of ALA-PDT, it is important to understand how the host organism identifies dying tumor cells and the molecular entities involved in this process. Research shows that during PDT oxidative stress damages the subcellular structures where photosensitizers accumulate, triggering the rapid expression, secretion, or exposure of specific molecules within the cells. These molecules act as "endogenous danger signals," which are recognized by the host, leading to the activation of phagocytic cells that migrate to the tumor site, creating a proinflammatory environment. These danger signals are known as damage-associated molecular patterns (DAMPs) [49]. DAMPs typically reside inside cells but become exposed or secreted when cellular damage or death occurs, thereby activating the immune system. DAMPs can be classified into three types: (1) DAMPs on the cell membrane, (2) DAMPs released into the extracellular space, and (3) DAMPs as end-stage degradation products.

In exploring the role of DAMPs in tumor treatment with ALA-PDT, the authors' group analyzed the expression of three key DAMPs—calreticulin (CRT), heat shock protein 70 (HSP70), and high mobility group box 1 (HMGB1)—in mouse skin squamous cell carcinoma tissues before and after ALA-PDT treatment. The results revealed distinct expression patterns of these DAMPs. Before PDT, HMGB1-positive cells were scarce and were located primarily within the nuclei of tumor cells. Following PDT treatment, HMGB1 levels increased in tumor tissues, with extracellular HMGB1 detected at 3 h, peaking at 6 h, and declining at 9 h. CRT, which was not expressed before PDT, became strongly positive at 6 h post-treatment and remained weakly positive at 9 and 12 h. HSP70 was not expressed before or 1 h after PDT, but weak positive expression was detected at 3 and 6 h, with no expression detected at 9 and 12 h post-PDT. Further cellular studies confirmed that ALA-PDT upregulated HMGB1, HSP70, and CRT in XL50 cells. PDT promoted the secretion of HMGB1 and HSP70, along with the membrane translocation of CRT and HSP70 [46]. This research highlights that ALA-PDT significantly induces the upregulation of DAMPs in squamous cell carcinoma cells.

The authors continued investigating the role of DAMPs in the immune activation triggered by ALA-PDT. They cocultured mouse XL50 cells treated with ALA-PDT with mouse bone marrow-derived DCs to assess DC maturation. Neutralizing antibodies were used to selectively inhibit HSP70, HMGB1, and CRT, and the effects on DC maturation were carefully monitored. The results showed that ALA-PDT-treated tumor cells induced DC maturation, increasing the expression of costimulatory molecules (MHC II, CD80, and CD86) on DCs and increasing their immune activity. When neutralizing antibodies were applied to inhibit these DAMPs, there was a marked decrease in the expression of these costimulatory molecules. This evidence highlights the crucial role of DAMPs in promoting DC maturation after PDT [46]. Moreover, the inhibition of individual DAMP molecules led to reduced INF-γ secretion by DCs, with a more significant reduction observed when all three molecules were inhibited simultaneously. This also resulted in decreased IL-12 secretion. These findings underscore that DAMPs are essential for the functional maturation of DCs in response to ALA-PDT-treated tumor cells. The simultaneous inhibition of HSP70, HMGB1, and CRT had the most significant suppressive effect on DC maturation [46].

The authors further examined the signaling pathways involved in ALA-PDT-induced damage-associated molecular patterns (DAMPs) by isolating activated DCs from mouse XL50 cells after ALA-PDT treatment. ALA-PDT-treated squamous cell carcinoma cells significantly increased the expression of TLR2, TLR4, IκB, p-IκB, and nuclear NF-κB in DCs. Inhibition of HSP70, HMGB1, or CRT, individually or together, reduced the expression of TLR2 and TLR4 in these cells. Additionally, inhibiting HSP70, HMGB1, or all three molecules led to decreased levels of IκB, p-IκB, and nuclear NF-κB in DCs.

In summary, ALA-PDT triggers the production of DAMPs in tumor cells, which activate DCs as endogenous danger signals. These DCs then process and present tumor-associated antigens to T cells, leading to the development of acquired immune memory against the tumor. The primary molecular mechanism by which DAMPs enhance tumor immunogenicity following ALA-PDT involves the activation of the TLR–NF-κB signaling pathway in DCs.

3.4.4 PDT-Induced Tertiary Lymphoid Structures Mediate Antitumor Immunity

Tertiary lymphoid structures (TLSs) are ectopic clusters of immune cells found in nonlymphoid tissues during chronic inflammation. They are particularly noticeable in tumor environments, microbial infections, transplant rejection, and autoimmune diseases. Like secondary lymphoid organs such as the lymph nodes, spleen, and mucosal immune system, TLSs represent ectopic lymphoid tissue. During tumor initiation and progression, the failure of the immune system to eliminate tumors effectively can result in chronic inflammation. A key characteristic of the local microenvironment in chronic inflammation is the infiltration of immune cells and the formation of TLSs, which may play crucial roles in activating the body's antitumor immune response [50].

TLSs act as central hubs for localized antigen-specific immune responses within tumor tissues. Its presence has been confirmed in various cancer types, including breast, lung, melanoma, and liver cancers. Notably, TLSs have also been identified in the metastatic lesions of certain tumors, potentially affecting lymphocyte infiltration at these sites. TLSs are highly organized aggregates of immune cells found in inflamed or infected tissues and are primarily composed of T-cell zones and B-cell zones. The peripheral T-cell zone contains clustered T cells, mature dendritic cells, and fibroblastic reticular cells. At the core of TLSs lies the B-cell zone, which features follicular-like structures and germinal center functions and is composed primarily of B cells, along with smaller populations of T cells, follicular dendritic cells, and macrophages. Moreover, TLSs are surrounded by high endothelial venules (HEVs), which serve as primary pathways for lymphocyte infiltration from the bloodstream into local tissues [50]. As illustrated in Fig. 3.8, within the tumor microenvironment, lymphocytes or stromal cells influenced by chronic inflammatory stimuli secrete CXCL13 and IL-7 to recruit lymphoid tissue-inducing cells. This series of cellular interactions draws lymphocytes into local tissue via high endothelial venules, facilitating the formation of TLSs. This coordinated process is crucial for exerting antitumor effects and preventing tumor micrometastasis.

PDT has the capacity to recruit various immune cells, including dendritic cells (DCs), T cells, B cells, and macrophages. In an investigation by the authors' group, after the administration of ALA-PDT, patients with skin squamous cell carcinoma exhibited the emergence of immature tertiary lymphoid structures (TLSs) in tumor tissue samples within 24 h. By the 48-h mark, a significant increase in the number of TLS struc-

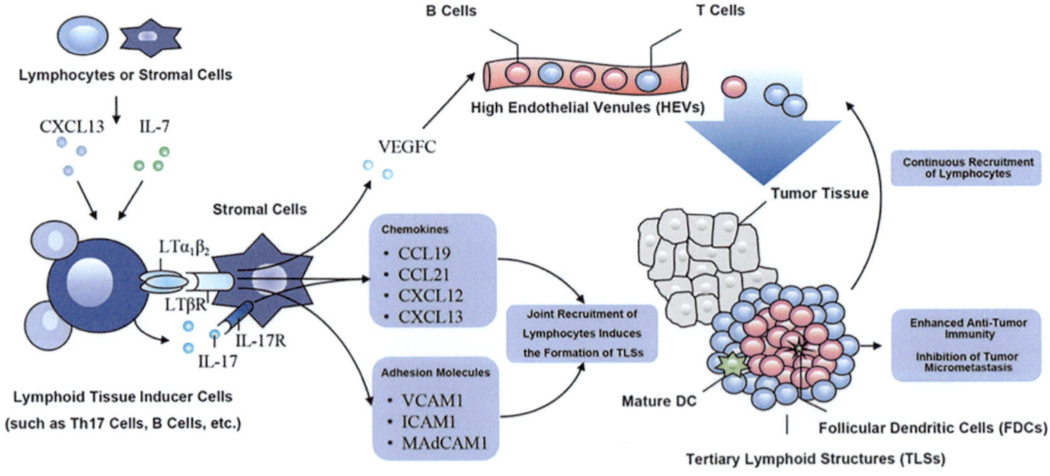

Fig. 3.8 Schematic diagram of the mechanism and main effects of tertiary lymphoid structures (TLSs)

tures was observed in the tumor tissues, revealing a discernible pattern of B-cell clustering around T cells and indicating enhanced structural maturity. These findings suggest that the antitumor immune response elicited by ALA-PDT involves not only immune cell recruitment but also the formation of TLS structures at the tumor tissue periphery. This process contributes to a sustained antitumor effect, as depicted in Fig. 3.9. However, the exact mechanisms underlying ALA-PDT-induced TLS formation require further investigation.

3.4.5 PDT and Antitumor Vaccines

Following PDT, tumor cells exhibit increased immunogenicity, contributing to the restoration of the host's antitumor immunity. The immunogenic response triggered by PDT-induced tumor cell inactivation is currently recognized as more effective than that triggered by other methods, such as ionizing radiation, freeze–thaw lysis, and ultraviolet irradiation. Building on this observation, whole-cell vaccines created from tumor cells treated with PDT have been developed. These vaccines have shown significant efficacy in preclinical studies, leading to progression into phase I clinical trials [51]. In research conducted by the authors' group, murine experiments demonstrated that tumor cells treated with ALA-PDT displayed vaccine-like characteristics, successfully preventing the development of skin squamous cell carcinoma (Fig. 3.10) [46].

DCs play a crucial role in orchestrating antitumor immunity by managing the effects of extracorporeal stimulation with tumor antigens and sensitizing DCs to create DC vaccines. This strategic method ensures efficient uptake and presentation of tumor antigens, along with the essential costimulatory signals needed to elicit a strong antitumor immune response. As a result, DC-based tumor vaccines have emerged as key players in anticancer applications because of

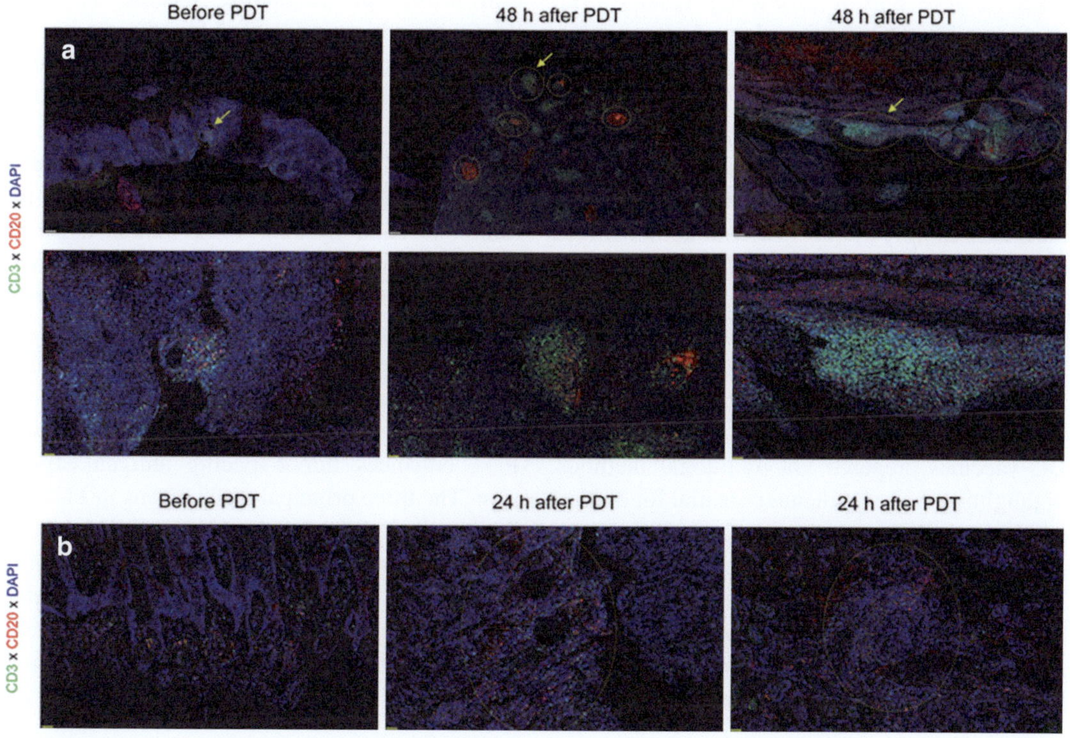

Fig. 3.9 Recruitment of TLSs in skin squamous cell carcinoma by ALA-PDT. (**a**) Mature TLSs appear 48 h after ALA-PDT and (**b**) TLSs begin to form 24 h after ALA-PDT

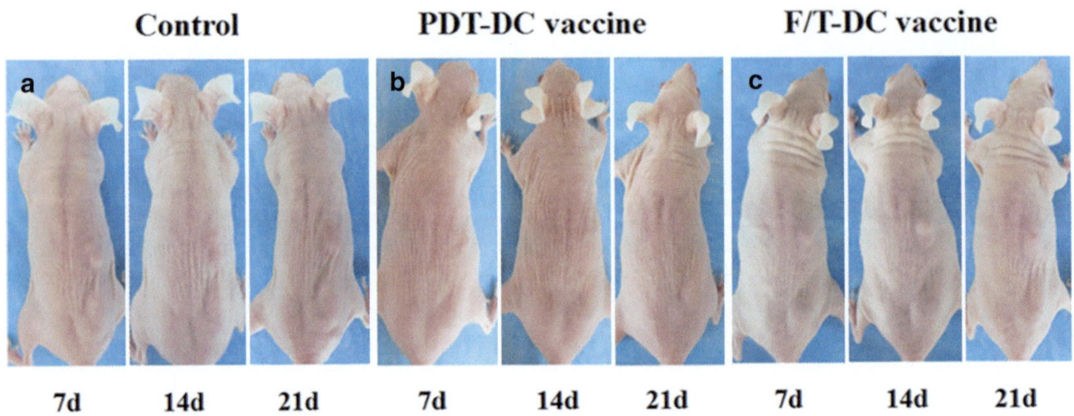

Fig. 3.10 ALA-PDT-sensitized DC vaccine prevents the occurrence of squamous cell carcinoma. (**a**) Mice were directly inoculated with tumor cells on the right back, and tumor growth was observed. (**b**) After ALA-PDT treatment of tumor cells sensitized DC cells, DC cells were inoculated into mice followed by tumor cells, and no tumor growth was observed. (**c**) After repeated freeze–thaw cycles of sensitized DC cells, DC cells were inoculated into mice followed by tumor cells, and tumor growth was observed

their high efficacy and low toxicity. Clinical trials targeting melanoma, renal cancer, and gynecological malignancies, as well as both preclinical and clinical investigations into nervous system cancers, have shown promising results [52]. Photodynamic DC vaccines have been successfully developed by exposing tumor cells to extracorporeal stimulation post-PDT and sensitizing DCs. Efficacy assessments indicate that these DC vaccines exhibit commendable tolerance, safety, and specificity. Notably, in animal studies focused on breast cancer, the DC vaccine demonstrated positive therapeutic effects. Building on the immunogenic apoptosis induced by ALA-PDT in tumor cells, the authors' group created ALA-PDT-based DC vaccines, which significantly prevented the onset of skin squamous cell carcinoma in animal models. This efficacy surpasses that of DC vaccines prepared via traditional methods, highlighting their significant potential for clinical applications [13].

PDT operates through a multifaceted set of mechanisms. It directly targets and eliminates specific cells, disrupts the microvascular circulation within tissues—leading to hypoxia and nutrient deprivation—and triggers an inflammatory response that promotes local immune cell aggregation, further activating the broader immune system (Fig. 3.11). In addition to its cytotoxic effects on tumor cells, PDT plays a critical role in stimulating specific antitumor immunity, which is essential for effectively controlling tumors and reducing the risk of recurrence. PDT induces immunogenic cell death in tumor cells, enhances the expression of endogenous danger signals, and increases tumor immunogenicity. Additionally, by compromising the tumor vascular system, PDT fosters a robust inflammatory response that recruits immune cells to the treatment site, initiating an antitumor immune response.

The potential for breakthroughs in tumor treatment lies in developing effective tumor vaccines that leverage the mechanisms by which PDT enhances tumor-specific antigen expression. The three principal mechanisms of PDT are interconnected, and recent research highlights the importance of immune mechanisms in tumor research. As the understanding of PDT mechanisms deepens and is applied judiciously, this therapy is expected to show improved clinical efficacy, offering greater hope for patients.

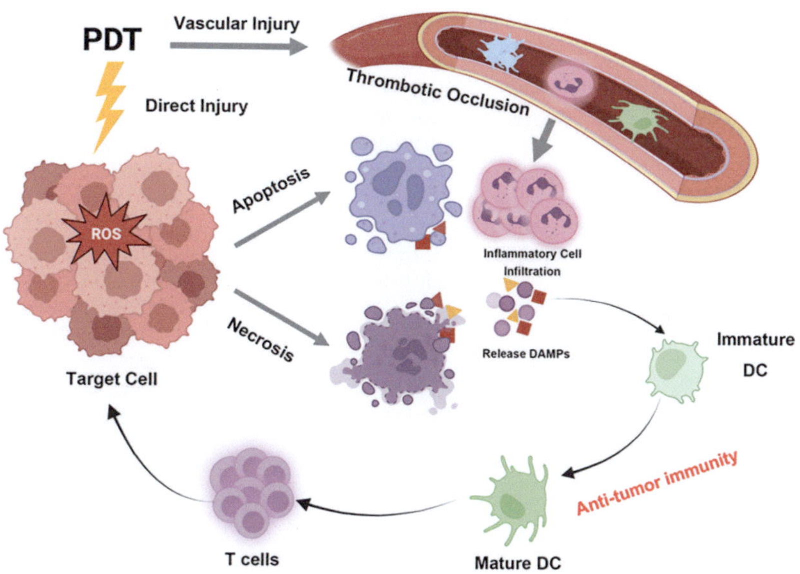

Fig. 3.11 Three main mechanisms of action of PDT

3.5 Research Models for PDT

The use of diverse cell and animal models is the primary approach for understanding the pathogenesis and treatment mechanisms of diseases in basic research. Over the past few decades, ALA-PDT has been extensively employed in dermatology for conditions such as skin photoaging, skin cancers, and moderate to severe acne [53]. Preclinical studies of these applications rely heavily on these cell and animal models.

3.5.1 Cells and Cell Lines

3.5.1.1 Skin Cancers

Cutaneous Squamous Cell Carcinoma (cSCC) SCC is primarily linked to DNA damage resulting from excessive ultraviolet (UV) exposure. However, the precise pathogenesis of cSCC remains incompletely understood. The establishment of relevant tumor cell lines is crucial for investigating the effects and mechanisms of action of new drugs and treatments. The advantages of using cell models include the following: (a) cell models minimize interference from the body's internal environment and individual variability, facilitating the analysis of various external factors on tumor cells. (b) They allow for the examination of carcinogenesis mechanisms at the gene and molecular levels. (c) They enable the study of drug resistance mechanisms in tumors and the screening of antitumor drugs. (d) These methods typically require a shorter experimental duration and are more economical and practical. Thus, cSCC cell lines are essential tools for investigating the mechanisms of carcinogenesis and potential interventions for cSCC. Common cSCC cell lines are summarized in Table 3.1.

Currently, there are numerous reports on the establishment of cSCC cell lines derived from the head, neck, mouth, and lung, but few have been developed from mouse skin. Building on previous postgraduate work, Dr. Ji Jie from the authors' group successfully isolated primary tumor cells from UV-induced cSCC in SKH-1 hairless mice with normal immunity, leading to the establishment of the XL50 cell line. This represents the first UV-induced mouse cSCC cell line.

Additionally, the authors' group introduced the murine-derived cSCC cell line PECA (RRID: CVCL_5859), which was isolated and established after the metastasis of primary mouse lung squamous cell carcinoma to the skin. PECA is now a commonly used cell line in cSCC research (Fig. 3.12).

Table 3.1 Common human and mouse cSCC cell lines

Cell line	Differentiation	Species	Source	Cytological characteristics
SCL-1	Poor	Human	74-year-old female with poorly differentiated facial cSCC [54]	Low level of keratinization and could grow into tumor nodules on collagen gel. Invasive growth and cSCC-like tumors when injected into immunosuppressed C3H mice and BALB/c nude mice
A431	Poor	Human	cSCC from an 85-year-old female patient [55]	High diopter and density, and cells can overlap each other on culture dish without obvious contact inhibition. Tumor formation after being injected into immunosuppressed mice
Colo-16	Poor	Human	59-year-old female patient with cSCC on left leg [56]	Cubic shape with obvious intercellular adhesion. The N/C ratio was nearly 1:1, and the cytoplasm was rich in soluble lipid vesicles. One X chromosome is missing and 9 h + polymorphism is present. Nodules formed after being transplanted into the skin of nude mice
HSC-1	Poor	Human	74-year-old Japanese male patient with cSCC on the right hand. The lesions recurred repeatedly after surgery, chemotherapy, and radiotherapy [57]	Cells are polygonal or elongated in shape and the majority are atypical with pyknotic nuclei. They showed mainly monolayer growth without obvious keratosis. After being injected into nude mice, tumor grew aggressively
SCC-12	Moderate		Facial cSCC of a 60-year-old male patient undergoing immunosuppressive therapy after kidney transplantation [58]	Colony formation was accelerated when cocultured with 3T3 cells. In nude mice, large, well-differentiated cyst-like structures containing cyst fluid could often be observed when inoculated, pathological examination showed a thin envelope of dermal connective tissue as the outermost layer of the tumor without invasive features
SCC-13	Moderate	Human	Facial cSCC of a 56-year-old female patient who had received multiple radiotherapy treatments [58]	Dependent on the feeding fibroblast layer. After inoculation into nude mice, moderately differentiated cyst-like structures could be observed with typical histopathological features of cSCC. Tumor was enveloped by a thin layer of dermal connective tissue, but did not show invasive growth
HSC-5	Moderate–high	Human	Ulcerative cSCC of the right back of a 74-year-old Japanese male, which recurred several times after surgery, chemotherapy, and radiotherapy [59]	It has a nearly round nucleus, tension filaments, microvilli, desmoid structure, and no obvious evidence of keratinization. When the cells were injected into BALB/c nude mice, no tumor growth was observed
XL50	Poor	SKH-1 mice	Ultraviolet-induced SKH-1 mice [60]	The polygonal cells varies in size, and heteromorphic nucleolus were obvious. Multiple mitosis figures, binuclear and multinucleate tumor giant cells could be observed under EM. Cytoplasm contains brown–yellow granules, CK expression was strongly positive, vimentin antigen was negative, suggesting its epithelial origin. cSCC tumors formed after being injected into the dermis of immunosuppressed mice or SKH-1 mice

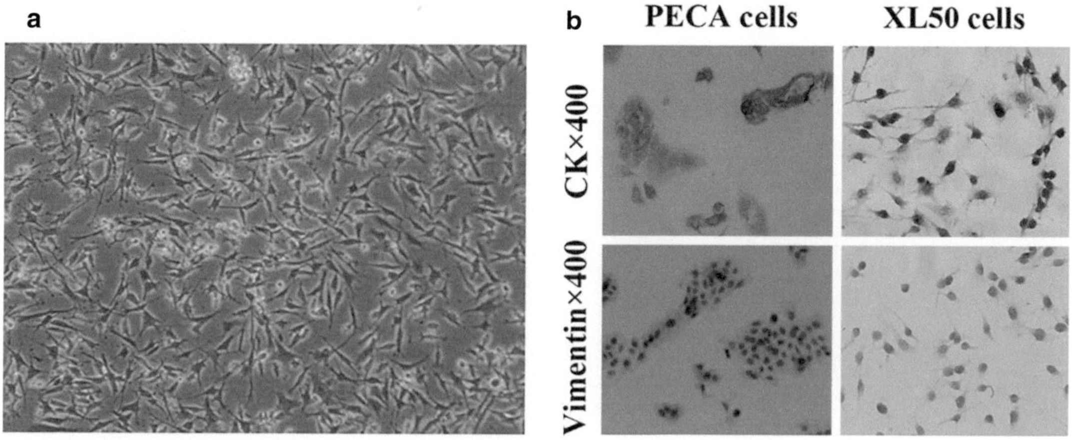

Fig. 3.12 Primary cSCC cell line derived from mice. (**a**) UV-induced mouse cSCC cell line XL50 and (**b**) surface markers of XL50

Leveraging this robust cell line platform, the authors' group and other research teams have conducted systematic and in-depth investigations into the establishment of PDT treatment parameters for cSCC, explored the treatment mechanisms, and identified efficacy enhancers (see Table 3.2). These studies provide valuable references and evidence for researching the mechanisms and clinical applications of PDT in cSCC treatment.

Basal Cell Carcinoma (BCC) Currently, BCC cell lines are relatively scarce in basic research. Epstein Jr. et al. in the United States reported the formation of BCC following long-term UVB exposure in Pach1 ± heterozygous mice. The resulting tumors were isolated, digested, cultured, and expanded to create the mouse basal cell carcinoma ASZ cell line [72]. Additionally, in a separate study, 6-week-old mice with Ptch1±, K14-CreER, and p53flox/flox genes were injected with tamoxifen, followed by a 5-Gy ion radiation dose at 8 weeks of age, leading to the isolation of the BSZ cell line from the resulting basal cell carcinoma [72]. Basal cell carcinoma also occurs in Ptch1±, K14-CrePR, and p53flox/flox mice after intracutaneous injection of RU486 without radiation, resulting in isolation of the CSZ cell line [72, 73]. The morphology and gene expression characteristics of these three cell types were similar to those of human BCC cells, although the BSZ and CSZ cell lines were found to be p53 deficient.

The clinical application of PDT for superficial BCC has demonstrated a high clearance rate with minimal damage to surrounding normal tissue. However, some patients still experience poor treatment efficacy or relapse. To address this clinical issue, Lucena et al. treated ASZ, BSZ, and CSZ cells with MAL-PDT and discovered a correlation between the expression and localization of intracellular PpIX and cell sensitivity to PDT. Tumor cells resistant to MAL-PDT exhibited a relatively low proliferation rate, high expression of the Wnt/β pathway-related protein Gsk3β, and strong tumorigenic potential [74]. Compared with parent cells, Mascaraque-treated ASZ and CSZ parental cells were subjected to MAL-PDT multiple times, resulting in daughter cells that presented significantly elevated aerobic glycolysis levels, ultimately affecting PpIX production following ALA treatment. Combining PDT with metformin was shown to inhibit the proliferation and decrease the survival rate of these resistant cells. Metformin inhibits the mitochondrial respiratory chain, causes mitochondrial membrane hyperpolarization, and suppresses intracellular glycolysis, leading to a significant increase in intracellular PpIX production, thus increasing the sensitivity of these daughter cells to PDT [75]. Furthermore, researchers have explored the development of new photosensitizers. Dabrzalska et al. utilized a methylene blue photosensitizer combined with a phosphor anionic polymer carrier, which was readily taken

Table 3.2 Researches on PDT using cSCC cell lines

Objective	Cell line	Key method	Conclusion
Parameter optimization of PDT	PECA [46][a]	PECA cells were treated with 0.1–10 mM ALA and the fluorescence intensity of PpIX was measured continuously within 24 h	The fluorescence intensity of PpIX in PECA cells peaks when ALA concentration was 0.5 mM with 5 h incubation, suggesting the best parameter for ALA-PDT treatment of PECA cells
	PECA,[a] A431, and SCC-13 [13, 61]	The cells were treated with different ALA concentrations and different light doses to measure the changes of cell viability	The cell viability decreased with total illumination dose increases, suggesting ALA concentration and total illumination dose are the key factors affecting the efficacy of PDT treatment on SCC
Direct mechanism of PDT in clearing cSCC	SCL-1 [62]	The invasion and metastasis ability of SCL-1 cells and MTSS1 expression and p63 gene pathway were measured after ALA-PDT treatment	ALA-PDT inhibits the invasion and metastasis of SCL-1 squamous cell through MTSS1 and p63 pathways
	Colo-16 [63]	The proliferation and apoptosis of Colo-16 cells and changes of STATA3 pathway were detected after ALA-PDT treatment	ALA-PDT inhibits the proliferation and promotes apoptosis of Colo-16 cells through STAT3 pathway
Indirect mechanism of PDT in clearing cSCC	PECA [64][a]	PECA cells were treated with ALA-PDT, exosomes of the supernatant were extracted to explore their activation on DC cells	Exosomes released by PECA cells after ALA-PDT treatment stimulated DC cells to mature, thus activating antitumor immunity
	A431, PECA [65][a]	IL-1r1 and IL-1β in mouse cSCC were significantly upregulated after ALA-PDT in gene profiling. A431, PECA, and CAF were measured. Expression and secretion of IL-1β in CAF after treatment with ALA-PDT were measured	Upregulation of IL-1β in cSCC induced by ALA-PDT is mainly related to CAF. ALA-PDT activates NLRP3 inflammasome and NFκB signaling pathway in CAF, thereby upregulating the expression and secretion of IL-1β
	PECA [60][a]	Gene profiling of human cSCC indicated that CCL8 was one of the most significantly upregulated cytokines after ALA-PDT treatment. The expression of CCL8 gene and protein in PECA cells and macrophages treated with ALA-PDT were measured	ALA-PDT stimulates PECA cells and macrophages to upregulate CCL8expression, and further inducing the polarization of macrophages toward M1 phenotype and enhances its migration ability
	PECA [13, 46, 66][a]	PECA cells were cocultured with DC cells after ALA-PDT treatment, and then DC cells were cocultured with T cells after 24 h. the changes of DAMPs-related molecular expression in PECA cells, the changes of DC cell surface marker expression and cytokine secretion, and the proliferation of T cells were measured to explore the related functional changes of each cell component	ALA-PDT induces PECA cells to release DAMPs-related molecules, which can induce DC cell activation. After coculture with activated DC cells, T-cell proliferation was significantly upregulated, suggesting that this process is a potential part in the antitumor immunity induced by ALA-PDT
	XL50 [67][a]	XL50 was cocultured with 3T3 cells to study the CAF phenotype of 3T3 cells, and to explore the effect of ALA-PDT treatment on CAF related phenotype of 3T3 cells	ALA-PDT inhibits the activation and migration of CAF in cSCC, destroying the tumor microenvironment

(continued)

Table 3.2 (continued)

Objective	Cell line	Key method	Conclusion
Resistance mechanism of cSCC to PDT therapy	A431 and SCC-13 [68]	cSCC cells were treated with CAF culture supernatant, TGFβ1 and TGFβ1 receptor inhibitor, respectively, and changes of morphology, vitality, apoptosis, and proliferation were measured	TGFβ1 secreted by CAF is one of the key factors inducing A431 cells to be resistant to PDT
Synergistic scheme of PDT combined therapy	A431 [69][a]	A431 was treated with ALA-PDT combined with PD-L1 monoclonal antibody, and expression of DAMPs-related molecules such as HSP70, ERp57, and CRT were measured	ALA-PDT combined with PD-L1 monoclonal antibody can significantly enhance expression of DAMPs in A431 cells, and the effect was superior to ALA-PDT alone
	SCL-1 [70][a]	Activity, migration, apoptosis, ROS production, and NRF2 pathway expression of SCL-1 cells were measured after treatment with ALA-PDT	The inhibitory effect of ALA-PDT on SCL-1 is enhanced by inhibiting NRF2 pathway
New photosensitizers	XL50 [71][a]	Cytotoxicity and induction of apoptosis of the novel nanomaterial on XL50 were investigated	It was confirmed that the H_2O_2 response nanoprobe had the potential in both diagnosis and treatment of cSCC due to its advantages of low cytotoxicity and good specificity

[a] Research from the authors' group

up by ASZ, BSZ, and CSZ cells. This approach produces a substantial amount of reactive oxygen species (ROS) upon excitation, effectively eliminating BCC cells. These in vitro studies utilizing BCC cell lines provide new strategies for treating patients with poor responses to PDT and recurrent BCC.

3.5.1.2 Keratinocytes

Human Immortalized Keratinocyte Cell Line HaCaT In 1988, Boukamp et al. first reported the establishment of the HaCaT cell line (RRID: CVCL_0038), which was isolated from peripheral normal skin lesions in a 62-year-old male patient with back melanoma. HaCaT cells maintain complete epidermal differentiation ability and stable expression of keratin markers such as KRT1, KRT10, and filaggrin. During in vitro culture, they undergo spontaneous immortalization, retaining a transforming phenotype while remaining nontumorigenic even after more than 140 generations. When transplanted into nude mice, HaCaT cells can form orderly structures and differentiate into epidermal tissue [76]. Recently, HaCaT cells have been utilized to construct 3D full-layer skin models in vitro, establishing them as ideal tools for studying epidermal keratinization regulation and physiological functions. The authors reported that after the external application of ALA, fluorescence was primarily concentrated in the epidermis and hair follicle sebaceous gland units, indicating that PDT directly targets these areas. When PDT-treated HaCaT cells were cocultured with fibroblasts, the expression of TGFβ1 in HaCaT cells was upregulated, stimulating collagen synthesis in fibroblasts [77]. In PDT-related studies, HaCaT cells serve not only to explore the direct effects of PDT on the epidermis but also as a control for various tumor cells. They are also used to evaluate the in vitro uptake, transformation, cytotoxicity, and other characteristics of new photosensitizers [78–80].

3.5.1.3 Fibroblasts

Mouse Embryonic Fibroblast Cell Line 3T3 In 1963, Todaro et al. isolated fibroblasts from Swiss mouse embryos and established the 3T3 cell line (RRID: CVCL_0120). This cell line is morphologically similar to primary fibroblasts and is capable of synthesizing and secreting collagen, as well as undergoing spontaneous immortalization during in vitro culture [81]. As one of the most commonly used fibroblast lines, 3T3 cells are extensively applied in basic research related to skin aging and wound healing. However, relatively few studies have specifically investigated PDT interventions in skin aging or wound healing, with primary human fibroblasts often serving as research subjects. The authors' group mixed 3 T3 cells with the mouse squamous cell line XL50 (see Table 3.1) at a 1:5 ratio and inoculated this mixture under the skin of SKH-1 mice with normal immunity. This approach resulted in an increased tumor formation rate in the mice.

Cancer-Associated Fibroblasts (CAFs) Among the stromal cells in the tumor microenvironment, CAFs are the most abundant. They play crucial roles in mediating extracellular matrix remodeling, inducing angiogenesis, regulating tumor metabolism, and interacting with tumor and immune cells to promote tumor initiation and progression. Additionally, CAFs can contribute to tumor cell resistance to various treatment strategies, making them potentially important targets for enhancing the sensitivity of patients to anticancer therapies.

Currently, reports on the role of CAFs in PDT are limited. Gallego-Rentero et al. demonstrated that treating A431 cells with CAF culture supernatant significantly increased their resistance to PDT. They proposed that TGFβ1 secreted by CAFs plays a key role in this enhanced tolerance, potentially inducing HO-1 overexpression in A431 cells via the upregulation of the p38MAPK and PI3K pathways. This, in turn, disrupts the heme synthesis pathway, adversely affecting the efficacy of PDT [68]. Conversely, the authors' group reported that coculturing 3 T3 cells with XL50 cells successfully induced a CAF phenotype, and ALA-PDT treatment reversed this phenotype while inhibiting CAF migration. These findings suggest that ALA-PDT may modify the tumor microenvironment and enhance tumor elimination [67]. The differing outcomes of these studies may stem from variations in experimental design, cell lines used, and treatment methods. While the former study indicated that CAFs could contribute to A431 resistance to PDT, the latter confirmed that PDT could transform the tumor microenvironment by reverting the CAF phenotype.

3.5.1.4 Human Sebaceous Gland Cells

Human Sebaceous Gland Cell Line SZ95 In 1999, Zouboulis et al. isolated sebaceous glands from the facial skin of an 87-year-old Caucasian female and infected them with simian vacuolated virus 40 (SV40), successfully establishing the immortalized human sebaceous gland cell line "SZ95" (RRID: CVCL_9803) [81]. These cells exhibit morphological, phenotypic, and functional characteristics similar to those of primary sebaceous cells, including epithelial-derived morphology, size variation, and the presence of lipid droplets. SZ95 is widely used in research on acne and other diseases related to hair follicles and sebaceous glands. Most studies on ALA-PDT treatments for skin conditions associated with sebaceous glands have utilized this cell line.

In 2006, Kosaka et al. extensively characterized ALA uptake and PpIX formation in the SZ95 cell line and reported that the fluorescence intensity of PpIX increased with increasing ALA concentration. These authors reported that PpIX fluorescence was significantly greater under aggregated growth conditions than under single-cell conditions; PpIX fluorescence was primarily localized to the cell membrane and mitochondria and dispersed within the cytoplasm [82]. Liu et al. demonstrated that rapamycin enhances the effects of ALA-PDT and inhibits SZ95 cell proliferation by downregulating the mTOR-P70 S6K pathway, while the mTOR pathway agonist IGF-1 counteracts this effect. Further analysis suggested that ALA-PDT inhibits SZ95 cell proliferation via the Akt/Erk-mTOR-p70S6K pathway [83]. Tuo et al. reported that the inhibitory effects of ALA-PDT on SZ95 proliferation and lipid synthesis were dose dependent. They reported that ALA-PDT significantly reduced the expression of p70S6K, SREBP-1, and PPARγ—key regulators of cell proliferation and lipid synthesis—while rapamycin enhanced this inhibition, and IGF-1 mitigated it. These findings indicate that PDT may downregulate lipid synthesis in SZ95 cells through the mTOR-SREBP-1/PPARγ and PRAS40-RagC-mTOR pathways [84].

These studies confirm that sebaceous glands are significant targets for ALA-PDT, elucidating the mechanisms by which PDT influences the proliferation, apoptosis, and physiological functions of sebaceous gland cells. These findings provide a foundation for further investigations into the mechanisms of ALA-PDT in sebaceous glands and establish a theoretical basis for its clinical application in treating sebaceous gland-related diseases.

Human Sebaceous Gland Cell Line XL-i-20 The authors' group has extensively researched ALA-PDT treatment for acne, demonstrating for the first time that ALA targets the pilosebaceous unit [85]. Randomized controlled clinical trials have shown that ALA-PDT is more effective than first-line oral isotretinoin in treating moderate to severe acne [86]. However, research into the mechanisms of ALA-PDT remains limited by the use of existing cell models, particularly the commonly utilized SZ95 cell line, which is derived from European and American populations and may not represent the characteristics of Chinese patients [87].

In 2020, Dr. Xu Detian and Dr. Liu Jia successfully isolated primary sebaceous gland cells from the facial skin of acne patients, establishing the first Chinese acne patient-derived immortalized sebaceous gland cell line, XL-i-20. This cell line was created through the overexpression of the telomerase reverse transcriptase (Tert) gene (Fig. 3.13, CN202011577037.2). Morphological assessments and surface marker expression confirmed that XL-i-20 cells resemble primary sebaceous cells. Nile red staining revealed the presence of abundant lipid droplets, confirming robust lipid metabolism and suggesting that this cell line exhibits biological characteristics similar to those of sebaceous cells in vivo and in primary culture. Consequently, XL-i-20 serves as a valuable research tool for studying acne and other sebaceous gland-related diseases.

Dr. Yang Jiayi from the authors' group reported that ALA-PDT inhibited the proliferation and lipid secretion of XL-i-20 cells while increasing the expression of the inflammatory factor CXCL8 via the p38MAPK pathway. Additionally, Dr. Liu Jia conducted single-cell sequencing and lipidomics studies on XL-i-20 cells after ALA-PDT treatment, confirming that ALA-PDT can activate inflammatory pathways in XL-i-20 through TNF-α/SREBP-1, thereby modulating various lipid metabolism pathways. This research offers new insights into the mechanisms by which ALA-PDT treats acne, as detailed in Chap. 13, Sect. 13.1.

3.5.1.5 Vascular Endothelial Cells

Port wine stain (PWS) is a capillary malformation disease, and heimbofen-PDT (HMME-PDT) has shown promising results in its treatment (see Chap. 17). However, basic research on this topic is limited. To investigate the mechanisms of HMME-PDT in treating PWS, human umbilical vein endothelial cells (HUVECs) serve as a suitable research model. The authors' group conducted fluorescence dynamics studies on cultured HUVECs to optimize HMME-PDT parameters. These findings confirmed that HMME-PDT effectively inhibits the proliferation and migration of HUVECs and significantly reduces their angiogenic capacity by downregulating the expression of KLF2 and VEGF.

3.5.2 Animal Models

3.5.2.1 Skin Cancer

Animal Models of cSCC The cSCC mouse model is among the most widely used and earliest animal models for research in this field. Common methods for generating cSCC models include UV induction, chemical induction, cell transplantation, and gene knockout (see Table 3.3). UV- or chemically induced cSCC models result in spontaneous cSCC development due to the impact of physical and chemical factors on mouse skin. These models closely mimic clinical pathological and physiological processes, although they have limitations such as long development times, varying tumor sizes

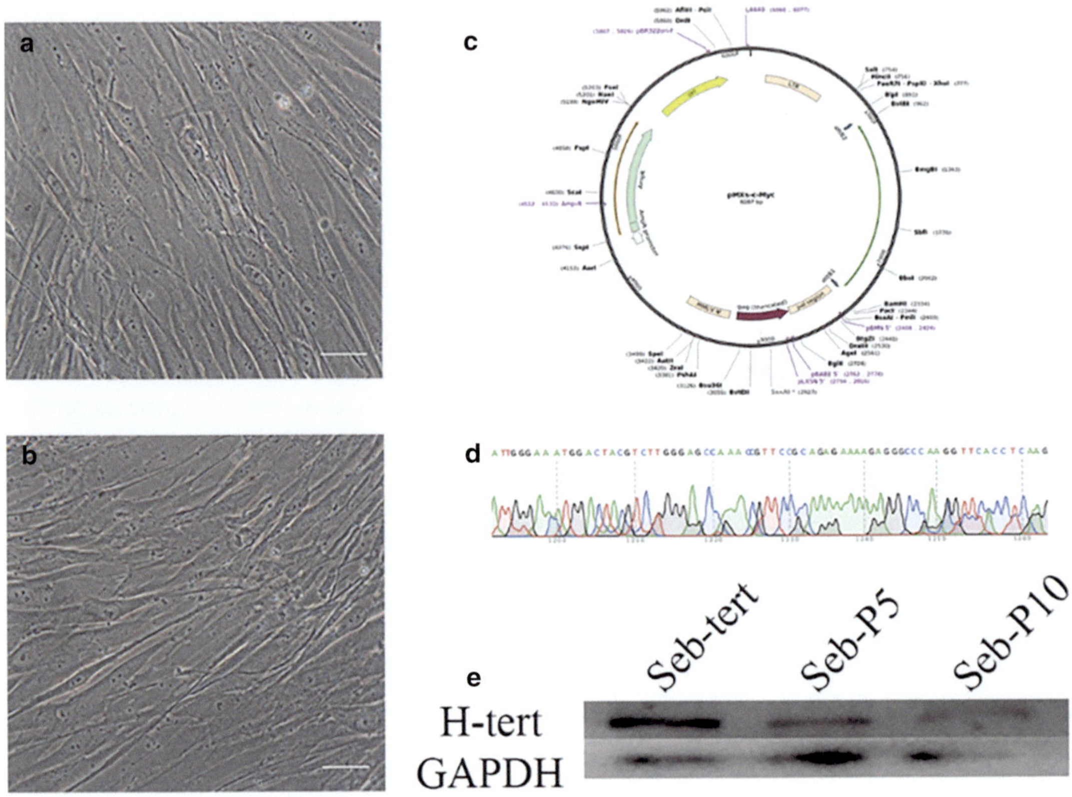

Fig. 3.13 Establishment of the human sebaceous gland cell line XL-i-20. (**a**) Primary human sebaceous gland cells. (**b**) Human sebaceous gland XL-i-20 cells. (**c**) Construction of the c.p-MXs-h-tert plasmid. (**d**) Constructing the plasmid sequence. (**e**) Expression levels of H-tert protein in immortalized and primary sebaceous cells

and numbers, and significant individual variability. Cell transplantation models, which use xenografts or allografts, have shorter development times and allow for control over tumor size and quantity, but they do not replicate the natural occurrence and progression of cSCC. Gene knockout models, on the other hand, conditionally knock out specific genes in the epidermis to explore the role of particular genes or pathways in cSCC. These three types of animal models are commonly employed in basic research on PDT for cSCC.

The SKH-1 mouse, a hairless strain with an albino background, was developed and bred by Charles River Laboratories in 1986. These mice have mutations or losses in genes related to hair traits, resulting in hairlessness or minimal hair, while maintaining normal immune function. SKH-1 mice are uniquely suited for studies on skin aging, skin tumors, and wound healing. In 2008, Lu Ting from the authors' group introduced this mouse strain from the United States and was the first to explore the establishment of UV-induced primary cSCC models in SKH-1 mice (Fig. 3.14). This mouse strain is housed in the Experimental Animal Center of Shanghai Public Health Center, affiliated with Fudan University, providing dermatology researchers with relevant animal models.

In addition to SKH-1 mice, other strains, such as C57BL/6, FVB, and BALB/c nude mice, are also used for cSCC modeling. Their respective modeling protocols, along with advantages and disadvantages, are detailed in Table 3.3.

In general, cSCC animal models are relatively well established, allowing for multilevel evalua-

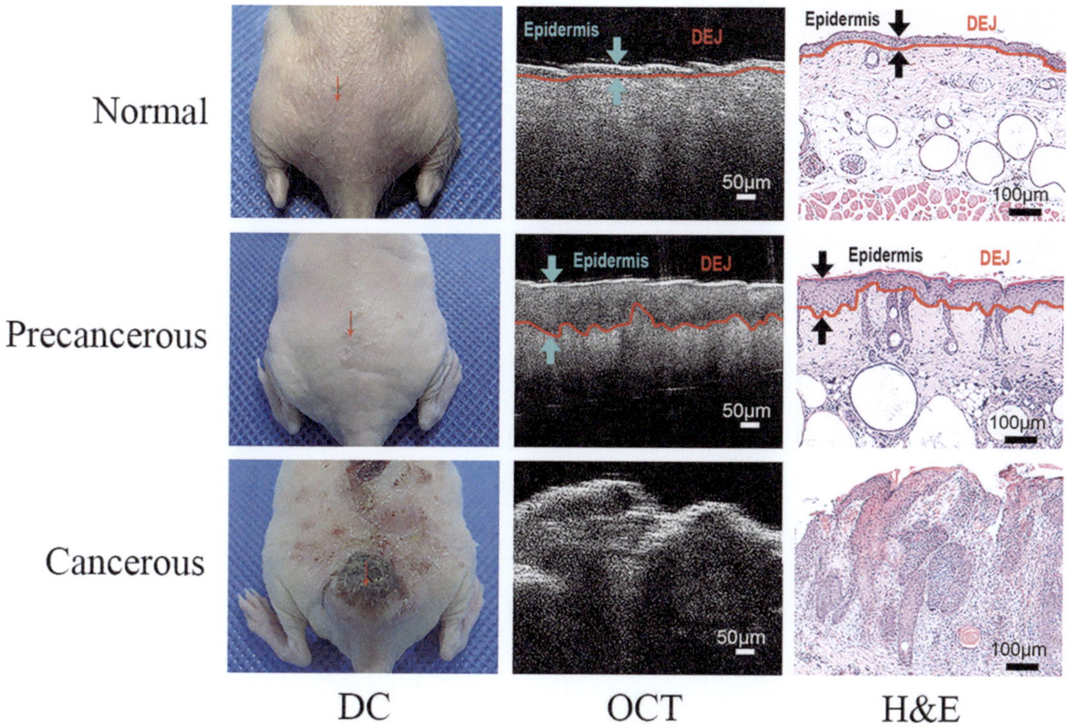

Fig. 3.14 Optical coherence tomography and pathological evaluation of normal, precancerous, and cancerous lesions in the SKH-1 mouse model of cSCC. (J Biophotonics. 2021, 14(6):e202000490)

tions at the system, organ, tissue, and cellular levels. These findings provide a foundation for in vivo exploration of the effects of PDT. Similar to studies on cell models, research using cSCC animal models for PDT can be categorized into the following areas: (1) confirmation of PDT efficacy; (2) optimization of PDT parameters; (3) explore the therapeutic mechanism of PDT; (4) combination therapy involving PDT; (5) new photosensitizer; (6) preventive role of PDT; and (7) resistance to PDT.

In 2008, the authors' group successfully established a UV-induced cSCC model using SKH-1 mice, with results published in 2011 [88]. This model is key for confirming the effectiveness of ALA-PDT in treating cSCC [33]. Since no prior studies have applied ALA-PDT to this model, the initial focus was on defining therapeutic parameters for PDT. The optimization of PDT parameters largely relies on the construction and application of a real-time fluorescence detection platform in vivo. By monitoring the fluorescence intensity of PpIX in cSCC lesions, key parameters such as drug concentration, application timing, and light dose were determined [33]. Further studies demonstrated that ALA-PDT could effectively delay cSCC development. Investigations into the therapeutic mechanisms of ALA-PDT revealed that its effects are multifaceted and include direct tumor cell killing, immune modulation, and regulation of the tumor microenvironment. Initially, ALA-PDT rapidly induced apoptosis in mouse cSCC and stimulated antitumor immunity, effectively preventing tumor formation. Dendritic cells (DCs) are crucial in this immune response. On the basis of these findings, Zhang Haiyan and Wang Xiaojie from the group developed an ALA-PDT-induced DC vaccine, offering a novel approach to immunotherapy for invasive and metastatic SCC [13, 46, 47, 66]. Additionally, Zhang Haiyan, Ji Jie, and Zhu Lude used a UV-induced SKH-1 mouse cSCC model to conduct gene chip analyses before and after ALA-PDT. They reported that ALA-PDT

Table 3.3 Establishment of cSCC mouse models

Methods	Strain	Carcinogenesis	Period	Characteristics of modeling process	Advantage and disadvantage
UV induction	SKH-1,[a] ICR	UV irradiation 4 times weekly, light dose was 90% MED in the first 2 weeks, 1MED in the third week, and then increased by 12.5% MED every week until the eighth week. Then, light dose remained unchanged [88]	16–24 weeks	Dorsal skin was thickened at 4 weeks after UV exposure, photoaging appears at 6–8 weeks, and papilloma appears after 10 weeks, some lesions spontaneously subside and rest continue to increase. Tumors measuring 5-8 mm with hyperkeratosis develop at 16 weeks	Advantage: simulating the carcinogenesis of human cSCC Disadvantages: time consuming, unpredictable tumor size and number, and individual variability
Chemical induction	SKH-1, FVB, C57BL/6	100 μg/200 μL DMBA propanol solution was applied once after shaving on the back, and TPA was applied 3 times a week	20–30 weeks	Papilloma gradually appeared after 10 weeks, some lesions continued to grow into tumors measuring 5–8 mm at 20–30 weeks	Advantages: easy to handle, high likelihood of tumor formation Disadvantages: time consuming, uncontrollable tumor size and number, contact carcinogenicity of the reagents
Cell transplantation	BALB/c nude	A431 cells were collected at logarithmic phase, 10^6 to 10^7/ml single-cell suspension was prepared, and 100 μl was injected subcutaneously into lateral hind leg of mice	7–10 days	Small papules develop after inoculation, some may spontaneously resolve. After approximately 1 week, hemispherical tumor develops measuring 5–8 mm	Advantages: short modeling period, size of the tumor is uniform Disadvantages: it is greatly affected by the growth state of tumor cells
	BALB/c nude, SKH-1[a]	XL50 cells were collected at logarithmic phase, 2×10^6/ml single-cell suspension was prepared, and 100 μl was injected subcutaneously	7–10 days		The percentage of tumor formation in normal immune mice is limited. Other advantages and disadvantages are the same as above
Gene knock-out	FVB-Rb1^{tm2Brn} Tg (KRT14-cre) 8Brn Trp53^{tm1Brn}	Conditionally knockout p53 gene or double knockout pRb, p53 gene in FVB mouse skin epidermal cells [89]	12–32 weeks	Papules appeared spontaneously on the face, neck and back of mice, followed by tumor enlargement	Advantages: it is beneficial to the study of specific genes and pathways related to cSCC occurrence and treatment Disadvantages: long period and high cost

[a] The authors' group established the mouse cSCC model for the first time in China

upregulated several cytokines, including CCL8, CXCL13, and IL-1β, in cSCC tissue. This leads to the recruitment and infiltration of immune cells such as neutrophils, macrophages, and T cells, which promote the functional maturation of various immune cells and alter the tumor immune microenvironment, contributing to tumor elimination [33, 60, 90].

To improve the efficacy of ALA-PDT, the authors' group recently proposed painless PDT or modified PDT. This approach reduces the production rate of reactive oxygen species and minimizes nerve stimulation by shortening the incubation period while extending the illumination time. The modification maintained the same therapeutic efficacy as traditional PDT while significantly reducing pain. Further studies revealed that painless PDT inhibited cSCC cell proliferation primarily through the PP2A/PP5-mediated MAPK pathway [91].

In addition to painless PDT, the authors explored various PDT combination therapies to enhance therapeutic effects and overcome the limitation of treatment depth. These efforts focused on increasing both the direct cytotoxic effects and the immunological impact of PDT, as well as improving photosensitizer absorption and PpIX conversion. Notably, the group pioneered the combination of ALA-PDT with PD-L1 therapy, which effectively eliminated implanted cSCC in SKH-1 mice. Compared with ALA-PDT alone, this combined approach also significantly reduced the tumor volume in untreated distal areas, with superior results. For UV-induced primary cSCC in SKH-1 mice, combination therapy not only efficiently removed tumors but also prevented those induced by chronic UV exposure. Further investigations revealed that this therapy significantly enhanced apoptosis and ferroptosis in cSCC and upregulated the expression of DAMP-related proteins, suggesting that the combination of ALA-PDT with a PD-L1 monoclonal antibody activates antitumor immunity via immunogenic cell death (ICD) [69]. Moreover, combining ALA-PDT with imiquimod, an immune adjuvant, significantly increased the levels of inflammatory factors such as CXCL8, TNF-α, and IFN-α in tumors, thereby improving the efficacy of ALA-PDT for treating mouse cSCC [92]. Anand et al. demonstrated that pretreatment with methotrexate significantly increased PpIX accumulation in tumors of both chemically induced and implanted cSCC models. Similarly, calcitriol showed a synergistic effect by upregulating porphyrin synthetase-coproporphyrinogen oxidase and downregulating iron chelatase, which increased local PpIX levels in tumors more than tenfold [93]. Another study revealed that dietary vitamin D3 significantly enhanced ALA-PDT efficacy in both mouse models and SCC patients without adverse effects [94, 95]. Various physical therapies have also been tested in combination with PDT to improve photosensitizer absorption and increase treatment depth. The authors reported that plum needle puncture significantly promoted the diffusion and absorption of ALA in the superficial dermis, with better results than a CO2 fractional laser [96].

To advance research on new photosensitizers and drug carriers that increase bioavailability, absorption, and penetration depth, various nanoparticles have been designed via nanotechnology, offering promising new avenues for clinical application. The cSCC mouse model plays a crucial role in these experimental studies. Shi Lei, from the authors' group, was the first to design and prepare polylactic glycolic acid nanoparticles (PLGANPs), which are biodegradable and nontoxic, to encapsulate and deliver ALA. This innovation significantly improved the bioavailability of the photosensitizer ALA [97]. Dr. Shi Lei also developed a novel X-ray-triggered PDT system mediated by scintillator nanoparticles, utilizing high-energy, deep-penetrating X-rays for photosensitizer activation, thus combining the effects of PDT and X-ray radiotherapy [98]. Additionally, Peiru Wang and Shuzhan Shen from the authors' group designed a new nanomaterial that not only enhanced the bioavailability and selectivity of ALA but also exhibited photothermal effects and could be used for photoacoustic imaging. These properties were confirmed in SCC mouse models, providing theoretical support for the noninvasive diagnosis and treatment of cSCC in clinical settings [71].

Since SCC is often the result of prolonged UV exposure, the UV-induced cSCC mouse model has been used to study the preventive effects of ALA-PDT. Liu et al. in Canada conducted an experiment in which SKH-1 hairless mice were irradiated with UV three times a week and treated with ALA-PDT once a week. The results demonstrated that ALA-PDT effectively prevented and delayed the onset of UV-induced SCC [99]. Like other antitumor therapies, some cSCC cases are resistant to ALA-PDT, although reports on this topic are limited. Recent studies suggest that certain cSCC tumors undergo metabolic reprogramming, enhancing aerobic glycolysis and weakening oxidative phosphorylation, which alters the response of tumors to PDT. Metformin has been shown to counteract this metabolic shift and improve the efficacy of ALA-PDT [100].

Animal Models of BCC The BCC mouse model consists primarily of transgenic mouse models and implanted tumor models. ALA-PDT is an effective therapy for treating superficial BCC and nodular BCC with invasion depths of less than 2 mm. However, basic research is limited, and the use of BCC mouse models remains restricted. Sunar et al. used the K5-Gli transgenic BCC mouse model to demonstrate that the spatial frequency domain imaging system could effectively detect the absolute fluorescence intensity of local PpIX in tumors after ALA incubation [101]. Rollakanti et al. employed a model involving 6-week-old mice with the Ptch1±, K14-CreER, and p53flox/flox genes and treated them with tamoxifen for three consecutive days followed by 4 Gy ionizing radiation at 8 weeks. This model typically resulted in the formation of multiple BCCs after 6–8 months. They reported that pretreatment with calcitriol increased local PpIX accumulation within tumors more than sixfold after ALA incubation. Calcitriol also promoted the differentiation, proliferation, and apoptosis of BCC cells, enhancing ALA-PDT efficacy [102]. More recently, Mascaraque et al. injected ASZ cells mixed with Matrigel into the skin of Foxn1nu nude mice. Within 7 days, implant tumors approximately 30 mm^3 in size formed. Their study revealed that metformin significantly increased the sensitivity of ASZ-treated cells to PDT. The combination of metformin and PDT enhances tumor cell apoptosis and necrosis, significantly reducing tumor volume [75].

Currently, many clinical studies on the use of PDT for the treatment of BCC exist. Although clinical studies have shown that ALA-PDT is comparable to surgery for superficial BCC and nodular BCC with less than 2 mm invasion depth and yields better cosmetic outcomes, challenges remain in practical application. Questions regarding how to further improve the efficacy of ALA-PDT and the specific mechanisms by which PDT treats BCC require further research.

Animal Models of Malignant Melanoma and Amelanotic Melanoma Commonly used experimental models of melanoma include genetically engineered mouse models, homologous transplanted tumor models, patient-derived xenotransplantation models, organoid melanoma models, and other in vitro melanoma models.

Genetically engineered mouse models: These models involve the introduction of one or more human melanoma driver genes into mice to simulate the pathological characteristics of human melanoma [103–105]. These models are useful for evaluating therapeutic effects and drug actions. With the emergence of immune checkpoint inhibitors, these models have also been applied to assess immune efficacy [106, 107]. Córdoba et al. conducted a study using transgenic mice carrying the MT-ret fusion gene and confirmed that melanoma cells from MT-I mice responded effectively to ALA-PDT in vitro. However, melanomas that spontaneously develop on mouse skin do not respond to ALA-PDT [108].

Homologous transplanted tumor model: The homologous transplanted tumor model was established by inoculating the mouse B16 cell line into immune-competent C57BL/6 mice [109]. This model is easy to generate, cost-effective, and time-efficient, making it a mainstay in preclinical studies. In one study, melanin in a B16 tumor model was photobleached with 420 nm violet light, which significantly improved the sensitivity of nonpigmented melanoma to PDT by reducing the protective effect of melanin. The inhibition of melanin production has been identified as an effective therapeutic target, enhancing the efficacy of PDT against advanced melanoma [110]. Schacht et al. compared the effects of ALA-PDT via systemic injection and topical administration in tumor-bearing Syrian golden hamsters. Their results indicated that topical administration had a stronger effect on tumor microcirculation than did systemic administration when patients were treated with high-energy PDT (100 J/cm^2) [111].

Patient-derived xenotransplantation models: These models are established by inoculating melanoma cells from patients into immunocompromised mice, providing a more comprehensive simulation of the clinical, histological, and genetic diversity of human melanoma than do genetically engineered mouse models [112, 113]. However, interactions between the tumor and its microenvironment can complicate the model, and owing to the immunosuppression of the host mice, these models are not suitable for monitoring immunotherapy.

Organoid melanoma model: This model involves organoid cultures derived from patient melanomas, which can mimic the original tumor morphology and function [114]. It effectively addresses some of the limitations found in mouse models. Recent studies indicate that these organoids can produce autoimmune cells, making them useful for evaluating immunotherapy [115].

On the basis of these models, the varying efficacy of ALA-PDT in treating melanoma in vivo may be due to several factors: (a) melanin particles in melanoma can obstruct light penetration during ALA-PDT and (b) melanoma tends to infiltrate deeply in vivo. Recent research has focused on improving photosensitizers and altering the wavelength and energy of the light source to overcome these challenges. Combining ALA-PDT with photothermal therapy has shown promising results in cultured melanoma cells and mouse models. The immunological effects of PDT are also a key area of ongoing research.

3.5.2.2 Photoaging

A skin photoaging model was established through long-term UV exposure. The authors' group utilized a UVA + UVB light source (275–380 nm, peak at 310–315 nm) while filtering out UVC (<290 nm). SKH-1 hairless mice were subjected to repeated irradiation for 5–10 weeks. The initial dose was 0.9 minimal erythema dose (MED), increasing by 0.5–1 MED/week up to 3 MED, with exposure 3 times per week until 10 weeks of cumulative irradiation. Other models using C57BL/6, BALB/c, or nude mice have also been employed [116], although these require frequent hair removal or immune deficiencies. SKH-1 mice, however, are naturally hairless and have intact immune function. Ting Lv from the authors' group successfully established this model, which is characterized by dry, scaly skin with thickening and deep wrinkles. Barrier dysfunction, including increased transdermal water loss and decreased hydration, was also observed. Histopathology revealed slight epidermal thickening and disorganized, broken collagen fibers in the dermis.

At the genetic level, the authors' group analyzed gene profiling data during phenotype induction in SKH-1 mice. They reported that UV dose-dependent changes in gene expression were concentrated in processes such as macromolecule metabolism, DNA methylation, cell cycle regulation, collagen metabolism, and extracellular matrix remodeling. These findings suggest that cell senescence plays a key role in UV-induced photoaging.

Additionally, Peiru Wang from the authors' group discovered that n-3 polyunsaturated fatty acids (PUFAs) protect against photoaging by maintaining skin homeostasis and barrier function. These effects include regulating PLA2 enzyme activity, inhibiting COX2 and PGE2 expression, downregulating the NF-κB and MAPK signaling pathways, reducing matrix metalloproteinase synthesis, curbing inflammatory responses, and inhibiting UV-induced skin collagen degradation [117, 118]. Proteomic analysis after n-3 PUFA supplementation revealed that differentially expressed proteins were enriched in adipogenesis and lipid metabolism. Lipidomic analysis confirmed that n-3 PUFAs increase the triglyceride content, a crucial component for skin barrier integrity [119].

The authors' group was the first to apply the SKH-1 photoaging mouse model in the study of ALA-PDT for skin photoaging. Research has confirmed that ALA-PDT effectively promotes collagen production and that multiple low-dose ALA-PDT treatments significantly improve collagen density and organization in photoaged skin tissue, thus promoting skin rejuvenation [120].

Further exploration revealed that PpIX fluorescence is primarily concentrated in the epidermis and sebaceous gland units of hair follicles and is unable to penetrate the basement membrane. These findings suggest that the effects of ALA-PDT are mainly confined to the epidermis. Interestingly, ALA-PDT induces TGF-β expression in epidermal keratinocytes, which, upon entering the dermis, upregulates the TGF-β signaling pathway in fibroblasts. This cascade reduces collagen degradation and promotes collagen synthesis in the dermis [77].

Additionally, Peiru Wang and Yuling Yang from the authors' group reported that lymphatic vessels, key components of the skin microenvironment, experience structural and functional degradation that may contribute to or accelerate skin aging [121]. ALA-PDT was shown to remodel lymphatic vessel structures, increasing their density and enhancing their filtration and collection functions, thereby improving the photoaging phenotype in SKH-1 mice.

3.5.2.3 Acne

The understanding of acne pathogenesis is constantly evolving. Four classical key pathogenic factors are involved in the development of acne: follicular hyperkeratinization, sebum production, microbial colonization, and the immune response. On the basis of these mechanisms, common experimental animals used for acne models include rabbits, rats, guinea pigs, Syrian hamsters, and mice. However, owing to anatomical differences, variations in sebum composition, and microbial diversity between animals and humans, no single animal model can replicate all four pathogenic factors simultaneously. Therefore, only certain aspects of acne pathology can be simulated. Table 3.4 summarizes the protocols for establishing the four common animal models of acne.

Numerous studies have demonstrated that ALA-PDT is an effective treatment for acne, particularly for moderate to severe inflammatory acne. The authors' group pioneered clinical and basic research on ALA-PDT for acne treatment in China, successfully establishing models such as the rabbit ear acne model, the rat ear acne-like inflammation model, and the sebaceous gland spot model in golden hamsters. These models simulate various pathological processes of acne, including acne formation, inflammation, and sebaceous gland hypertrophy. Using these models, further research revealed that ALA-PDT increases ROS levels in sebaceous gland cells, significantly reducing the volume of sebaceous glands after treatment, indicating that the sebaceous gland is a primary target of ALA-PDT [45, 125]. Additionally, ALA-PDT downregulated lipid metabolism-related transcription factors, such as SREBP-1, and the AMPK pathway, suggesting that ALA-PDT may inhibit sebaceous gland hyperplasia and sebum production through the AMPK/SREBP-1 pathway [125].

It is now widely accepted that inflammation plays a role throughout the acne process. Although ALA-PDT is known to regulate local inflammatory responses in acne treatment, its precise mechanism remains unclear. Zhang Linglin from the authors' group reported that inflammation-related genes were significantly upregulated 24 h after ALA-PDT treatment, as confirmed in three acne models. This led to the novel hypothesis that ALA-PDT may rapidly recruit neutrophil-dominated acute inflammatory cells, amplifying the inflammatory response and disrupting the "sticky state" of chronic inflammation, which aids in clearing abnormal matter from skin lesions and gradually resolving inflammation. These findings present a new perspective on the mechanism underlying the effect of ALA-PDT on acne.

In addition to mechanistic insights, these animal models help optimize treatment parameters. Early ALA-PDT treatments for acne often cause

Table 3.4 Establishment of animal models of acne

Animal models	Method	Characteristics of the model
Rabbit ear	Human sebum was applied daily to the external ear canal of rabbits for 2 weeks	Epithelial hyperplasia could be seen in sebaceous duct and hair follicle. Keratin buildup leads to dilation of sebaceous ducts and hair follicles, resulting in microcomedone or comedones. There are various inflammatory changes, such as follicular pustules and dermal infiltration of mononuclear and polymorphonuclear leukocytes
	2% coal tar was applied to medial ears of New Zealand rabbits 5 times a week for 2 weeks [122]	Comedonal lesions are induced after repeated application of coal tar. Epithelium epithelial hyperplasia occurs in pilosebaceous ducts, which is similar to the pathological manifestations of human acne
	Suspension of *C. acnes* is injected into medial ear of New Zealand rabbits followed by application of 50% oleic acid (70% propylene glycol, 30% ethanol) once daily for 4 weeks [123]	Papular and comedonal lesions could be induced in this model. Chemical agents are usually thought to be superior to sebum in inducing acne
Acneiform inflammation model on mouse ear	Suspension of C. Acnes is injected to the auricle skin of ICR mice or Sprague–Dawley rats [124]	This mouse ear model of acneiform inflammation can simulate the inflammation of granulomatous acne after damage and rupture of hair follicles. Attention should be given to the activity of *C. acnes* activity on modeling and evaluation of subsequent experimental efficacy
Sebaceous gland model on golden hamster	Depilation and expose the sebaceous glands on the back of golden hamsters	The sebaceous glands of golden hamsters are androgen-dependent organs with abundant sebaceous glands. Sebaceous plaques of golden hamsters are usually symmetrical, so it is easy to set self-control group and conduct quantitative evaluation by morphological method. It is an ideal model to study the anti-sebaceous gland hyperplasia effect of drugs or other treatments
Acne model on $hr^{rh}hr^{rh}$ mice	$hr^{rh}hr^{rh}$ mice from Jackson Laboratory	Short period of hair growth after birth. Four weeks later, the hair of $hr^{rh}hr^{rh}$ mice is irreversibly shed, and become hairless mice. The pilosebaceous unit remain after shedding and histologically mimic open comedones in human, and thus can be used as a disease model for comedonal acne

adverse reactions, such as pain and post-treatment erythema. To address this, Kosaka et al. conducted ALA-PDT treatments on a mouse model using different ALA concentrations and application times. They reported that lower ALA concentrations (2.5–5.0%) and shorter application times (1–2 h) resulted in better efficacy, with significantly fewer adverse reactions than the traditional protocol did [126]. These findings provide a scientific basis for controlling and minimizing adverse reactions in clinical ALA-PDT treatment for acne.

3.5.2.4 Port Wine Stain

The rooster comb, with its rich capillary network and histological structure similar to that of port wine stains, is frequently used as an animal model for studying this condition. The authors' group utilized this model to optimize the therapeutic parameters of HMME-PDT through fluorescence dynamic studies. They reported that the number of upper dermal capillaries decreased and that vascular shrinkage occurred immediately after treatment. Histological examinations revealed thrombus formation in the dermal capillary layer one week post-treatment, with a significant reduction in the number of blood vessels 2 weeks later. Further molecular studies indicated that HMME-PDT significantly downregulated the expression of the KLF2 and VEGF genes and proteins in combination, thereby inhibiting angiogenesis in the treated area.

3.5.2.5 Hypertrophic Scars

ALA-PDT has also been applied for the treatment of hypertrophic scars, with the New Zealand rabbit ear scar model being a classic choice for studying this condition [127]. To investigate the efficacy of ALA-PDT on hypertrophic scars and clarify its therapeutic mechanism, Wang et al. selected 2.0–2.5 kg New Zealand rabbits and created four wounds on the inner ear via a 1 cm^2 trephine. After approximately 3 weeks of healing, hypertrophic scars developed at the incision site, rising 2 mm above the normal skin surface. Histopathological analysis and RT–PCR studies before and after ALA-PDT treatment confirmed that the therapy effectively inhibited hypertrophic scar formation. The mechanism may be related to the increased ratio of matrix metalloproteinases (MMPs) to tissue inhibitors of metalloproteinases (TIMPs) in the scar, which is associated with accelerated fibroblast senescence and the degradation of collagen and the extracellular matrix [128]. Recent studies have also explored PDT using modified photosensitizing agents for hypertrophic scars. For example, Yu et al. reported a new nanomaterial supported by near-infrared IR-808 that reaches the dermis, significantly enhancing PDT efficacy by inducing fibroblast apoptosis and remodeling collagen fibers, thereby improving the appearance of hypertrophic scars [129]. Similarly, Chen et al. designed a transdermal nanomaterial, HA/ES-ALA, which synergistically delivers ALA deep into hypertrophic scars and is absorbed by fibroblasts, improving ALA utilization and enhancing PDT efficacy [130].

3.5.2.6 Psoriasis

Demerjian et al. induced psoriasis-like skin hyperplasia in mice by applying adhesive tape twice daily for 5 days to cause mechanical superficial peeling on the dorsal skin [131]. Another method involved applying 5% imiquimod cream topically for 5 days after hair removal to BALB/c mice, which successfully induced a psoriasis phenotype. Psoriatic lesions can also develop in some transgenic mice, such as K14-VEGF transgenic mice. Yi et al. modified the clinical psoriasis severity score to assess skin lesions in an imiquimod-induced psoriasis model, scoring erythema, scales, and skin thickness on a scale from 0 to 4 (0: none, 1: slight, 2: moderate, 3: significant, 4: very significant), with the final score being the sum of these components [132].

On the basis of the findings of animal studies, topical ALA-PDT can be used to treat large psoriatic lesions with good efficacy and safety [133]. ALA-PDT was found to potentially alleviate psoriatic lesions in mice by promoting SOCS1/3 and inhibiting JAK1/2 [132]. Additionally, Chen et al. reported that systemic ALA-PDT via intraperitoneal injection significantly reduced the expression of IL-17 and IFN-γ in lesions, improving the psoriasis-like phenotype of K14-VEGF transgenic mice and reducing the infiltration of neutrophils, dendritic cells, and T lymphocytes [134]. However, owing to the hyperplastic nature of psoriasis lesions, the penetration depth of ALAs is a key factor in determining PDT efficacy. To improve ALA absorption, Wang et al. developed lipid-soluble cell nanovesicles that specifically accumulate in lesions, providing a synergistic photodynamic/photothermal effect under near-infrared irradiation to regulate the local immune state, reduce the release of imbalanced inflammatory factors, and alleviate psoriasis symptoms [135]. Yi et al. reported that the use of methotrexate-ALA nanoparticles with chitosan/hyaluronic acid as a carrier effectively improved the skin condition in imiquimod-induced psoriasis models, reducing the levels of key proinflammatory factors such as TNF-α and IL-17 [136].

Moreover, clinical studies from the authors' group demonstrated that brick–red fluorescence could be detected in psoriasis lesions via Wood's lamp fluorescence diagnosis, suggesting that this technique has potential for diagnosing psoriasis and assessing disease progression [137].

In summary, studying ALA-PDT in various skin disease-related cells and animal models enables the optimization of PDT parameters and improves treatment outcomes. This research provides the foundation for uncovering the mechanisms of ALA-PDT in different skin diseases. With advances in modern medicine, further development of cell and animal models will help optimize and standardize ALA-PDT in dermatology.

References

1. Wang X, Wang H, Huang Z. The application of 5-aminolevulinic acid photodynamic therapy in dermatology. Chin J Dermatol. 2009;5:368–70.
2. Miki Y, Akimoto J, Moritake K, Hironaka C, Fujiwara Y. Photodynamic therapy using talaporfin sodium induces concentration-dependent programmed necroptosis in human glioblastoma T98G cells. Lasers Med Sci. 2015;30(6):1739–45. https://doi.org/10.1007/s10103-015-1783-9.
3. D'Arcy MS. Cell death: a review of the major forms of apoptosis, necrosis and autophagy. Cell Biol Int. 2019;43(6):582–92. https://doi.org/10.1002/cbin.11137.
4. Soriano J, Mora-Espi I, Alea-Reyes ME, Perez-Garcia L, Barrios L, Ibanez E, et al. Cell death mechanisms in tumoral and non-tumoral human cell lines triggered by photodynamic treatments: apoptosis, necrosis and parthanatos. Sci Rep. 2017;7:41340. https://doi.org/10.1038/srep41340.
5. Coupienne I, Fettweis G, Rubio N, Agostinis P, Piette J. 5-ALA-PDT induces RIP3-dependent necrosis in glioblastoma. Photochem Photobiol Sci. 2011;10(12):1868–78. https://doi.org/10.1039/c1pp05213f.
6. Wang H, Wang X, Guo M, Yu Y. 5-Aminolevulinic acid photodynamic therapy for the treatment of precancerous skin lesions and skin carcinoma in situ. Chin J Dermatol. 2006;3:137–9.
7. Wang XL, Wang HW, Guo MX, Xu SZ. Treatment of skin cancer and precancer using topical ALA-PDT–a single hospital experience. Photodiagn Photodyn Ther. 2008;5(2):127–33. https://doi.org/10.1016/j.pdpdt.2008.05.003.
8. Zhang C, Wang X, Xu S, Zhu X, Xia W. Δ-Aminolevulinic acid photodynamic therapy for the treatment of male urethral condyloma acuminatum. In: The 1st national conference on integrated Chinese and Western andrology, Xi'an, China, 2001, pp. 308–310.
9. Wang X, Wang H, Zhang C. Discussion on the mechanism of δ-aminolevulinic acid photodynamic therapy in the treatment of condyloma acuminatum. Chin J Dermatol Venereol. 2001;4:234–7.
10. Wang XL, Wang HW, Wang HS, Xu SZ, Liao KH, Hillemanns P. Topical 5-aminolaevulinic acid-photodynamic therapy for the treatment of urethral condylomata acuminata. Br J Dermatol. 2004;151(4):880–5. https://doi.org/10.1111/j.1365-2133.2004.06189.x.
11. Li J, Lv T, Wang H, Wang P, Wang X. Study on the mechanism of Aminolevulinic acid photodynamic therapy in the treatment of skin squamous cell carcinoma in SKH-1 mice. Chin J Dermatol. 2014;47(03):181–5.
12. Lv T, Wang X, Zhou W, Wang H, Miao F, Li J. Establishment of a mouse model of UV-induced skin squamous cell carcinoma. Chin J Dermatol. 2011;3:174–7.
13. Ji J, Fan Z, Zhou F, Wang X, Shi L, Zhang H, et al. Improvement of DC vaccine with ALA-PDT induced immunogenic apoptotic cells for skin squamous cell carcinoma. Oncotarget. 2015;6(19):17135–46. https://doi.org/10.18632/oncotarget.3529.
14. Agarwal ML, Clay ME, Harvey EJ, Evans HH, Antunez AR, Oleinick NL. Photodynamic therapy induces rapid cell death by apoptosis in L5178Y mouse lymphoma cells. Cancer Res. 1991;51(21):5993–6.
15. Inoue H, Kajimoto Y, Shibata MA, Miyoshi N, Ogawa N, Miyatake S, et al. Massive apoptotic cell death of human glioma cells via a mitochondrial pathway following 5-aminolevulinic acid-mediated photodynamic therapy. J Neuro-Oncol. 2007;83(3):223–31. https://doi.org/10.1007/s11060-006-9325-8.
16. Miao F. Study on the mechanism of ALA photodynamic induction of apoptosis in HPV16 E7-transfected keratinocytes. Master's (degree), Yangzhou University.
17. Miao F, Wang X, Wang H, Ding H, Lv T, Zhang L. Establishment of a stable human papillomavirus type 16 E7 protein-expressing HaCaT cell line. Chin J Dermatol. 2011;5:310–3.
18. Li Z, Teng M, Wang Y, Wang Q, Feng Y, Xiao Z, et al. The mechanism of 5-aminolevulinic acid photodynamic therapy in promoting endoplasmic reticulum stress in the treatment of HR-HPV-infected HeLa cells. Photodermatol Photoimmunol Photomed. 2021;37(4):348–59. https://doi.org/10.1111/phpp.12663.
19. Mizushima N, Komatsu M. Autophagy: renovation of cells and tissues. Cell. 2011;147(4):728–41. https://doi.org/10.1016/j.cell.2011.10.026.
20. Kessel D, Oleinick NL. Initiation of autophagy by photodynamic therapy. Methods Enzymol. 2009;453:1–16. https://doi.org/10.1016/S0076-6879(08)04001-9.
21. Signorelli S, Tarkowski LP, Van den Ende W, Bassham DC. Linking autophagy to abiotic and biotic stress responses. Trends Plant Sci. 2019;24(5):413–30. https://doi.org/10.1016/j.tplants.2019.02.001.
22. Liu X, Ding S, Liu P. The roles of Gasdermin D in coronavirus infection and evasion. Front Microbiol. 2021;12:784009. https://doi.org/10.3389/fmicb.2021.784009.
23. Li N, Wang Y, Wang X, Sun N, Gong YH. Pathway network of pyroptosis and its potential inhibitors in acute kidney injury. Pharmacol Res. 2022;175:106033. https://doi.org/10.1016/j.phrs.2021.106033.
24. Su X, Wang WJ, Cao Q, Zhang H, Liu B, Ling Y, et al. A carbonic anhydrase IX (CAIX)-anchored rhenium(I) photosensitizer evokes Pyroptosis for enhanced anti-tumor immunity. Angew Chem Int Ed Engl. 2022;61(8):e202115800. https://doi.org/10.1002/anie.202115800.
25. Lu Y, Xu F, Wang Y, Shi C, Sha Y, He G, et al. Cancer immunogenic cell death via photopyroptosis with light-sensitive Indoleamine 2,3-dioxygenase

inhibitor conjugate. Biomaterials. 2021;278:121167. https://doi.org/10.1016/j.biomaterials.2021.121167.
26. Li L, Song D, Qi L, Jiang M, Wu Y, Gan J, et al. Photodynamic therapy induces human esophageal carcinoma cell pyroptosis by targeting the PKM2/caspase-8/caspase-3/GSDME axis. Cancer Lett. 2021;520:143–59. https://doi.org/10.1016/j.canlet.2021.07.014.
27. Kagan VE, Mao G, Qu F, Angeli JP, Doll S, Croix CS, et al. Oxidized arachidonic and adrenic PEs navigate cells to ferroptosis. Nat Chem Biol. 2017;13(1):81–90. https://doi.org/10.1038/nchembio.2238.
28. Meng X, Deng J, Liu F, Guo T, Liu M, Dai P, et al. Triggered all-active metal organic framework: ferroptosis machinery contributes to the apoptotic photodynamic antitumor therapy. Nano Lett. 2019;19(11):7866–76. https://doi.org/10.1021/acs.nanolett.9b02904.
29. Zhu T, Shi L, Yu C, Dong Y, Qiu F, Shen L, et al. Ferroptosis promotes photodynamic therapy: supramolecular photosensitizer-inducer nanodrug for enhanced cancer treatment. Theranostics. 2019;9(11):3293–307. https://doi.org/10.7150/thno.32867.
30. Castellani A, Pace GP, Concioli M. Photodynamic effect of hematoporphyrin on blood microcirculation. J Pathol Bacteriol. 1963;86:99–102. https://doi.org/10.1002/path.1700860111.
31. Yi W, Xu HT, Tian DF, Wu LQ, Zhang SQ, Wang L, et al. Photodynamic therapy mediated by 5-aminolevulinic acid suppresses gliomas growth by decreasing the microvessels. J Huazhong Univ Sci Technolog Med Sci. 2015;35(2):259–64. https://doi.org/10.1007/s11596-015-1421-6.
32. Star WM, Marijnissen HP, van den Berg-Blok AE, Versteeg JA, Franken KA, Reinhold HS. Destruction of rat mammary tumor and normal tissue microcirculation by hematoporphyrin derivative photoradiation observed in vivo in sandwich observation chambers. Cancer Res. 1986;46(5):2532–40.
33. Wang H, Li J, Lv T, Tu Q, Huang Z, Wang X. Therapeutic and immune effects of 5-aminolevulinic acid photodynamic therapy on UVB-induced squamous cell carcinomas in hairless mice. Exp Dermatol. 2013;22(5):362–3. https://doi.org/10.1111/exd.12132.
34. Semenza GL. Hypoxia-inducible factors in physiology and medicine. Cell. 2012;148(3):399–408. https://doi.org/10.1016/j.cell.2012.01.021.
35. Zhang A, Zu D, Yang L, Wang L. Photodynamic therapy with 5-aminolevulinic acid for 28 cases of hemangioma. Chin J Aesth Med. 2007;4:541–2.
36. Chen H, Zou X, Zhang Y, Qu L, Guo X, Lin H. Recent advances in photodynamic therapy for the treatment of hemangioma. Chin J Dermatol Venereol. 2014;28(6):631–3. https://doi.org/10.13735/j.cjdv.1001-7089.2014.0631.
37. Wen L, Hyoju R, Wang P, Shi L, Li C, Li M, et al. Hydrogen-peroxide-responsive protein biomimetic nanoparticles for Photothermal-photodynamic combination therapy of melanoma. Lasers Surg Med. 2021;53(3):390–9. https://doi.org/10.1002/lsm.23292.
38. Zhang Y, Miao F, Wang H, Lv T, Li J, Wang X. Study on the local immune response in the treatment of Condyloma Acuminatum with Aminolevulinic acid photodynamic therapy. Chin J Dermatol. 2013;5:309–12.
39. Miao F, Lv T, Zhang Y, Huang Z, Wang X, Wang H. Induction of apoptosis in HPV16 E7 transfected human keratinocyte by ALA-mediated photodynamic therapy. Photodiagn Photodyn Ther. 2016;13:205–10. https://doi.org/10.1016/j.pdpdt.2015.07.004.
40. Zaenglein AL. Acne vulgaris. N Engl J Med. 2018;379(14):1343–52. https://doi.org/10.1056/NEJMcp1702493.
41. Zhang L, Wang X, Wang H, Su L, Guo M. Photodynamic therapy with 5-aminolevulinic acid for the treatment of acne. Chin J Dermatol. 2009;2:78–80.
42. Ma L, Xiang LH, Yu B, Yin R, Chen L, Wu Y, et al. Low-dose topical 5-aminolevulinic acid photodynamic therapy in the treatment of different severity of acne vulgaris. Photodiagn Photodyn Ther. 2013;10(4):583–90. https://doi.org/10.1016/j.pdpdt.2013.06.007.
43. Zaenglein AL, Pathy AL, Schlosser BJ, Alikhan A, Baldwin HE, Berson DS, et al. Guidelines of care for the management of acne vulgaris. J Am Acad Dermatol. 2016;74(5):945–73. https://doi.org/10.1016/j.jaad.2015.12.037.
44. Shi L, Yang J, Zhang L, Zhang Y, Yan G, Zhang H, et al. A prospective study of adverse reactions of ALA-PDT for acne vulgaris. Photodiagn Photodyn Ther. 2022;38:102752. https://doi.org/10.1016/j.pdpdt.2022.102752.
45. Zhang L, Yang J, Liu X, Xu D, Shi L, Liu J, et al. 5-Aminolaevulinic acid photodynamic therapy amplifies intense inflammatory response in the treatment of acne vulgaris via CXCL8. Exp Dermatol. 2021;30(7):923–31. https://doi.org/10.1111/exd.14357.
46. Wang X, Ji J, Zhang H, Fan Z, Zhang L, Shi L, et al. Stimulation of dendritic cells by DAMPs in ALA-PDT treated SCC tumor cells. Oncotarget. 2015;6(42):44688–702. https://doi.org/10.18632/oncotarget.5975.
47. Ji J, Zhang Y, Chen WR, Wang X. DC vaccine generated by ALA-PDT-induced immunogenic apoptotic cells for skin squamous cell carcinoma. Onco Targets Ther. 2016;5(6):e1072674. https://doi.org/10.1080/2162402X.2015.1072674.
48. Demidova TN, Hamblin MR. Macrophage-targeted photodynamic therapy. Int J Immunopathol Pharmacol. 2004;17(2):117–26. https://doi.org/10.1177/039463200401700203.
49. Garg AD, Krysko DV, Verfaillie T, Kaczmarek A, Ferreira GB, Marysael T, et al. A novel pathway

combining calreticulin exposure and ATP secretion in immunogenic cancer cell death. EMBO J. 2012;31(5):1062–79. https://doi.org/10.1038/emboj.2011.497.
50. Sautes-Fridman C, Petitprez F, Calderaro J, Fridman WH. Tertiary lymphoid structures in the era of cancer immunotherapy. Nat Rev Cancer. 2019;19(6):307–25. https://doi.org/10.1038/s41568-019-0144-6.
51. Gollnick SO, Brackett CM. Enhancement of anti-tumor immunity by photodynamic therapy. Immunol Res. 2010;46(1-3):216–26. https://doi.org/10.1007/s12026-009-8119-4.
52. Schuler G, Schuler-Thurner B, Steinman RM. The use of dendritic cells in cancer immunotherapy. Curr Opin Immunol. 2003;15(2):138–47. https://doi.org/10.1016/s0952-7915(03)00015-3.
53. Shi L, Wang H, Chen K, Yan J, Yu B, Wang S, et al. Chinese guidelines on the clinical application of 5-aminolevulinic acid-based photodynamic therapy in dermatology (2021 edition). Photodiagn Photodyn Ther. 2021;35:102340. https://doi.org/10.1016/j.pdpdt.2021.102340.
54. Boukamp P, Tilgen W, Dzarlieva RT, Breitkreutz D, Haag D, Riehl RK, et al. Phenotypic and genotypic characteristics of a cell line from a squamous cell carcinoma of human skin. J Natl Cancer Inst. 1982;68(3):415–27.
55. Giard DJ, Aaronson SA, Todaro GJ, Arnstein P, Kersey JH, Dosik H, et al. In vitro cultivation of human tumors: establishment of cell lines derived from a series of solid tumors. J Natl Cancer Inst. 1973;51(5):1417–23. https://doi.org/10.1093/jnci/51.5.1417.
56. Moore GE, Merrick SB, Woods LK, Arabasz NM. A human squamous cell carcinoma cell line. Cancer Res. 1975;35(10):2684–8.
57. Kondo S, Aso K. Establishment of a cell line of human skin squamous cell carcinoma in vitro. Br J Dermatol. 1981;105(2):125–32. https://doi.org/10.1111/j.1365-2133.1981.tb01196.x.
58. Rheinwald JG, Beckett MA. Tumorigenic keratinocyte lines requiring anchorage and fibroblast support cultured from human squamous cell carcinomas. Cancer Res. 1981;41(5):1657–63.
59. Hozumi Y, Kondo S, Shimoura T, Aso K. Human squamous cell carcinoma from skin: establishment and characterization of a new cell line (HSC-5). J Dermatol. 1990;17(3):143–8. https://doi.org/10.1111/j.1346-8138.1990.tb01615.x.
60. Ji J, Wang P, Zhou Q, Zhu L, Zhang H, Zhang Y, et al. CCL8 enhances sensitivity of cutaneous squamous cell carcinoma to photodynamic therapy by recruiting M1 macrophages. Photodiagn Photodyn Ther. 2019;26:235–43. https://doi.org/10.1016/j.pdpdt.2019.03.014.
61. Novak B, Heesen L, Schary N, Lübbert H. The influence of different illumination parameters on protoporphyrin IX induced cell death in squamous cell carcinoma cells. Photodiagn Photodyn Ther. 2018;21:385–92. https://doi.org/10.1016/j.pdpdt.2018.02.007.
62. Ye T, Chen T, Jiang B, Yang L, Liu X, Chen B, et al. 5-aminolevulinic acid photodynamic therapy inhibits invasion and metastasis of SCL-1 cells probably via MTSS1 and p63 gene related pathways. Photodiagn Photodyn Ther. 2020;32:102039. https://doi.org/10.1016/j.pdpdt.2020.102039.
63. Qiao L, Mei Z, Yang Z, Li X, Cai H, Liu W. ALA-PDT inhibits proliferation and promotes apoptosis of SCC cells through STAT3 signaling pathway. Photodiagn Photodyn Ther. 2016;14:66–73. https://doi.org/10.1016/j.pdpdt.2016.01.008.
64. Zhao Z, Zhang H, Zeng Q, Wang P, Zhang G, Ji J, et al. Exosomes from 5-aminolevulinic acid photodynamic therapy-treated squamous carcinoma cells promote dendritic cell maturation. Photodiagn Photodyn Ther. 2020;30:101746. https://doi.org/10.1016/j.pdpdt.2020.101746.
65. Nie S, Wang X, Wang H. NLRP3 Inflammasome mediated interleukin-1β production in cancer-associated fibroblast contributes to ALA-PDT for cutaneous squamous cell carcinoma. Cancer Manag Res. 2019;11:10257–67. https://doi.org/10.2147/cmar.S226356.
66. Zhang H, Wang P, Wang X, Shi L, Fan Z, Zhang G, et al. Antitumor effects of DC vaccine with ALA-PDT-induced immunogenic apoptotic cells for skin squamous cell carcinoma in mice. Technol Cancer Res Treat. 2018;17:1533033818785275. https://doi.org/10.1177/1533033818785275.
67. Li S, Wang P, Zhang G, Ji J, Lv T, Wang X, et al. The effect of ALA-PDT on reversing the activation of cancer-associated fibroblasts in cutaneous squamous cell carcinoma. Photodiagn Photodyn Ther. 2019;27:234–40. https://doi.org/10.1016/j.pdpdt.2019.05.043.
68. Gallego-Rentero M, Gutiérrez-Pérez M, Fernández-Guarino M, Mascaraque M, Portillo-Esnaola M, Gilaberte Y, et al. TGFβ1 secreted by cancer-associated fibroblasts as an inductor of resistance to photodynamic therapy in squamous cell carcinoma cells. Cancer. 2021;13(22):5613. https://doi.org/10.3390/cancers13225613.
69. Zeng Q, Yang J, Ji J, Wang P, Zhang L, Yan G, et al. PD-L1 blockade potentiates the antitumor effects of ALA-PDT and optimizes the tumor microenvironment in cutaneous squamous cell carcinoma. Onco Targets Ther. 2022;11(1):2061396. https://doi.org/10.1080/2162402x.2022.2061396.
70. Lv T, Zeng Q, Huang J, Wu M, Wang H, Wang X. Halofuginone enhances the anti-tumor effect of ALA-PDT by suppressing NRF2 signaling in cSCC. Photodiagn Photodyn Ther. 2021;2021:102572. https://doi.org/10.1016/j.pdpdt.2021.102572.
71. Wang P, Yang W, Shen S, Wu C, Wen L, Cheng Q, et al. Differential diagnosis and precision therapy of two typical malignant cutaneous tumors leveraging their tumor microenvironment: a photomedicine

strategy. ACS Nano. 2019;13(10):11168–80. https://doi.org/10.1021/acsnano.9b04070.
72. Therefore PL, Langston AW, Daniallinia N, Hebert JL, Fujimoto MA, Khaimskiy Y, et al. Long-term establishment, characterization and manipulation of cell lines from mouse basal cell carcinoma tumors. Exp Dermatol. 2006;15(9):742–50. https://doi.org/10.1111/j.1600-0625.2006.00465.x.
73. Aszterbaum M, Epstein J, Oro A, Douglas V, LeBoit PE, Scott MP, et al. Ultraviolet and ionizing radiation enhance the growth of BCCs and trichoblastomas in patched heterozygous knockout mice. Nat Med. 1999;5(11):1285–91. https://doi.org/10.1038/15242.
74. Gracia-Cazaña T, Mascaraque M, Lucena SR, Vera-Álvarez J, González S, Juarranz Á, et al. Biomarkers of basal cell carcinoma resistance to methyl-aminolevulinate photodynamic therapy. PLoS One. 2019;14(4):e0215537. https://doi.org/10.1371/journal.pone.0215537.
75. Mascaraque M, Delgado-Wicke P, Nuevo-Tapioles C, Gracia-Cazaña T, Abarca-Lachen E, González S, et al. Metformin as an adjuvant to photodynamic therapy in resistant basal cell carcinoma cells. Cancer. 2020;12(3):668. https://doi.org/10.3390/cancers12030668.
76. Boukamp P, Petrussevska RT, Breitkreutz D, Hornung J, Markham A, Fusenig NE. Normal keratinization in a spontaneously immortalized aneuploid human keratinocyte cell line. J Cell Biol. 1988;106(3):761–71. https://doi.org/10.1083/jcb.106.3.761.
77. Wang P, Han J, Wei M, Xu Y, Zhang G, Zhang H, et al. Remodeling of dermal collagen in photoaged skin using low-dose 5-aminolevulinic acid photodynamic therapy occurs via the transforming growth factor-β pathway. J Biophotonics. 2018;11(6):e201700357. https://doi.org/10.1002/jbio.201700357.
78. Suciu M, Porav S, Radu T, Rosu MC, Lazar MD, Macavei S, et al. Photodynamic effect of light emitting diodes on E. Coli and human skin cells induced by a graphene-based ternary composite. J Photochem Photobiol B. 2021;223:112298. https://doi.org/10.1016/j.jphotobiol.2021.112298.
79. Zhao M, Leggett E, Bourke S, Poursanidou S, Carter-Searjeant S, Po S, et al. Theranostic near-infrared-active conjugated polymer nanoparticles. ACS Nano. 2021;15(5):8790–802. https://doi.org/10.1021/acsnano.1c01257.
80. Nowak-Perlak M, Bromke MA, Ziółkowski P, Woźniak M. The comparison of the efficiency of Emodin and aloe-Emodin in photodynamic therapy. Int J Mol Sci. 2022;23(11):6276. https://doi.org/10.3390/ijms23116276.
81. Todaro GJ, Green H. Quantitative studies of the growth of mouse embryo cells in culture and their development into established lines. J Cell Biol. 1963;17(2):299–313. https://doi.org/10.1083/jcb.17.2.299.
82. Kosaka S, Kawana S, Zouboulis CC, Hasan T, Ortel B. Targeting of sebocytes by aminolevulinic acid-dependent photosensitization. Photochem Photobiol. 2006;82(2):453–7. https://doi.org/10.1562/2005-08-08-ra-643.
83. Liu W, Wang Q, Tuo J, Chang Y, Ying J, Jiang M, et al. ALA-PDT suppressed the cell growth by Akt-/Erk-mTOR-p70 s6k pathway in human SZ95 sebocytes in vitro. Photodiagn Photodyn Ther. 2018;24:1–6. https://doi.org/10.1016/j.pdpdt.2018.06.024.
84. Tuo J, Wang Q, Zouboulis CC, Liu Y, Ma Y, Ma L, et al. ALA-PDT suppressing the cell growth and reducing the lipogenesis in human SZ95 sebocytes by mTOR signaling pathway in vitro. Photodiagn Photodyn Ther. 2017;18:295–301. https://doi.org/10.1016/j.pdpdt.2017.03.006.
85. Ding HL, Wang XL, Wang HW, Huang Z. Successful treatment of refractory facial acne using repeat short-cycle ALA-PDT: case study. Photodiagn Photodyn Ther. 2011;8(4):343–6. https://doi.org/10.1016/j.pdpdt.2011.07.003.
86. Linglin Zhang XW, Wang H, Lina S, Guo M. Topical aminolevulinic acid-photodynamic therapy in acne. Chin J Dermatol. 2009;42(2):78–80.
87. Zouboulis CC, Seltmann H, Neitzel H, Orfanos CE. Establishment and characterization of an immortalized human sebaceous gland cell line (SZ95). J Invest Dermatol. 1999;113(6):1011–20. https://doi.org/10.1046/j.1523-1747.1999.00771.x.
88. Ting Lv XW, Zhou W, Wang H, Miao F, Li J. Establishment of mouse model for cutaneous squamous cell carcinoma induced by ultraviolet. Chin J Dermatol. 2011;44(3):174–7. https://doi.org/10.3760/cma.j.issn.0412-4030.2011.03.008.
89. Martínez-Cruz AB, Santos M, Lara MF, Segrelles C, Ruiz S, Moral M, et al. Spontaneous squamous cell carcinoma induced by the somatic inactivation of retinoblastoma and Trp53 tumor suppressors. Cancer Res. 2008;68(3):683–92. https://doi.org/10.1158/0008-5472.Can-07-3049.
90. Zhu L, Zhang G, Wang P, Zhang L, Ji J, Liu X, et al. The effect of C-X-C motif chemokine ligand 13 in cutaneous squamous cell carcinoma treated with aminolevulinic acid-photodynamic therapy. Photodiagn Photodyn Ther. 2019;26:389–94. https://doi.org/10.1016/j.pdpdt.2019.04.018.
91. Liu J, Yan G, Chen Q, Zeng Q, Wang X. Modified 5-aminolevulinic acid photodynamic therapy (M-PDT) inhibits cutaneous squamous cell carcinoma cell proliferation by targeting PP2A/PP5-mediated MAPK signaling pathway. Int J Biochem Cell Biol. 2021;137:106036. https://doi.org/10.1016/j.biocel.2021.106036.
92. Bhatta AK, Wang P, Keyal U, Zhao Z, Ji J, Zhu L, et al. Therapeutic effect of Imiquimod enhanced ALA-PDT on cutaneous squamous cell carcinoma. Photodiagn Photodyn Ther. 2018;23:273–80. https://doi.org/10.1016/j.pdpdt.2018.07.010.

93. Anand S, Honari G, Hasan T, Elson P, Maytin EV. Low-dose methotrexate enhances aminolevulinate-based photodynamic therapy in skin carcinoma cells in vitro and in vivo. Clin Cancer Res. 2009;15(10):3333–43. https://doi.org/10.1158/1078-0432.Ccr-08-3054.
94. Anand S, Wilson C, Hasan T, Maytin EV. Vitamin D3 enhances the apoptotic response of epithelial tumors to aminolevulinate-based photodynamic therapy. Cancer Res. 2011;71(18):6040–50. https://doi.org/10.1158/0008-5472.Can-11-0805.
95. Anand S, Rollakanti KR, Horst RL, Hasan T, Maytin EV. Combination of oral vitamin D3 with photodynamic therapy enhances tumor cell death in a murine model of cutaneous squamous cell carcinoma. Photochem Photobiol. 2014;90(5):1126–35. https://doi.org/10.1111/php.12286.
96. Chen J, Zhang Y, Wang P, Wang B, Zhang G, Wang X. Plum-blossom needling promoted PpIX fluorescence intensity from 5-aminolevulinic acid in porcine skin model and patients with actnic keratosis. Photodiagn Photodyn Ther. 2016;15:182–90. https://doi.org/10.1016/j.pdpdt.2016.06.012.
97. Wang X, Shi L, Tu Q, Wang H, Zhang H, Wang P, et al. Treating cutaneous squamous cell carcinoma using 5-aminolevulinic acid polylactic-co-glycolic acid nanoparticle-mediated photodynamic therapy in a mouse model. Int J Nanomedicine. 2015;10:347–55. https://doi.org/10.2147/IJN.S71245.
98. Shi L, Liu P, Wu J, Ma L, Zheng H, Antosh MP, et al. The effectiveness and safety of X-PDT for cutaneous squamous cell carcinoma and melanoma. Nanomedicine. 2019;14(15):2027–43. https://doi.org/10.2217/nnm-2019-0094.
99. Liu Y, Viau G, Bissonnette R. Multiple large-surface photodynamic therapy sessions with topical or systemic aminolevulinic acid and blue light in UV-exposed hairless mice. J Cutan Med Surg. 2004;8(2):131–9. https://doi.org/10.1007/s10227-004-0117-5.
100. Mascaraque-Checa M, Gallego-Rentero M, Nicolás-Morala J, Portillo-Esnaola M, Cuezva JM, González S, et al. Metformin overcomes metabolic reprogramming-induced resistance of skin squamous cell carcinoma to photodynamic therapy. Mol Metab. 2022;60:101496. https://doi.org/10.1016/j.molmet.2022.101496.
101. Sunar U, Rohrbach DJ, Morgan J, Zeitouni N, Henderson BW. Quantification of PpIX concentration in basal cell carcinoma and squamous cell carcinoma models using spatial frequency domain imaging. Biomed Opt Express. 2013;4(4):531–7. https://doi.org/10.1364/boe.4.000531.
102. Rollakanti K, Anand S, Maytin EV. Topical calcitriol prior to photodynamic therapy enhances treatment efficacy in nonmelanoma skin cancer mouse models. Proc SPIE Int Soc Opt Eng. 2015;9308:93080q. https://doi.org/10.1117/12.2077296.
103. Marsh Durban V, Deuker MM, Bosenberg MW, Phillips W, McMahon M. Differential AKT dependency displayed by mouse models of BRAFV600E-initiated melanoma. J Clin Invest. 2013;123(12):5104–18. https://doi.org/10.1172/jci69619.
104. Bonet C, Luciani F, Ottavi JF, Leclerc J, Jouenne FM, Boncompagni M, et al. Deciphering the role of oncogenic MITFE318K in senescence delay and melanoma progression. J Natl Cancer Inst. 2017;109(8):340. https://doi.org/10.1093/jnci/djw340.
105. Florell SR, Clayton F, Rahman H, Holmen S, Burd C, Grossman D. Characterization of amelanotic melanomas from genetically engineered mouse models. J Invest Dermatol. 2019;139(5):S139.
106. Pérez-Guijarro E, Yang HH, Araya RE, El Meskini R, Michael HT, Vodnala SK, et al. Multimodel preclinical platform predicts clinical response of melanoma to immunotherapy. Nat Med. 2020;26(5):781–91. https://doi.org/10.1038/s41591-020-0818-3.
107. Galvani E, Mundra PA, Valpione S, Garcia-Martinez P, Smith M, Greenall J, et al. Stroma remodeling and reduced cell division define durable response to PD-1 blockade in melanoma. Nat Commun. 2020;11(1):853. https://doi.org/10.1038/s41467-020-14632-2.
108. Córdoba F, Braathen LR, Weissenberger J, Vallan C, Kato M, Nakashima I, et al. 5-aminolaevulinic acid photodynamic therapy in a transgenic mouse model of skin melanoma. Exp Dermatol. 2005;14(6):429–37. https://doi.org/10.1111/j.0906-6705.2005.00303.x.
109. Meeth K, Wang JX, Micevic G, Damsky W, Bosenberg MW. The YUMM lines: a series of congenic mouse melanoma cell lines with defined genetic alterations. Pigment Cell Melanoma Res. 2016;29(5):590–7. https://doi.org/10.1111/pcmr.12498.
110. Ma LW, Nielsen KP, Iani V, Moan J. A new method for photodynamic therapy of melanotic melanoma – effects of depigmentation with violet light photodynamic therapy. J Environ Pathol Toxicol Oncol. 2007;26(3):165–72. https://doi.org/10.1615/jenvironpatholtoxicoloncol.v26.i3.10.
111. Schacht V, Szeimies RM, Abels C. Photodynamic therapy with 5-aminolevulinic acid induces distinct microcirculatory effects following systemic or topical application. Photochem Photobiol Sci. 2006;5(5):452–8. https://doi.org/10.1039/b514128a.
112. Sanmamed MF, Chester C, Melero I, Kohrt H. Defining the optimal murine models to investigate immune checkpoint blockers and their combination with other immunotherapies. Ann Oncol. 2016;27(7):1190–8. https://doi.org/10.1093/annonc/mdw041.
113. Tasdogan A, Faubert B, Ramesh V, Ubellacker JM, Shen B, Solmonson A, et al. Metabolic heterogeneity confers differences in melanoma metastatic potential. Nature. 2020;577(7788):115–20. https://doi.org/10.1038/s41586-019-1847-2.

114. Tuveson D, Clevers H. Cancer modeling meets human organoid technology. Science. 2019;364(6444):952–5. https://doi.org/10.1126/science.aaw6985.
115. Votanopoulos KI, Forsythe S, Sivakumar H, Mazzocchi A, Aleman J, Miller L, et al. Model of patient-specific immune-enhanced organoids for immunotherapy screening: feasibility study. Ann Surg Oncol. 2020;27(6):1956–67. https://doi.org/10.1245/s10434-019-08143-8.
116. Wang M, Yang X, Chang L, Chen J, Luo J, Wu Y, et al. Low-level PDT treatment modulated photoaging mediated by UVA irradiation through regulating Bach2. Photodiagn Photodyn Ther. 2020;29:101606. https://doi.org/10.1016/j.pdpdt.2019.101606.
117. Yuting X, Han J, Wang X. Protective effect of n-3 polyunsaturated fatty acids on acute skin photodamage in SKH-1 mice. Chin J Dermatol. 2018;51(8):586–91. https://doi.org/10.3760/cma.j.issn.0412-4030.2018.08.006.
118. Peiru Wang HX, Wang X. The role of n-3 polyunsaturated fatty acids in skin photoaging. Chin J Dermatovenereol. 2021;35(7):721–6. https://doi.org/10.13735/j.cjdv.1001-7089.202010063.
119. Wang P, Yan G, Xue H, Shen S, Cao Y, Zhang G, et al. Proteomics and lipidomics reveal the protective mechanism of dietary n-3 PUFA supplementation for photoaging. Food Funct. 2021;12(17):7883–96. https://doi.org/10.1039/d0fo03228j.
120. Lv T, Huang ZF, Wang HW, Lin JQ, Chen GN, Chen XW, et al. Evaluation of collagen alteration after topical photodynamic therapy (PDT) using second harmonic generation (SHG) microscopy–in vivo study in a mouse model. Photodiagn Photodyn Ther. 2012;9(2):164–9. https://doi.org/10.1016/j.pdpdt.2011.12.006.
121. Gur-Cohen S, Yang H, Baksh SC, Miao Y, Levorse J, Kataru RP, et al. Stem cell-driven lymphatic remodeling coordinates tissue regeneration. Science. 2019;366(6470):1218–25. https://doi.org/10.1126/science.aay4509.
122. DeYoung L, Ballaron S, Epstein W. Transglutaminase activity in human and rabbit ear comedogenesis: a histochemical study. J Invest Dermatol. 1984;82(3):275–9. https://doi.org/10.1111/1523-1747.ep12260366.
123. Kwon TR, Choi EJ, Oh CT, Bak DH, Im SI, Ko EJ, et al. Targeting of sebaceous glands to treat acne by microinsulated needles with radio frequency in a rabbit ear model. Lasers Surg Med. 2017;49(4):395–401. https://doi.org/10.1002/lsm.22599.
124. De Young LM, Young JM, Ballaron SJ, Spires DA, Puhvel SM. Intradermal injection of Propionibacterium acnes: a model of inflammation relevant to acne. J Invest Dermatol. 1984;83(5):394–8. https://doi.org/10.1111/1523-1747.ep12264715.
125. Yang J, Shi L, Xu D, Liu J, Zhang L, Liu X, et al. 5-Aminolaevulinic acid photodynamic therapy suppresses lipid secretion of primary sebocytes through AMPK/SREBP-1 pathway. Photodiagn Photodyn Ther. 2021;36:102537. https://doi.org/10.1016/j.pdpdt.2021.102537.
126. Kosaka S, Miyoshi N, Akilov OE, Hasan T, Kawana S. Targeting of sebaceous glands by δ-aminolevulinic acid-based photodynamic therapy: an in vivo study. Lasers Surg Med. 2011;43(5):376–81. https://doi.org/10.1002/lsm.21062.
127. Kloeters O, Tandara A, Mustoe TA. Hypertrophic scar model in the rabbit ear: a reproducible model for studying scar tissue behavior with new observations on silicone gel sheeting for scar reduction. Wound Repair Regen. 2007;15(Suppl 1):S40–5. https://doi.org/10.1111/j.1524-475X.2007.00224.x.
128. Wang Q, Dong Y, Geng S, Su H, Ge W, Zhen C. Photodynamic therapy inhibits the formation of hypertrophic scars in rabbit ears by regulating metalloproteinases and tissue inhibitor of metalloproteinase-1. Clin Exp Dermatol. 2014;39(2):196–201. https://doi.org/10.1111/ced.12265.
129. Yu Z, Meng X, Zhang S, Wang X, Chen Y, Min P, et al. IR-808 loaded nanoethosomes for aggregation-enhanced synergistic transdermal photodynamic/photothermal treatment of hypertrophic scars. Biomater Sci. 2021;10(1):158–66. https://doi.org/10.1039/d1bm01555a.
130. Chen Y, Zhang Z, Xin Y, Zhou R, Jiang K, Sun X, et al. Synergistic transdermal delivery of nanoethosomes embedded in hyaluronic acid nanogels for enhancing photodynamic therapy. Nanoscale. 2020;12(28):15435–42. https://doi.org/10.1039/d0nr03494k.
131. Demerjian M, Man MQ, Choi EH, Brown BE, Crumrine D, Chang S, et al. Topical treatment with thiazolidinediones, activators of peroxisome proliferator-activated receptor-gamma, normalizes epidermal homeostasis in a murine hyperproliferative disease model. Exp Dermatol. 2006;15(3):154–60. https://doi.org/10.1111/j.1600-0625.2006.00402.x.
132. Yi F, Zheng X, Fang F, Zhang J, Zhou B, Chen X. ALA-PDT alleviates the psoriasis by inhibiting JAK signaling pathway. Exp Dermatol. 2019;28(11):1227–36. https://doi.org/10.1111/exd.14017.
133. Fang YP, Huang YB, Wu PC, Tsai YH. Topical delivery of 5-aminolevulinic acid-encapsulated ethosomes in a hyperproliferative skin animal model using the CLSM technique to evaluate the penetration behavior. Eur J Pharm Biopharm. 2009;73(3):391–8. https://doi.org/10.1016/j.ejpb.2009.07.011.
134. Chen T, Zhang LW, Fu LX, Wu YB, Liu XY, Guo ZP. Systemic ALA-PDT effectively blocks the development of psoriasis-like lesions and alleviates leucocyte infiltration in the K14-VEGF transgenic mouse. Clin Exp Dermatol. 2017;42(8):849–56. https://doi.org/10.1111/ced.13148.
135. Wang H, Su D, Huang R, Shu F, Cheng F, Zheng G. Cellular nanovesicles with bioorthogonal targeting enhance photodynamic/photothermal therapy in

psoriasis. Acta Biomater. 2021;134:674–85. https://doi.org/10.1016/j.actbio.2021.07.068.
136. Wang Y, Fu S, Lu Y, Lai R, Liu Z, Luo W, et al. Chitosan/hyaluronan nanogels codelivering methotrexate and 5-aminolevulinic acid: a combined chemo-photodynamic therapy for psoriasis. Carbohydr Polym. 2022;277:118819. https://doi.org/10.1016/j.carbpol.2021.118819.
137. Wang B, Xu YT, Zhang L, Zheng J, Sroka R, Wang HW, et al. Protoporphyrin IX fluorescence as potential indicator of psoriasis severity and progression. Photodiagn Photodyn Ther. 2017;19:304–7. https://doi.org/10.1016/j.pdpdt.2017.05.016.

4 Pain During Photodynamic Therapy

Zhijie Ruan, Xiuli Wang, and Bo Wang

4.1 Introduction

ALA-PDT is widely used to treat various skin diseases, but pain during and after therapy remains a common and significant adverse event, often hindering its clinical use. Effective pain management during PDT is crucial for enhancing patient comfort and broadening ALA-PDT applications. Recent research from the authors' group investigated the associations between pain perception and various factors, including photosensitizer concentration, treatment duration, light dose, and light source selection. These findings revealed that daylight photodynamic therapy (DL-PDT) and modified 5-aminolevulinic acid photodynamic therapy (M-PDT) are superior in maintaining therapeutic effectiveness while minimizing pain. These explorations not only revealed the potential to achieve patient comfort during PDT but also expanded the use of PDT in clinical practice.

Z. Ruan · X. Wang
Institute of Photomedicine, Shanghai Skin Disease Hospital, School of Medicine, Tongji University, Shanghai, China
e-mail: zhijieRuan@tongji.edu.cn; wangxiuli_1400023@tongji.edu.cn

B. Wang (✉)
Avera Medical Group Dermatology, Aberdeen, SD, USA

University of South Dakota, Vermillion, SD, USA
e-mail: makiwang@med.umich.edu

4.2 Mechanism of Pain Production in PDT

Pain refers to an unpleasant sensation and emotional experience associated with actual or potential tissue damage. When nociceptors sense stimulation, they convert pain stimuli to electrical signals by opening ion channels. Cumulative voltage changes result in action potential firing on nociceptive fibers, which relay to the cerebral sensory cortex and are perceived as painful. Pain during PDT is the main adverse effect of PDT and can be classified as pain during illumination and pain after treatment. Pain during illumination is the primary factor affecting treatment experience and hindering PDT treatment. It usually appears in the first few seconds of illumination, manifesting as sensations of burning, electric shock, sore and tingling, and typically decreases after light exposure ends.

As mentioned earlier, the acute phase of pain occurs within a few seconds of illumination and typically peaks within 1 min. It usually diminishes in intensity within several hours before progressing into chronic pain. The chronic phase refers to pain persisting for more than 1 day after PDT. The specific mechanisms of pain at each stage of PDT remain unclear. Ongoing research from the authors' group proposed four theories that may provide valuable insight (Fig. 4.1) [1].

X. Wang, B. Wang (eds.), *Photodynamic Therapy in Dermatology*,
https://doi.org/10.1007/978-981-96-8915-6_4

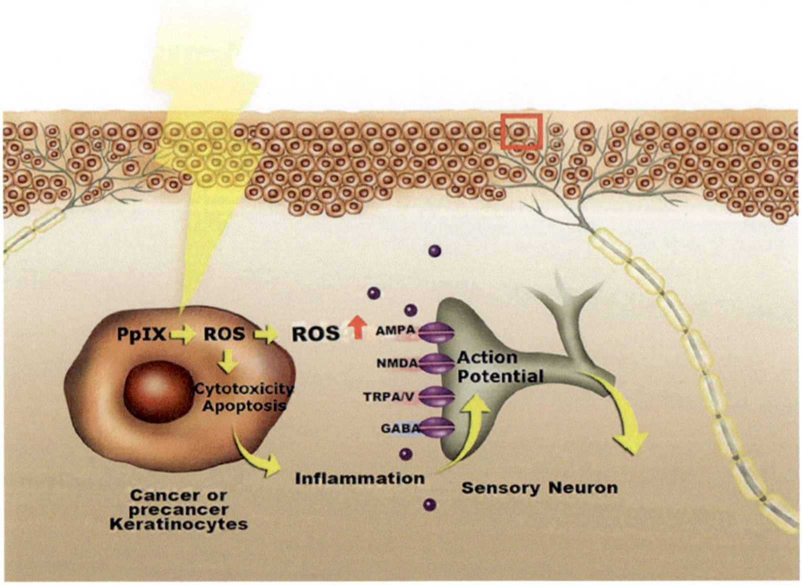

Fig. 4.1 Potential mechanisms of pain experience during photodynamic therapy [1]. *AMPA* a-amino3-hydroxy-5-methyl-4-isoxazole propionic acid, *GABA* c-aminobutyric acid, *NMDA* N-methyl-D-aspartate receptor, *TRPA/V* transient receptor potential cation channel, subfamilies A and V, *PpIX* protoporphyrin IX

4.2.1 Reactive Oxygen Species

The primary mechanism of pain during PDT is likely initiated during the photoactivation stage when protoporphyrin IX (PpIX) generates reactive oxygen species (ROS). Previous studies have shown that ROS can directly activate nerve endings, leading to increased phosphorylation of N-methyl-D-aspartate (NMDA) and α-amino-3-hydroxy-5-methyl-4-isoxazole propionic acid (AMPA) receptors while decreasing γ-aminobutyric acid (GABA) release [2–4]. This process results in increased firing of nociceptive neurons. Consequently, the ROS generated by PpIX initiates pain transmission and activates nociceptive neurons, resulting in the sensation of pain. Supporting evidence includes studies indicating a positive correlation between the PpIX fluorescence intensity and the severity of pain associated with PDT.

4.2.2 Inflammatory Pain

Inflammatory pain may be the main contributor to chronic pain during PDT. The ROS generated during PDT can mediate tissue damage and stimulate the production of proinflammatory cytokines, such as interleukin (IL)-1, IL-2, and tumor necrosis factor (TNF)-α, which can increase the sensitivity of sensory neurons to capsaicin, resulting in a state of inflammatory pain [5, 6]. Nonsteroidal anti-inflammatory drugs (NSAIDs), ibuprofen, and opioid analgesics have been shown to be effective in the management of inflammatory pain. A previous study by Huang et al. revealed that the administration of oxycodone at 5 mg/acetaminophen 325 mg did not reduce pain during PDT illumination; however, it alleviated PDT-induced chronic pain [7]. These findings suggest that inflammatory pain may play a role in the underlying mechanism of chronic pain during PDT. However, since inflammation is crucial to the therapeutic effect of PDT, further investigation is warranted to determine whether inhibiting the inflammatory response might diminish the therapeutic efficacy of PDT.

4.2.3 Transient Receptor Potential (TRP) Channels

TRP channels are a family of nonselective cation channels that are expressed in various cells, such as sensory neurons and keratinocytes. Members of this family, including TRPA1, TRPM8, and TRPV1, are closely related to nociceptive sensation and the response to various pain stimuli.

TRPA1 and TRPM8 are associated with thermal and cold sensations, respectively. TRPV1, also known as the capsaicin receptor, is the most studied TRP channel and can be activated by various intrinsic and extrinsic stimuli: (1) temperatures >43 °C; (2) acidity; and (3) capsaicin. PDT can generate localized heat and subsequently trigger the activation of TRPV1 channels. In addition, ROS can sensitize TRPV1 by modifying its covalent cysteine [8]. Thus, the authors' group speculated that TRPV1 may be a key mediator of chronic pain during PDT [1].

4.2.4 Genetic Variance and Pain Sensitivity

Nociception is a complex multifactorial process, and its mechanisms are still not fully understood. Clinical observations have revealed significant individual differences in pain perception during PDT, where the same painful stimulation can elicit different nociceptions and responses among different individuals. A recent study involving monozygotic twins investigated the effect of DNA methylation on pain sensitivity [9]. They reported that increased TRPA1 promoter methylation and decreased TRPA1 expression were strongly associated with decreased pain tolerability. A similar result was also found for TRPV3 channels. With the advancement of next-generation sequencing, more gene modifiers related to pain sensitivity will be revealed. The ultimate goal of pain management is to enable personalized pain management. By predicting a patient's propensity toward pain on the basis of genetic profiling, clinicians could tailor pain management strategies to each individual, increasing treatment efficacy and patient comfort.

4.3 Factors that Affect the Production of Pain During PDT

Factors affecting the occurrence and severity of pain during PDT include photosensitizers, light sources, fluorescence intensity, irradiation dose, and lesion characteristics.

4.3.1 Photosensitizers

Previous studies have suggested that different photosensitizers can influence pain during PDT. ALA and methyl aminolevulinate (MAL) are the two most commonly used photosensitizer prodrugs in dermatology. Previously, some studies reported a mild increase in pain intensity with ALA-PDT compared with MAL-PDT [10–15]. One possible explanation for this phenomenon is attributed to the reduced tissue specificity of ALA relative to MAL. This disparity causes a noticeable accumulation of protoporphyrin IX (PpIX) in noncancerous cells, consequently resulting in increased pain sensation in patients undergoing PDT.

4.3.2 Light Sources

The choice of light source is a crucial factor in PDT, affecting both therapeutic efficacy and the level of pain experienced. For example, pulsed light produces less pain than continuous light during PDT; green light causes less pain than red light when applied, although its clinical efficacy is inferior. Thus, clinicians should consider the impact of different light sources on effectiveness and pain during PDT when selecting appropriate light sources for PDT [16, 17].

4.3.3 Fluence Rate and Light Dose

Previous studies have shown inconsistent evidence regarding a positive correlation between the fluence rate and light dose with pain severity during PDT [18–22]. The authors' group proposed a threshold theory for pain during PDT: it is positively correlated with the fluence rate and dose below a certain threshold (rate of ~60 mW cm^2, dose of ~50 J cm^2). When this threshold is surpassed, pain intensity no longer increases [1], a concept supported by Cottrell et al. [23]. It is possible that increased light doses and fluence rates accelerate ROS generation and nerve stimulation, resulting in more severe pain during PDT. However, once the threshold is reached, the pain plateaus, possibly due to the saturation of ROS generation or desensitization of nociceptors and ion channels.

4.3.4 Lesion Characteristics

- Location: Lesions on the scalp and face are typically the most painful in PDT [12, 24]. However, Wiegell et al. reported that after adjusting for PpIX fluorescence, pain scores were not dependent on lesion localization [25], which could be explained by the different densities of nerve endings across different body regions.
- Size: Pain intensity was found to be associated with lesion size [24, 26, 27]. Larger lesions produce more severe pain during PDT.
- Type of disease: Pain intensity per unit area varies among different skin conditions, with actinic keratosis causing the most pain, followed by acne and condyloma acuminatum [28, 29].

4.4 Pain Management During PDT

4.4.1 Pain Assessment

The NRS is a convenient method with high reliability and validity that is clinically used to assess pain levels during PDT. It consists of 11 numerical values, ranging from 0 to 10, where patients describe the specific intensity of pain. Higher numbers indicate more severe pain: 0 denotes no pain; 1–3 indicates mild pain; 4–6 represents moderate pain; 7–9 signifies severe pain (the patient cannot sleep or wakes up due to pain); and 10 indicates unbearable pain. During PDT, clinicians use the NRS to gauge pain and implement appropriate pain management strategies accordingly.

4.4.2 Pain Management

Pain management during PDT should prioritize the patient's subjective experience and aim to minimize discomfort. This involves considering the patient's baseline condition and NRS score grading and selecting the best personalized treatment to relieve pain. In this section, we discuss common pain management strategies.

- Cooling: Cooling is the most commonly used method in PDT pain management. It effectively reduces pain intensity, shortens post-PDT erythema duration, and improves patient satisfaction with PDT. The cooling methods include the use of electric fans, coolers, and cold sprays during illumination and the application of ice packs post-treatment (2–3 times a day for approximately 15 min each). However, the impact of cooling on PDT efficacy is not fully understood. Juzeniene et al. and Tyrrell et al. suggested that cooling might reduce the effectiveness of PDT by affecting PpIX photobleaching [30, 31]. Owing to limited evidence, more investigations are needed to clarify this issue and determine whether measures need to be taken to compensate for the potential impact of cooling on PDT efficacy.
- Oral analgesics: Tramadol is recommended to be orally administered 45 min prior to PDT because of its low potential for addiction and minimal adverse reactions, providing moderate pain control. In addition, the administration of 800 mg ibuprofen 30 min before PDT was recommended by Gholam [32–34]. However, since acute pain is not primarily mediated by inflammation, more research is needed to explore the effectiveness of these methods.
- Local infiltration anesthesia: Lidocaine and bupivacaine are used for local infiltration anesthesia during PDT. They block sodium channels, preventing nociceptive neurons from firing and thereby decreasing pain. Lidocaine with epinephrine takes effect after 5 min and lasts for 1.5 h, whereas bupivacaine takes effect after 4 min and lasts for 2–6 h. Articaine with epinephrine should be used with caution because of its potential to reduce blood circulation and the oxygen content in the lesion, which can influence PDT efficacy.
- Nerve block: Nerve block provides superior pain relief compared with cooling [35–37] and can be further enhanced when combined with cold air and oral analgesics. However,

nerve blocks pose potential risks of thrombosis or nerve damage and require experienced operators.

- Two-step irradiance schedule: This method reduces pain during PDT without significantly increasing treatment time. It involves low-power density red light irradiation to quench most of the PpIX, followed by high-power density irradiation to complete the remaining required light dose [38]. However, it shows limited effectiveness for thicker skin lesions such as hypertrophic AK and BCC, likely due to the limited penetration depth from the light source.
- Compared with conventional PDT (C-PDT), daylight photodynamic therapy (DL-PDT) uses sunlight as the light source, which has lower fluence rates and light doses [39]. It reduces the local concentration of ROS and minimizes stimulation to nerve endings, thereby reducing the degree of pain experienced. Currently, immediately exposing the treated area to sunlight for 2–2.5 h after the application of photosensitizers and chemical sunscreens is recommended. This approach can achieve satisfactory treatment outcomes. For example, a study in China by Wang et al. revealed that, compared with cPDT, DL-PDT has a similar overall efficacy in treating acne with significantly less pain [40]. However, DL-PDT is highly dependent on weather conditions. Therefore, the treatment protocol needs to be adjusted accordingly.
- General anesthesia: General anesthesia included inhalational anesthesia and intravenous anesthesia. Inhalational anesthesia offers quicker onset and recovery, making it suitable for moderate pain during PDT. On the other hand, intravenous anesthesia is more suitable for patients with severe pain and extensive lesions, as it provides more effective pain relief. However, intravenous anesthesia is associated with increased costs and increased risks. General anesthesia is commonly used in hemoporfin-mediated PDT (HMME-PDT) and hematoporphyrin derivative PDT (HpD-PDT), and it requires evaluation and management by anesthesiologists.

The authors' group suggested the following approaches for pain management during PDT: (1) mild pain: the use of cooling methods such as electric fans, cold air machines, and cold sprays; (2) moderate pain: the use of oral analgesics, local infiltration anesthesia, nerve block anesthesia, and a two-step irradiance schedule; and (3) severe pain: the use of oral tramadol or morphine, topical fentanyl patches, and even general anesthesia (Fig. 4.2). Close monitoring of the patient's vital signs is crucial. If necessary, the PDT treatment should be terminated.

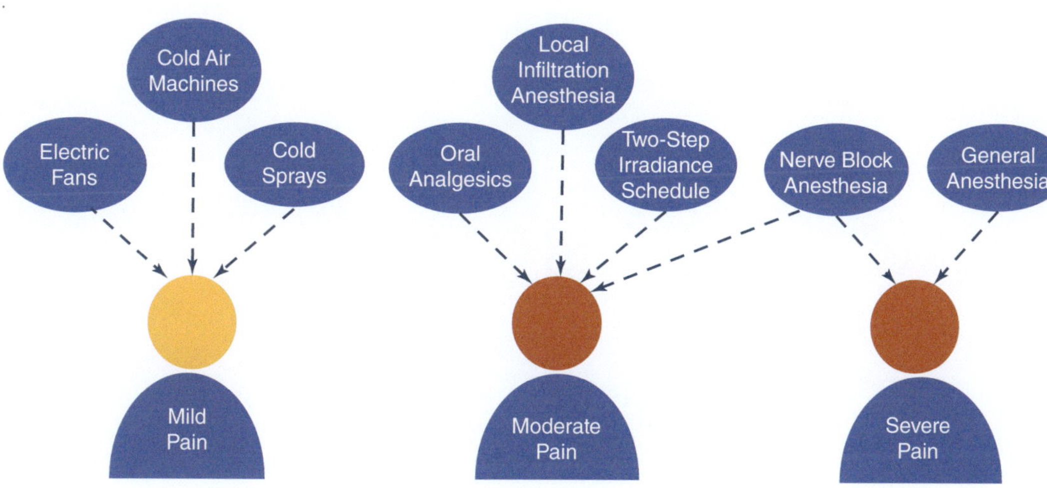

Fig. 4.2 Pain management during photodynamic therapy

4.5 Modified Photodynamic Therapy Protocol

Pain during PDT is a significant factor that prevents patients from pursuing treatment. To address this, the authors proposed a modified photodynamic therapy protocol (M-PDT) in 2020. By reducing the incubation time and increasing the light dose, M-PDT effectively alleviates pain during PDT while maintaining its efficacy.

In a 2020 prospective, randomized, self-controlled study by the authors, M-PDT (using 20% ALA, incubation for 30 min, light dose of 300 J/cm^2) achieved equivalent clinical efficacy to C-PDT (20% ALA, incubation for 3 h, light dose of 100 J/cm2) in treating condyloma acuminatum. The M-PDT group experienced significantly less pain, with some patients reporting no pain at all [41]. In 2021, another study from the authors' group published in the *Journal of the American Academy of Dermatology* highlighted the benefits of M-PDT in treating acne. This prospective, randomized, half-face-controlled study ($n = 20$) revealed that M-PDT (5% ALA, incubation for 30 min, light dose of 150 J/cm^2) was as effective as C-PDT (5% ALA, incubation for 90 min, light dose of 50 J/cm^2). Notably, the M-PDT group reported significantly reduced pain levels (Fig. 4.3) [42]. These studies demonstrated the pain-relieving effects of M-PDT as well as its equivalent treatment efficacy, highlighting its vast potential for application. However, further investigations are needed to explore the optimal parameters for M-PDT across various disease entities.

In 2022, Wang et al. further demonstrated the superior therapeutic effect of M-PDT and reduced pain compared with C-PDT in a mouse model of cSCC [43]. They attributed the reduced pain to the different patterns of ROS production between the two therapies. In C-PDT, substantial amounts of ROS accumulate rapidly, damaging tumor cells and triggering pain. Conversely, M-PDT led to a slower accumulation of ROS, thereby preventing immediate pain induction. Over the extended duration of light exposure in M-PDT,

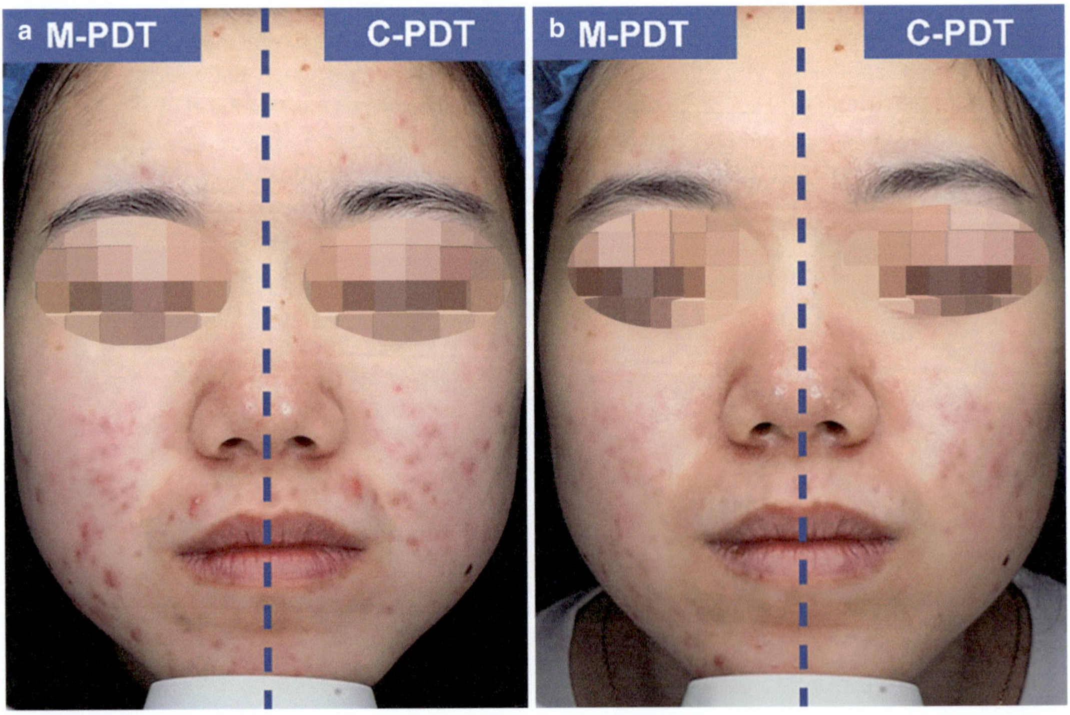

Fig. 4.3 Comparison of the efficacy of M-PDT and C-PDT in acne treatment [42]. (**a**) Before treatment with photodynamic therapy. (**b**) Four weeks after treatment with photodynamic therapy

more ROS are ultimately produced, resulting in equivalent or better therapeutic effects with only mild or no pain.

These findings underscore the potential of M-PDT to alleviate pain while maintaining or even enhancing therapeutic efficacy, offering a promising solution for broader application and promotion of PDT, particularly among patients with low pain tolerance. Further research is needed to optimize the M-PDT parameters for different disease entities.

References

1. Wang B, Shi L, Zhang YF, Zhou Q, Zheng J, Szeimies RM, Wang XL. Gain with no pain? Pain management in dermatological photodynamic therapy. Br J Dermatol. 2017;177(3):656–65. https://doi.org/10.1111/bjd.15344.
2. Yowtak J, Lee KY, Kim HY, Wang J, Kim HK, Chung K, Chung JM. Reactive oxygen species contribute to neuropathic pain by reducing spinal GABA release. Pain. 2011;152(4):844–52. https://doi.org/10.1016/j.pain.2010.12.034.
3. Lee DZ, Chung JM, Chung K, Kang M-G. Reactive oxygen species (ROS) modulate AMPA receptor phosphorylation and cell-surface localization in concert with pain-related behavior. Pain. 2012;153(9):1905–15. https://doi.org/10.1016/j.pain.2012.06.001.
4. Gao X, Kim HK, Mo Chung J, Chung K. Reactive oxygen species (ROS) are involved in enhancement of NMDA-receptor phosphorylation in animal models of pain. Pain. 2007;131(3):262–71. https://doi.org/10.1016/j.pain.2007.01.011.
5. Westlund KN, Kochukov MY, Lu Y, McNearney TA. Impact of central and peripheral TRPV1 and ROS levels on proinflammatory mediators and nociceptive behavior. Mol Pain. 2010;6:46. https://doi.org/10.1186/1744-8069-6-46.
6. Hackel D, Pflücke D, Neumann A, Viebahn J, Mousa S, Wischmeyer E, Rittner HL. The connection of monocytes and reactive oxygen species in pain. PLoS One. 2013;8(5):e63564. https://doi.org/10.1371/journal.pone.0063564.
7. Huang N, Zeng J, Liang J, Qiu H, Wang Y, Gu Y. A randomized, double-blind, placebo-controlled study of oral oxycodone plus acetaminophen for the treatment of pain in photodynamic therapy on port wine stains. Photodiagn Photodyn Ther. 2014;11(2):134–40. https://doi.org/10.1016/j.pdpdt.2014.03.004.
8. Chuang H, Lin S. Oxidative challenges sensitize the capsaicin receptor by covalent cysteine modification. Proc Natl Acad Sci USA. 2009;106(47):20097–102. https://doi.org/10.1073/pnas.0902675106.
9. Bell JT, Loomis AK, Butcher LM, Gao F, Zhang B, Hyde CL, Spector TD. Differential methylation of the TRPA1 promoter in pain sensitivity. Nat Commun. 2014;5:2978. https://doi.org/10.1038/ncomms3978.
10. Wiegell SR, Stender I-M, Na R, Wulf HC. Pain associated with photodynamic therapy using 5-aminolevulinic acid or 5-aminolevulinic acid methylester on tape-stripped normal skin. Arch Dermatol. 2003;139(9):1173–7. https://doi.org/10.1001/archderm.139.9.1173.
11. Steinbauer JM, Schreml S, Babilas P, Zeman F, Karrer S, Landthaler M, Szeimies R-M. Topical photodynamic therapy with porphyrin precursors–assessment of treatment-associated pain in a retrospective study. Photochem Photobiol Sci. 2009;8(8):1111–6. https://doi.org/10.1039/b823378k.
12. Gaál M, Otrosinka S, Baltás E, Ocsai H, Oláh J, Kemény L, Gyulai R. Photodynamic therapy of non-melanoma skin cancer with methyl aminolaevulinate is associated with less pain than with aminolaevulinic acid. Acta Derm Venereol. 2012;92(2):173–5. https://doi.org/10.2340/00015555-1223.
13. Ko D-Y, Kim K-H, Song K-H. Comparative study of photodynamic therapy with topical methyl aminolevulinate versus 5-aminolevulinic acid for facial actinic keratosis with long-term follow-up. Ann Dermatol. 2014;26(3):321. https://doi.org/10.5021/ad.2014.26.3.321.
14. Schleyer V, Radakovic-Fijan S, Karrer S, Zwingers T, Tanew A, Landthaler M, Szeimies RM. Disappointing results and low tolerability of photodynamic therapy with topical 5-aminolaevulinic acid in psoriasis. A randomized, double-blind phase I/II study. J Eur Acad Dermatol Venereol. 2006;20(7):823–8. https://doi.org/10.1111/j.1468-3083.2006.01651.x.
15. Wiegell SR, Wulf HC. Photodynamic therapy of acne vulgaris using 5-aminolevulinic acid versus methyl aminolevulinate. J Am Acad Dermatol. 2006;54(4):647–51. https://doi.org/10.1016/j.jaad.2005.12.033.
16. Babilas P, Knobler R, Hummel S, Gottschaller C, Maisch T, Koller M, Szeimies R-M. Variable pulsed light is less painful than light-emitting diodes for topical photodynamic therapy of actinic keratosis: a prospective randomized controlled trial. Br J Dermatol. 2007;157(1):111–7. https://doi.org/10.1111/j.1365-2133.2007.07959.x.
17. Morton CA, Whitehurst C, Moore JV, MacKie RM. Comparison of red and green light in the treatment of Bowen's disease by photodynamic therapy. Br J Dermatol. 2000;143(4):767–72. https://doi.org/10.1046/j.1365-2133.2000.03773.x.
18. Algermissen B, Osterloh D, Philipp CM, Berlien H-P. Management of ALA-PDT induced pain sensations. Med Laser Appl. 2003;18(1):57–64. https://doi.org/10.1078/1615-1615-00088.
19. Apalla Z, Sotiriou E, Panagiotidou D, Lefaki I, Goussi C, Ioannides D. The impact of different fluence rates on pain and clinical outcome in patients with actinic keratoses treated with photo-

dynamic therapy. Photodermatol Photoimmunol Photomed. 2011;27(4):181–5. https://doi.org/10.1111/j.1600-0781.2011.00595.x.
20. Attili SK, Lesar A, McNeill A, Camacho-Lopez M, Moseley H, Ibbotson S, Ferguson J. An open pilot study of ambulatory photodynamic therapy using a wearable low-irradiance organic light-emitting diode light source in the treatment of nonmelanoma skin cancer. Br J Dermatol. 2009;161(1):170–3. https://doi.org/10.1111/j.1365-2133.2009.09096.x.
21. Ericson MB, Sandberg C, Stenquist B, Gudmundson F, Karlsson M, Ros A-M, Rosdahl I. Photodynamic therapy of actinic keratosis at varying fluence rates: assessment of photobleaching, pain and primary clinical outcome. Br J Dermatol. 2004;151(6):1204–12. https://doi.org/10.1111/j.1365-2133.2004.06211.x.
22. Ibbotson SH. Irradiance is an important determinant of pain experienced during topical photodynamic therapy. J Am Acad Dermatol. 2011;65(1):201–2. https://doi.org/10.1016/j.jaad.2010.11.060.
23. Cottrell WJ, Paquette AD, Keymel KR, Foster TH, Oseroff AR. Irradiance-dependent photobleaching and pain in delta-aminolevulinic acid-photodynamic therapy of superficial basal cell carcinomas. Clin Cancer Res. 2008;14(14):4475–83. https://doi.org/10.1158/1078-0432.CCR-07-5199.
24. Miller IM, Nielsen JS, Lophaven S, Jemec GBE. Factors related to pain during routine photodynamic therapy: a descriptive study of 301 patients. J Eur Acad Dermatol Venereol. 2011;25(11):1275–81. https://doi.org/10.1111/j.1468-3083.2010.03964.x.
25. Wiegell SR, Skiveren J, Philipsen PA, Wulf HC. Pain during photodynamic therapy is associated with protoporphyrin IX fluorescence and fluence rate. Br J Dermatol. 2008;158(4):727–33. https://doi.org/10.1111/j.1365-2133.2008.08451.x.
26. Buinauskaite E, Zalinkevicius R, Buinauskiene J, Valiukeviciene S. Pain during topical photodynamic therapy of actinic keratoses with 5-aminolevulinic acid and red light source: randomized controlled trial. Photodermatol Photoimmunol Photomed. 2013;29(4):173–81. https://doi.org/10.1111/phpp.12044.
27. Middelburg TA, Nijsten T, Neumann MHA, de Haas ERM, Robinson DJ. Red light ALA-PDT for large areas of actinic keratosis is limited by severe pain and patient dissatisfaction. Photodermatol Photoimmunol Photomed. 2013;29(5):276–8. https://doi.org/10.1111/phpp.12055.
28. Clark C, Bryden A, Dawe R, Moseley H, Ferguson J, Ibbotson SH. Topical 5-aminolaevulinic acid photodynamic therapy for cutaneous lesions: outcome and comparison of light sources. Photodermatol Photoimmunol Photomed. 2003;19(3):134–41. https://doi.org/10.1034/j.1600-0781.2003.00024.x.
29. Grapengiesser S, Ericson M, Gudmundsson F, Larkö O, Rosén A, Wennberg A-M. Pain caused by photodynamic therapy of skin cancer. Clin Exp Dermatol. 2002;27(6):493–7. https://doi.org/10.1046/j.1365-2230.2002.01065.x.
30. Juzeniene A, Juzenas P, Bronshtein I, Vorobey A, Moan J. The influence of temperature on photodynamic cell killing in vitro with 5-aminolevulinic acid. J Photochem Photobiol B. 2006;84(2):161–6. https://doi.org/10.1016/j.jphotobiol.2006.02.009.
31. Tyrrell J, Campbell SM, Curnow A. The effect of air cooling pain relief on protoporphyrin IX photobleaching and clinical efficacy during dermatological photodynamic therapy. J Photochem Photobiol B Biol. 2011;103(1):1–7. https://doi.org/10.1016/j.jphotobiol.2010.12.011.
32. Gholam P, Denk K, Sehr T, Enk A, Hartmann M. Factors influencing pain intensity during topical photodynamic therapy of complete cosmetic units for actinic keratoses. J Am Acad Dermatol. 2010;63(2):213–8. https://doi.org/10.1016/j.jaad.2009.08.062.
33. Gholam P, Weberschock T, Denk K, Enk A. Treatment with 5-aminolaevulinic acid methylester is less painful than treatment with 5-aminolaevulinic acid nanoemulsion in topical photodynamic therapy for actinic keratosis. Dermatology. 2011;222(4):358–62. https://doi.org/10.1159/000329025.
34. Gholam P, Fink C, Uhlmann L, Enk A. Pain reduction in patients after applying a nitrous oxide/oxygen mixture (Livopan) during photodynamic therapy: study protocol for an observational study (Livopan study). BMJ Open. 2015;5(3):e006412. https://doi.org/10.1136/bmjopen-2014-006412.
35. Halldin CB, Gonzalez H, Wennberg A-M, Lepp M. Patients' experiences of pain and pain relief during photodynamic therapy on actinic keratoses: an interview study. Acta Derm Venereol. 2013;93(4):433–7. https://doi.org/10.2340/00015555-1500.
36. Klein A, Karrer S, Horner C, Werner A, Heinlin J, Zeman F, Kerscher C. Comparing cold-air analgesia, systemically administered analgesia and scalp nerve blocks for pain management during photodynamic therapy for actinic keratosis of the scalp presenting as field cancerization: a randomized controlled trial. Br J Dermatol. 2015;173(1):192–200. https://doi.org/10.1111/bjd.13547.
37. Serra-Guillen C, Hueso L, Nagore E, Vila M, Llombart B, Requena Caballero C, Guillen C. Comparative study between cold air analgesia and supraorbital and supratrochlear nerve block for the management of pain during photodynamic therapy for actinic keratoses of the frontotemporal zone. Br J Dermatol. 2009;161(2):353–6. https://doi.org/10.1111/j.1365-2133.2009.09184.x.
38. Zeitouni NC, Paquette AD, Housel JP, Shi Y, Wilding GE, Foster TH, Henderson BW. A retrospective review of pain control by a two-step irradiance schedule during topical ALA-photodynamic therapy of nonmelanoma skin cancer. Lasers Surg Med. 2013;45(2):89–94. https://doi.org/10.1002/lsm.22118.
39. Morton CA, Braathen LR. Daylight photodynamic therapy for actinic keratoses. Am J Clin Dermatol. 2018;19(5):647–56. https://doi.org/10.1007/s40257-018-0360-y.

40. Zhang L, Zhang Y, Liu X, Shi L, Wang P, Zhang H, Wang X. Conventional versus daylight photodynamic therapy for acne vulgaris: a randomized and prospective clinical study in China. Photodiagn Photodyn Ther. 2020;31:101796. https://doi.org/10.1016/j.pdpdt.2020.101796.
41. Zhang H, Shi L, Zhang Y, Wang P, Zhang G, Cao Y, Wang X. Modified photodynamic therapy to minimize pain in the treatment of condylomata acuminata: a prospective, randomized, self-controlled study. Photodiagn Photodyn Ther. 2020;32:101915. https://doi.org/10.1016/j.pdpdt.2020.101915.
42. Zhang Y, Zhang H, Zhang L, Wang P, Shi L, Zhang G, Wang X. Modified 5-aminolevulinic acid photodynamic therapy to reduce pain in the treatment of moderate to severe acne vulgaris: a prospective, randomized, split-face study. J Am Acad Dermatol. 2021;84(1):218–20. https://doi.org/10.1016/j.jaad.2020.04.146.
43. Zeng Q, Zhou C, Zhang Y, Yan G, Wang X. Modified 5-aminolevulinic acid photodynamic therapy reduces pain and improves therapeutic effects in cutaneous squamous cell carcinoma mouse model. Lasers Surg Med. 2022;54(5):804–12. https://doi.org/10.1002/lsm.23516.

5 ALA-PDT in Nonmelanoma Skin Cancer

Guolong Zhang, Peiru Wang, Chunxiao Li, Zijun Zhao, Jiandan Li, Qihang Chang, Bo Wang, and Xiuli Wang

5.1 ALA-PDT in Actinic Keratosis

5.1.1 Introduction

Actinic keratosis (AK), also known as solar keratosis, primarily occurs in sun-exposed areas and predominantly affects elderly individuals, individuals with fair skin, and those with extensive sun exposure. AK is considered a precancerous lesion with the potential to progress into cutaneous squamous cell carcinoma (cSCC). Owing to the aging population, the incidence of AK is increasing globally. In the United States, AK is one of the diseases most commonly treated by dermatologists [1]. In Shanghai, China, an epidemiological study reported a 3.08% prevalence of AK among 2038 individuals over the age of 60, with the incidence increasing with age [2]. Additionally, 5-year statistics from Beijing and Xi'an hospitals in 2015 revealed that AKs accounted for 0.52% of the 1.59 million outpatients, with an average age of 69.8 ± 11.8 years. Among these patients, 50% had multiple AKs. A broader cross-sectional study, which screened 72,437 patients, reported a 1.05% AK diagnosis rate [3].

5.1.1.1 Clinical Manifestations

AK predominantly appears on sun-exposed areas such as the cheeks, temples, neck, dorsal hands, and forearms. Lesions can be either single or multiple, with the latter being more common. Clinically, they present as erythematous or reddish-brown papules and plaques with rough surfaces, which may be associated with adherent scales. In severe cases, erosion, ulcers, or even cutaneous horns may occur. The surrounding skin often shows signs of photodamage, including mottled pigmentation, telangiectasia, and skin atrophy. Most AK patients are asymptomatic, although some may experience mild pain and itching. Because early AKs may be subtle, they are often overlooked. Photodamaged skin surrounding multiple AKs frequently contains subclinical AK lesions, forming what is known as "field cancerization" (Fig. 5.1) [4]. Therefore, AK treatment should consider the entire affected area. To guide treatment, the Olsen grading system is commonly used to classify AKs into three levels on the basis of lesion thickness and the degree of keratinization (Table 5.1).

On the basis of its clinical morphology, AKs can be categorized into hypertrophic, pigmented, atro-

G. Zhang · P. Wang · C. Li · Z. Zhao · J. Li · Q. Chang
X. Wang (✉)
Institute of Photomedicine, Shanghai Skin Disease Hospital, School of Medicine, Tongji University, Shanghai, China
e-mail: wangxiuli_1400023@tongji.edu.cn

B. Wang
Avera Medical Group Dermatology, Aberdeen, SD, USA

University of South Dakota, Vermillion, SD, USA
e-mail: makiwang@med.umich.edu

X. Wang, B. Wang (eds.), *Photodynamic Therapy in Dermatology*,
https://doi.org/10.1007/978-981-96-8915-6_5

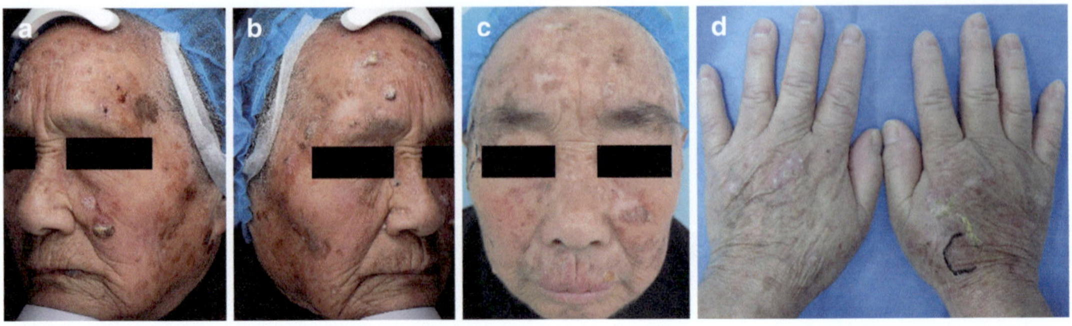

Fig. 5.1 (**a**, **b**) Multiple actinic keratosis of the face with field cancerization and hyperkeratotic papules. (**c**, **d**) Field cancerization on the face and dorsal hands

Table 5.1 Olsen clinical grading of AK [5, 6]

Grade	Clinical manifestations
I	Mild: Pink to grayish papules and plaques with mildly palpable scales, but hard to visualize
II	Moderate: Erythematous plaques with moderately palpable and visible scales
III	Severe: Thick scales, significant hyperkeratosis, difficult to distinguish from early cSCC
Field cancerization	Multiple AK lesions merging into plaques (more than a few centimeters)

phic, cutaneous horns, and actinic cheilitis (AC) [7]. AC is a specific type of AK that primarily affects the lower lip and presents with symptoms such as peeling, cracking, ulcers, and/or focal hyperkeratosis. Owing to the greater risk of progression to cSCC, approximately 10–30%, AC requires a proactive approach in management. About 95% of lip cSCC cases originate from the AC.

The diagnosis of AK is often made through a combination of patient history, clinical evaluation, and physical examination, but histopathology remains the gold standard, especially when malignancy is suspected. The pathological features of AK include dysplastic keratinocytes in the epidermis, presenting a spectrum of changes from hyperkeratosis to parakeratosis. When dysplasia involves the full thickness of the epidermis, it may resemble cutaneous squamous cell carcinoma in situ. Varying degrees of lymphocytic infiltration, sometimes in a lichenoid pattern, may also be observed.

In recent years, noninvasive diagnostic methods such as dermatoscopy and reflectance confocal microscopy (RCM) have gained clinical importance in the diagnosis of AK. They are used for screening, diagnosis, determining the location for biopsy, and post-treatment follow-up. The authors' group recommended the use of dermatoscopy for lesion localization before photodynamic therapy and for observing treatment effectiveness and follow-up, providing more precise guidance for treatment [8].

Dermatoscopic findings are related to the severity and grade of skin lesions. The typical dermatoscopic patterns include Grade I: red pseudonetwork. Grade II: strawberry pattern, follicular plugging, surrounding white halo, and visible pinpoint and irregular linear vessels. Grade III: significant hyperkeratosis appearing as a yellow-white structureless area with conspicuous follicular plugs (Fig. 5.2). The appearance of yellow-white structureless areas, ulcerations, or atypical vascular patterns, such as coarse vessels around hair follicles, radiating glomerular-like vessels, and irregular linear vessels, may indicate progression to cSCC, warranting histopathological confirmation [9].

In RCM, the most characteristic feature of AK is the disordered arrangement of epidermal spinous cell layers, leading to the loss of the normal honeycomb structure. It can show features such as dysplastic keratinocytes of varying sizes and irregularly high-refractive borders, resembling target-shaped cells (Fig. 5.3). However, RCM is limited in detecting thickened AK lesions because of its superficial focus.

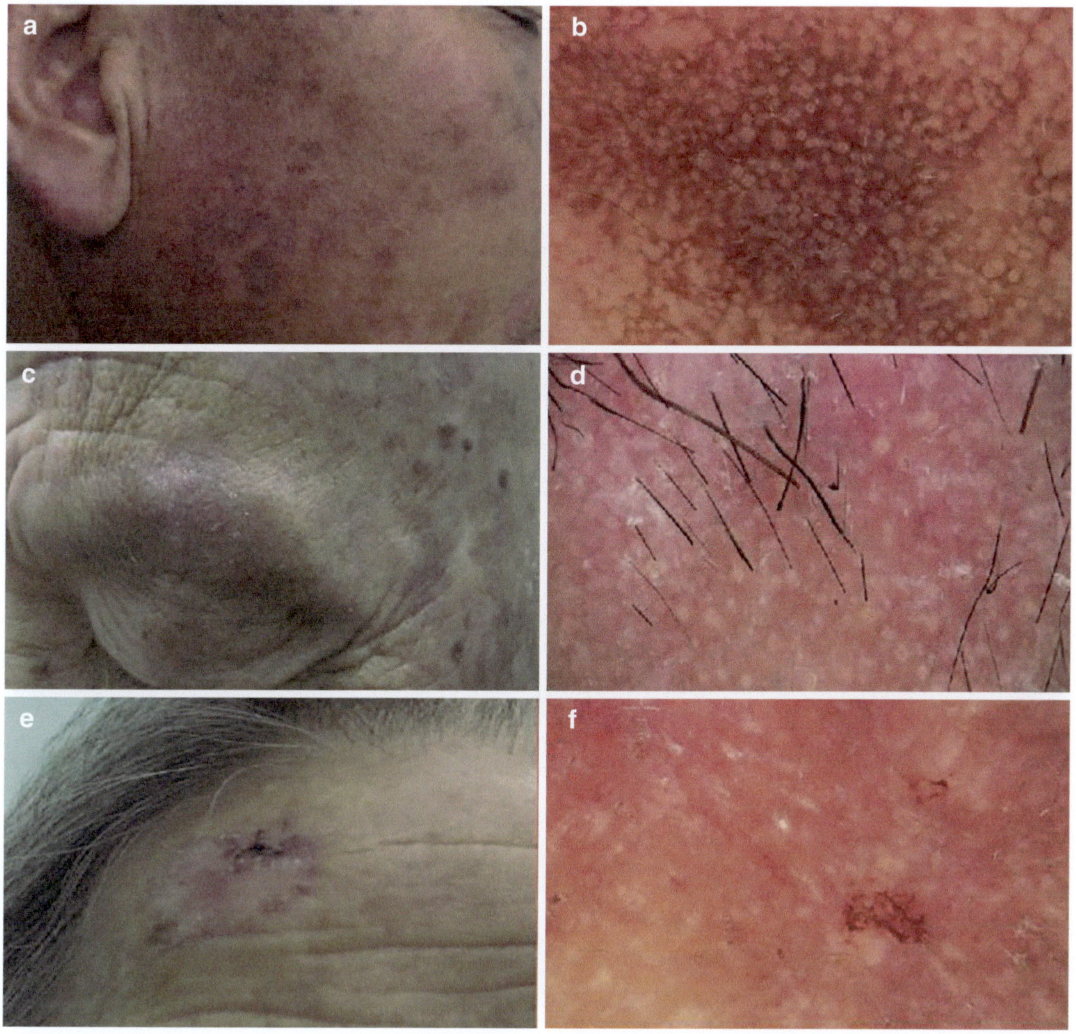

Fig. 5.2 Clinical and dermatoscopic manifestations of different grades of AK. (**a**, **b**) Clinical grade I lesions can be palpated. Dermatoscopy reveals a red pseudoreticular structure, scattered white scales, and a reticular distribution of punctate or linear perifollicular blood vessels. (**c**, **d**) Clinical grade II. Dermatoscopic findings include a strawberry pattern with yellowish to whitish dilated hair follicles on an erythematous background; white halos around the hair follicle opening and dotted and irregular linear vessels can be seen. (**e**, **f**) Clinical grade III, obvious visible thickening of the lesions. Dermatoscopic findings include apparent hyperkeratosis, a yellow–white structureless area, and enlarged follicular plugging that is covered with yellowish-white scales

5.1.1.2 Pathogenesis and Prognosis

The most significant risk factor for developing AK is prolonged exposure to ultraviolet (UV) radiation. UV radiation can induce genetic mutations, promote chronic skin inflammation, suppress the immune system, and ultimately lead to abnormal keratinocyte proliferation. Individuals with fair skin (Fitzpatrick skin types I and II) are at greater risk for AKs, whereas the incidence of AKs in skin types III and IV is similarly lower [10, 11]. Immunosuppressed individuals, such as organ transplant recipients or those on long-term cytotoxic medications, are also at increased risk for AK, which may increase their risk of developing cSCC [12]. The probability of an AK lesion progressing to cSCC within 1 year is 0.60%, which increases to 2.57% after 4 years. Approximately 60% of cSCC patients have a his-

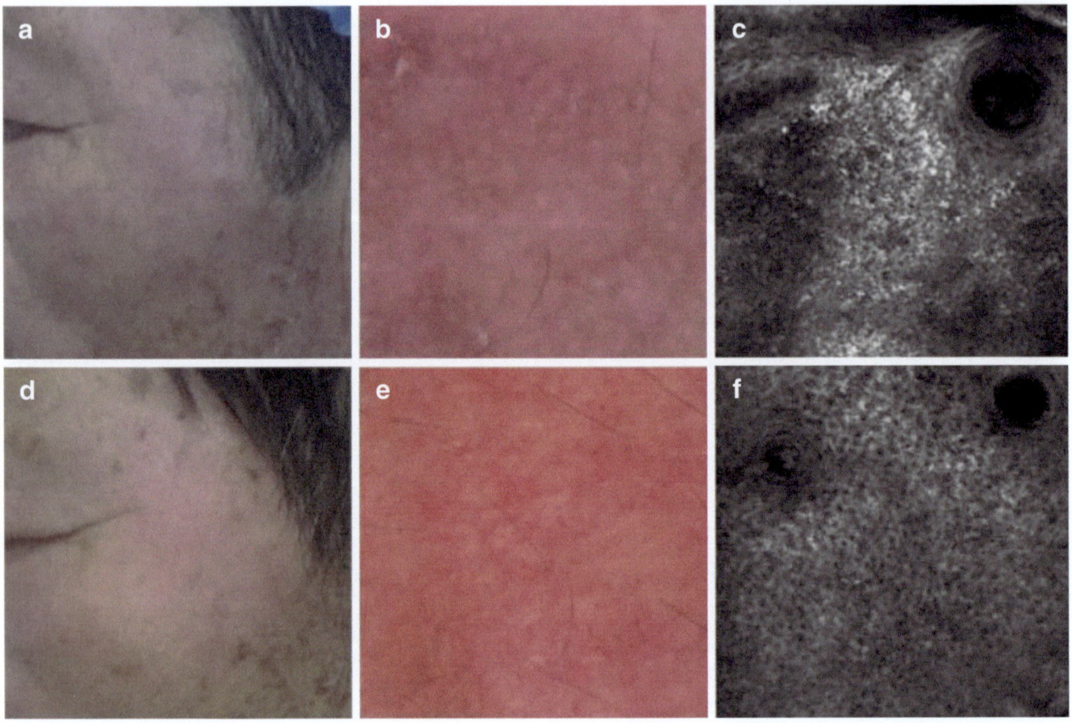

Fig. 5.3 Clinical, dermatoscopic, and RCM manifestations of AK before and after PDT treatment. (**a**) Left temporal AK before treatment. (**b**) Perifollicle yellow halo, numerous rose petal signs, and few white scales. (**c**) Disordered basal cells, abnormal target cells, and phagocytic pigment particles. (**d**) After two ALA-PDT treatments. (**e**) A small amount of yellow around the hair follicle, no rose petal sign, and a few irregular blood vessels. (**f**) The epidermal cells were regularly arranged, and no abnormal target cells or phagocytic pigment particles were found

tory of AK [13]. The risk of malignant transformation is significantly greater in individuals with multiple AK lesions than in those with a single lesion, and this risk increases with age [14].

5.1.1.3 Diagnosis and Treatment

AK is a chronic progressive disease with the potential for malignant transformation and is often associated with other nonmelanoma skin tumors. Both domestic and international guidelines recommend managing AKs as soon as lesions are identified [15]. Initially, the authors' group used ALA-PDT for individual AK lesions. However, clinical experience has revealed that AK typically presents with multiple lesions and widespread photodamage in sun-exposed skin, making the treatment of isolated lesions insufficient. Considering that ALA-PDT has a "field-clearance" effect, it removes both AK lesions and reverse photodamage in the surrounding skin, providing a more comprehensive approach. Drawing from ALA-PDT's success in genital warts and its "field-clearance" effect on subclinical and latent infections, the author's group initiated a randomized study on full-face ALA-PDT for AK in 2017. International scholars have recognized this phenomenon, coining the term "field-directed PDT" for AK treatment. In 2021, the authors' group led the development of the "Expert Consensus on Clinical Diagnosis and Treatment of Chinese Actinic Keratosis (2021)," emphasizing "field-directed treatment for AK and lifelong follow-up" for high-risk AK patients, including those with multiple or recurrent lesions, advanced age, immunosuppression, a history of nonmelanoma skin cancers, and mucosal or hypertrophic lesions.

Local treatments for AK include topical medications such as imiquimod, 5-fluorouracil, and diclofenac, as well as physical therapies such as cryotherapy, laser therapy, electrocautery, curettage, and surgical excision. Systemic treatments, such as oral retinoids (see Table 5.2), are used for more widespread or high-risk cases. Given the occurrence of regional carcinogenesis in multiple AK lesions, it is crucial to perform field-directed treatment for the entire significantly photodamaged area in addition to treating existing lesions. This approach helps reduce the incidence and recurrence of AK. Physical therapies primarily target existing AKs, whereas photodynamic therapy and topical medications are effective for both lesion removal and field-directed treatment. Systemic treatment is recommended for field-directed treat-

Table 5.2 Common treatment methods for AK

Therapy	Protocol	Advantage	Limitation
ALA-PDT	10–20% ALA Conventional red light-PDT: incubation time: 3 h ~ 6 h, LED red light: 100–150 J/cm^2 Daylight-PDT: Incubation time 0.5 h, daylight 2 h (summer treatment time should be reduced as appropriate) Modified PDT: incubation time 0.5 h, energy density 150 J/cm^2	Minimally invasive, good cosmetic effect, field treatment, reduce recurrence and new lesion, can be repeated	Erythema, edema, itching, burning sensation, pigmentary changes, etc. The pain of conventional red light-PDT is significant
Cryotherapy	Spray or cotton swab liquid nitrogen application, freezing time is 5–10 s, the end reaction is skin lesions, white and hard can be pinched in both hands	The effect of local skin lesion is good, inexpensive	Pain, erythema, blisters and infection, hypopigmentation, scar, etc. The treatment endpoint was poorly controllable
Surgery	Curettage or surgical excision	Direct removal of skin lesions Effective for hypertrophic AK and clinically suspicious cSCC lesions and other treatment-resistant AK	Risk of infection and scarring
Laser therapy	Ablative fractional laser, such as CO_2 laser	Direct destruction, preferred for hypertrophic AK	Risk of infection, hypopigmentation, and scarring
Topical medication	5% 5-fluorouracil is recommended for AK on the head, back, and forearm Twice daily for no more than 4 weeks	Easy to use and field therapy	Longer treatment course requiring continuous use. Erythema, blisters, erosion, ulcers, scabs, burning sensation, itching, pain, and photosensitivity and pigmentary changes
	Imiquimod: 5% imiquimod, 3 times weekly for 4–16 weeks, each use area <25 cm^2	Easy to use and field therapy	The course of treatment is longer and needs continuous use. Fever, erythema, scab, erosion/ulcers, itching, pain, and hypopigmentation
	Diclofenac: 2.5% hyaluronic acid gel containing 3% diclofenac, twice daily for at least 60–90 days	Convenient to use	Less effective and irritating
System medication	Acitretin 20–25 mg/d for more than 3 weeks	The number of AK can be effectively reduced in patients with multiple AK, high-risk or immunosuppressed patients	Hepatotoxic, hyperlipemia, xerosis, erythema, alopecia, teratogenesity, etc.

ment in cases of regional carcinogenesis in patients with multiple AK lesions or for high-risk patients.

AK prevention requires long-term sun protection. International guidelines recommend the use of both sunscreen and physical barriers. Broad-spectrum sunscreen with an SPF greater than 15 is suggested [16, 17]. The daily application of high-efficiency UVB/UVA sunblocks (SPF30, PA+++) to the face, neck, and ears (at 2 mg/cm^2) can inhibit the development of UV-induced carcinogenesis, reducing the incidence of new AKs in individuals with normal or compromised immunity. This also lowers the risk of AK progressing to cSCC and the cSCC recurrence rate [18–21].

PDT is recommended as the preferred therapy for AK lesions in various guidelines, including the "Expert Consensus on Clinical Diagnosis and Treatment of Chinese Actinic Keratosis (2021)" [15], the "Clinical Application Guidelines of Aminolevulinic Acid Photodynamic Therapy in Dermatology (2021)" [22], and the "European Guidelines for the Use of PDT (2019)" [23]. PDT is particularly suitable for facial and scalp lesions or multiple and extensive AK lesions. ALA-PDT not only clears AK and actinic cheilitis lesions but also reverses photodamage, yielding superior cosmetic outcomes.

5.1.2 ALA-PDT

Nonmelanoma skin cancer was one of the earliest applications of PDT. In 1996, the authors' group applied ALA-PDT to treat Bowen's disease and superficial basal cell carcinoma (BCC). They later expanded its use to treat precancerous lesions such as AK, erythroplasia, and bowenoid papulosis [24–27]. In 2000, Levulan (ALA formulation) was officially approved by the U.S. FDA for AK treatment, marking the first global indication for ALA-PDT. In 2001, Metvix (ALA-methyl ester) received approval for AK treatment in the European Union. By 2003, Metvix was promoted and clinically applied worldwide, including in more than 30 countries such as EU member states, Australia, New Zealand, and Brazil. Network meta-analysis revealed that ALA-PDT offers excellent long-term efficacy (beyond 12 months) for nonsurgical interventions in AK, making it one of the best treatment options for AK [28]. As a result, AK has become the earliest and most widely applicable indication for ALA-PDT in dermatology.

5.1.2.1 Mechanism of ALA-PDT in AK

Direct Killing ALA is a natural hydrophilic small molecule and a precursor in the heme synthesis pathway. When exogenous ALA is absorbed through the skin, it is selectively taken up by tumor cells and other rapidly proliferating cells at rates 10 times greater than those in normal cells. These aberrant cells undergo a series of enzymatic reactions, resulting in the accumulation of a photosensitive substance called protoporphyrin IX (PpIX) within mitochondria. Upon exposure to specific wavelengths of light, PpIX undergoes a photochemical reaction that generates reactive oxygen species (ROS), such as singlet oxygen ($^1O_2$). ROS are highly reactive and can damage key biomolecules, including unsaturated fatty acids, proteins, and nucleic acids, causing destruction of cell membranes, mitochondria, and DNA. This causes abnormal keratinocytes to undergo necrosis, apoptosis, pyroptosis, and autophagy, thereby effectively treating AK [29].

Immune Regulation In addition to directly eliminating atypical cells, PDT induces a local inflammatory response, releasing cytokines and chemokines that attract immune cells such as neutrophils, T cells, dendritic cells (DCs), and B cells. This further enhances the body's immune response [29]. PDT can trigger immunogenic cell death, promote the expression of endogenous danger signals, increase tumor immunogenicity, elicit specific antitumor immunity, and help prevent the recurrence and relapse of AK [30].

5.1.2.2 Therapeutic Parameters

Concentration and Time of ALA Application In 1997, Jeffes et al. explored the optimal concentration of ALA for AK treatment and reported no statistically significant difference in the clearance rate of AK lesions after 8 weeks of single treatment with different ALA concentrations (10%, 20%, or 30%) [31]. Similarly, the authors reported no significant difference in efficacy or adverse reactions between 10% and 20% ALA cream [32]. Several studies have investigated the effect of application time on PpIX accumulation in tissues. In 2000, Ormrod et al. reported that the PpIX level peaked at 11 hours, with a half-life of 30 h [33]. In 2010, Warren et al. reported a linear correlation between PpIX accumulation and application time within the first 2 h, with significantly greater accumulation of PpIX occurring in all skin lesions at 2 h [34]. Although the FDA recommends an application time of 14–18 h, such longer durations can increase adverse reactions in ALA-PDT. Numerous studies have confirmed that a 3-hour application time yields similar therapeutic effects on AK. In 2007, a clinical report revealed no significant difference in AK clearance with different application times (1–3 h) [35]. In 2009, Braathen et al. reported no significant difference in AK clearance rates between 1-h and 3-h application times for superficial and moderately thick lesions [36]. Melanie Palm et al. suggested no absolute correlation between PpIX accumulation and efficacy, suggesting a 1-h application time for thinner AKs and up to 3 h for thicker or larger AKs [37]. For individualized treatment response to ALA-PDT, some experts have proposed that personalized parameters can balance efficacy and adverse reactions [38]. In 2005, Radankovic et al. tested different light doses of 70 J/cm^2, 100 J/cm^2, and 140 J/cm^2 for a single red light-PDT session, with clearance rates of 89%, 92%, and 81%, respectively, after 1 month and 81%, 77%, and 69%, respectively, after 3 months, without significant differences [39]. On the basis of available evidence, Chinese guidelines for photodynamic therapy recommend the use of ALA concentrations of 10–20% with an application time of 3–6 h and a light dose of 100–150 J/cm^2 for traditional red light-PDT. For daylight-PDT (DL-PDT), a 0.5 h application time and 2 h of sunlight exposure are recommended [22]. In recent years, the authors' group developed modified photodynamic therapy (M-PDT) by shortening the application time of ALA to relieve pain during PDT. In 2020, Mordon et al. compared mask-style LED red light-PDT with a 0.5-h ALA application time to traditional red light-PDT with a 3-hour application. After 1–2 sessions, the efficacy for grade I–II AK was comparable, with clearance rates at 3 months of 79.3% and 80.7%, respectively [40].

ALA Formulations ALA is available in emulsions, gels, or cream forms for treating AK, with cream offering the highest drug absorption efficiency. ALA methyl ester (MAL), which has better skin permeability due to its hydrophilic nature, is widely used in Europe and the United States. In recent years, a 7.8% ALA gel (BF-200 ALA, biofrontera bioscience GmbH, Leverkusen, Germany) and ALA patch (2 × 2 cm, containing 8 mg ALA) have also been used in clinical practice. Studies have shown no significant difference in the efficacy of these formulations compared with traditional methods. The patch is convenient, requires no light avoidance, and can be used with home light sources or D-PDT.

Light Sources ALA can be activated by various light sources, including IPL (400–1200 nm), red light (630–635 nm), blue light (405–420 nm), pulsed dye lasers (585 nm or 595 nm), and sunlight. For skin cancer treatment, red light is preferred because of its deeper penetration. Red LED light is the primary light source for AK treatment. Compared with traditional red light-PDT, DL-PDT is nearly painless and causes fewer acute adverse reactions, such as redness. In 2019, the authors developed an M-PDT method that significantly reduced pain while maintaining treatment efficacy.

Pretreatment PDT requires three elements: photosensitizers, light, and oxygen. The depth of ALA penetration and distribution, along with the depth of light source radiation, are critical to the clinical efficacy of PDT. Pretreatment of AK lesions, such as the use of plum-blossom needles, microneedles, curettes, or CO_2 fractional lasers, promotes photosensitizer absorption and conversion, especially for hypertrophic and grade II–III AK lesions. The authors' group used plum-blossom needles as a pretreatment before ALA-

PDT and observed greater effectiveness in a single session than in the no pretreatment group, significantly reducing the treatment duration [41]. Furthermore, using animal models and clinical trials, the authors compared the efficacy of plum-blossom needle pretreatment and CO_2 fractional laser pretreatment. They reported that plum-blossom needle pretreatment resulted in greater ALA penetration and conversion, without tissue carbonization, which could hinder ALA absorption, making it more suitable for primary healthcare facilities (Fig. 5.4) [42]. However, for thinner skin areas, pretreatment should be performed with caution to avoid skin ulcers and scarring [43].

Field-Directed Treatment In the past, ALA-PDT for AK was focused solely on individual lesions. During treatment, freshly prepared 10% ALA cream was applied to the skin lesions and the surrounding 0.5–1 cm area, but normal-looking areas were not treated. The concept of "field cancerization" was introduced in 1953 and refers to the presence of subclinical tumor changes, with gene mutations in clinically normal peritumoral skin. This surrounding area can eventually evolve into visible tumors. In elderly individuals with AKs on their head and face, AKs often accompany field cancer, with a progressively deteriorating trajectory. If treatment targets only visible lesions, patients are at increased risk of developing new AKs in untreated areas, often requiring repeat interventions, leading to increased patient burden. The situation with AK is similar to that with condyloma acuminatum, where high recurrence rates are due to subclinical and latent infections around warts. In 2006, the authors' group conducted a comparative study on the efficacy of ALA-PDT versus CO_2 laser therapy for external genital condyloma acuminatum. The results demonstrated that ALA-PDT selectively targeted warts and surrounding subclinical and latent infections, achieving a "field clearance" effect, whereas traditional CO_2 lasers only produced a "spot clearance" effect. ALA-PDT "field clearance" was associated with higher cure

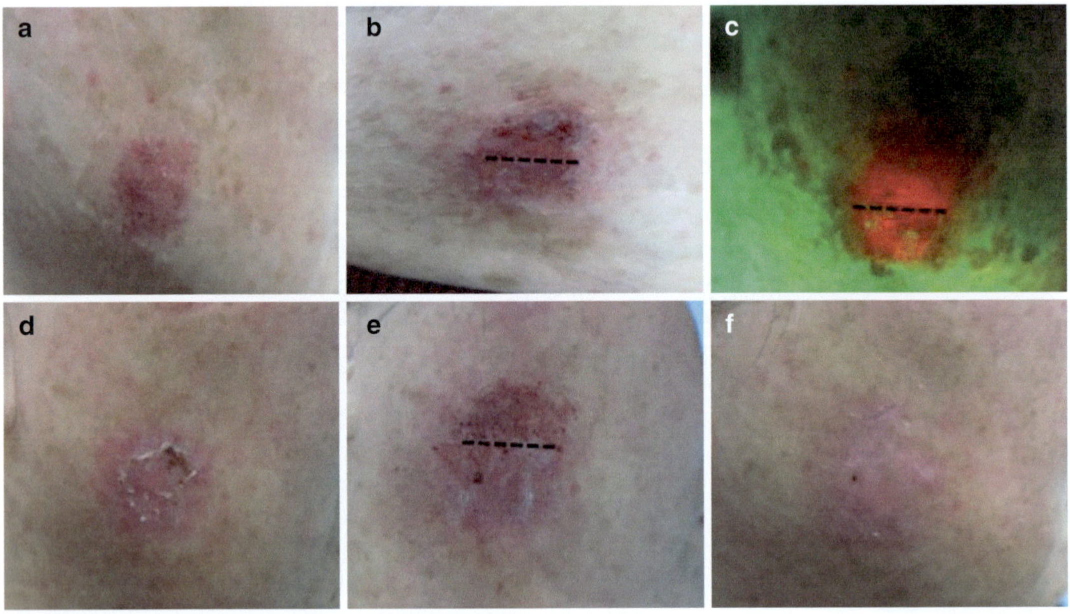

Fig. 5.4 PDT treatment of AK through plum-blossom needle or CO_2 ablative fraction laser pretreatment. (**a**) Before treatment. (**b**) After the first pretreatment session, the area above the dotted line was treated with a plum-blossom needle with the endpoint of pinpoint bleeding; the area below the line was treated with a CO_2 ablative fraction laser (deep mode, dose 17.5 mJ/cm^2, density 5%). (**c**) Fluorescence photographs taken after external application of 10% ALA for 3 h. (**d**) 2 weeks after the first PDT. (**e**) Pretreatment before the second PDT. (**f**) 2 weeks after the second PDT

rates and lower recurrence rates [44, 45]. This was the first time the concept of "field clearance" with PDT was proposed, illustrating its positive therapeutic and preventive effects on subclinical lesions around treated skin. This concept was later extended to "field-directed treatment" for AK associated with field cancer. PDT has since become a crucial method for reducing the incidence and incidence of AK.

Previous studies have shown that compared with cryotherapy and 5-fluorouracil, PDT is more effective at treating multiple AK lesions [46]. In 2005, a multicenter study evaluating MAL-PDT in the treatment of NMSC in 81 organ transplant recipients reported that 1 year post-treatment, the incidence of new lesions in treated areas was lower than that in untreated areas. These findings indicate that MAL-PDT is an effective treatment for field cancer [44]. The 2007 International Consensus on PDT for NMSCs also stated that PDT for treating AK with regional cancer has a high clearance rate [47]. In 2008, Wennberg et al. suggested that repetitive PDT for field-directed treatment effectively prevents the development of new AK lesions in transplant recipients [48]. For immunocompetent patients, a randomized, placebo-controlled trial showed that ALA-PDT for field cancerization in NMSCs significantly delayed the appearance of new lesions and reduced the total number of new lesions, especially AK lesions [49]. PDT offers high cure rates, rapid treatment outcomes, and good cosmetic effects, making it a significantly advantageous option for field-directed treatment of AK.

5.1.2.3 Clinical Efficacy (Table 5.3)

Blue Light-PDT In 2000, blue light was approved by the US FDA as the light source for treating AK with ALA-PDT. A multicenter phase IV clinical study in the United States revealed that, after a single treatment with 20% ALA blue light-PDT, the clearance rate of AK lesions on the head and face was 76% after 1 month. With 1–2 sessions, a 12-month follow-up demonstrated a sustained clearance rate of 78% [51]. For AK lesions on the upper limbs, the clearance rate was 69% after 1–2 treatments and a 2-month follow-up [50].

Red Light-PDT Red light is currently the most commonly used light source for ALA-PDT treatment, both in China and internationally (Fig. 5.5). In 2002, Professor Szeimies conducted a study involving 193 patients with multiple AK lesions. These patients were randomly divided into two groups and received either MAL-PDT or a single session of cryotherapy. The cure rates were 69% and 75%, respectively, with MAL-PDT resulting in significantly better cosmetic outcomes [57]. The authors' group used ALA-PDT to treat 31 AK patients, with clearance achieved after 2–6 sessions. During the 3–6-month follow-up, three patients experienced recurrence, yielding a recurrence rate of 14%. These recurrent cases were successfully retreated with ALA-PDT. All patients achieved excellent cosmetic results, with no scarring or adverse reactions [68]. The group also applied ALA-PDT to treat AK in special areas, such as the nose and eyelids, and the results revealed that ALA-PDT was safe and effective without causing damage to surrounding tissues. However, ALA-PDT had less favorable results for hypertrophic AK lesions, and the treatment efficacy for limb lesions was not as good as that for lesions on the head or face (Fig. 5.6) [69–71]. A multicenter study involving 121 patients with 1343 limb lesions revealed that the efficacy of a single treatment was 78%, which was comparable to that of the cryotherapy control group. However, some studies reported a cure rate as low as 45% [31, 56]. A multicenter prospective randomized controlled study published in the *New England Journal of Medicine* revealed that for field-directed therapy of multiple grade I–III AK lesions, the 3-month lesion clearance rate after a single treatment with red light MAL-PDT was 76%, whereas it was 90.6% with 5% FU cream, 75.8% with 5% imiquimid cream, and 67.3% with 0.015% ingenol mebutate [52].

Modified Painless PDT Conventional PDT (C-PDT) often causes varying degrees of pain, making it difficult for patients to endure and limiting their widespread application. To overcome this issue, the authors' group explored modified painless PDT (M-PDT). Through a combination of animal experiments, clinical research, and

Table 5.3 Clinical studies on PDT for the treatment of AK

PDT type	Authors	Case number, location	Treatment protocol					Efficacy
			Groups	Photosensitizer, incubation time	Light source	Treatment parameters	Treatment and follow-up time	
Blue light-PDT	Brian Jiang et al. [50]	269, upper limb	ALA-PDT vs placebo-PDT	20% ALA, 3 h	Blue light, 417 ± 5 nm	10 mW/cm^2, 10 J/cm^2	1–2 sessions, 8-week interval; 12-week follow-up	Blue light-PDT effectively removes AK from the upper limb (mean AK clearance at 12 weeks was 69%)
	Tschen et al. [51]	101, face and head	ALA-PDT	20% ALA, 14–18 h	Blue light, 417 ± 4 nm	10 mW/cm^2, 10 J/cm^2	1–2 sessions, 8-week interval; 1-year follow-up	Blue light-PDT is safe and effective in treating head and face AK (the clearance rate is 86.2% in 4 months and 78.3% in 1 year); histopathological recurrence rate over 1 year is 19%

Red light-PDT	Zhang et al. [32]	59, face	10% ALA group and 20% ALA group	10% or 20% ALA, 3 h	Red light, 630 ± 5 nm	100 J/cm^2	3 sessions, 1-month interval; 1-year follow-up	There was no significant difference between 10% ALA-PDT and 20% ALA-PDT for AK
	Jansen et al. [52] Jansen et al. [52]	624, head	5% 5-FU, 5% imiquimod , MAL-PDT, 0.015% IM	MAL, 3 h	Red light, 635 ± 18 nm	75 J/cm^2	1–2 sessions, 12-week interval; 15-month follow-up	AK lesion clearance rate at 3 months was 5%FU > MAL-PDT > 5% imiquimod cream >0.015%IM
	Holzer et al. [53]	28, face and head	ALA-PDT group, 35% TCA group	20%ALA, 4 h	Metal halide lamp, 600–740 nm	75 mW/cm^2, 75 J/cm^2	14 sessions, 1-month interval; 1-year follow-up	ALA-PDT has better clinical results than TCA for extensive field cancerization and multiple AK
	Cai et al. [54]	42, face	ALA-PDT	20% ALA, 5 h	Red light 630 nm	100 mW/cm^2, 180 J/cm^2	1–3 sessions, 2-week interval; 6-month follow-up	The complete clearance rate of AK lesion after 1 month was 85.71% with good cosmetic effect
	Szeimies et al. [55]	122, face and head	BF-200 ALA-PDT group and placebo-PDT group	ALA, placebo, 3 h	ALA group: 630 ± 20 nm; placebo group: 580–1400 nm	ALA group: 37 J/cm^2; placebo group: 170 J/cm^2	1–2 sessions, 12-week interval; 12-week follow-up	The total clearance rate of AK was 64% in BF-200 ALA-PDT and 11% in control group. Total clearance rate of AK lesions was 81% for BF-200 ALA-PDT and 22% for control group
	Kaufmann et al. [56]	121, limbs	MAL-PDT group and cryotherapy group	MAL, 3 h	Red light, 630 nm	37 J/cm^2	1 session, 24-week follow-up	The effective of MAL-PDT was inferior to cryotherapy in nonface/scalp lesions (78% vs. 88%, respectively). MAL-PDT has better cosmetic results and patient satisfaction
	Szeimies et al. [57]	193, face and head	MAL-PDT group and cryotherapy group	MAL, 3 h	Red light, 570–670 nm	70–200 mW/cm^2, 75 J/cm^2	1–2 sessions, 1-week interval, 3-month follow-up	MAL-PDT has similar efficacy with cryotherapy (69% vs. 75%), MAL-PDT has better cosmetic results and patient satisfaction

(continued)

Table 5.3 (continued)

PDT type	Authors	Case number, location	Treatment protocol					Efficacy
			Groups	Photosensitizer, incubation time	Light source	Treatment parameters	Treatment and follow-up time	
Daylight-PDT	Dirschka et al. [58]	52, face and head	BF-200 ALA group MAL group	BF-200ALA: 7.8%, MAL: 16%	Daylight	2 h	1 session, 1-year follow-up	The efficacy of BF-200 ALA DL-PDT was not inferior to MAL DL-PDT; recurrence rate was significantly reduced after 1 year (19.9% and 31.6%, respectively)
	Zhu et al. [59]	55, face	DL-PDT group and C-PDT group	10%ALA; DL-PDT group: 30 min, C-PDT group: 3 h	Daylight; Red light: 630 nm	Daylight: 2 h; Red light: 100 J/cm^2	1–3 sessions, 2-week interval; 1-month follow-up	Compared with C-PDT, DL-PDT was effective, better tolerated, and almost painless in Chinese AK patients (1-month clearance rate of DL-PDT and C-PDT was 95.5% and 96.8%)
	Lacour et al. [60]	107, face and head	DL-PDT group and C-PDT group	MAL	Daylight: 2 h; red light	Red light: 37 J/cm^2	1 session 12-week follow-up	MAL DL-PDT is effective for mild to moderate AK (DL-PDT and C-PDT have a total lesion complete response rate of 70% and 74%), with better tolerability and satisfaction
	Rubel et al. [61]	100, face and head	Half-face control: DL-PDT side, red light-PDT side	MAL; DL-PDT side: 2.5 h, red-PDT side: 3 h	Daylight: 2.5 h Red light	Red light	1 session, 24-week follow-up	Efficacy of DL-PDT in the treatment of mild AK is comparable to red light PDT (clearance of 89.2% and 92.8%), and better tolerated, almost painless, and more convenient for patients.

Patch-PDT	Bai-Habelski et al. [62]	20, hand and arm	Patch-PDT	ALA, 4 h ± 10 min	Red light, 630 ± 5 nm	37 J/cm^2	2 sessions, 1–2-week interval, 12-week follow-up	Patch-PDT is an effective method for mild and moderate AK on the hands and arms, 78% of AK are completely cleared
	Szeimies et al. [63]	316, face and head	Patch-PDT group, placebo-PDT group, cryotherapy group	ALA, 4 h	Red light, 630 ± 3 nm	37 J/cm^2	1 session, 1-year follow-up	A single session for mild to moderate AK was superior to placebo and cryotherapy, the recurrence rate after 1 year was lower than cryotherapy
	Hauschild et al. [64]	449, head	Patch-PDT group, placebo-PDT group, cryotherapy group	ALA, 4 h	Red light, 630 ± 3 nm	37 J/cm^2	1 session, 12-week follow-up	A single session for mild to moderate AK was superior to placebo and cryotherapy, and did not require pretreatment
	Hauschild et al. [64]	149, face and head	Patch-PDT with 0.5 h/1 h/2 h/4 h incubation	ALA, 0.5 h/1 h/2 h/4 h	Red light, 630 ± 3 nm	37 J/cm^2	1 session, 8-week follow-up	After patch-PDT treatment with a 4-h patch, 86% of AK lesions (74% of patients) were completely cleared
IPL-PDT	Abrouk et al. [65]	214 (88 AK), face	Different light sources(PDL, PDL + blue light, IPL, IPL + blue light) + PDT	20%ALA, 2 h	PDL, PDL + blue, IPL, IPL + blue	6–12 J/cm^2	1 session, 1-month follow-up	Rate of lesion elimination in IPL was 70.8%, IPL+ blue light was 84.4%, PDL was 70.5%, and PDL+ blue light was 69.3%
	Kohl et al. [66]	37, dorsum of hand	MAL-IPL-PDT group and placebo-IPL-PDT group	Mal, 3 h	IPL	16.2 J/cm^2	3 sessions, 6-week interval, 10-week follow-up	AK clearance rate of each hand after IPL-MAL-PDT was 54.5% versus 3.0% for placebo, and the total AK clearance rate was 69% and 15%
	Ruiz Rodriguez et al. [67]	17, face	IPL-PDT	20%ALA, 4 h	IPL	40 J/cm^2	2 sessions, 1-month interval, 3-month follow-up	AK lesion clearance was 87%, with no pigment changes or scarring

IM ingenol mebutate, which is currently off the market due to tumor risk, *TCA* trichloroacetic acid

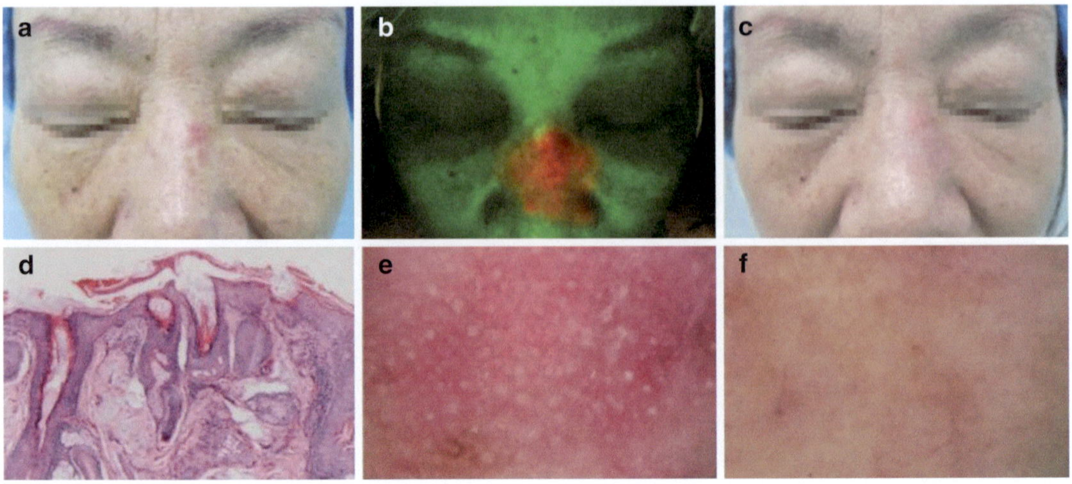

Fig. 5.5 Treatment of nasal AK with red light-PDT. AK lesions subsided after three sessions. (**a**) Before treatment. (**b**) Red fluorescence at the nasal dorsum after ALA incubation. (**c**) After three sessions of red light-PDT treatment. (**d**) Pretreatment histopathological findings revealed hyperkeratosis and atypical cells in the basal layer with budding and significant background elastosis. (**e**) Pretreatment dermoscopy image showing a perifollicular yellow halo and numerous rosettes. (**f**) Post-treatment dermoscopy showing no rosette sign after three sessions of red light-PDT

equipment improvements, they identified the optimal drug application time and light dosage to minimize pain during PDT. In a prospective split-face controlled study, patients with severe regional cancer and hyperplastic AKs were treated with 10% ALA-PDT once every 2 weeks. The incubation time was shortened, and the irradiation energy density increased. After 1 month and three treatments, the total lesion clearance rate was 89.0% for C-PDT and 91.6% for M-PDT. M-PDT achieved a 100% lesion clearance rate for grade I lesions earlier than C-PDT did, with M-PDT requiring only two treatments compared with C-PDT's three treatments. For grade III lesions, the M-PDT yielded a significantly higher clearance rate than did the C-PDT (86.5% vs. 72.0%, $p < 0.05$) (Fig. 5.7) [72]. Mordon et al. conducted a randomized, multicenter, self-controlled clinical study involving 47 patients. One side of the face received MAL application for 3 h, followed by LED red light treatment (12.3 mW/cm^2, 37 J/cm^2). The other side received MAL application for 0.5 h and low-dose LED red light via a mask for 2.5 h (1.3 mW/cm^2, 12 J/cm^2). The results revealed similar clearance rates for grade I and II AK lesions on both sides. After one treatment, the efficacy at 3 months was 79.3% and 80.7%, respectively. For lesions that did not clear initially, two additional sessions achieved efficacies of 94.2% and 94.9% at 6 months [73].

Daylight-PDT (DL-PDT) In 2007, Batchelor reported the initial DL-PDT case of a 90-year-old male patient with widespread scalp AK, and scalp AKs were completely cleared after 10 weeks, with no recurrence after 11 months of follow-up [74]. A summary analysis of 17 published studies on DL-PDT involved a total of 559 patients, and the results revealed that the complete clearance rate of AK ranged from 46% to 89.2% [75]. The DL-PDT was found to be as effective and safe as the C-PDT, with significantly less pain [76]. A multicenter randomized phase III clinical study in Europe reported a 3-month clearance rate of 70% for DL-PDT and 74% for C-PDT, confirming that daylight can be a safe and effective light source for PDT, regardless of weather conditions (except rainy days), with increased patient tolerability and satisfaction [60, 77, 78].

DL-PDT continuously produces small doses of PpIX locally, reducing irritation to normal skin, resulting in less pain and improved compliance. In 2015, Togsver Bo treated 16 immuno-

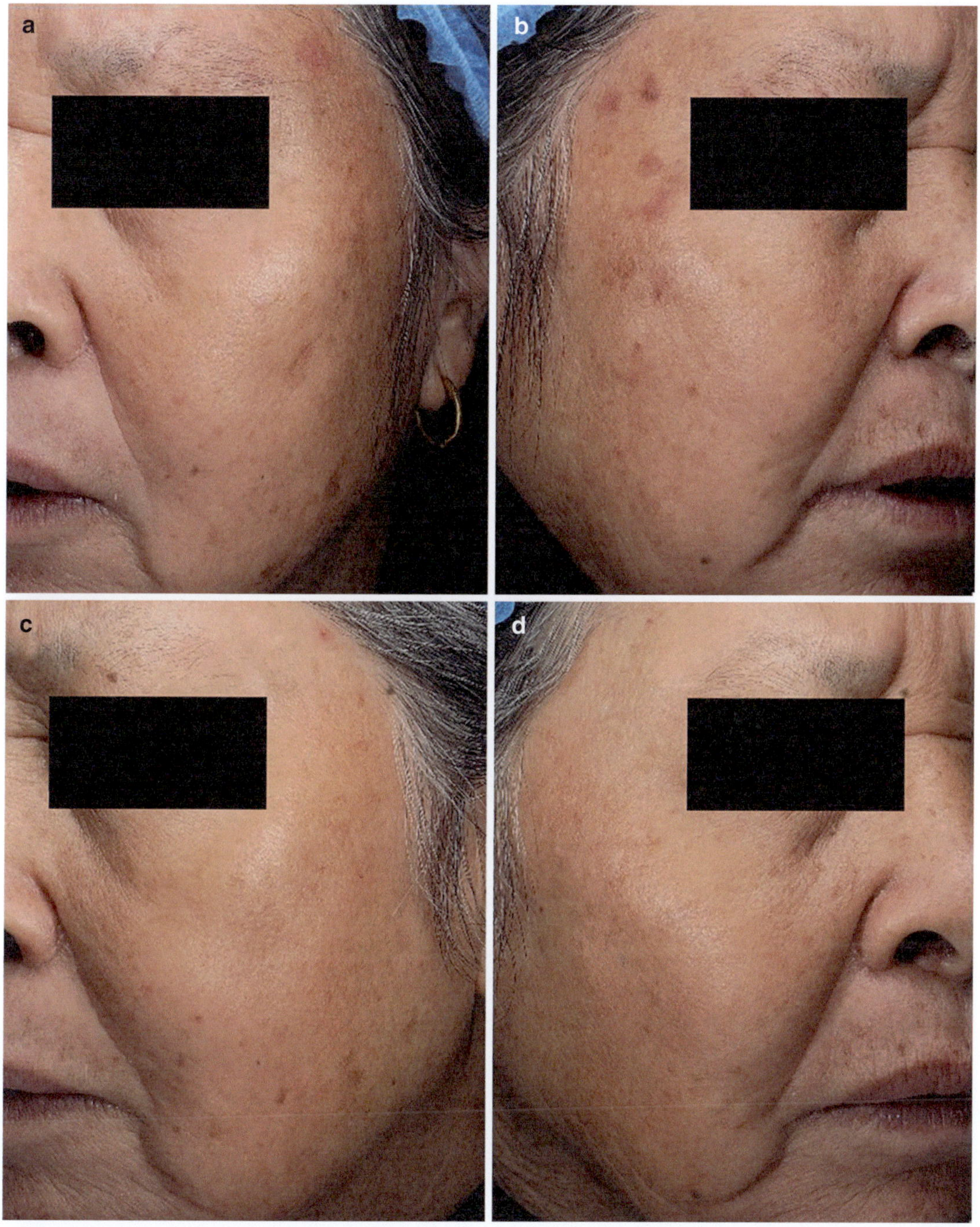

Fig. 5.6 A 69-year-old woman with multiple facial AKs accompanied by photoaging received full-face ALA-PDT (20% ALA, 3 h, red light irradiation, once every 2 weeks, 3 times in total). (**a**, **b**) Before treatment. (**c**, **d**) After three sessions of ALA-PDT

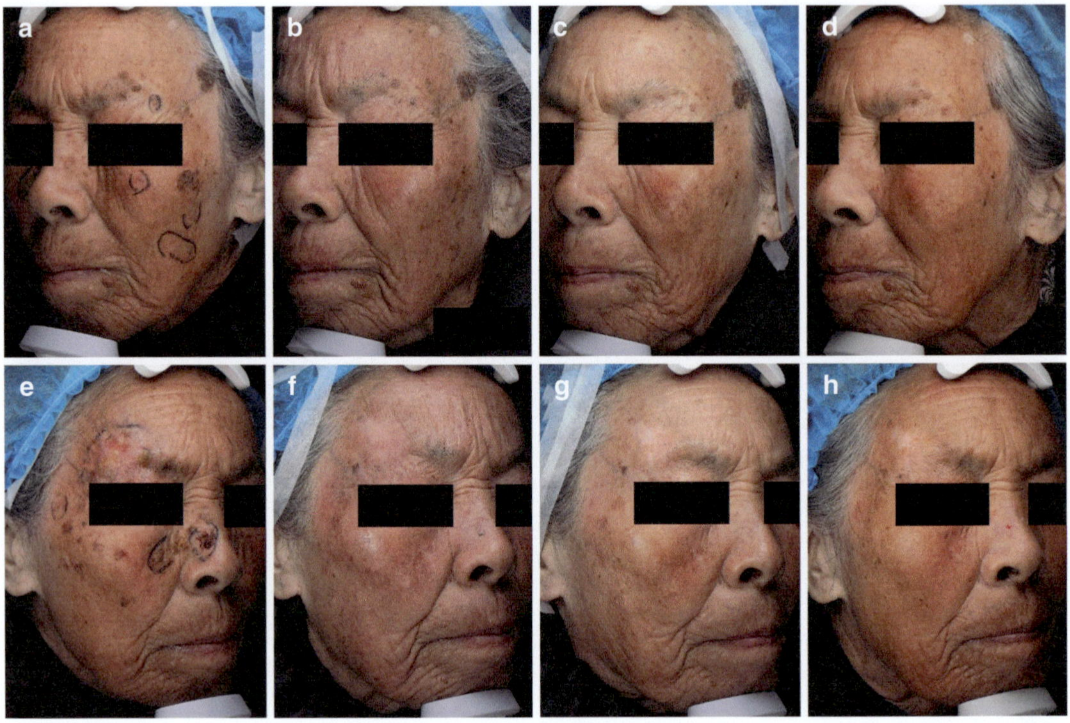

Fig. 5.7 Half-face-controlled study comparing M-PDT and C-PDT for multiple AKs. The top row (**a–d**) shows the C-PDT, whereas the bottom row (**e–h**) shows the M-PDT. Both groups demonstrated comparable efficacy, with the M-PDT significantly reducing pain during treatment. (**a**, **e**) Before treatment. (**b**, **f**) 1 month after three sessions of ALA-PDT. (**c**, **g**) Three months after three sessions of ALA-PDT. (**d**, **h**) 8 months after three sessions of ALA-PDT treatments

compromised AK patients and reported no statistically significant difference in efficacy between DL-PDT and C-PDT after 3 months, with clearance rates of 46% and 50%, respectively [79]. In 2018, a prospective randomized controlled study by the authors' group used 10% ALA-PDT to treat grade I–III AK. After three treatments, the complete clearance rate at the 1-month follow-up was 96.8% for the C-PDT and 95.5% for the DL-PDT. For grade I and II AK, the DL-PDT achieved 100% clearance, whereas for grade III AK, the DL-PDT had slightly lower efficacy than the C-PDT, with rates of 82.1% and 88.9%, respectively (Fig. 5.8) [59].

ALA Patch-PDT A clinical study revealed that the optimal duration for ALA patches in a single PDT session with a fixed light dose (37 J/cm^2) and wavelength (≈630 nm) was 4 h. After patch-PDT, the AK clearance rate reached 86% after 2 months [64]. Two randomized phase III clinical studies comparing the clinical efficacy and safety of patch-PDT with those of placebo PDT or cryotherapy compared the efficacy and safety of patch-PDT with those of placebo C-PDT and cryotherapy in a total of 449 AK patients. After a single treatment session, the AK clearance rates were 82%, 19%, and 77%, respectively, after 3 months [80]. A noninferiority study over 12 months demonstrated the superior performance of patch-PDT over cryotherapy, with AK clearance rates of 79% and 63% and a lower recurrence rate of 11% compared with 18% for cryotherapy [63].

Intense Pulsed Light-PDT (IPL-PDT) Compared with the continuous red light exposure used in C-PDT, IPL-PDT causes less discomfort and is better tolerated while offering comparable efficacy [81]. In 2002, Ruiz Rodriguez et al. evaluated the combined use of ALA-PDT and IPL for treating facial AK. After two sessions of IPL-

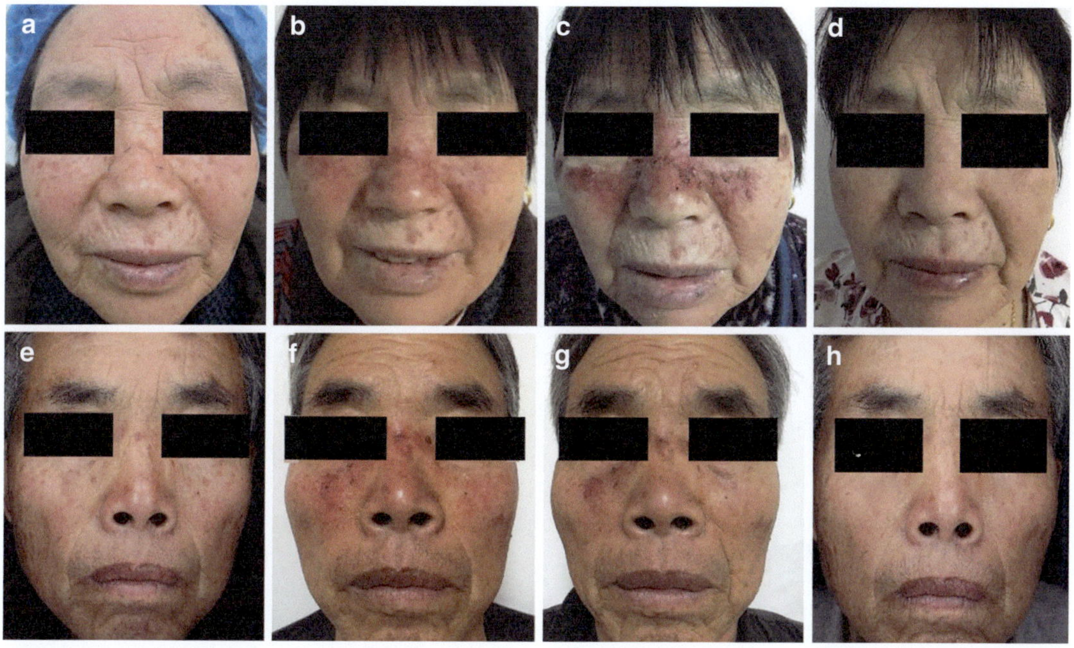

Fig. 5.8 Randomized controlled study comparing DL-PDT and C-PDT for multiple AKs. The top row (**a**–**d**) shows the C-PDT, whereas the bottom row (**e**–**h**) shows the DL-PDT. (**a**, **e**) Before treatment. (**b**, **f**) 1 day post-treatment. (**c**, **g**) 5 days post-treatment. (**d**, **h**) 6 months after three sessions of ALA-PDT treatments. The efficacy in both groups was similar, but the degree of pain and postoperative redness in the DL-PDT group were significantly lower than those in the other groups

ALA-PDT spaced 1 month apart, 87% of AKs were cleared at the 3-month follow-up [67]. In 2017, Kohl et al. conducted a prospective randomized controlled study assessing IPL-MAL-PDT versus placebo IPL for treating AK on the dorsal hand. The complete clearance rates after 10 weeks were 54.5% for IPL-MAL-PDT and 3.0% for placebo IPL. Both treatments significantly improved photoaging and promoted collagen regeneration [66]. Studies have shown that higher IPL light doses provide better results in treating AK and photoaging with ALA-PDT [82].

5.1.2.4 Recommendations

The authors' group recommended ALA-PDT for AK via the use of 10–20% ALA cream, gel, or solution as a photosensitizer and incubation with light protection for 3–6 h. Red light (wavelengths of 630–635 nm) can be used as a light source as it penetrates deeper into the skin. LED light sources are commonly used with recommended power densities of 60–120 mW/cm^2 and energy densities of 100–150 J/cm^2 (Table 5.4). For M-PDT, the application time for the photosensitizer is reduced to 0.5 h, with a recommended power density of 40 mW/cm^2 and energy densities of 200–300 J/cm^2. In DL-PDT, sunscreen (SPF 20–30) is applied to the exposed areas (including lesions), followed by the photosensitizer to the lesion and suspected areas, with 30 min of light protection before 2 h of daylight exposure (excluding rainy days). Treatments are repeated every 1–2 weeks until lesion clearance. Dermoscopy and RCM can be used to monitor treatment endpoints and follow-up when available.

Adverse reactions associated with ALA-PDT include pain, redness, swelling, exudation, itching, and a burning sensation. Post-treatment adverse events during recovery may include dry skin, scabbing, and pigmentation changes. Pain, the most frequent adverse reaction during treatment, can be managed through local skin cooling, adjusting light power density, or the use of pain relievers and anesthetics, depending on the

Table 5.4 Recommended ALA-PDT protocol for AK

PDT modality	Pretreatment	ALA	Light source	Application time	Illumination dose	
C-PDT	Plum-blossom needle, microneedling, dot matrix laser, repeat tape stripping, scraping	10–20% cream, gel, or solution	Red light	3–6 h	60–120 mW/cm^2	100–150 J/cm^2
M-PDT	As above	As above	As above	0.5 h	40 mW/cm^2	200–300 J/cm^2
DL-PDT	As above	As above	As above	0.5 h	2 h	All except rainy days

severity of the pain [22]. Although DL-PDT generally results in less pain than does conventional PDT, it must be performed under medical supervision [59].

5.2 ALA-PDT in Bowen's Disease

5.2.1 Introduction

Bowen's disease (BD), also known as cutaneous squamous cell carcinoma in situ, is now recognized as an intraepidermal carcinoma rather than a precancerous lesion as it was once mistakenly believed. BD results from long-term exposure to arsenics or chronic sun damage and can also be associated with viral infections, immunosuppression, and chronic skin diseases [65, 83, 84].

5.2.1.1 Clinical Manifestations

BD commonly affects elderly individuals over 60 years of age, with a slight predominance in women. BD typically presents as a well-demarcated erythematous scaly patch or plaque, often found in sun-exposed areas, such as the head, neck, and extremities. Less commonly, it can appear in non-sun-exposed areas such as the perineal, palm, genitalia, perianal, lips, nipples, and mucous membranes. The lesion is generally singular but can be multiple and, in rare cases, widespread. Symptoms are usually absent, although larger lesions may cause pruritus. The disease progresses slowly, taking years or even decades.

If BD lesions become erosive, ulcerate, or grow rapidly, progression to invasive cutaneous squamous cell carcinoma (cSCC) may occur. Between 3% and 5% of BD lesions may progress to cSCC, and if this occurs, there is a 20% risk of distant metastasis [83–85]. Compared with the general population, patients with BD are 16 times more likely to develop aggressive cSCC within 1 year of diagnosis [85].

5.2.1.2 Histopathology

Under a microscope, BD is characterized by hyperkeratosis, parakeratosis, acanthosis, and broad rete ridges. Disordered atypical keratinocytes and dyskeratosis can be observed in the full-thickness epidermis. The nuclei of typical keratinocytes are hyperchromatic, vary in size, and exhibit mitotic features. Dyskeratotic cells appear large and round, with a uniformly red cytoplasm and pyknosis or karyolysis. The dermal–epidermal boundary is well defined, with an intact basement membrane. Moderate lymphocytic inflammatory infiltrates around the superficial dermal vessels were observed.

5.2.2 Treatment

Surgery remains the preferred treatment method for BD. However, surgery can affect tissue structure and function, particularly in cosmetically or functionally sensitive areas or those with large lesions. Alternative treatment methods include medications, cryotherapy, electrodeiccation and curettage, lasers, and radiotherapy. These methods, however, have variable clinical efficacy, high recurrence rates, and can be traumatic.

5.2.2.1 ALA-PDT

Kennedy et al. first used ALA-PDT in the treatment of skin cancers in 1990, including 80 cases of basal cell carcinoma (BCC), 6 cases of BD, 2 cases of invasive cSCC, 10 cases of AK, and 4 cases of metastatic breast cancer. They applied a 20% ALA emulsion for 3–6 h, followed by red light exposure (≥600 nm) at a power density of 150–300 mW/cm^2 and an energy density of 15–150 J/cm^2. The complete response rate of BCC and AK lesions after a single treatment was 90%. All BD and early invasive cSCC lesions achieved a complete response with good cosmetic effects and high patient satisfaction [86].

In 1996, Professor Shizheng Xu and Professor Xiuli Wang introduced ALA-PDT for the treatment of skin cancer in China. In 1999, the authors' group published the first clinical report on "5-aminolevulinic acid photodynamic therapy for Bowen Disease" in the *Chinese Journal of Laser Medicine*, where five BD cases completely resolved after up to four sessions of ALA-PDT, with normal skin lines restored. In 2015 and 2021, the authors' group led the Photodynamic Therapy Research Center of the Dermatology and Venereology Branch of the Chinese Medical Association and developed the "Expert Consensus on Clinical Application of Photodynamic Therapy with 5-aminolevulinic acid" and "Guidelines for Clinical Application of 5-aminolevulinic acid Photodynamic Therapy Dermatology (2021 version)," recommending ALA-PDT for patients who cannot or do not want surgery for cosmetic or functional reasons. ALA-PDT is recognized as the preferred treatment for BD lesions under 2 cm with evidence level I [87–89].

The 2014 "British Association of Dermatologists' Guidelines for the Treatment of In Situ Squamous Cell Carcinoma/BD Disease" recommended PDT for BD over cryotherapy and 5-fluorouracil, especially for larger lesions (>3 cm) or for those located on legs or other special areas, given its effectiveness and superior cosmetic properties [83]. The United States "Photodynamic Therapy: Clinical Consensus Guidelines" (2016) advise a 4-h ALA incubation with red light irradiation and an energy density ≥100 J/cm^2 for 2–3 sessions. Methyl aminolevulinate (MAL) PDT with a 3-h incubation and red light energy density of 70–100 J/cm^2 is recommended [90]. The 2019 "European Dermatology Forum Guidelines on Local Photodynamic Therapy" recommended 16% MAL incubation for 3 h with 570–670 nm red light irradiation with an energy density of 75 J/cm^2 or narrow wave 630 nm red light irradiation with a density of 37 J/cm^2. Both protocols include two sessions with a 7-day interval, followed by 3-month evaluation and potentially repeated treatment of residual lesions [23]. These guidelines and the consensus consistently recommend PDT as a first-line treatment for BD, with the highest recommendation level (A) and evidence level (I) [23, 83, 90].

The mechanism of ALA-PDT in BD mainly includes the following: (1) ROS production that directly kills tumor cells. (2) The destruction of the microvascular circulatory system results in hypoxia or nutrient deficiency in cancer cells, leading to indirect death. (3) The activation of the acute inflammatory response and local immune cell aggregation enhance antitumor immunity.

Clinical Application The authors' group has conducted multiple studies on ALA-PDT for BD since 1996 [24, 26, 27, 41, 68]. They initially applied ALA-PDT to treat large BD lesions (up to 4.5 × 3.0 cm). ALA cream (20%) was incubated for 3 h, followed by irradiation with a 632.8 nm He–Ne laser for 8–15 min at an energy density of 60–100 J/cm^2. After 1–4 sessions, all five patients achieved a complete response without recurrence over the 1-year follow-up period [26]. Morton et al. further demonstrated that ALA-PDT effectively treated large (≥2 cm) and multiple (lesions ≥3, ≤2 cm) BD lesions. After 1–3 sessions (20% ALA cream with 3–4 h of incubation followed by red light (630 nm) irradiation with an energy density of 125 J/cm^2 and a power density of 20–86 mW/cm^2), 88% (35/44) of the large BC lesions were cleared. Among them, four BD lesions recurred within 12 months, resulting in a 78% total effective rate. For patients with multiple BD lesions, the ALA-PDT clearance rate was 98%. Among them, four BD lesions recurred within 12 months, with a total effective rate of 89% [91], suggesting that while ALA-PDT is highly effective, recurrence is more likely in lesions over 2 cm in diameter.

The authors' group also used the same ALA-PDT parameters for treating special anatomical locations, such as perinasal, periauricular, and periorbital areas where surgical treatment would be challenging (Fig. 5.9). One study revealed that nine patients achieved a complete response after 1–4 sessions, with excellent cosmetic outcomes [27]. In a patient with multiple BDs, the lesions were located on the ventral side of the left thumb (2.5 × 2 cm) and the right palmar margin (1 × 1.5 cm), with both clinical and pathological findings consistent with BD (Fig. 5.10). The patient had undergone surgery for BD in the right knee and right shoulder, leaving scars of 6.5 cm × 5.5 cm and 11 cm, respectively. After three sessions of ALA-PDT, the two new lesions were successfully treated without scarring or functional impairment of the hand joints. This case demonstrated the safety, efficacy, and noninvasive nature of ALA-PDT for treating multiple BDs [92]. Furthermore, ALA-PDT was applied to 8 BD patients who had not responded to previous treatments, including medications, lasers, cryotherapy, or surgery. Among them, only one patient with perianal lesions achieved a partial response after four sessions and ultimately opted for surgical treatment. The other seven patients achieved a complete response after 4–8 ALA-PDT sessions, with a follow-up period of 8–32 months. Only one patient experienced recurrence at 4 months post-treatment, but they achieved a complete response after additional ALA-PDT [24]. Therefore, ALA-PDT remains a viable and effective option for patients with treatment-resistant or recurrent BD, with surgery as a complementary approach when necessary.

The authors' group also reported a successful case of topical ALA-PDT treatment in a female

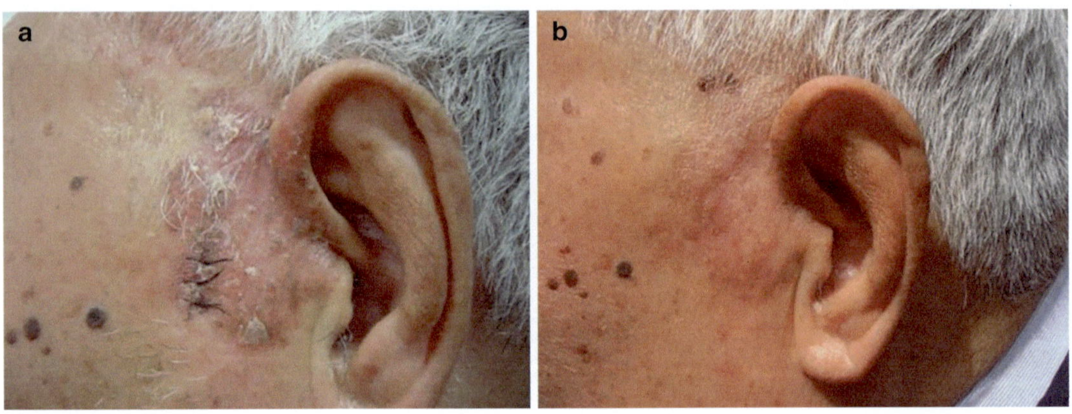

Fig. 5.9 ALA-PDT treatment of large facial BD lesions. (**a**) 4 × 5 cm well-demarcated erythematous scaly plaque over the preauricular skin and helix. Multiple sessions of cryotherapy failed, and BD was confirmed by histopathology. (**b**) Complete clearance of the BD lesion after five sessions of ALA-PDT, with no scarring or recurrence during the 2-year follow-up and a great cosmetic effect

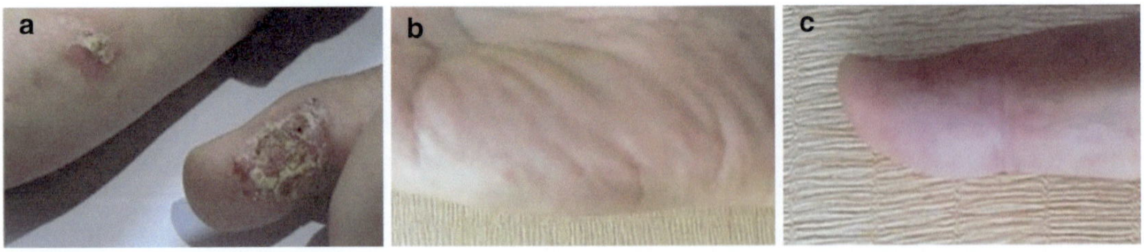

Fig. 5.10 ALA-PDT treatment of multiple hand BD lesions. (**a**) The ventral aspect of the left thumb (2.5 × 2 cm) and margin of the right palm (1 × 1.5 cm) showed well-demarcated erythematous scaly plaques with yellowish crusts and exudation, and BD was confirmed by histopathology. (**b**, **c**) Complete response after three sessions of ALA-PDT, with no scarring, recurrence, or functional impairment at the 3-year follow-up

BD patient who also had systemic lupus erythematosus (SLE) and diabetes (Fig. 5.11). After incubation with 20% ALA cream for 3 h and 630 nm red light irradiation (energy density 100 J/cm^2, power density 100 mW/cm^2) once a month for a total of four sessions, the skin lesions completely resolved systemic photosensitivity [93]. In contrast, a 1993 case involved an SLE patient with a stable condition who underwent HPD-PDT for recurrent HPV infection in the larynx. After treatment, the patient developed erythema, edema, and blisters on the exposed parts of the face and hands, and laboratory results indicated SLE activation [94]. Therefore, photosensitive diseases such as porphyria and SLE are clinically contraindicated for PDT treatment. However, the authors' group demonstrated that ALA, as a precursor compound of PpIX, is not inherently photosensitive. Its small molecular weight makes it suitable for local transdermal drug delivery, and with standardized operation, protection of nontreatment areas, and photoprotection post-treatment, ALA-PDT can be safely used. This case suggests that ALA-PDT could serve as an alternative treatment for skin tumors in patients with photosensitive diseases such as SLE. Additionally, the group applied ALA-PDT to an epidermodysplasia verruciformis patient with multiple AK and BD lesions. After incubation with 10% ALA for 4 h, followed by 20 or 40 min of 630 nm red light irradiation (power density of 90 mW/cm^2) every 2 weeks for a total of eight sessions, all lesions were cleared with good cosmetic results and without affecting functionality [95].

Considering that some patients do not respond after three sessions of ALA-PDT, the authors attributed this to the limited absorption depth of the photosensitizer [68]. To address this, they studied the combination of plum-blossom needles and ALA-PDT in treating BD. In this initial study, three patients were treated with ALA-PDT alone, whereas another three received plum-blossom needles to induce pinpoint bleeding prior to ALA-PDT. The results showed that plum-blossom needle pretreatment improved the efficacy of ALA-PDT (Fig. 5.12) [41]. A larger prospective study followed, with

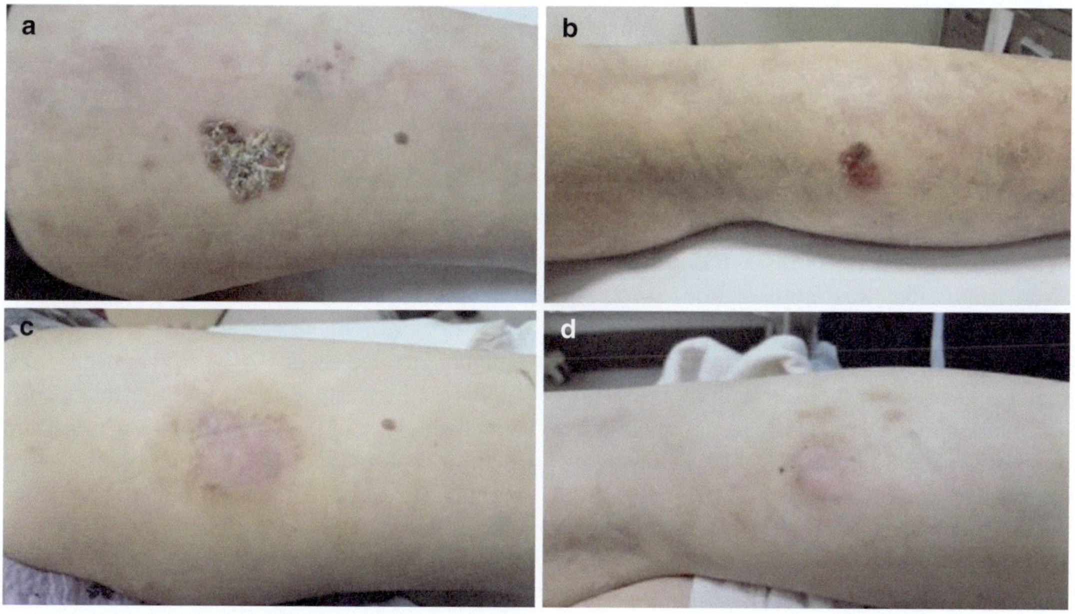

Fig. 5.11 BD lesions in SLE patients treated with ALA-PDT. (**a**, **b**) The left flexural thigh and left posterior calf: irregular well-demarcated erythematous scaly plaques with yellow scabbing and BD were confirmed by histopathology. (**c**, **d**) Complete clearance after four sessions of ALA-PDT, with no photosensitivity or systemic symptoms observed, and no recurrence at the 2-month follow-up

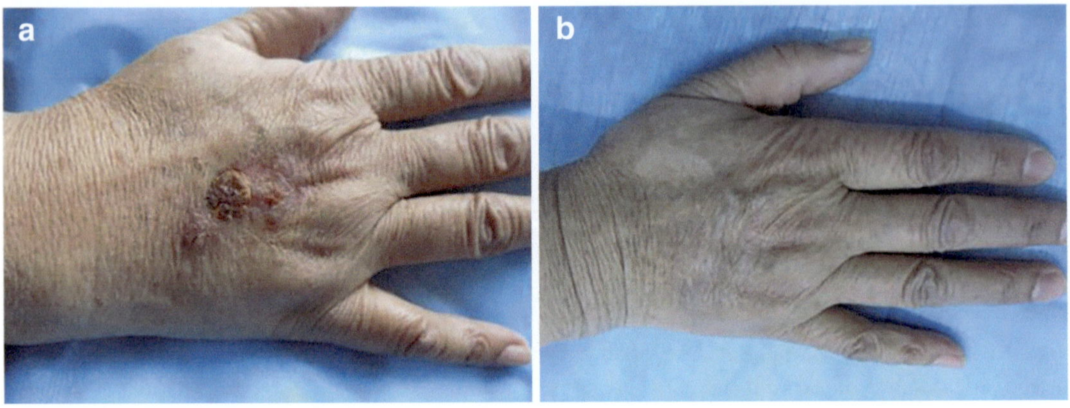

Fig. 5.12 Treatment of BD lesions with plum-blossoming needles combined with ALA-PDT. (**a**) Scaly erythematous plaques on the right dorsal hand measuring 3.5 × 2 cm; histopathology confirmed BD. (**b**) ALA-PDT treatment followed by pretreatment with a plum-blossom needle resulted in no local recurrence at the 1-year follow-up

43 BD lesions randomly assigned to two groups. The control group was treated with 10% ALA and a 633 nm LED (energy density 100–200 J/cm^2, power density 20–86 mW/cm^2), whereas the experimental group received plum-blossom needles prior to ALA incubation. Compared with the control group (3.4 ± 0.7 courses), the experimental group required fewer courses to achieve a complete response (2.9 ± 0.8 courses), indicating that plum-blossom needles enhance ALA penetration and efficacy in treating BD [96]. Another study by Yang et al. explored skin dermabrasion combined with ALA-PDT for BD treatment. Nineteen patients were divided into two groups: the ALA-PDT group and the dermabrasion + ALA-PDT group. After a 5-h incubation with 20% ALA solution, 635 nm He–Ne laser irradiation was applied for 8–15 min (power density of 100 mW/cm^2) once a week for three sessions. The combined treatment group showed a better response, with 8 out of 10 patients achieving a complete response, whereas 5 out of 9 patients in the ALA-PDT-only group achieved a complete response [97]. Recently, the authors' group conducted a retrospective analysis of 122 BD lesions treated with ALA-PDT, revealing a total clearance rate of 89.3% and a recurrence rate of 4.1% after a median follow-up time of 36 months. These results underscore the long-term efficacy of ALA-PDT in most BD patients.

In a phase III clinical study, 40 BD patients were randomly assigned to two treatment groups. One group received 5-FU cream for 4 weeks, whereas the other group was treated with 20% ALA applied 3–4 h before illumination with 100 J/cm^2 narrowband red light (630 ± 15 nm). If necessary, a repeat treatment cycle was performed after 6 weeks. The results revealed that 88% of the lesions treated with PDT achieved a complete initial response, whereas 67% of those treated with 5-FU achieved a complete initial response. After 12 months, there were two recurrences in the PDT group and six in the 5-FU group, resulting in complete clinical clearance rates of 82% for PDT and 48% for 5-FU. Seven lesions developed severe eczematous reactions, three had ulcerations, and two had erosions, whereas no such reactions occurred following PDT [93, 98]. In a separate survey of 95 BD patients treated with ALA-PDT, over 90% expressed high satisfaction with the treatment's effectiveness, and the side effects were reported as mild. The most common side effects were a burning sensation (21%) and crusting or scabbing (14%) [99]. A 2020 meta-analysis of randomized controlled trials evaluating the efficacy of PDT in BD patients revealed that PDT demonstrated superior efficacy, lower recurrence rates, and better cosmetic outcomes than did cryotherapy and topical 5-FU. Additionally, combining treatments, such as the use of an ablative fractional CO_2 laser, has been shown to increase the efficacy of PDT in the treatment of BD [100].

Both domestic and international guidelines recommend PDT as a first-line treatment for BD, particularly for patients who cannot tolerate surgery or for those with lesions in sensitive locations [87, 88]. Combining PDT with pretreatment, such as a curette, plum-blossom needle, microneedling, or CO_2 laser, can further improve the therapeutic effect of ALA-PDT. Importantly, large (>2 cm) BD lesions should undergo comprehensive clinical evaluation, and if necessary, multiple scouting biopsies should be performed to rule out invasive cSCC. For aggressive cSCC or metastatic disease, surgery and additional adjuvant therapy are recommended [87, 88].

5.2.2.2 Recommended Treatment

According to the "Clinical Application Guide of Dermatology for Photodynamic Therapy of amino-ketovalerate (2021 edition)," the following recommendations are made for ALA-PDT in treating BD (Table 5.5) [87–89].

Pretreatment: The lesion and the surrounding area (5 cm around the lesion) were cleaned and disinfected with povidone-iodine and normal saline. Depending on the skin characteristics, an appropriate technique, such as a curette, plum-blossom needle, CO_2 laser, ablative fractional laser, microneedle, or fire needle, can be selected to improve the transdermal absorption of ALA.

ALA incubation: ALA cream was applied to cover the lesions and extend 1 cm beyond the lesion borders.

Interval: Administer treatment every 2 weeks.

Assessment of efficacy: If there was no improvement in the skin lesions within 2 weeks after completing two sessions, alternative treatment methods were considered. If there was only partial improvement, the treatment was repeated.

Special considerations: Pretreatment, particularly with a plum-blossom needle, is highly recommended. For pain relief, local anesthesia and cooling devices are recommended. Follow-up should be scheduled every 6 months after the last treatment, and regular lifelong follow-up is recommended to monitor for recurrences or new lesions.

5.2.2.3 Other PDT Treatments

In addition to ALA combined with red light, the photosensitizers commonly used in BD treatment include MAL and ALA nanoemulsion gel (BF-200 ALA) and ALA combined with blue light. Retrospective studies from the past 5 years (summarized in Table 5.6 [101–109]) reported overall lesion clearance rates ranging from 52% to 100% [106], which are comparable to those of ALA combined with red light.

According to the literature, there is no significant difference in the clinical efficacy of ALA and MAL in the treatment of BD. Some scholars have enhanced clinical efficacy by using ALA nanoemulsions, extending the incubation time, increasing the number of treatment sessions, increasing the energy density, prolonging the illumination time, etc. The recommended parameters include a total energy density of ≥100 J/cm² for ALA and ≥75 J/cm² for MAL, with at least two treatment sessions. The follow-up time should be extended to more than 5 years.

In summary, although BD is an in situ cSCC, it carries the risk of progressing to invasive cSCC and metastasis, thus warranting active treatment. ALA-PDT is recommended as a level A treatment with level I evidence for BD, especially for patients unable to tolerate surgery, those in specific anatomical locations, and those with multiple or recurrent BD. ALA-PDT is highly effective, provides excellent cosmetic outcomes, and has high patient satisfaction. To further optimize clinical efficacy, the combination of a plum-blossom needle and a CO_2 laser as pretreatment is recommended.

Table 5.5 Recommended ALA-PDT treatment for BD

ALA			Illumination dose	
Formulation	Concentration (%)	Incubation time (h)	Energy density (J/cm²)	Power density (mW/cm²)
Solution/cream	10–20	3–6	100–200	60–150

Table 5.6 Retrospective study on PDT treatment of BD

Author	Publication year and country	Number of lesions	Photosensitizer	Parameters	Sessions and interval	Follow-up time	Final clearance rate	Factors of effection
Jose et al.	2021, the United States	12	BF-200 ALA	3 h, red light, 37 J/cm^2, 10 min	2–4, 10 d	4 w	100%	–
Nour et al.	2020, the United States	68	20% ALA	1–16.5 h, blue light, 10 J/cm^2	1–4, 1–8 m	≥33.4 m	67.60%	Lesion size ($d \geq 2$ cm), location, incubation time
Clara et al.	2019, Spain	21	16% MAL	3 h, 630 nm, 75 J/cm^2, 10 min	3, 4 w	12 m	100%	Not identified
Sergio et al.	2019, Spain	191	MAL/ BF-200ALA	3 h, 635 nm, 37 J/cm^2, 8 min	2, 0.5 w	52 w	55.15% 84.75%	–
Miguel et al.	2019, Spain	537	MAL	3 h, 630 nm, 37 J/cm^2, 10 min	2, 1 w	3–136 m	71.5% (no recurring survival rate)	Location (upper limb), lesion size (S>300 mm^2, $d \geq 21$ mm)
Zaar et al.	2017, Sweden	423	MAL	630 nm, 37 J/cm^2	1–2, –	0.2–151 m	63.40%	Number of PDT treatments (1 session), lesion size ($d \geq 20$ mm)
Tamara et al.	2017, Spain	68	MAL	3 h, 630 nm, 37 J/cm^2	1–3, –	35.96 ± 23.46 m (mean follow-up time 间)	77.90%	Location(nose), use of local anesthetics, higher pain scores
Maud et al.	2017, the Netherlands	241	ALA/MAL	630 nm	2, 1 w	0–87 m	22.3% (overall recurrence rate)	–
Hmbly et al.	2017, Ireland	82	MAL	630 nm, 37 J/cm^2/570–730 nm, 50 J/cm^2	2, 1 w	≥2 y	10.98% (overall recurrence rate)	Not identified

min minute, *h* hour, *w* week, *m* month, *J* Joule, *nm* nanometer, *mm* nanometer, *cm* centimeter, *d* diameter, *S* area

5.3 ALA-PDT for the Treatment of Erythroplasia

5.3.1 Overview of Erythroplasia

Erythroplasia of Queyrat (EQ), also known as proliferative erythema, is a type of carcinoma in situ that affects the mucosal epithelium. The pathogenesis of EQ is unknown. However, it is often linked to chronic local irritation, HPV infection, and other factors. EQ commonly appears on the glans and prepuce and has the potential to progress into invasive squamous cell carcinoma (SCC), accounting for approximately 10% of all penile malignancies.

5.3.2 Clinical Manifestations

EQ typically affects middle-aged and older men, particularly those with redundant prepuce or phimosis. The most common sites are the glans, prepuce, coronal sulcus, and urinary meatus, although lesions can also occur in other areas, such as the oral mucosa, female genitalia, and anus. EQ usually presents as a solitary lesion but can sometimes appear in multiple locations. EQs typically manifest as well-demarcated, round or irregular bright erythematous patches or plaques, with slightly raised indurated borders and shiny adherent gray-white scales. Some EQ lesions may appear as velvety plaques. The development of indurated nodules, papillomatous hyperplasia, erosion, ulceration, scabbing, or bleeding typically signals progression to invasive SCC. In contrast to Bowen's disease (BD), EQ has a greater risk of squamous carcinogenesis and invasive growth, with 10–33% of patients developing invasive carcinoma and 20% experiencing metastases [110]. Conversely, approximately 3% of BD patients progress to invade the skin, and 10% progress in the genital region [111].

5.3.3 Histopathology

The histopathological characteristics of EQ are similar to those of BD, presenting as full-thickness atypia with mitotic figures, and median to dense lymphocytic perivascular infiltrates around superficial dermal vessels, plasma cells, and histiocytes can also be observed. EQ differs from BD in its greater occurrence in the mucosa of the glans, where parakeratosis is less prominent. Additionally, the superficial dermis in EQ patients has increased vascular and endothelial cell proliferation.

5.3.4 Treatment Methods

Currently, there are no definitive treatments or established clinical guidelines for EQ, and the available treatment options are primarily based on case studies and small-scale clinical trials. Treatment approaches include medications, physical therapies, and surgery, but these conventional methods often compromise the structural integrity of the tissue and result in functional loss of the affected organ, which may negatively impact the patient's physical and mental health.

5.3.4.1 Medication Therapy

Topical medications such as imiquimod and 5-fluorouracil (5-FU) are commonly used to treat EQ. However, these treatments often require prolonged use, can cause localized irritation, and have uncertain efficacy, frequently leading to recurrence. Thus, they are often combined with other treatments for enhanced results. Imiquimod activates Toll-like receptor-7, exerting immunomodulatory, antiviral, and anticancer effects. Side effects include localized erythema, swelling, erosion, and pain upon topical application. A study revealed that 53% (17 out of 32) of EQ patients achieved total remission, 8% (3 patients) achieved partial remission, and 38% (12 patients) achieved no improvement. One case of recurrence was noted in both the total remission group and the partial remission group [112]. 5-FU, an antipyrimidine compound that inhibits DNA synthesis, is another option for treating precancerous skin lesions. Like imiquimod, it has side effects such as localized irritation. In one study, 5-FU ointment was applied to eight EQ patients, with five achieving total remission, two showing partial remission, and one showing no effect. After an average follow-up of

34 months, none of the five patients who achieved total remission experienced recurrence, yielding an effective rate of 62.5% [113].

5.3.4.2 Physical Therapy

For smaller EQ lesions, physical treatments such as lasers and cryotherapy are viable options. Laser therapy is relatively simple and can quickly remove lesions, but there is a risk of triggering cancerous changes and promoting metastasis. In a study in which a CO_2 laser and Nd:YAG laser were used to treat 19 EQ patients, approximately 26% of the patients experienced recurrence after 32 months of follow-up [114]. Clinical vigilance is necessary when lasers are used for EQ treatment to minimize the risk of cancer progression.

5.3.4.3 Surgical Treatment

Surgical treatments for treating EQ include excision, partial or total penectomy, and Mohs surgery. For invasive lesions or those involving the urethra, partial or total penectomy may be necessary. Although surgical removal of the lesion is definitive, it results in loss of genital anatomy and function, which can have profound psychological impacts on the patient. Mohs surgery is a highly effective treatment for EQ as it completely removes the lesion while preserving as much normal tissue as possible, reducing the risk of recurrence. However, the procedure is technically complex and not widely available because of its specific requirements.

5.3.5 ALA-PDT

ALA-PDT offers several benefits, including the targeted elimination of cancer cells while preserving the integrity and functionality of normal tissues. This treatment is well tolerated and repeatable, making it suitable for patients with lesions in unique locations, extensive areas, or multiple areas of focal damage. Its precision and effectiveness make it a superior option for EQ.

5.3.5.1 Treatment Mechanism

The primary mechanism of action of PDT in the treatment of EQ is similar to its use in treating BD. ALA is selectively absorbed by tumor cells and converted into PpIX within the mitochondria. When exposed to light at a specific wavelength, PpIX generates large amounts of singlet oxygen, free radicals, and other reactive agents that target and destroy tumor cells. This process not only leads to the destruction of tumor tissues but also stimulates a local antitumor immune response, which reduces the recurrence rate of the disease.

5.3.5.2 Clinical Applications

Given the specific accumulation of PpIX in EQ lesions, ALA-PDT was pioneered in 1999 to treat EQs. Four EQ patients underwent 20% ALA incubation for 3 h, followed by irradiation with 630 nm red light at 100 J/cm^2 energy density or 400–700 nm white light at 125 J/cm^2 energy density. The treatment regimen was repeated 1–2 times. The results revealed that two patients with limited lesions were clinically cured, with one patient remaining recurrence-free after 36 months and the other experiencing a small recurrence after 18 months. The two patients with larger lesions had a significant reduction in lesion size [110]. Since then, several clinical studies have confirmed the efficacy of ALA-PDT in treating EQ. In another study, two patients with EQ in the glans area achieved complete remission using light sources of 600–730 nm, with an energy density of 40–65 J/cm^2 and a power density of 40–65 mW/cm^2. Both patients showed no recurrence after follow-ups of 35 and 40 months [115]. The authors' group investigated the efficacy of ALA-PDT in seven EQ patients. They were treated with 20% ALA cream or 10% ALA solution, incubated for 3–5 h, and then irradiated with 635 nm LED red light at a power density of 60 mW/cm and an energy density of 80–100 J/cm^2. The treatment interval was 2 weeks, and patients underwent 2–7 courses. Except for one patient whose 90% of glans involved did not achieve complete remission, all six patients achieved complete remission, with an effective rate of 85.7%, with a 1-year follow-up showing no recurrence and a normal tissue appearance with no scarring (Figs. 5.13 and 5.14) [68]. In a study conducted in 2019 involving eight EQ patients, seven achieved complete remission, and one achieved partial remission after 3–6 courses

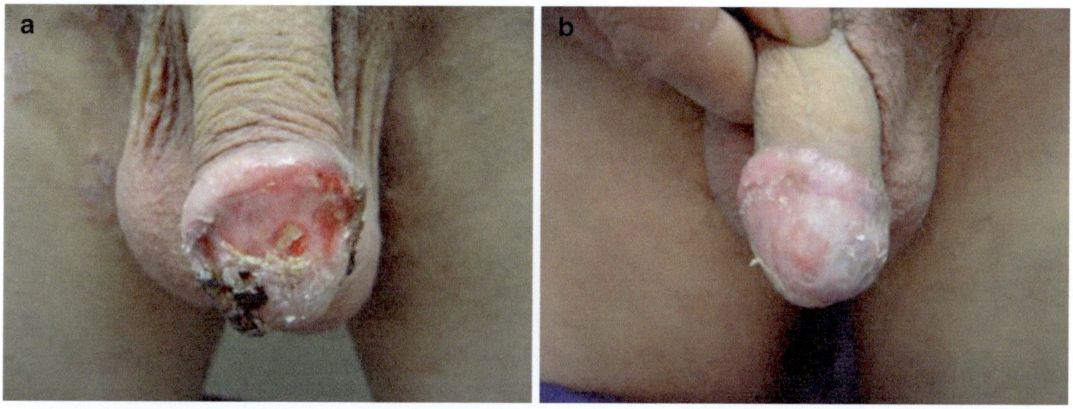

Fig. 5.13 ALA-PDT for EQ. (**a**) A 36-year-old male patient with EQ. Before ALA-PDT treatment, EQ presents as an infiltrative red scaly plaque on the glans, with surface vesiculation and curstings. (**b**) After three sessions of ALA-PDT, the lesions were cleared

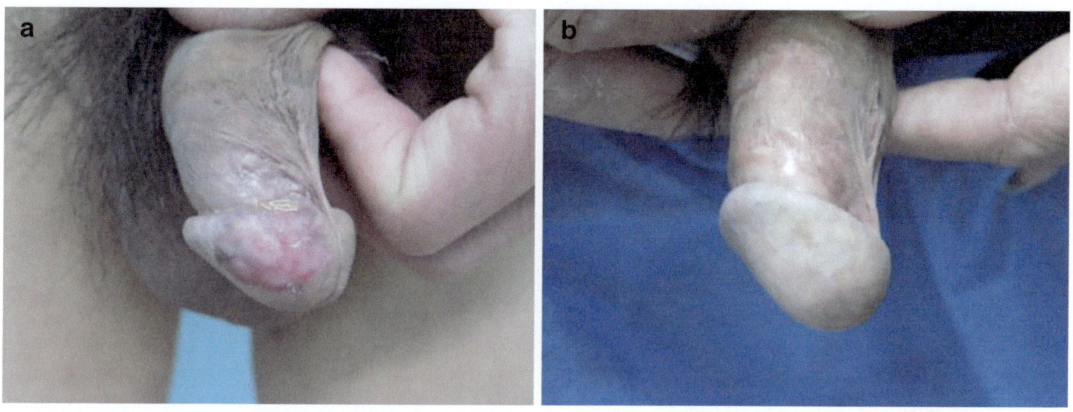

Fig. 5.14 ALA-PDT treatment for EQ. (**a**) A 63-year-old male patient with EQ, presenting with a well-demarcated infiltrative erythematous plaque in the coronal sulcus and foreskin, with a slightly raised margin, scaling, and hyperpigmentation. (**b**) The lesions were cleared after 14 ALA-PDT sessions, and there was no recurrence after 6 months of follow-up

of ALA-PDT (20% ALA solution, with 3–4 h incubation, followed by 633 nm red light irradiation for 20–25 min at a power density of 100 mW/cm^2, with a treatment interval of 1 week, for a total of 3–6 times) [116]. In 2023, another study described a 68-year-old man with EQ with HPV-16 infection in the urethra and glans. Following five courses of ALA-PDT (20% ALA with a 4-h incubation at the urethral orifice and 635-nm red light irradiation for 20 min at a power density of 60 mW/cm^2), the patient experienced no recurrence after 2 years [117]. A review and analysis of ALA-PDT for EQ treatment revealed that its clinical efficacy depends on several factors, including the size of the lesion, incubation time, light dose, number of treatments, and physician experience [118]. Therefore, an appropriate PDT protocol is essential for ensuring effective treatment. Compared with surgery, ALA-PDT may require multiple treatments and is more expensive than topical medications or physical therapies. The 2021 Chinese guidelines on the clinical application of ALA-PDT in dermatology, led by Professor Xiuli Wang, suggest attempting ALA-PDT when other therapeutic methods are ineffective or challenging to implement. However, clinicians must remain cautious about the risk of progression to invasive cSCC [89].

In addition to ALA-PDT, international clinical studies have also examined MAL-PDT for treating EQ. A 2012 study treated a 50-year-old patient with EQ via the MAL-PDT. Despite an initial reduction in lesion size, the lesion eventually expands, progresses to invasive squamous cell carcinoma, and requires partial penile resection [119]. Further studies revealed more favorable outcomes, such as a study by Fai Dario et al., where 19 of 23 EQ patients achieved complete remission after two treatments, with no recurrence after an average follow-up of 18 months [120]. A review of 67 EQ patients treated with PDT revealed that the overall effective rate of MAL-PDT was 62.5%, whereas that of ALA-PDT was 58.3% [121]. Interestingly, some patients treated with MAL-PDT experienced delayed complete remission, suggesting a therapeutic follow-up effect [122]. A 60-year-old EQ patient was treated with five sessions of MAL-PDT at 2-week intervals, achieving complete remission and no recurrence after 6 years of follow-up [123]. The adverse effects of MAL-PDT are similar to those of ALA-PDT, including pain, discomfort, and burning sensations during treatment, as well as edema and local hyperpigmentation [121, 124].

5.4 ALA-PDT in the Treatment of Basal Cell Carcinoma

5.4.1 Introduction

Basal cell carcinoma (BCC) is the most common type of malignant skin tumor, accounting for 75–80% of all nonmelanoma skin cancers. It is currently believed that BCC originates from hair follicles, and its development is associated with the Hedgehog signaling pathway and gene mutations such as those in PTCH1 and SMO [125]. BCC typically grows slowly and is dependent on the surrounding stroma, resulting in most cases being locally invasive and causing tissue damage but with a very low metastasis rate (0.0028–0.55%) [126]. The incidence is approximately twice as high in males as in females and is associated with risk factors such as prolonged intermittent sun exposure, fair skin, immunosuppression, family history of tumors, and advanced age.

5.4.2 Clinical Manifestations

BCC subtypes include: (1) nodular BCC: the most common subtype, appearing as waxy, shiny nodules with superficial, branching capillaries, and ulceration as the tumor enlarges. (2) Superficial BCC: This type of BCC is often observed in younger males in nonexposed areas and is characterized by one or more erythematous or scaly patches with mild infiltration, rolled edges, and melanin deposition, gradually expanding at the periphery. (3) Morpheaform BCC: A rare form presenting as flat or indurated, poorly defined pink or white lesions resembling scars or morphea patches. (4) Fibroepithelioma-type BCC: Also known as Pinkus' fibroepithelioma, a rare subtype manifesting as skin-colored or pink patches or pedunculated papules/nodules with a smooth surface, often appearing on the waist and back. BCC is also linked with genetic syndromes, including basal cell nevus syndrome (Gorlin–Goltz syndrome), linear unilateral basal cell nevus, and Bazex syndrome.

5.4.3 Histopathology

All BCC subtypes share common pathological features, including basaloid cells, palisading of peripheral cells, and tumor masses often separated by clefts from the surrounding stroma. Varying degrees of cellular atypia and mitotic activity are also observed. Histologically, BCC can be classified into several types: superficial, nodular, fibroepithelioma-type, morpheaform, micronodular, infiltrative, and differentiated. Most cases are undifferentiated, but some show differentiation toward skin appendages: keratinizing BCCs differentiate toward hair follicles; cystic BCCs differentiate toward sebaceous glands; adenoid BCCs differentiate toward sweat glands; and basaloid squamous carcinomas differentiate toward spinous cells. Histological type is a factor for predicting clinical recurrence risk, with superficial BCC, nodular BCC, and low-risk growth patterns (e.g., keratinizing, cystic, and fibroepithelioma-type BCC) considered lower risk [127].

5.4.4 Treatment Methods

5.4.4.1 Common Methods

Treating BCC requires a thorough evaluation of individual patient and tumor characteristics to determine the risk of recurrence. Key tumor factors include size (greater or less than 2 cm), location (higher risk of recurrence in the facial H-zone), clinical margin clarity, whether the tumor is primary or recurrent, histological type, and any aggressive features such as perineural or vascular involvement [128]. On the basis of these factors, BCC can be classified into low-risk and high-risk types. Most BCCs encountered clinically are low risk, whereas locally advanced or metastatic BCCs are considered high risk, necessitating different treatment strategies. Low-risk BCC has a low recurrence risk, and common treatment options include curettage, electrodessication, and standard excision, with recommended surgical margins of 2–5 mm, potentially combined with flap reconstruction or skin grafting. Local nonsurgical therapies include cryotherapy, CO_2 laser treatment, ALA-PDT, topical imiquimod, or 5% 5-fluorouracil cream. High-risk BCC local treatments primarily involve Mohs micrographic surgery, followed by standard excision, with a recommended margin of 5–15 mm [129]. The cure rate of standard excision is 90–93% for primary BCC, whereas it is only 80.1% for recurrent cases; the 5-year cure rate of Mohs micrographic surgery can reach 99% for primary BCC and over 95% for recurrent cases [130]. While Mohs surgery is highly effective, it is expensive, time intensive, and requires significant expertise in both surgical and pathological evaluation, making it less accessible in primary care settings.

Although locally advanced BCC incidence is 0.001%, and metastatic BCC incidence is 0.0028–0.55%, these cases necessitate more than just local treatment and often require systemic therapy. Currently, specific inhibitors of the Hedgehog pathway protein Smoothened, including vismodegib and sonidegib, have been approved by the U.S. Food and Drug Administration and the European Medicines Agency for the treatment of locally advanced BCC that recurs or is unsuitable for surgery or radiotherapy. Vismodegib can also treat metastatic BCC, with a global safety study showing 68.5% efficacy for locally advanced cases and 36.9% efficacy for metastatic cases after a median follow-up of 17.9 months [131]. A prospective, randomized, double-blind trial revealed that continuous 12-month treatment with sonidegib, at a dose of 200 mg orally once daily, had a 57.6% effective rate for locally advanced BCC and a 7.7% effective rate for metastatic BCC [132]. However, most patients experienced adverse events such as muscle spasms, taste changes, hair loss, fatigue, and weight loss during treatment with vismodegib and sonidegib, with 30% discontinuing treatment owing to intolerance. In July 2021, phosphate sorafertinib was approved for treating locally advanced BCC in China, becoming the first targeted therapy available domestically. Its long-term effectiveness and side effect profile are still under investigation because of its recent introduction.

Patients with a history of BCC have a significantly greater risk of recurrence, with a 3-year cumulative risk ranging from 33% to 77%. Both surgical and nonsurgical treatments carry risks of residual tumor cells leading to recurrence, and extensive surgery may result in scar formation and functional deformity. Radiotherapy is reserved for patients over 60 years of age who cannot undergo surgery, but it involves a longer treatment course and increases the risk of future skin cancers. Traditional treatments may have limitations for certain patients or tumor locations, making it challenging to achieve optimal outcomes.

5.4.4.2 ALA-PDT

In 1990, Kennedy first introduced ALA-PDT for the treatment of superficial BCC [86]. In 1999, ALA-PDT was used in China by Shizheng Xu, Xiuli Wang, and colleagues treated 11 BCC patients in China via ALA-PDT and achieved complete remission in all patients after 2–6 treatments. While temporary pigmentation or hypopigmentation occurred, no scarring was noted, and blood, urine, and liver function remained normal, establishing the efficacy and safety of ALA-PDT. This foundation paves the way for its use in treating nonmelanoma skin cancers in China. In 2008, the authors' group summarized ALA-PDT for 76 cases of nonmelanoma skin cancer since 1996, including BCC, SCC, Bowen's disease, and breast and extramammary Paget disease [68]. The treatment proved effective, even for recurrent cases, such as a superficial BCC on the temporal area that regressed after two ALA-PDT treatments. A comparative study by Fang et al. on BCC misdiagnosed as pigmented nevi reported similar recurrence rates between ALA-PDT and surgical excision but with less trauma and greater cosmetic satisfaction with ALA-PDT than with other methods [133]. Current guidelines recommend ALA-PDT for superficial BCC and thin nodular BCC (thickness <2 mm), with cure rates exceeding 87% for superficial BCC and 53% for nodular BCC, with higher cure rates for scalp and facial BCC with repeated treatment [23]. Combining ALA-PDT with other treatments enhances the cure rate and reduces recurrence, offering selective tumor cell targeting, minimal trauma, and good cosmetic outcomes, particularly for elderly or anatomically challenging patients. For example, Lu et al. treated periocular BCC with surgical excision followed by ALA-PDT, maintaining eyelid function without recurrence for more than 2.5 years [134]. Similarly, Zhao and colleagues treated facial and neck BCCs via excision followed by ALA-PDT, achieving cures [135].

Mechanism of Action

Currently, there is limited research on the mechanisms of ALA-PDT for BCC. Previous studies have suggested that ALA-PDT generates reactive oxygen species (ROS) that induce oxidative reactions with adjacent biomacromolecules, selectively destroying subcellular structures that absorb a large amount of photosensitizer, thereby achieving direct targeting and killing of cancer cells.

Clinical Application

ALA concentration and formulation: Active treatment for BCC is recommended for a 20% ALA concentration. Although recent studies have proposed 10% ALA for BCC, changes in concentration typically reflect improvements in drug formulation. Conventional ALA preparations (mixed with sterilized injectable water, cream, or gel) are less stable and degrade quickly, often necessitating higher concentrations for clinical effectiveness. An optimized formulation, BF-200 ALA, combines ALA with a nanoemulsion to stabilize it for up to 24 months. In Europe in 2017, this 10% ALA nanoemulsion gel effectively treats superficial and nodular BCC but is not yet available in China [136]. A phase III clinical trial (EudraCT No. 2013–003241-42) comparing BF-200 ALA-PDT with MAL-PDT in 281 noninvasive BCC patients reported cure rates of 93.4% for BF-200 ALA-PDT and 91.8% for MAL-PDT, with the BF-200 group showing a lower recurrence rate after 1 year.

Light source selection: Various light sources, such as filtered xenon arc and metal halide lamps, LEDs, and semiconductor lasers, can be used for ALA-PDT. Although protoporphyrin IX (PpIX) has peak absorption at 410 nm, most PDT light sources use red light (~630 nm) to enhance tissue penetration. Sunlight is another accessible light source for PDT and is used in daylight-PDT (DL-PDT), where lesions incubated with a photosensitizer for 0.5 h are exposed to sunlight for 2 h, followed by the application of sunscreen to the surrounding skin. While DL-PDT can reduce treatment-related pain, its use in BCC treatment is limited, and its recurrence rate for superficial BCC within 1 year is relatively high, at approximately 21% [137].

Lesion pretreatment: Pretreatment of lesions can improve ALA absorption, addressing the limited penetration depth of the treatment light. In 2015, the authors proposed the use of traditional Chinese medicine characteristic plum-blossom needle tapping as a pretreatment to increase the clinical efficacy in treating BCC [138]. Common pretreatment methods include the following:

1. Minimally invasive transdermal method pretreatment: After the lesion surface is cleaned with paraffin oil, tools such as plum-blossom needles, microneedles, or curettes can be used to tap or curettage the surface, increasing

ALA permeability (Fig. 5.15). This method is suitable for superficial and thin nodular BCCs (≤3 mm thickness).

2. Laser pretreatment: After local anesthesia, CO_2, erbium, or holmium lasers ablate the tumor mass, a method suited to superficial and nodular BCC (≤5 mm thickness).
3. Surgical pretreatment: Dermoscopy and ultrasonography were used to mark the size and depth of the tumor, the tumor was excised, the wound was left open, and ALA-PDT was administered. This approach is ideal for thicker low-risk BCCs or debulking in locally advanced BCCs.

Clinical Efficacy

For superficial BCC with a lesion thickness under 2 mm, ALA-PDT achieves cure rates ranging from 81% to 100% after 1–2 treatments, with follow-up periods ranging from 12 to 24 months and a recurrence rate ranging from 6% to 18%. No skin atrophy or pigmentation has been reported at the treatment site [139]. However, nodular BCC absorbs ALA less efficiently and unevenly, resulting in lower clinical efficacy with ALA-PDT than with superficial BCC. To address this, a 10-year histological study revealed that pretreatment with a curette and the penetration enhancer dimethyl sulfoxide improved ALA absorption. In a study of 60 nodular BCC lesions (thickness <3.5 mm), the primary cure rate was 63% after one ALA-PDT session, which increased to 90% after two sessions [140]. Another prospective clinical study reported no significant difference in cure rates for superficial and nodular BCC between surgery and ALA-PDT after 25 months of follow-up ($P = 0.64$), with ALA-PDT demonstrating good cosmetic outcomes at 12 months [141]. On the basis of these findings, guidelines in various countries recommend ALA-PDT with grade A and level I evidence for treating superficial BCC and nodular BCC (thickness <2 mm).

ALA-PDT offers selective tumor cell targeting, is minimally invasive, and provides good cosmetic results; however, pain during treatment remains a common side effect, often limiting patient tolerance for multiple sessions. While local anesthesia and oral analgesics are common pain-relief measures, they are not always effective. Some studies suggest that DL-PDT offers comparable clinical efficacy to traditional photodynamic therapy with milder pain, but factors such as season, region, and weather affect its consistency. To improve pain management, the authors developed M-PDT, which reduces pain by shortening the ALA incubation time and extending irradiation, allowing slower, continuous PpIX generation and avoiding the intense inflammatory response from rapid PpIX accumulation [142]. For example, a 75-year-old man with more than 55 BCC lesions in the H-zone of the face was successfully treated with a combination of curettage and M-PDT (Fig. 5.16). After three PDT sessions, the lesions were fully resolved without visible scarring, and the patient reported low pain scores (VAS scores of 1–2) and good comfort [143]. In another case, a 91-year-old patient with locally advanced BCC on the scalp (invasion to the galea aponeurotica) showed

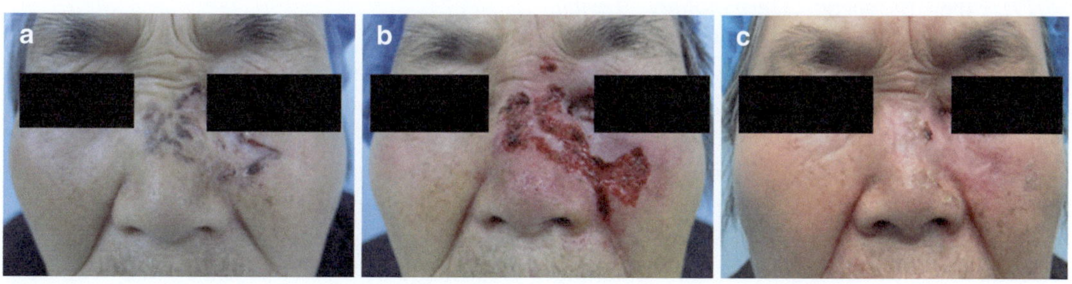

Fig. 5.15 Pretreatment of BCC on the left nasal dorsum and medial canthus with a curette and CO_2 laser before PDT. (**a**) Before treatment, (**b**) pretreatment of BCC lesions with a curette and CO_2 laser after local infiltration anesthesia, and (**c**) 1 month after four sessions of ALA-PDT

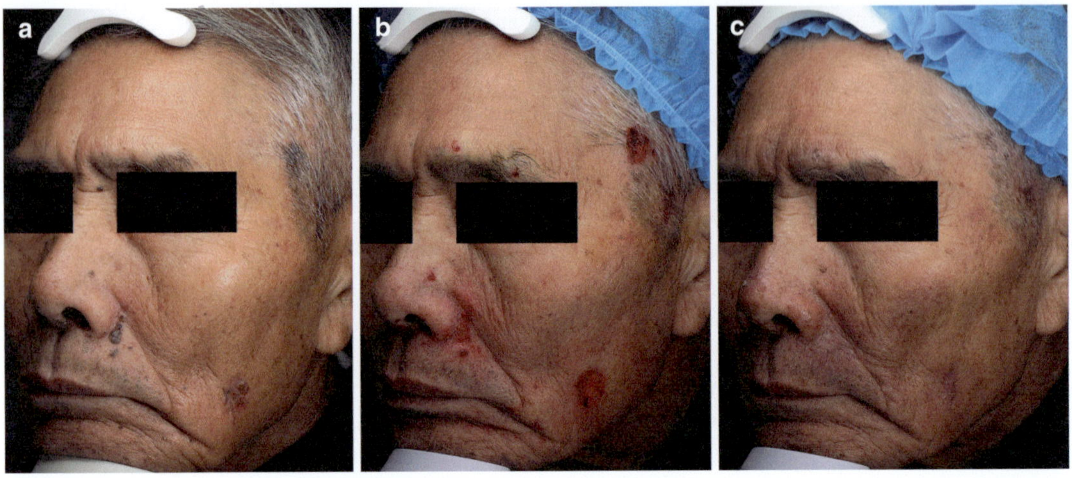

Fig. 5.16 Treatment of multiple facial BCCs with curettage combined with M-PDT: (**a**) before treatment, (**b**) after curettage, and (**c**) after modified painless ALA-PDT treatment

no recurrence after 1 year following M-PDT combined with a holmium laser and photofrin-PDT, with hair regrowth noted in the treated area (Fig. 5.17) [144]. This approach avoids anesthesia and disfigurement risks associated with extensive resection and skin grafting. M-PDT, combined with surgical excision, CO_2 lasers, and other therapies, shows promise for treating advanced BCC in patients older than 80 years, with clinical cases supporting its safety, efficacy, and minimally invasive benefits.

Scope of Indications

Currently, the primary indications for ALA-PDT are superficial BCC and nodular BCC with thicknesses of less than 2 mm. This recommendation is supported by the *European Consensus on the Diagnosis and Treatment of Basal Cell Carcinoma (2019)*, the *European Dermatology Forum Guidelines on Photodynamic Therapy (2019)*, and the *Chinese Expert Consensus on the Diagnosis and Treatment of Cutaneous Basal Cell Carcinoma (2021)*, all of which endorse PDT with a grade A evidence level. The secondary indications for ALA-PDT include thick low-risk BCC, locally advanced BCC, and the selection of metastatic BCC cases for debulking purposes. For these types, PDT is typically combined with other therapies, such as laser treatment, surgery, or Smoothened inhibitors.

Treatment Steps

- Pretreatment education and signing of informed consent. The patient was instructed to assume a comfortable position and prepare the skin lesion for treatment.
- The prepared ALA was applied evenly to the patient's skin lesion and surrounding skin, and the patient was asked to rest with the lesion covered to prevent light exposure.
- A Wood's lamp was used to observe ALA absorption in the treated area, and the light power density was measured with a power meter.
- An appropriate light source and dosage were selected, the light beam was positioned over the treated area, and the patient was monitored for discomfort, providing symptomatic relief as needed.

Precautions

Before treatment, if significant bleeding occurred during pretreatment of the BCC lesion, invasive procedures were halted, and a thick layer of gauze soaked in saline was applied for 10–20 min to manage bleeding.

During treatment, sensitive areas such as the eyes should be protected. Unnecessary exposure of the surrounding normal skin is limited by covering it with black cloth. The patient was observed for symptoms of pain and high skin temperature,

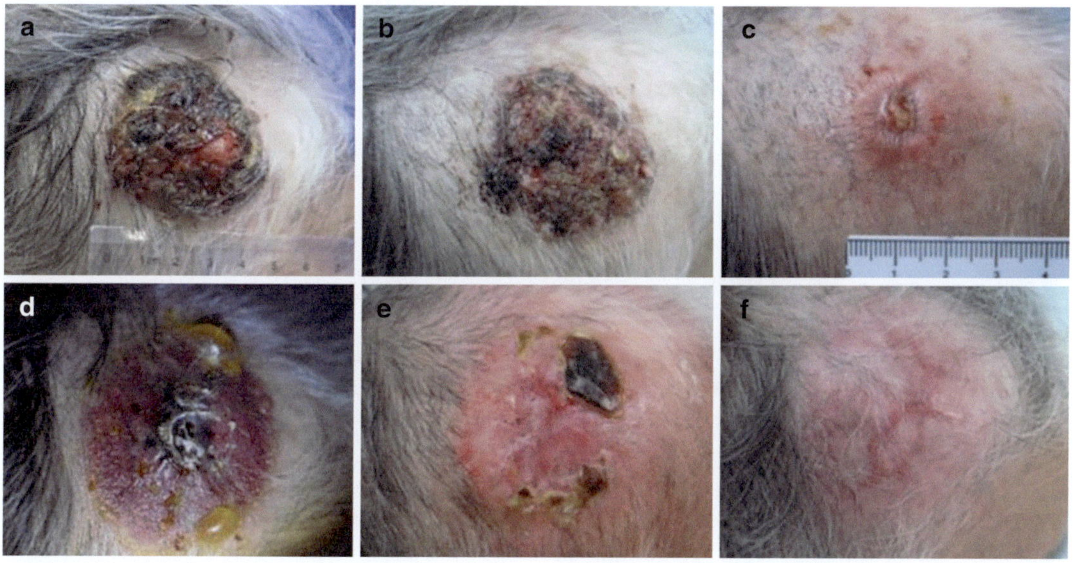

Fig. 5.17 ALA-PDT combined with a holmium laser and Hyporfin-PDT for the treatment of locally advanced BCC on the scalp of a 91-year-old patient. (**a**) Before treatment. (**b**) 2 weeks after two sessions of ALA-PDT and one session of holmium laser treatment. (**c**) After six sessions of ALA-PDT sessions and three sessions of holmium laser treatments, the exophytic tumor basically disappeared. (**d**) Local erythema and blisters appeared 4 days after Hyporfin-PDT treatment. (**e**) Scar formation and black scab formation were visible after 1.5 months of Hyporfin-PDT treatment. (**f**) No tumor recurrence was found at follow-up 6 months after the last treatment

and symptomatic management was provided as necessary.

After treatment, the patient was advised to avoid sun exposure, and if necessary, antibiotic ointment was applied to protect the wound. The next follow-up appointment was scheduled.

Adverse Reactions and Management

During and after ALA-PDT treatment, various degrees of adverse reactions may occur. It is necessary to educate and communicate with patients before treatment and provide timely management.

Local skin redness and exudation: A local cold compress was applied immediately after treatment. For significant exudates, saline or compound berberine solution was used as a wet compress twice daily.

Local skin pigmentation: Pigmentation may develop post-treatment. Sun avoidance is recommended for the treated area; pigmentation usually fades over time.

Pain: Pain during PDT varies among individuals. M-PDT can help reduce pain levels, but additional cooling measures, such as fans or air coolers, oral analgesics, or localized anesthesia, can be provided if pain is severe.

Recommended Protocol

Interval: treated every 2 weeks.

Number of treatments: complete elimination of skin lesions.

Effectiveness evaluation: combinations with noninvasive diagnostic techniques, such as dermatoscopy, reflectance confocal microscopy, and skin ultrasound, are used to observe treatment outcomes.

While surgery is the primary treatment for localized BCC, lesions often appear on the head and face, where multiple or extensive lesions can limit surgical options. In cases where BCC occurs in challenging anatomical areas on the head or face or in elderly or frail patients who may not be suitable candidates for surgery, ALA-PDT offers a viable alternative (Table 5.7). ALA-PDT is both safe and effective, making it a valuable option for broader clinical application.

Table 5.7 Recommended ALA-PDT protocol for BCC treatment

Pretreatment method	ALA-PDT protocol	ALA formulation		Application time (H)	Irradiation dose	
		ALA form	ALA concentration (%)		Energy density (J/cm^2)	Power density (mW/cm^2)
Plum-blossom needle, microneedle, curettage, laser, surgery	Traditional ALA-PDT	Cream or solution	10–20	3–6	100–200	60–150
	Modified painless ALA-PDT	Cream or solution	10–20	0.5–1	200	28

5.5 ALA-PDT in the Treatment of Cutaneous Squamous Cell Carcinoma

Cutaneous squamous cell carcinoma (cSCC) is a malignant tumor arising from epidermal or appendageal keratinocytes with varying degrees of keratinization, often progressing from actinic keratosis (AK) or Bowen's disease (BD) [145].

5.5.1 Epidemiology

In Caucasian populations in Europe and America, cSCC is the second most common nonmelanoma skin cancer, following basal cell carcinoma (BCC). The BCC-to-cSCC ratio is approximately 4:1 in the United States, Australia, and the United Kingdom and 6:1 in Norway. From 2013 to 2015 in the United Kingdom, the incidence of cSCC was 62.7% in men, with a median age of 80 years and an annual increase rate of 5% [146, 147]. US data revealed a 263% increase in the incidence of cSCC from 1976–1984 to 2000–2010, with the most significant increase in women and people under 40 years of age [148]. Large-scale epidemiological data from China are limited. However, a 2006 study by Gao Tianwen's team revealed that cSCC accounted for 29.4% of skin cancers, with an annual incidence increase of 2.6% [149]. In 2011, the authors' group conducted an epidemiological survey in a cohort of 2038 elderly individuals over 60 years of age and reported 76 precancerous and malignant skin tumors, including 3 cSCC cases, with the incidence increasing with age and peaking in individuals over 75 years of age. Most tumors appeared on the head and neck and were highly correlated with long-term UV exposure ($P < 0.05$) [150].

5.5.2 Pathogenesis Mechanism

The exact mechanisms of cSCC development remain unclear, although multiple studies have revealed factors such as UV radiation, HPV infection, chemical exposure, and immunosuppression. UV radiation induces mutations in the p53 tumor suppressor gene on chromosome 17p13.1 in keratinocytes, leading to loss of tumor suppression, increased cell proliferation, genetic instability, and cSCC development [151]. Additionally, UV exposure has been linked to mutations in the CDKN2A and Ras genes, further promoting cSCC [152, 153]. In 2021, Dr. Zhang Guolong from the authors' group conducted single-cell sequencing on cSCC and photoaged skin and reported significant upregulation of the FABP5, S100, and SPRR gene families in cSCC. Knocking out FABP5 or S100A9 significantly slowed cSCC progression. In a UV-induced cSCC mouse model, Rorα emerged as a critical transcription factor for progression from photoaging to invasive cSCC, likely by downregulating S100A9 and Sprr2f in cSCC cells, suggesting promising targets for prevention and treatment [154, 155].

5.5.3 Clinical Manifestations

Most cSCC lesions develop on the head, neck, or exposed limbs but can also arise from chronic wounds, scars, or radiodermatitis. Early cSCC presents as an infiltrative papule or plaque that may evolve into nodules, plaques, or verrucous lesions. These lesions are firm, may ulcerate, and often have a cauliflower-like appearance with a poorly defined, infiltrative base and red–yellow margins. The surrounding tissue is often hyperemic, with a dark yellow–red margin that may be pruritic or tender, but most patients remain asymptomatic. As cSCC progresses, the lesions may ulcerate into wide, raised edges become crateriform, often with foul-smelling, purulent discharge and necrotic tissue. Advanced tumors, exceeding 2 cm in diameter, may invade deeper tissues, become immobile, and metastasize through lymphatic spread, causing enlarged, firm, and painless regional lymph nodes; distant metastasis via hematogenous routes is rare. Advanced cSCC may also present with systemic symptoms such as fever, weight loss, and cachexia, particularly in mobile or sensitive areas such as the lips or genitals, where recurrent and challenging ulcers may develop.

5.5.4 Histopathology

Histopathological examination is essential for diagnosing cSCC. Key features include invasive clusters or cords of epidermal tumor cells that break through the basement membrane into the dermis, sometimes involving skin appendages, blood vessels, or nerves. Tumor cells show varying levels of differentiation, from well-differentiated squamous cells with polygonal shapes, abundant cytoplasm, intercellular bridges, multinucleation, and mitoses to poorly differentiated atypical cells with spindle shapes, minimal cytoplasm, and deeply stained nuclei. In well-differentiated cells, keratinization increases near the center, forming keratin pearls and areas of parakeratosis. Poorly differentiated cells lack these features, with more mitotic figures and greater potential for malignancy. The Broders system grades cSCC into four levels on the basis of poorly differentiated cells: grade I: less than 25% poorly differentiated cells, confined to the sweat gland level, with abundant keratin pearls and significant dermal inflammation. Grade II: 25–50% poorly differentiated cells with poorly defined clusters, few keratin pearls, incomplete keratinization, and mild inflammation. Grade III: 50–75% poorly differentiated cells, minimal keratinization, absence of keratin pearls, and minimal inflammation. Grade IV: more than 75% poorly differentiated cells with numerous mitoses, no intercellular bridges, and nearly no keratinization.

5.5.5 Risk Assessment

On the basis of recent relevant domestic and international literature and guidelines such as the “Clinical Practice Guidelines for Cutaneous Squamous Cell Carcinoma 2021.1” published by the National Comprehensive Cancer Network (NCCN), the “European Interdisciplinary Guidelines for Cutaneous Invasive Squamous Cell Carcinoma,” and the “ Consensus on Diagnosis and Treatment of Cutaneous Squamous Cell Carcinoma (2021)” of China, risk factors for cSCC are based on clinical features (e.g., tumor size, site, and nerve involvement), pathological features (e.g., tumor thickness, depth of invasion, differentiation, histological subtype, and vascular or lymphatic infiltration), and patient factors (e.g., immunosuppression, radiotherapy history). On the basis of these criteria, cSCC can be categorized into very high-risk, high-risk, and low-risk types, as shown in Table 5.8 [156]. This classification reflects the choice of treatment, the need for sentinel lymph node biopsy, and the follow-up strategy. Low-risk: Annual follow-up for 5 years. High-risk and very high-risk: Follow-up every 3–6 months for the first 2 years, every 6 months for the next 3 years, and then every 6–12 months thereafter, with lifelong follow-up recommended.

5.5.6 Treatment Methods

cSCC treatment should be tailored to the patient’s age, health, tumor location, depth, size, and aesthetic preferences. Treatment approaches include surgery, laser therapy, cryotherapy, radiochemotherapy, and topical

Table 5.8 cSCC risk assessment

Risk level	Clinical features		Pathological feature
	Lesion feature	High-risk factors	
Very high-risk[a]	Diameter ≥4 cm (any site)		Histologically poorly differentiated, desmoplastic type, tumor infiltration depth ≥6 mm or beyond subcutaneous fat, deep dermis or nerve sheath with tumor cells diameter ≥0.1 mm, vascular or lymphatic involvement
High-risk[b]	Diameter 2–<4 cm Primary lesion located on the trunk and limbs, or head, neck, hands, feet, anterior tibial, perianal genital (any size), unclear boundaries	Recurrent tumor; immunosuppressed state, history of local radiotherapy or chronic inflammation, rapid tumor growth, nerve involvement symptoms	High-risk histological subtypes (acantholytic type, adenosquamous carcinoma, sarcomatoid differentiation type, fusiform cell type); perineural invasion
Low-risk	Diameter less than 2 cm primary lesion located on the trunk or limbs, clear boundaries	Primary tumor; no immunosuppressed state, history of local radiotherapy or chronic inflammation, rapid tumor growth, nerve involvement symptoms	Well-differentiated or moderately differentiated tumors, non-high-risk histological subtypes; tumor thickness ≤6 mm and infiltration not exceeding the subcutaneous fat layer, without perineural invasion; no vascular or lymphatic invasion

[a] Possessing any of the abovementioned very high-risk clinical or pathological features qualifies as very high-risk cSCC, with more risk factors leading to a higher risk of recurrence

[b] Possessing any of the abovementioned high-risk clinical or pathological features qualifies as high-risk cSCC, with more risk factors leading to a higher risk of recurrence or metastasis

medications. Newer options, such as PDT and biologics, are being explored for early cSCC and advanced palliative care. cSCC metastasizes to lymph nodes and distant sites in 2–5% of cases postsurgery, and metastatic cSCC shows a limited response to chemotherapy, with a mortality rate of 40%, posing a serious health risk [157].

5.5.6.1 Surgical Excision

Surgical excision, including standard excision and Mohs micrographic surgery, is the primary treatment for cSCC. However, surgeries on areas such as the head, neck, and genitalia can cause significant tissue and structural loss, leading to scarring and psychological effects. Igal Leibovitch's 2005 study on 1263 cSCC patients who underwent Mohs surgery revealed a 3.9% recurrence rate over 5 years, with most tumors being located on the head and neck [158]. Mohs surgery is complex, has limited indications, and requires consideration of tumor progression, patient preferences, and overall health.

5.5.6.2 Physical Therapy

Physical therapies, such as lasers and cryotherapy, are effective and straightforward for treating superficial early-stage cSCC or as adjunct therapies. Commonly used lasers include Nd:YAG lasers and CO_2 fractional lasers. In 1998, in a study by Humphrey et al., pulsed CO_2 laser therapy was administered to 17 BCC patients and 13 in situ SCC patients; laser therapy effectively cleared BCC but was less successful for thicker in situ SCC lesions [159], suggesting that laser and cryotherapy alone may not be suitable for thicker malignant tumors.

5.5.6.3 Drug Therapy

Imiquimod is an immunomodulator that locally activates antitumor immunity, with common side effects such as redness, erosion, and pain. In a study by Ketty Peris et al., 5% imiquimod was applied to 10 patients with BD and cSCC lesions for 8–16 weeks. The clinical cure rate for cSCC was 71.4%, with no recurrences after a 31-month follow-up [160].

Molecular-targeted therapies, particularly immune checkpoint inhibitors, have become significant options for treating skin cancers. Key agents include anti-programmed death-1 (PD-1) human monoclonal antibodies and their ligands (PD-L1) inhibitors, vascular endothelial growth factor receptor (VEGFR) monoclonal antibodies, etc. A 2018 New England Journal of Medicine study reported phase I and II trials showing a 47–50% response rate for PD-1 inhibitors in advanced cSCC, although with a 15% adverse event rate [161]. While effective, targeted drugs are primarily used in palliative care because of their high costs and limited efficacy in locally advanced and metastatic cSCC.

5.5.6.4 Radiotherapy/Chemotherapy

Radiotherapy and chemotherapy are options for patients who are unsuitable for surgery due to disease progression, multiple complications, or preference, or when the anatomy prevents radical surgery. Although platinum-based chemotherapy is a previous standard, its low efficacy has led to the use of targeted therapies such as PD-1 inhibitors. Modern radiotherapy, delivered via external beam or brachytherapy, offers effective local treatment but may cause side effects such as acute radiation dermatitis and chronic skin changes such as depigmentation and telangiectasia. Stratigos et al. combined cetuximab with radiotherapy in five cSCC patients and achieved partial response in four patients after 2 months [162]. Radiotherapy, especially in combination with other treatments, can provide clinical benefits, although it is complex, costly, and limited in application owing to equipment needs.

5.5.7 ALA-PDT Treatment

5.5.7.1 Development Overview

ALA-PDT was first used in 1990 by Kennedy to treat superficial cSCC and precancerous lesions. It has since gained popularity in Europe and the United States for treating nonmelanoma skin cancer (NMSC), backed by substantial clinical evidence. The 2007 *European Guidelines on Photodynamic Therapy for NMSC* recommended PDT for AK, BD, and superficial and nodular BCC, noting superior clinical efficacy and cosmetic outcomes compared with standard treatments, as well as its effectiveness in preventing NMSC recurrence [154]. In 1996, professors Shizheng Xu and Xiuli Wang introduced ALA-PDT for BD, BCC, and cSCC treatment in China, achieving promising results [163]. Since then, ALA-PDT has been widely applied in China for AK, erythroplasia of Queyrat (EQ), and mammary and extramammary Paget's disease (MPD and EMPD), with satisfactory results [89, 164]. European and Chinese guidelines now endorse PDT as a first-line treatment for AK and BD. On the basis of two decades of experience, the *Expert Consensus on Aminolevulinic Acid Photodynamic Therapy Clinical Application* (2015) and the *Guidelines for Clinical Application of Photodynamic Therapy in Dermatology (2021)* further established China's standing in ALA-PDT research, with the latter guideline published internationally.

5.5.7.2 Treatment Mechanism

ALA-PDT treats tumors by converting ALA, which is selectively absorbed by tumor cells, into photosensitive protoporphyrin IX (PpIX) in the mitochondria. When exposed to light, PpIX generates reactive oxygen species (ROS), including singlet oxygen and free radicals, which destroy tumor cells and the tumor's vascular system and stimulate local antitumor immunity [165]. PDT can directly induce cell death processes such as apoptosis, pyroptosis, autophagy, and ferroptosis, as described in other chapters.

In 2007, the authors introduced a UV-induced cSCC model in SKH-1 hairless mice and conducted foundational studies to support the clinical application of ALA-PDT [166]. By 2013, they demonstrated that ALA-PDT could induce localized antitumor immunity involving dendritic cells (DCs), CD8+ T cells, B cells, and macrophages [165, 167]. DCs play a critical role in antitumor immunity by presenting antigens, and DC vaccines are used for solid tumor immunotherapy. In 2015, the team showed that cSCC cells treated with ALA-PDT released DAMPs such as HSP70 and HMGB1, which promoted DC maturation and the secretion of IL-12 and IFN-γ, enhancing their antigen-presentation ability. Injecting these mature DCs into cSCC-bearing mice significantly inhibited tumor growth and increased CD4+ and CD8+ T-cell infiltration in tumor tissues [168]. By 2018, the team demonstrated that preventive injections of these ALA-PDT-induced mature DCs inhibited tumor formation in mice, increased CD4+ and CD8+ T cells in the spleen, and confirmed the potential of ALA-PDT-induced DCs as a cSCC vaccine [169].

Tertiary lymphoid structures (TLSs) are critical sites for local immune responses and are composed of immune cells such as DCs, T cells, B cells, and macrophages. The authors' group reported a marked increase in TLSs in the tumor tissues of cSCC patients 48 h after ALA-PDT, indicating that TLSs may mediate the antitumor immunity induced by ALA-PDT. To further explore this mechanism, they conducted transcriptomic analysis, which identified 828 genes whose expression was altered 6 h after PDT. Enrichment analysis linked these genes to pathways involved in immune regulation, including the NF-κB, TLR, PI3K-Akt, TNF, and MAPK signaling pathways.

The effectiveness of PDT in inducing antitumor immunity depends on both DC activation and immune cell recruitment to the tumor microenvironment (TME), with chemokines playing a central role. Studies have revealed that MCP-2/CCL8, which is highly expressed in the TME post-PDT, directs macrophages to transform into the M1 type, which chemoattracts DCs to suppress cSCC progression [170]; the authors observed elevated expression of CXCL13 in cSCC post-PDT, which binds to CXCR5 to attract B cells, follicular helper T cells (Tfhs), DCs, and M1 macrophages, reinforcing antitumor immunity. After ALA-PDT, cancer-associated fibroblasts (CAFs) in the TME increase CXCL13 secretion, further promoting B-cell recruitment and enhancing the immune response [171]. The team noted that ALA-PDT inhibited CAF activation and migration, reducing tumor growth in coculture studies with cSCC cells [172]. In addition, ALA-PDT-treated cSCC cells release a high volume of exosomes into the TME, which are absorbed by DCs and promote their maturation, further supporting an antitumor immune response [173].

In summary, ALA-PDT enhances cSCC treatment by activating DCs through DAMPs, stimulating tumor vaccine effects, and recruiting immune cells to tumors, leading to the formation of TLSs that aid in tumor immunity. Chemokines and exosomes released in the TME post-ALA-PDT draw immune cells and activate DCs, effectively killing tumor cells and preventing recurrence. However, the full induction mechanism remains unclear, and further investigation is needed to identify additional sensitizing targets to optimize PDT efficacy.

5.5.7.3 Clinical Application

PDT treatment parameters for skin cancer focus on photosensitizers, light sources, and combination therapies. The key advantages of PDT include the following: (1) selective targeting: PDT selectively kills tumor cells and inhibits "regional carcinogenesis" while preserving surrounding tissue; (2) tissue preservation: it spares normal tissue structure and can be used on various body areas, preserving both tissue function and cosmetic appearance; (3) low side effects: PDT can be repeated with minimal side effects, making it suitable for all ages, particularly elderly patients; (4) flexible treatment: it can be applied alone or in combination with other treatments, such as lasers, surgery, cryotherapy, or topical imiquimod; and (5) applicability for multiple lesions: it is viable for patients with large, multiple lesions or contraindications to surgery or radiotherapy. Despite these benefits, PDT is limited by the penetration depth of photosensitizers and light sources, which restricts treatment depth, and some patients experience treatment-related pain.

5.5.7.4 Photosensitizer Selection

Common photosensitizers for cSCC include topical ALA, methyl aminolevulinate (MAL), and BF-200 ALA, as well as systemic hematoporphyrin injection (HpD). ALA and MAL are second-generation photosensitizers, with MAL commonly used at a fixed 16.8% cream concentration in Europe and the United States, and are typically incubated for 3–6 h to improve penetration. HpD, an intravenous photosensitizer, has been used in recent cSCC treatments because of its greater degree of tissue absorption and deeper penetration, although no standard protocol exists for its clinical use (see Chap. 6, Sect. 6.2 for details). Case reports suggest that ALA-PDT and MAL-PDT may benefit invasive cSCC patients who are unable to undergo surgery, although efficacy data remain limited.

PDT is recommended for patients who cannot tolerate surgery. Pathological evaluation and long-term follow-up after PDT are recommended. A randomized controlled study reported that the cure rates of MAL-PDT for BD and early cSCC ranged from 54% to 74% [174]. Most suboptimal clinical cases pathologically show deep-invasive cSCC, suggesting that tumor depth is the main factor in PDT for cSCC. PDT can be considered for thin nonmelanoma skin cancers (thickness <2–3 mm) [175]. The authors' group reported successful lesion clearance using ALA-PDT on lower-lip lesions, with long-term follow-up showing low recurrence (20% ALA, 3-h incubation, 630 nm red light, light dose of 100 J/cm^2, 50 mW/cm^2, 2–7 sessions) [176]. Similarly, Fargnoli reported remission in a microinvasive SCC patient treated with MAL-PDT, with no recurrence at 24 months (16.8% MAL, 3 h incubation, 635 nm red light, light dose of 37 J/cm^2, 2 sessions) [177]. Li et al. described successful weekly MAL-PDT treatment for a cSCC patient with a lesion depth of 5.5 cm (weekly MAL-PDT for 7 consecutive weeks, total light dose of 791 J/cm^2) [175]. Previous clinical studies regarding ALA and MAL have shown comparable clinical efficacy for NMSC and similar side effects [178]. However, a meta-analysis suggested that ALA-PDT may yield a slightly higher remission rate than MAL-PDT for Bowen's disease [179]. On the basis of the literature reports and previous studies, tumor depth may not be an absolute factor affecting clinical efficacy. Studies indicate that combining PDT with immunomodulators such as imiquimod enhances clinical outcomes, particularly through antitumor immune responses [175, 180, 181].

BF-200 ALA, approved by the FDA as Ameluz®, is a 7.8% ALA nanoemulsion gel that improves stability and epidermal permeability, enhancing safety and tolerance [182]. PpIX fluorescence intensity after photosensitizer incubation can indicate permeability; studies have shown that BF-200 ALA produces stronger PpIX fluorescence than 20% ALA cream does, indicating greater permeability and promising application potential [183].

5.5.7.5 Light Source Selection

Two primary wavelengths are used in PDT for NMSC: blue light (410 nm) and red light (630 nm), on the basis of the PpIX absorption peaks. Blue light penetrates skin depths of 1–2 mm [184], whereas red light penetrates 2–5 mm, reaching dermal fibroblasts and skin appendages [185]. Blue light-PDT, which is common in the United States, uses a 20% ALA solution (LevulanKerastick®) with an FDA-recommended energy density of 10 J/cm^2 at wavelengths of 400–450 nm [186]. Owing to its deeper penetration, red light is widely applied in ALA-PDT and MAL-PDT globally, with treatment parameters adjusted according to the light source [23]. For blue light-PDT, the energy density typically ranges from 1.8 to 48 J/cm^2 with a power density of 10–40 mW/cm^2 [178]. In contrast, red light-PDT, as outlined in the Chinese Guidelines for Photodynamic Therapy, is administered with an energy density of 100–200 J/cm^2 and a power density of 60–150 mW/cm^2 [89]. While clinical studies suggest similar efficacy and side effects for red and blue light in AK and BCC treatments, red light tends to cause more discomfort for patients [187, 188]. The choice of light source depends on both the photosensitizer and the characteristics of the lesion. Prior to irradiation, any necrotic tissue or secretions on the lesion surface should be removed, and the tumor's fluorescence border should be mapped with Wood's lamp. The light should cover the entire tumor area and extend beyond its edges; for larger or more extensive lesions, multipoint or partitioned irradiation may be used. The PDT irradiation time for protruding tumors should be based on the tumor size and laser power.

Following treatment, tumor tissue may degenerate and necrose. Once necrotic tissue falls off, PDT can be repeated if residual tumor remains.

5.5.7.6 Combined Treatment

PDT is a safe, effective, and straightforward treatment option that is used either alone or alongside other treatments for cSCC. It can serve as a debulking step before surgery for aggressive cSCC or as an adjuvant treatment following CO_2 laser or surgical procedures. As such, refining strategies and protocols for combined PDT treatment of cSCC is valuable. According to the 2007 European Guidelines on Photodynamic Therapy, evidence supporting the use of PDT in cSCC remains limited (evidence level 4, grade C) [47]. Owing to its metastatic potential, cSCC treatment generally prioritizes surgery, with Mohs surgery achieving a 5-year cure rate of 97.4% for early SCC [158]. Given its uncertain efficacy in treating deep or aggressive cSCC, PDT alone is typically not recommended in clinical settings. However, studies suggest that pretreatment with PDT alone or in combination with other drugs or physical or surgical treatments may enhance clinical outcomes.

Pretreatment before PDT involves removing any scabs and abrading the tumor surface to improve photosensitizer penetration. Haedersdal and colleagues employed CO_2 fractional laser pretreatment to increase photosensitizer absorption [189]. However, this approach creates a carbonization zone, which can impede penetration. To address this, the authors' group used a traditional Chinese plum-blossoming needle to enhance penetration without creating a carbonization zone, proving to be more effective and economical than laser pretreatment [42]. Other researchers have employed microneedling to prepare skin cancers for ALA-PDT [190].

A common pharmacological combination with ALA-PDT is imiquimod. In 2018, the authors' group applied plum-blossom needle-assisted ALA-PDT with imiquimod in a 96-year-old patient with cSCC. After nine PDT sessions and 3 months of imiquimod, the lesion achieved complete remission with no recurrence at 18 months of follow-up (Fig. 5.18) [180]. A follow-up mouse model study revealed that combining ALA-PDT and imiquimod enhanced CD8+ T-cell infiltration and tumor cell apoptosis in cSCC, indicating that local imiquimod administration can stimulate an immune response, creating a favorable immune microenvironment for PDT and achieving superior efficacy to single-agent treatments. The authors' group also achieved complete remission in two patients with scalp and lower-lip cSCC after three and six combined treatments, respectively [181]. Building on these findings, they initiated a single-center clinical study involving 33 cSCC patients who were not surgical candidates. After plum-blossom needle pretreatment, the patients received ALA-PDT with imiquimod, resulting in complete remission

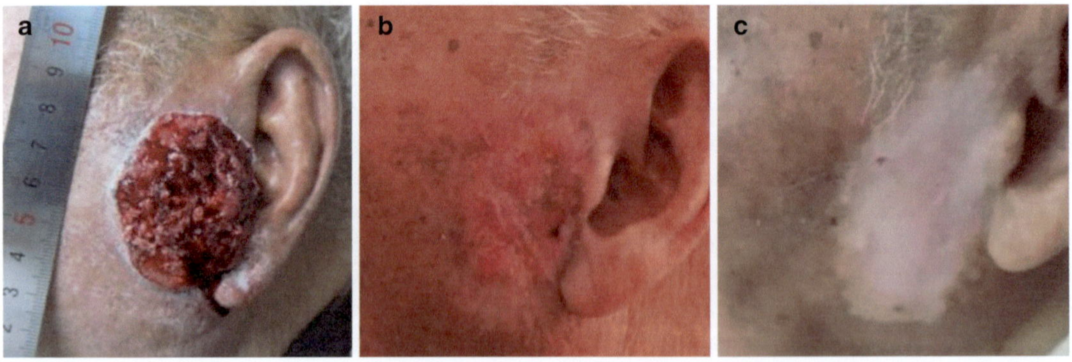

Fig. 5.18 ALA-PDT combined with imiquimod for the treatment of cSCC in elderly patients. (**a**) Before treatment. (**b**) After nine sessions of ALA-PDT combined with plum-blossom needle pretreatment, the tumor regressed. (**c**) After 3 months of imiquimod treatment, no recurrence was observed during an 18-month follow-up, and local vitiligo-like hypopigmentation occurred

for five patients, partial remission with quality-of-life improvement for 24 patients, and four patients lost to follow-up [191]. The 2021 "Chinese guidelines on the clinical application of 5-aminolevulinic acid-based photodynamic therapy in dermatology (2021 edition)" elevated the evidence level for cSCC to level II, with a grade B recommendation [89]. Additional research has explored drugs combined with PDT for AK treatment for potential use in cSCC. Sanjay Anand's team reported that combining 5-fluorouracil (5-FU) with ALA-PDT effectively increases PpIX levels, increasing cSCC cell death [192]. Methotrexate (MTX) was identified early on for its role in the upregulation of coproporphyrinogen oxidase (CPO), which increases PpIX accumulation. In vitro studies have shown that MTX enhances ALA-PDT cytotoxicity in cSCC cells by upregulating CPO, further enriching PpIX within tumor cells [193].

In recent years, PD-1 monoclonal antibodies, a newer class of molecularly targeted drugs, have been introduced for clinical use, although their response rate in cSCC remains modest. Since PDT can stimulate local antitumor immunity, it is hypothesized that combining it with PD-L1 monoclonal antibodies could yield synergistic effects, offering a potential palliative treatment for advanced cSCC. In 2022, the authors reported that cSCC cells express PD-L1 and that combining PD-L1 with ALA-PDT induced apoptosis and ferroptosis in these cells while recruiting lymphocytes to infiltrate and form tertiary lymphoid structures in the tumor stroma, enhancing antitumor immunity and improving ALA-PDT efficacy [194]. Clinical trials are needed to validate the combined use of PD-1 monoclonal antibodies and ALA-PDT for treating cSCC.

For cSCC lesions with high tumor volume and deep infiltration, ultrasound-guided tumor excision followed by PDT of the exposed wound can target the remaining tumor tissue and enhance treatment efficacy. Wenbo Bu and colleagues combined surgery with PDT for a 90-year-old patient with a large facial cSCC, excised the visible tumor, and then applied PDT to reduce the tumor boundary, followed by radical surgery, with no recurrence noted over 6 months [195]. In another case, the authors' group treated two patients with well-differentiated cSCC on the lower lip, first surgically removing the visible tumor and then performing PDT on the open wound to selectively destroy residual tissue, aiming to minimize trauma while preserving normal tissue. After three PDT sessions, the lesion cleared with minimal scarring [196]. Wang and colleagues similarly achieved complete lesion clearance with minimal scarring via curettage followed by ALA-PDT for a lower lip cSCC, with no recurrence after 1 year (Figs. 5.19 and 5.20) [197]. In a retrospective study of 68 patients with skin tumors, Chen Zhang and colleagues reported that combining surgery with ALA-PDT provided a clear clinical benefit and favorable prognosis compared with surgery alone. The authors' group also applied CO_2 laser ablation combined with ALA-PDT to treat a 6 × 5 cm well-differentiated scalp cSCC. After laser ablation, three ALA-PDT sessions resulted in full clinical remission without recurrence after 1 year (Fig. 5.21) [198]. In summary, for treating cSCC in complex sites or special populations, initial debulking via surgery or CO_2 laser ablation followed by ALA-PDT can enhance treatment outcomes by maximizing efficacy while minimizing harm to surrounding tissue.

5.5.7.7 Modified Painless Photodynamic Therapy

Pain is a frequent adverse effect during or after conventional PDT, and local anesthesia or painkillers often provide insufficient relief. The most commonly used topical photosensitizers, ALA and MAL, cause similar pain levels under standard treatment conditions. Research suggests that pain severity is correlated with PpIX accumulation and reactive oxygen species (ROS) production. Modifying treatment parameters—such as the photosensitizer incubation time and the light source's power density—can reduce patient pain. When the power density is kept under 60 mW/cm^2 and the energy density is under 50 J/cm^2, PDT-related pain is significantly reduced [199, 200]. Cottrell et al. applied a 633 nm wavelength light source at a power density of 10–40 mW/cm^2, which was effective and produced minimal

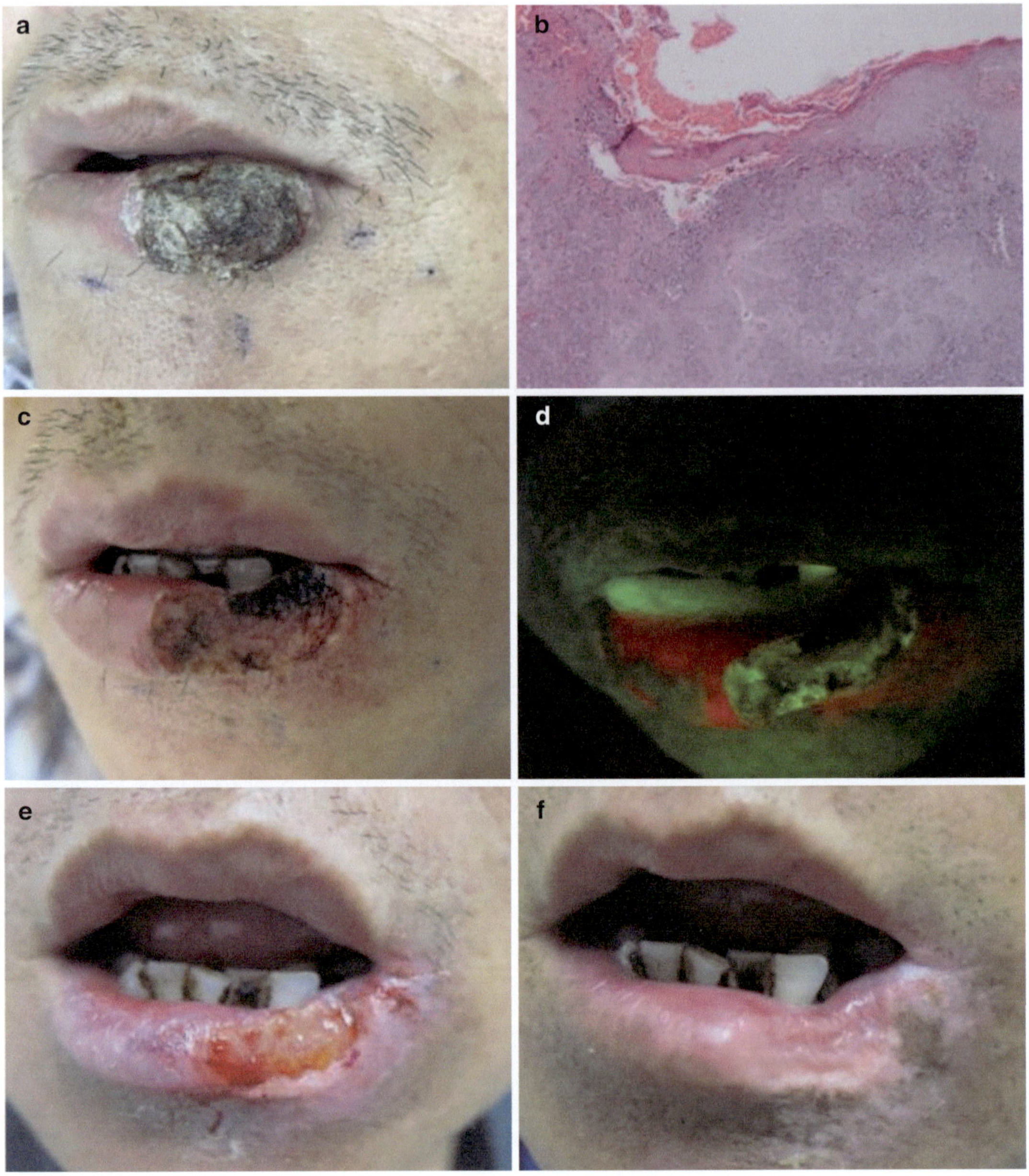

Fig. 5.19 Surgery combined with ALA-PDT for lower lip cSCC. (**a**) Before treatment. (**b**) Histopathology showing well-differentiated cSCC. (**c**) Secondary wound healing postsurgery. (**d**) Fluorescence image of the lower lip after ALA application. (**e**), After three sessions of ALA-PDT. (**f**) After eight sessions of ALA-PDT, the patient was followed up for 2 months, and the image showed complete clinical results with mild scarring and preservation of anatomical structures

pain. After 90% of the PpIX was bleached, a second round of irradiation at 150 mW/cm^2 was used to maintain efficacy and reduce discomfort [201]. By optimizing PDT parameters, the authors improved patient comfort by shortening the ALA application time to reduce PpIX accumulation, lowering the light source power density, and extending the irradiation time to reach a higher total energy density than traditional PDT, maintaining efficacy [142]. Although PDT shows

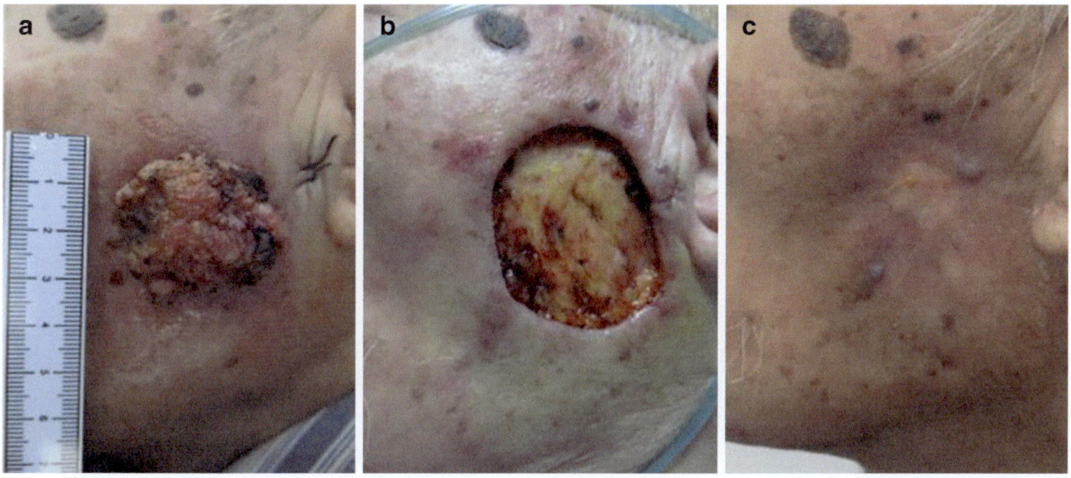

Fig. 5.20 Surgery combined with ALA-PDT for the treatment of facial cSCC. (**a**) Before treatment. (**b**) Secondary wound healing postsurgery. (**c**) After six sessions of ALA-PDT postoperatively, complete clinical remission at the 1-month follow-up

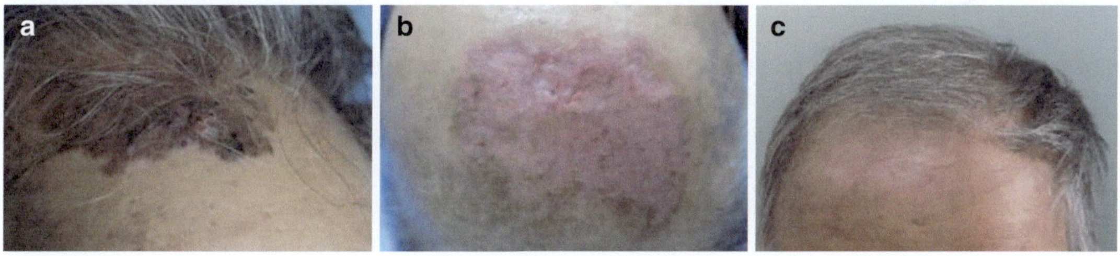

Fig. 5.21 Laser combined with ALA-PDT for giant cSCC. (**a**) Before treatment. (**b**) 2 weeks after laser treatment, the visible lesion was removed. (**c**) 1 year after a session of laser treatment and three sessions of ALA-PDT, no recurrence was found

promise for cSCC, further research is needed to reduce PDT-related pain without compromising therapeutic outcomes, thereby enhancing patient tolerance.

Application Scope

(a) Recommendations for early minimally invasive cSCC.
(b) Suitable for well-differentiated cSCC in specific locations, with multiple lesions or challenging traditional treatment options; evidence-based level II and clinical recommendation grade B.
(c) Palliative treatment of advanced cSCC when other options are unsuitable or ineffective aims to improve quality of life.

Treatment Steps (Table 5.9)

(a) Clean and disinfect the area with disinfectant and gauze.
(b) For lesions with scabs, thick tissue, or deeper damage, pretreatment options (e.g., scab removal, plum-blossom needle tapping, or rolling microneedles) are considered to increase photosensitizer penetration.
(c) ALA cream was prepared and applied to the treatment area and surrounding skin, avoiding the eyes and keeping it protected from light.
(d) Before irradiation, the ALA was gently washed off, ensuring that both the patient and doctor wore protective goggles.

Table 5.9 Recommended ALA-PDT protocol for cSCC treatment

Pretreatment method	Recommended combined therapy	ALA formulation		Application time (h)	Light dose	
		ALA form	ALA concentration (%)		Energy density (J/cm^2)	Power density (mW/cm^2)
Remove necrotic tissue and secretions, plum-blossom needle tapping	Surgery, laser, imiquimod, PD-1 monoclonal antibody	Cream	20	3–6	100–200	60–150

(e) Select the appropriate light source and parameters for PDT and provide symptomatic treatment for discomfort, such as pain.
(f) After treatment, local cold compresses were applied as needed to relieve symptoms.

- Interval: Once every 2 weeks.
- Number of treatments: Until complete clearance of the skin lesions.
- Classic evaluation of therapeutic outcomes: If there is no significant improvement after 2 treatments, other treatment options are recommended; if the skin lesions improve but are not completely clear, repeated treatment is recommended.
- Attention: Even after a clinical cure, regular follow-up is recommended on the basis of risk assessment, and lifelong follow-up is advocated. For immunosuppressed patients, shortened follow-up is warranted, and biopsy should be performed for suspicious lesions.

In summary, with an aging population and increasing number of cSCC cases in China, the role of PDT in treating cSCC is advancing but remains limited to in situ and early superficial cases as an alternative treatment. The ongoing development of new photosensitizers, nanotechnology applications, optimized PDT techniques, and combination treatment protocols will drive further breakthroughs, expanding the role of PDT in cSCC management.

5.6 ALA-PDT for the Treatment of EMPD

5.6.1 Introduction

Extramammary Paget disease (EMPD), also known as extramammary eczema-like cancer, is a relatively rare neoplastic disease with a global prevalence of 0.1–2.4 people per million people. The incidence in Asian populations is four times greater, and the 5-year survival rate is approximately 72–87% [202–204]. The prevalence of sex differences between Western and Asian populations. In studies of Caucasian populations, EMPD has a female predominance, with male-to-female ratios ranging from 1:2 to 1:7. In contrast, a male predominance has been reported in Asian studies [205]. Invasive EMPD is prone to lymph node metastasis or distant metastasis, with a high mortality rate, with a 5-year survival rate after metastasis of only 7%. The exact pathogenesis of EMPD is unknown. Primary EMPD is thought to originate from the malignant transformation of pluripotent keratinocyte stem cells in situ or from the metastasis of apocrine gland ductal carcinoma from the apocrine gland epidermis, whereas secondary EMPD is associated with subcutaneous or distant tumors of the cervix, colorectum, or urinary system [202, 206].

5.6.1.1 Clinical Features

EMPD typically affects areas with abundant apocrine sweat glands, such as the scrotum, penis, labia minora, vagina, perianal area, groin, and axilla [206]. Lesions present as well-demarcated erythematous patches or infiltrative plaques with white adhesive scales, crusting, erosion, or exudates. In the early stages, lesions appear nonspecifically eczematous. Lesions are usually asymptomatic or accompanied by varying degrees of pruritus, pain, or burning. Lesions are often misdiagnosed as eczema or tinea cruris because of their nonspecific symptoms and slow progression over several months to years. Misdiagnosis contributes to tumor persistence and progression.

5.6.1.2 Etiology

The origin of primary EMPD is inconclusive, but it has been speculated that Paget cells arise from apocrine sweat gland-opening cells, pluripotent cells derived from differentiation into apocrine sweat glands, sweat duct epithelium migrating to the epidermis, or intraepidermal keratinocytes and Toker cells.

5.6.1.3 Histopathology

Under a microscope, EMPD presents as hyperkeratosis or parakeratosis and acanthosis. The number of infiltrating tumor cells varies. Typically, Paget cells, which are large, round, clear to pale cells with abundant eosinophilic cytoplasm, are present in the epidermis. The nucleoli of Paget cells are prominent and round or slightly irregular with occasional mitosis. Paget cells typically cluster in the center and lower parts of the epidermis. Atypical Paget cells exhibit vacuolar changes; affected sweat glands can be partially or completely replaced by Paget cells. The basal cell layer can be flattened between Paget cell nests and the basement membrane. Paget cells can also invade epidermal appendages, especially the epithelium of hair follicles or exocrine sweat ducts, and even invade the dermis. Common immunohistochemical markers include CK7+, CK20+/−, CEA+, and EMA+. CK7 and CK20 are the most commonly used markers to distinguish between primary and secondary EMPDs, with CK7 being a sensitive marker for EMPD and CK20 suggesting gastrointestinal and urinary tract tumor origin. CK7+ and CK20− suggest primary EMPD, whereas CK7+ and CK20+ suggest secondary EMPD [207].

5.6.2 Treatment

There is no unified or internationally recognized disease staging system for EMPD. A TNM staging system has been proposed according to disease characteristics to guide treatment and prognostic evaluation. Murad Alam et al. reviewed 483 articles and 23,493 cases from 1990 to 2019 and proposed the latest evidence-based clinical practice guidelines for EMPD, which focus on diagnosis, screening, treatment, and follow-up management [203, 208]. The main goals of EMPD treatment are complete resection, clear surgical margins, preservation of function, and aesthetics. All treatment plans should be individualized on the basis of clinical manifestations, medical history, and patient preferences.

Surgery is the preferred treatment for EMPD, but the recurrence rate of wide local excision is as high as 37.0%, and margin-controlled surgery, such as Mohs micrographic surgery, has advantages over traditional surgery or extended resection [203, 208]. For secondary EMPD, the primary lesions should also be treated. Other treatments include electrodeiccation, curettage, lasers, 5% imiquimod cream, radiation therapy, and local chemotherapy, which have limited efficacy, high recurrence rates, and significant adverse reactions, making them less favorable options [209, 210]. While Mohs micrographic surgery remains the first-line treatment, it has several challenges. EMPD often presents with large, multifocal lesions and poorly defined boundaries, making surgery difficult, destructive, and prone to postoperative recurrence. Factors such as tumor location, patient age, tumor size, and comorbidities can make some patients unsuitable for surgery, highlighting the need for alternative therapies.

5.6.3 ALA-PDT

In 1999, Henta et al. first applied ALA-PDT to treat a 74-year-old woman with vulvar EMPD who was not a surgical candidate and had lymph node and lung metastases. After the tumor was reduced by 60% with etoposide (VP16, 100 mg) and 5000 cGy electron beam irradiation, residual tumor tissue was treated with ALA-PDT, leading to near-complete remission [211]. Many recent reviews have recommended ALA-PDT as an alternative or palliative treatment for EMPD [212, 213]. Additionally, photodynamic diagnosis (PDD) can noninvasively identify tumor margins and potential metastatic foci, thereby reducing the recurrence rate. ALA-PDT combined with other therapies has shown promise in improving the cure rate and reducing recurrence, especially for elderly patients or those with lesions in difficult anatomical areas. ALA-PDT offers selective tumor cell destruction, minimal trauma, and good cosmetic effects.

5.6.3.1 Mechanism

ALA-PDT works by generating reactive oxygen species (ROS) that directly kill tumor cells and disrupt tissue microvascular circulation. It also induces local immune cell aggregation and activates the antitumor immune response.

5.6.3.2 Clinical Application

ALA is mixed with ALA at a concentration of 10–20% in sterilized injection water or cream. Owing to the instability of ALA, it should be prepared fresh and used within 3 h.

Light source: The recommended light source is red light at approximately 630 nm, and LED or semiconductor lasers are used.

Pretreatment significantly increased ALA absorption and light penetration. The following pretreatment methods were identified:

For transdermal pretreatment, liquid paraffin is used to clean the tumor surface, followed by plum-blossom needles, microneedles, or curettage to increase the permeability of ALA, which is suitable for skin lesions ≤4 mm thick.

Laser pretreatment: After local infiltration anesthesia, a CO_2 laser, erbium laser, or holmium laser are used to ablate thickened lesions, which are suitable for pretreating lesions ≥4 mm thick.

Surgical pretreatment: The size and depth of EMPD lesions were marked via ultrasound. After local infiltration or general anesthesia, the tumor was removed along the positioning marker, followed by hemostasis and subsequent ALA-PDT. Patients with EMPD nodules, sclerotic lesions, and some locally advanced EMPD lesions are suitable.

Clinical Efficacy In 2002, Shizheng Xu, Xiuli Wang et al. reported two cases of MPD and eight EMPD patients treated with ALA-PDT, and the results indicated that ALA-PDT could improve MPD and EMPD lesions, although the lesions could not be cured by ALA-PDT alone [27] (Figs. 5.22 and 5.23). Hu et al. treated five EMPD patients with PDT [214]. Three patients were treated with one session of PDT followed by surgery, and all recovered well without recurrence during follow-up. One patient was treated with two sessions of PDT, resulting in a significant reduction in lesion size. Another patient was treated with 12 sessions of PDT, which resulted in a substantial reduction in the area of erythema. Shieh et al. treated 16 lesions in five male EMPD patients with ALA-PDT [215]. Most lesions have recurred after previous treatment with laser ablation or resection. ALA (20%) was applied for 18–24 h, followed by red light irradiation (37 J/cm^2) applied 12 times at 2-week intervals. After 6 months of treatment, the complete response rate was 50%, with preserved tissue structure and function post-treatment. Rosanna et al. applied MLA-PDT in 32 patients with vaginal EMPD, 16 of whom had lesions involving the perineum and perianal area. After three sessions of MAL-PDT, 3 patients experienced complete clearance of lesions, 25 experienced partial clearance, and 4 patients experienced no improvement. Also, 18 patients experienced relapse, 16 of whom received further PDT treatment [216]. The authors' group applied ALA-PDT to a patient with giant secondary vulvar EMPD. Red light irradiation (10%, 100 J/cm^2) was used. After three sessions of ALA-PDT at 2-week intervals, the lesions improved, and a slight burning sensation was the main adverse reaction. Although the secondary EMPD was not completely eradicated, her symptoms significantly improved. Organ function was preserved, and patients' quality of life improved [217] (Fig. 5.24). PDT has several advantages, including good selectivity, the ability to eliminate occult lesions, minimal trauma, and preservation

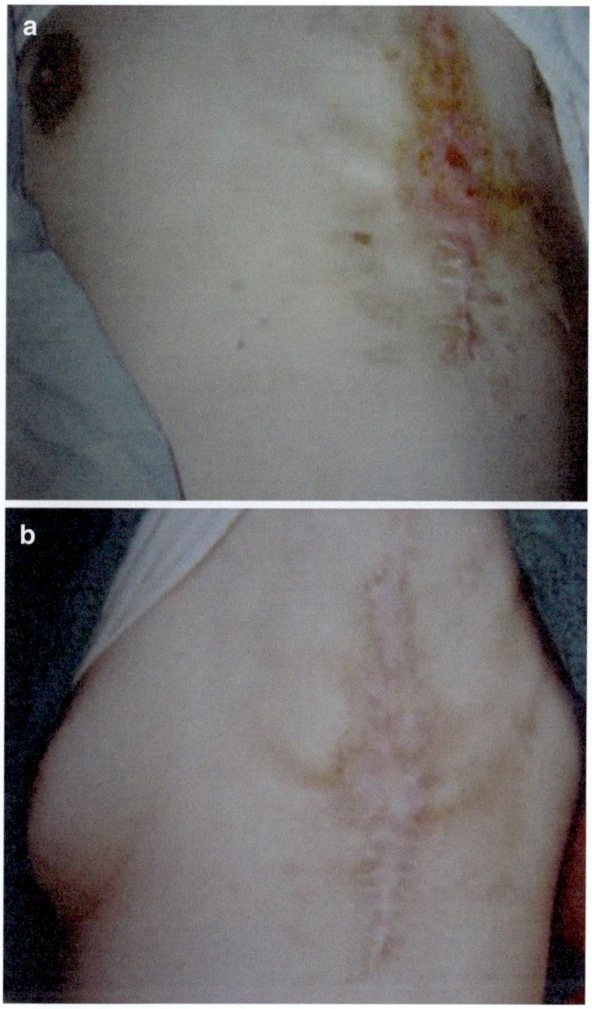

Fig. 5.22 MPD before and after ALA-PDT treatment. (**a**) Clinical manifestations of recurrent MPD in a 28-year-old woman 1 year postmastectomy, (**b**) 4 months after ALA-PDT treatment, the lesion was completely cleared without recurrence

of tissue and organ function. PDT is not only a therapy for early-stage tumors and recurrent lesions but also a measure to improve the quality of life of patients with advanced tumors.

5.6.3.3 Recommended Protocols

ALA-PDT is increasingly used to treat EMPD, and on the basis of clinical experience and research data, the following treatment protocols are recommended (Table 5.10).

- Interval: 2 weeks, with efficacy evaluation before each treatment.
- Frequency: At least three sessions are recommended and treated until the endpoint is achieved.
- Efficacy evaluation: In addition to recording the lesion area, ultrasound evaluation of lesion depth is essential:
  - Complete response (CR): no lesion observed and normal structures shown on ultrasound;
  - Partial response (PR): ≥50% reduction in the total lesion area or ≥50% reduction in lesion depth.
  - Stable disease (SD): the lesion area or depth is reduced but not enough to be categorized as a PR or is increased but not enough to be categorized as PD.
  - Progressive disease (PD): lesion size or depth increased by ≥20% or new lesions observed.

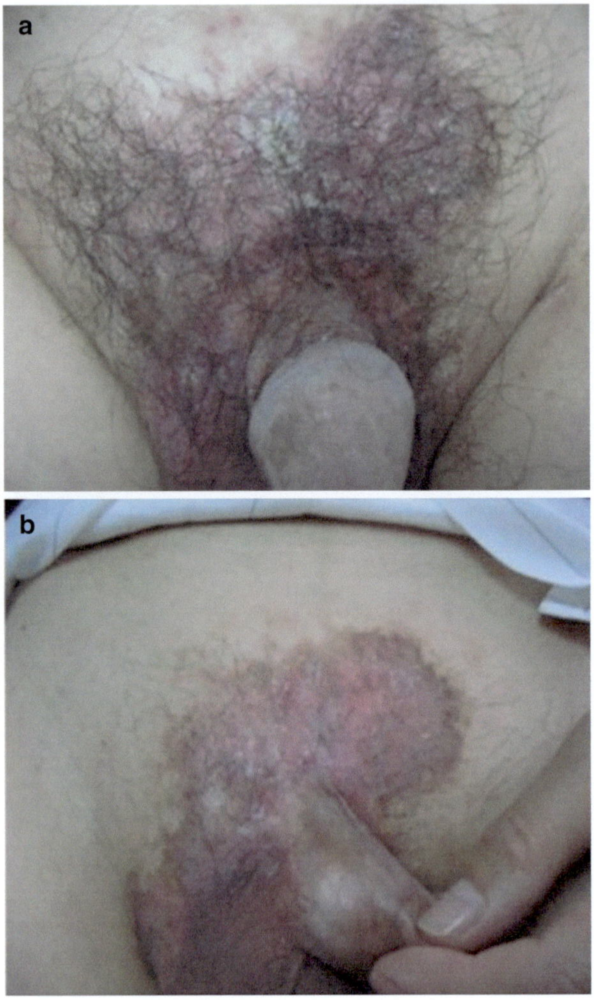

Fig. 5.23 EMPD before and after ALA-PDT treatment. (**a**) Clinical manifestations of a 66-year-old male patient with EMPD before treatment. (**b**) Improvement after three sessions of ALA-PDT

- The endpoints are as follows: treatment can be stopped when a CR is achieved, and combination with other therapies can be considered when PD occurs.
- Precautions: pretreatment, such as plum-blossom needling, should be applied before treatment; for pain and other side reactions, local anesthesia is recommended, and systemic analgesics can be applied if necessary; lifelong follow-up after treatment is necessary.

5.6.4 Combination Therapy

For aggressive lesions with deep infiltration, ALA-PDT alone may not achieve the desired effect because of limited photosensitizer penetration. Therefore, ALA-PDT can be applied in combination with other therapies to treat EMPD.

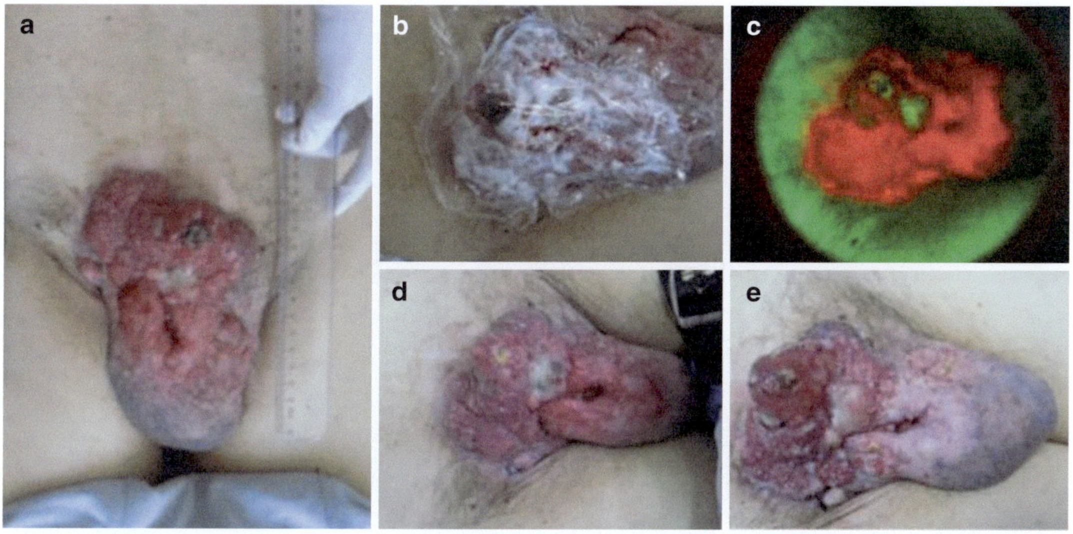

Fig. 5.24 Clinical manifestations of EMPD before and after ALA-PDT treatment. (**a**) 78-year-old male EMPD patients before treatment. (**b**) Incubation of penoscrotal lesions with 10% ALA. (**c**) After 3 h of incubation, the lesions showed red fluorescence. (**d**) After one session of ALA-PDT. (**e**) Improvement after two sessions of ALA-PDT

Table 5.10 Recommended protocols for the sequential treatment of EMPD with ALA-PDT and surgery

Mainly pretreatment	ALA		Incubation time (h)	Dosage of light	
	ALA formulation	ALA concentration (%)		Power density (mW/cm^2)	Energy density (J/cm^2)
Plum-blossom microneedling, fractional laser, holmium laser	Cream	20	3–6	80–150	100–200

5.6.4.1 Combining Surgery

In 2013, the authors compared the efficacy of the combination of ALA-PDT and surgery with that of surgery alone in 13 patients with EMPD. The recurrence rate was 25% in the surgery-only group but 9.1% in the combined ALA-PDT and surgery group, with superior efficacy and recurrence rates. Preoperative PDT can eliminate small surrounding lesions, reduce the tumor area, and make the lesion boundary clearer since PDeD can identify surgical margins. PDT combined with surgery is one of the recommended treatments for EMPD [218].

In recent years, therapies combining Mohs micrographic surgery with methods such as preoperative PDD, fluorescent labeling, multisite biopsy, or adjuvant chemoradiotherapy have been shown to improve functional sequelae and wound healing. In 2014, Yang Gao et al. treated 38 patients with EMPD in the scrotum and penis. Thirty-one patients underwent surgical excision followed by ALA-PDT, and seven were treated with ALA-PDT alone because of refusal of surgery or inability to perform surgery. Postsurgery PDT (120 J/cm^2 for 15 min with a 635-nm laser) was applied three times after surgery, and there was no recurrence in the PDT + surgery group, whereas on patient in the PDT alone group experienced recurrence within 6 months. All patients were able to complete the treatment with good structural preservation and no moderate-to-severe adverse reactions [219].

5.6.4.2 Combining with a Laser

Limited photosensitizer penetration is one reason for the poor efficacy of ALA-PDT. Combining ALA-PDT with ablative lasers can improve outcomes. The authors' group treated a patient with recurrent and invasive perineal EMPD (2.5 mm deep) via a holmium laser combined with ALA-

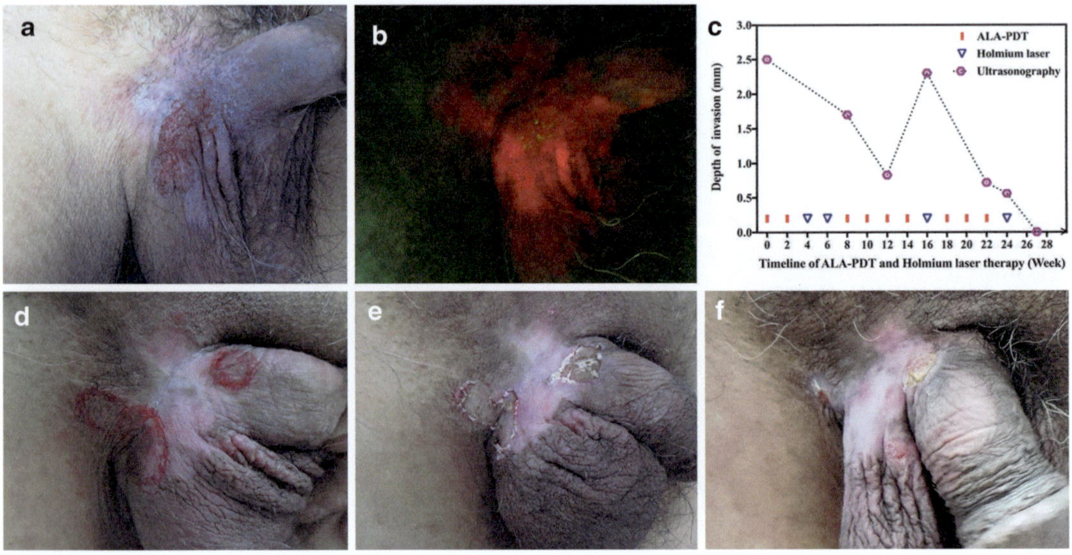

Fig. 5.25 Relapsed EMPD lesions before and after ALA-PDT combined with holmium laser treatment. (**a**) Relapsed EMPD lesions in the scrotum and penis of a 71-year-old male patient with erythema before treatment. (**b**) Red fluorescence of the lesions after 3 h of incubation with 20% ALA. (**c**) Changes in the depth of the lesions detected by ultrasound at visit. (**d**) Ultrasound at the red circle indicates residual skin lesions after 9 ALA-PDT + 3 holmium laser treatments. (**e**) Manifestation after 9 ALA-PDT + 4 holmium laser treatments. (**f**) Three weeks after 9 ALA-PDT + 4 holmium laser treatments, the lesions were completely cleared, and scarring and hypopigmentation were observed

PDT. After holmium laser (0.5–2.5 J) pretreatment, 20% ALA was applied for 3–4 h, followed by 100 J/cm^2 red light irradiation. After nine sessions of ALA-PDT and four sessions of holmium laser irradiation, the lesions were completely removed, and skin ultrasound revealed complete clearance of the hypoechoic lesions [220] (Fig. 5.25).

5.6.4.3 Combining Topical Medications

Imiquimod, a Toll-like receptor-7 activator with immunomodulatory effects, has been used as a single agent for treating EMPD, although its efficacy is limited [221]. Wang et al. used six sessions of ALA-PDT combined with topical imiquimod to treat two patients with recurrent EMPD lesions in the penoscrotal and groin areas. After six sessions of ALA-PDT, a complete response was achieved, and there was no recurrence at the 24- and 36-month follow-ups [222]. Bauman et al. treated a patient with secondary scrotal EMPD [223] via a combination of ALA-PDT and 5% imiquimod ointment. The patient received imiquimod five times per week, gradually reducing the frequency over 6 months, after which imiquimod was discontinued, and the patient continued quarterly PDT. The appearance of the lesion significantly improved, and pathology revealed no residual disease. The patient has remained disease-free for more than 5 years.

In summary, the efficacy of PDT alone in treating EMPD is limited, primarily due to the deep and extensive nature of tumor tissue in many patients. However, combining ALA-PDT with surgery or other therapies improves the treatment efficacy and reduces the recurrence rate.

References

1. Salasche SJ. Epidemiology of actinic keratoses and squamous cell carcinoma. J Am Acad Dermatol. 2000;42(1):4–7. https://doi.org/10.1067/mjd.2000.103342.
2. Tu Q, Lv T, Lai Y, Zhang L, Shi L, Li J, et al. Epidemiological study of elderly skin tumors in

a community in Shanghai. Gerontol Health Care. 2013;19(3):142–5. https://doi.org/10.3969/j.issn.1008-8296.2013-05.
3. Zhao Y, Li C, Wen C, Wei Y, Li R, Wang G, et al. The prevalence of actinic keratosis in patients visiting dermatologists in two hospitals in China. Br J Dermatol. 2016;174(5):1005–10. https://doi.org/10.1111/bjd.14344.
4. Vatve M, Ortonne JP, Birch-Machin MA, Gupta G. Management of field change in actinic keratosis. Br J Dermatol. 2007;157(Suppl 2):21–4. https://doi.org/10.1111/j.1365-2133.2007.08268.x.
5. Olsen E, Abernethy M, Kulp-Shorten C, Callen J, Glazer S, Huntley A, et al. A double-blind, vehicle-controlled study evaluating masoprocol cream in the treatment of actinic keratoses on the head and neck. J Am Acad Dermatol. 1991;24:738–43. https://doi.org/10.1016/0190-9622(91)70113-g.
6. de Berker D, McGregor J, Mohd Mustapa M, Exton L, Hughes B. British Association of Dermatologists' guidelines for the care of patients with actinic keratosis 2017. Br J Dermatol. 2017;176(1):20–43. https://doi.org/10.1111/bjd.15107.
7. Reinehr C, Bakos R. Actinic keratoses: review of clinical, dermoscopic, and therapeutic aspects. An Bras Dermatol. 2019;94(6):637–57. https://doi.org/10.1016/j.abd.2019.10.004.
8. Yang XQ, Hu C, Wen L, Xu YT, Keyal U, Zhang GL, et al. Dermoscopic monitoring for treatment and follow-up of actinic keratosis with 5-aminolaevulinic acid photodynamic therapy. Technol Cancer Res Treat. 2018;17:1533033818820091. https://doi.org/10.1177/1533033818820091.
9. Hu C, Yang X, Liu X, Zhang G, Cao Z, Wen L, et al. Dermoscopic features of solar keratosis of different grades and cutaneous squamous cell carcinoma. Gerontol Health Care. 2018;24(5):511–4. https://doi.org/10.3969/j.issn.1008-8296.2018.05.011.
10. Fargnoli M, Altomare G, Benati E, Borgia F, Broganelli P, Carbone A, et al. Prevalence and risk factors of actinic keratosis in patients attending Italian dermatology clinics. J Eur J Dermatol. 2017;27(6):599–608. https://doi.org/10.1684/ejd.2017.3126.
11. Chetty P, Choi F, Mitchell T. Primary care review of actinic keratosis and its therapeutic options: a global perspective. Dermatol Ther. 2015;5(1):19–35. https://doi.org/10.1007/s13555-015-0070-9.
12. Lopes M, Silva Júnior F, Lima K, Oliveira P, Silveira É. Clinicopathological profile and management of 161 cases of actinic cheilitis. An Bras Dermatol. 2015;90(4):505–12. https://doi.org/10.1590/abd1806-4841.20153848.
13. Criscione V, Weinstock M, Naylor M, Luque C, Eide M, Bingham S. Actinic keratoses: natural history and risk of malignant transformation in the veterans affairs topical tretinoin chemoprevention trial. Cancer. 2009;115(11):2523–30. https://doi.org/10.1002/cncr.24284.
14. Dodson J, DeSpain J, Hewett J, Clark D. Malignant potential of actinic keratoses and the controversy over treatment. A patient-oriented perspective. Arch Dermatol. 1991;127(7):1029–31. https://doi.org/10.1001/archderm.1991.01680060103013.
15. Dermatology Rehabilitation Committee of Chinese Rehabilitation Medical Association and Photomedical Treatment Equipment Group of Dermatology and Cosmetology Branch of Chinese Medical Equipment Association. Expert consensus on clinical diagnosis and treatment of Chinese actinic keratosis. Chin J Dermatol. 2021;54(12):561. https://doi.org/10.35541/cjd.20210561.
16. Glanz K, Saraiya M, Wechsler H. Guidelines for school programs to prevent skin cancer. MMWR Recomm Rep. 2002;51(4):1–18.
17. Eisen DB, Asgari MM, Bennett DD, Connolly SM, Dellavalle RP, Freeman EE, et al. Guidelines of care for the management of actinic keratosis. J Am Acad Dermatol. 2021;85(4):e209–33. https://doi.org/10.1016/j.jaad.2021.02.082.
18. Thompson SC, Jolley D, Marks R. Reduction of solar keratoses by regular sunscreen use. N Engl J Med. 1993;329(16):1147–51. https://doi.org/10.1056/Nejm199310143291602.
19. Naylor MF, Boyd A, Smith DW, Cameron GS, Hubbard D, Neldner KH. High sun protection factor sunscreens in the suppression of actinic neoplasia. Arch Dermatol. 1995;131(2):170–5. https://doi.org/10.1001/archderm.131.2.170.
20. Ulrich C, Jurgensen JS, Degen A, Hackethal M, Ulrich M, Patel MJ, et al. Prevention of non-melanoma skin cancer in organ transplant patients by regular use of a sunscreen: a 24 months, prospective, case-control study. Br J Dermatol. 2009;161:78–84. https://doi.org/10.1111/j.1365-2133.2009.09453.x.
21. Kunimoto K, Furukawa F, Uede M, Mizuno M, Yamamoto Y. The continued use of sunscreen prevents the development of actinic keratosis in aged Japanese subjects. Exp Dermatol. 2016;25(Suppl 3):34–40. https://doi.org/10.1111/exd.13081.
22. Photodynamic Therapy Research Center, Chinese Medical Association, Dermatology Rehabilitation Committee, Light medical treatment Equipment Group, Chinese Medical Equipment Association. Clinical application guidelines of aminolevulinic acid photodynamic therapy in dermatology. Chin J Dermatol. 2021;54(1):1–9.
23. Morton CA, Szeimies RM, Basset-Seguin N, Calzavara-Pinton P, Gilaberte Y, Haedersdal M, et al. European dermatology forum guidelines on topical photodynamic therapy 2019 part 1: treatment delivery and established indications - actinic keratoses, Bowen's disease and basal cell carcinomas. J Eur Acad Dermatol Venereol. 2019;33(12):2225–38. https://doi.org/10.1111/jdv.16017.
24. Wang H, Wang X, Guo MX, Yu Y. Topical 5-aminolaevnlinie aeid-photodynamie therapy in the treatment of precancerous changes and olla of the skin in

situ. Chin J Dermatol. 2006;39(3):137–9. https://doi.org/10.3760/j.issn:0412-4030.2006.03.006.
25. Xu S, Wang X, Zhang C, Zheng W, Xiao W. 5-Aminoketovalerate photodynamic therapy for skin basal cell carcinoma and squamous cell carcinoma. Chin J Dermatol. 1999;32(3):185–6. https://doi.org/10.3760/j.issn:0412-4030.1999.03.023.
26. Wang X, Xu S, Zhang C, Zheng W, Xiao W. Photodynamic therapy of Bowen's disease using 5-aminolevulinic acid. Chin J Laser Med. 1999;1:9–11. https://doi.org/10.3969/j.issn.1003-9430.1999.01.004.
27. Xu S, Wang X, Xu W, Xia Y, Zhang C. Evaluation of photodynamic therapy of skin cancers with δ-aminolevulinic acid. Chin Med J. 2002;115(8):1141–5. https://doi.org/10.3760/j.issn:0366-6999.2002.08.005.
28. Steeb T, Wessely A, Petzold A, Brinker TJ, Schmitz L, Leiter U, et al. Evaluation of long-term clearance rates of interventions for actinic keratosis: a systematic review and network meta-analysis. JAMA Dermatol. 2021;157(9):1066–77. https://doi.org/10.1001/jamadermatol.2021.2779.
29. Wachowska M, Muchowicz A, Demkow U. Immunological aspects of antitumor photodynamic therapy outcome. Cent Eur J Immunol. 2015;40(4):481–5. https://doi.org/10.5114/ceji.2015.56974.
30. Ji J, Zhang Y, Chen WR, Wang X. DC vaccine generated by ALA-PDT-induced immunogenic apoptotic cells for skin squamous cell carcinoma. Onco Targets Ther. 2016;5(6):e1072674. https://doi.org/10.1080/2162402X.2015.1072674.
31. Jeffes EW, McCullough JL, Weinstein GD, Fergin PE, Nelson JS, Shull TF, et al. Photodynamic therapy of actinic keratosis with topical 5-aminolevulinic acid. A pilot dose-ranging study. Arch Dermatol. 1997;133(6):727–32.
32. Zhang G, Cao Z, Wang P, Zhu L, Zhang L, Zho Z, et al. Comparison of efficacy, adverse effects and costs between 20% ALA-PDT and 10% ALA-PDT for the treatment of actinic keratosis in Chinese patients. Photodiagn Photodyn Ther. 2020;31:101605. https://doi.org/10.1016/j.pdpdt.2019.101605.
33. Ormrod D, Jarvis B. Topical aminolevulinic acid HCl photodynamic therapy. Am J Clin Dermatol. 2000;1(2):133–9.
34. Warren CB, Lohser S, Wene LC, Pogue BW, Bailin PL, Maytin EV. Noninvasive fluorescence monitoring of protoporphyrin IX production and clinical outcomes in actinic keratoses following short-contact application of 5-aminolevulinate. J Biomed Opt. 2010;15(5):051607. https://doi.org/10.1117/1.3484255.
35. Touma D, Yaar M, Whitehead S, Konnikov N, Gilchrest BA. A trial of short incubation, broad-area photodynamic therapy for facial actinic keratoses and diffuse photodamage. Arch Dermatol. 2004;140(1):33–40. https://doi.org/10.1001/archderm.140.1.33.
36. Braathen LR, Paredes BE, Saksela O, Fritsch C, Gardlo K, Morken T, et al. Short incubation with methyl aminolevulinate for photodynamic therapy of actinic keratoses. J Eur Acad Dermatol Venereol. 2009;23(5):550–5.
37. Nissen CV, Heerfordt IM, Wiegell SR, Mikkelsen CS, Wulf HC. Increased protoporphyrin IX accumulation does not improve the effect of photodynamic therapy for actinic keratosis: a randomized controlled trial. Br J Dermatol. 2017;176(5):1241–6. https://doi.org/10.1111/bjd.15098.
38. Tyrrell JS, Campbell SM, Curnow A. The relationship between protoporphyrin IX photobleaching during real-time dermatological methyl-aminolevulinate photodynamic therapy (MAL-PDT) and subsequent clinical outcome. Lasers Surg Med. 2010;42(7):613–9. https://doi.org/10.1002/lsm.20943.
39. Radakovic-Fijan S, Blecha-Thalhammer U, Kittler H, Honigsmann H, Tanew A. Efficacy of 3 different light doses in the treatment of actinic keratosis with 5-aminolevulinic acid photodynamic therapy: a randomized, observer-blinded, intrapatient, comparison study. J Am Acad Dermatol. 2005;53(5):823–7. https://doi.org/10.1016/j.jaad.2005.06.010.
40. Mordon S. Painless and efficient ALA-PDT and MAL-PDT of actinic keratosis can be achieved by drastically reducing the drug-light interval. Dermatol Ther. 2020;33(3):e13423.
41. Wang P, Zhang L, Zhou Z, Wei M, Shi L, Ji J, et al. Plum-blossom needle tapping enhances the efficacy of aminolevulinic acid-based photodynamic therapy for actinic keratosis, basal cell carcinoma and squamous cell carcinoma. Chin J Dermatol. 2015;48(2):80–4. https://doi.org/10.3760/cma.j.issn.0412-4030.2015.02.003.
42. Chen J, Zhang Y, Wang P, Wang B, Zhang G, Wang X. Plum-blossom needling promoted PpIX fluorescence intensity from 5-aminolevulinic acid in porcine skin model and patients with actnic keratosis. Photodiagn Photodyn Ther. 2016;15:182–90. https://doi.org/10.1016/j.pdpdt.2016.06.012.
43. Shi L, Zhou C, Li C, Hu C, Wang P, Zhang G, et al. Ulceration occurring after ALA-PDT combined with plum-blossom needle percussion for the treatment of pretibial Bowen's disease: a case report. Photodiagn Photodyn Ther. 2020;32:101958. https://doi.org/10.1016/j.pdpdt.2020.101958.
44. Wennberg A, Schmook T, Keohane SJPPP. A multicentre study of photodynamic therapy with methyl aminolaevulinate (MAL-PDT) in immunocompromised organ transplant recipients with non-melanoma skin cancer. Transplantation. 2005;21:218.
45. Wang H, Wang X, Guo M, Liu F. 5-aminolevulinic acid-photodynamic therapy and CO_2 laser for condylomata acuminata. J Clin Dermatol. 2006;35:674–5.
46. Morton CA. Methyl aminolevulinate: actinic keratoses and Bowen's disease. Dermatol

Clin. 2007;25(1):81. https://doi.org/10.1016/j.det.2006.09.009.
47. Braathen LR, Szeimies RM, Basset-Seguin N, Bissonnette R, Foley P, Pariser D, et al. Guidelines on the use of photodynamic therapy for nonmelanoma skin cancer: an international consensus. J Am Acad Dermatol. 2007;56(1):125–43. https://doi.org/10.1016/j.jaad.2006.06.006.
48. Wennberg AM, Stenquist B, Stockfleth E, Keohane S, Lear JT, Jemec G, et al. Photodynamic therapy with methyl aminolevulinate for prevention of new skin lesions in transplant recipients: a randomized study. Transplantation. 2008;86(3):423–9. https://doi.org/10.1097/TP.0b013e318180731e.
49. Apalla Z, Sotiriou E, Chovarda E, Lefaki I, Devliotou-Panagiotidou D, Ioannides D. Skin cancer: preventive photodynamic therapy in patients with face and scalp cancerization. A randomized placebo-controlled study. Br J Dermatol. 2010;162(1):171–5. https://doi.org/10.1111/j.1365-2133.2009.09492.x.
50. Brian Jiang SI, Kempers S, Rich P, Marcus S, Houlihan A, Piacquadio D, et al. A randomized, vehicle-controlled phase 3 study of aminolevulinic acid photodynamic therapy for the treatment of actinic keratoses on the upper extremities. Dermatologic Surg. 2019;45(7):890–7. https://doi.org/10.1097/DSS.0000000000001760.
51. Tschen EH, Wong DS, Pariser DM, Dunlap FE, Houlihan A, Ferdon MB, et al. Photodynamic therapy using aminolaevulinic acid for patients with nonhyperkeratotic actinic keratoses of the face and scalp: phase IV multicentre clinical trial with 12-month follow up. Br J Dermatol. 2006;155(6):1262–9. https://doi.org/10.1111/j.1365-2133.2006.07520.x.
52. Jansen M, Kessels J, Nelemans P, Kouloubis N, Arits A, van Pelt H, et al. Randomized trial of four treatment approaches for actinic keratosis. N Engl J Med. 2019;380(10):935–46. https://doi.org/10.1056/NEJMoa1811850.
53. Holzer G, Pinkowicz A, Radakovic S, Schmidt JB, Tanew A. Randomized controlled trial comparing 35% trichloroacetic acid peel and 5-aminolaevulinic acid photodynamic therapy for treating multiple actinic keratosis. Br J Dermatol. 2017;176(5):1155–61. https://doi.org/10.1111/bjd.15272.
54. Cai H, Wang YX, Sun P, Yang ZY, Tian R, Liu XY, et al. Photodynamic therapy for facial actinic keratosis: a clinical and histological study in Chinese patients. Photodiagn Photodyn Ther. 2013;10(3):260–5. https://doi.org/10.1016/j.pdpdt.2012.12.003.
55. Szeimies RM, Radny P, Sebastian M, Borrosch F, Dirschka T, Krahn-Senftleben G, et al. Photodynamic therapy with BF-200 ALA for the treatment of actinic keratosis: results of a prospective, randomized, double-blind, placebo-controlled phase III study. Br J Dermatol. 2010;163(2):386–94. https://doi.org/10.1111/j.1365-2133.2010.09873.x.
56. Kaufmann R, Spelman L, Weightman W, Reifenberger J, Szeimies RM, Verhaeghe E, et al. Multicentre intraindividual randomized trial of topical methyl aminolaevulinate-photodynamic therapy vs. cryotherapy for multiple actinic keratoses on the extremities. Br J Dermatol. 2008;158(5):994–9. https://doi.org/10.1111/j.1365-2133.2008.08488.x.
57. Szeimies RM, Karrer S, Radakovic-Fijan S, Tanew A, Calzavara-Pinton PG, Zane C, et al. Photodynamic therapy using topical methyl 5-aminolevulinate compared with cryotherapy for actinic keratosis: a prospective, randomized study. J Am Acad Dermatol. 2002;47(2):258–62.
58. Dirschka T, Ekanayake-Bohlig S, Dominicus R, Aschoff R, Herrera-Ceballos E, Botella-Estrada R, et al. A randomized, intraindividual, non-inferiority, phase III study comparing daylight photodynamic therapy with BF-200 ALA gel and MAL cream for the treatment of actinic keratosis. J Eur Acad Dermatol Venereol. 2019;33(2):288–97. https://doi.org/10.1111/jdv.15185.
59. Zhu L, Wang P, Zhang G, Zhang L, Liu X, Hu C, et al. Conventional versus daylight photodynamic therapy for actinic keratosis: a randomized and prospective study in China. Photodiagn Photodyn Ther. 2018;24:366–71. https://doi.org/10.1016/j.pdpdt.2018.10.010.
60. Lacour JP, Ulrich C, Gilaberte Y, Von Felbert V, Basset-Seguin N, Dreno B, et al. Daylight photodynamic therapy with methyl aminolevulinate cream is effective and nearly painless in treating actinic keratoses: a randomised, investigator-blinded, controlled, phase III study throughout Europe. J Eur Acad Dermatol Venereol. 2015;29(12):2342–8. https://doi.org/10.1111/jdv.13228.
61. Rubel DM, Spelman L, Murrell DF, See JA, Hewitt D, Foley P, et al. Daylight photodynamic therapy with methyl aminolevulinate cream as a convenient, similarly effective, nearly painless alternative to conventional photodynamic therapy in actinic keratosis treatment: a randomized controlled trial. Br J Dermatol. 2014;171(5):1164–71. https://doi.org/10.1111/bjd.13138.
62. Bai-Habelski JC, Ko A, Ortland C, Stocker M, Ebeling A, Reinhold U. 5-ALA loaded self-adhesive patch-PDT is effective and safe in the treatment of actinic keratoses on hands and arms. Exp Dermatol. 2022;31(9):1385–91. https://doi.org/10.1111/exd.14606.
63. Szeimies RM, Stockfleth E, Popp G, Borrosch F, Bruning H, Dominicus R, et al. Long-term follow-up of photodynamic therapy with a self-adhesive 5-aminolaevulinic acid patch: 12 months data. Br J Dermatol. 2010;162(2):410–4. https://doi.org/10.1111/j.1365-2133.2009.09377.x.
64. Hauschild A, Popp G, Stockfleth E, Meyer KG, Imberger D, Mohr P, et al. Effective photodynamic therapy of actinic keratoses on the head and face with a novel, self-adhesive 5-aminolaevulinic acid

patch. Exp Dermatol. 2009;18(2):116–21. https://doi.org/10.1111/j.1600-0625.2008.00770.x.
65. Abrouk M, Gianatasio C, Li YM, Waibel JS. Prospective study of intense pulsed light versus pulsed dye laser with or without blue light in the activation of PDT for the treatment of actinic keratosis and photodamage. Lasers Surg Med. 2022;54(1):66–73. https://doi.org/10.1002/lsm.23492.
66. Kohl E, Popp C, Zeman F, Unger P, Koller M, Landthaler M, et al. Photodynamic therapy using intense pulsed light for treating actinic keratoses and photoaged skin of the dorsal hands: a randomized placebo-controlled study. Br J Dermatol. 2017;176(2):352–62. https://doi.org/10.1111/bjd.14970.
67. Ruiz-Rodriguez R, Sanz-Sanchez T, Cordoba S. Photodynamic photorejuvenation. Dermatologic Surg. 2002;28(8):742–4. https://doi.org/10.1097/00042728-200208000-00019.
68. Wang XL, Wang HW, Guo MX, Xu SZ. Treatment of skin cancer and pre-cancer using topical ALA-PDT - a single hospital experience. Photodiagn Photodyn Ther. 2008;5(2):127–33. https://doi.org/10.1016/j.pdpdt.2008.05.003.
69. Toledo-Alberola F, Belinchon-Romero I, Guijarro-Llorca J, Albares-Tendero P. Photodynamic therapy as a response to the challenge of treating actinic keratosis in the eyelid area. Actas Dermosifiliogr. 2012;103(10):938–9. https://doi.org/10.1016/j.ad.2011.10.021.
70. Han J, Wang P, Wang X. Clinical effect and safety of 5-aminolevulinic acid photodynamic therapy in the treatment of nose actinic keratosis. Chin J Ophthal Otolaryngol. 2018;18(3):175–7. https://doi.org/10.14166/j.issn.1671-2420.2018.03.011.
71. Zhang YF, Zhang GL, Yang DG, Lai YX, Zhang LL, Wang PR, et al. Egg membrane may protect eyes from ALA photodynamic therapy for eyelid actinic keratosis: two case reports. Photodiagn Photodyn Ther. 2016;15:156–8. https://doi.org/10.1016/j.pdpdt.2016.06.005.
72. Li J, Zhang Y, Zhang G, Zhang L, Zhou Z, Wang P, et al. Modified painless photodynamic therapy for facial multiple actinic keratosis in China: a prospective split-face control study. Lasers Surg Med. 2023;55(10):871–9. https://doi.org/10.1002/lsm.23728.
73. Mordon S, Vignion-Dewalle AS, Abi-Rached H, Thecua E, Lecomte F, Vicentini C, et al. The conventional protocol vs. a protocol including illumination with a fabric-based biophotonic device (the Phosistos protocol) in photodynamic therapy for actinic keratosis: a randomized, controlled, noninferiority clinical study. Br J Dermatol. 2020;182(1):76–84. https://doi.org/10.1111/bjd.18048.
74. Batchelor RJ, Stables GI, Stringer MR. Successful treatment of scalp actinic keratoses with photodynamic therapy using ambient light. Br J Dermatol. 2007;156(4):779–81. https://doi.org/10.1111/j.1365-2133.2007.07755.x.
75. Fitzmaurice S, Eisen DB. Daylight photodynamic therapy: what is known and what is yet to be determined. Dermatologic Surg. 2016;42(3):286–95. https://doi.org/10.1097/Dss.0000000000000633.
76. Wiegell SR, Haedersdal M, Philipsen PA, Eriksen P, Enk CD, Wulf HC. Continuous activation of PpIX by daylight is as effective as and less painful than conventional photodynamic therapy for actinic keratoses; a randomized, controlled, single-blinded study. Br J Dermatol. 2008;158(4):740–6. https://doi.org/10.1111/j.1365-2133.2008.08450.x.
77. Wiegell SR, Fabricius S, Stender IM, Berne B, Kroon S, Andersen BL, et al. A randomized, multicentre study of directed daylight exposure times of 1(1/2) vs. 2(1/2) h in daylight-mediated photodynamic therapy with methyl aminolaevulinate in patients with multiple thin actinic keratoses of the face and scalp. Br J Dermatol. 2011;164(5):1083–90. https://doi.org/10.1111/j.1365-2133.2011.10209.x.
78. Wiegell SR, Heydenreich J, Fabricius S, Wulf HC. Continuous ultra-low-intensity artificial daylight is not as effective as red LED light in photodynamic therapy of multiple actinic keratoses. Photodermatol Photoimmunol Photomed. 2011;27(6):280–5. https://doi.org/10.1111/j.1600-0781.2011.00611.x.
79. Togsverd-Bo K, Lei U, Erlendsson AM, Taudorf EH, Philipsen PA, Wulf HC, et al. Combination of ablative fractional laser and daylight-mediated photodynamic therapy for actinic keratosis in organ transplant recipients - a randomized controlled trial. Br J Dermatol. 2015;172(2):467–74. https://doi.org/10.1111/bjd.13222.
80. Hauschild A, Stockfleth E, Popp G, Borrosch F, Bruning H, Dominicus R, et al. Optimization of photodynamic therapy with a novel self-adhesive 5-aminolaevulinic acid patch: results of two randomized controlled phase III studies. Br J Dermatol. 2009;160(5):1066–74. https://doi.org/10.1111/j.1365-2133.2009.09040.x.
81. Babilas P, Knobler R, Hummel S, Gottschaller C, Maisch T, Koller M, et al. Variable pulsed light is less painful than light-emitting diodes for topical photodynamic therapy of actinic keratosis: a prospective randomized controlled trial. Br J Dermatol. 2007;157(1):111–7. https://doi.org/10.1111/j.1365-2133.2007.07959.x.
82. Haddad A, Santos IDDO, Gragnani A, Ferreira LM. The effect of increasing fluence on the treatment of actinic keratosis and photodamage by photodynamic therapy with 5-aminolevulinic acid and intense pulsed light. Photomed Laser Surg. 2011;29(6):427–32. https://doi.org/10.1089/pho.2009.2733.
83. Morton CA, Birnie AJ, Eedy DJ. British Association of Dermatologists' guidelines for the management of squamous cell carcinoma in situ (Bowen's disease) 2014. Br J Dermatol. 2014;170(2):245–60. https://doi.org/10.1111/bjd.12766.

84. Neagu TP, Tiglis M, Botezatu D, Enache V, Cobilinschi CO, Valcea-Precup MS, et al. Clinical, histological and therapeutic features of Bowen's disease. Romanian J Morphol Embryol. 2017;58(1):33–40.
85. Tokez S, Wakkee M, Louwman M, Noels E, Nijsten T, Hollestein L. Assessment of cutaneous squamous cell carcinoma (cSCC) in situ incidence and the risk of developing invasive cSCC in patients with prior cSCC in situ vs the general population in The Netherlands, 1989-2017. JAMA Dermatol. 2020;156(9):973–81. https://doi.org/10.1001/jamadermatol.2020.1988.
86. Kennedy JC, Pottier RH, Pross DC. Photodynamic therapy with endogenous protoporphyrin IX: basic principles and present clinical experience. J Photochem Photobiol B. 1990;6(1–2):143–8. https://doi.org/10.1016/1011-1344(90)85083-9.
87. Photodynamic Therapy Research Center. Expert consensus on clinical application of photodynamic therapy with 5-aminolevulinic acid. Chin J Dermatol. 2015;48(10):675–8. https://doi.org/10.3760/cma.j.issn.0412-4030.2015.10.001.
88. Photodynamic Therapy Research Center, Chinese Medical Association, Dermatology Rehabilitation Committee, Light medical treatment Equipment Group, Chinese Medical Equipment Association. Guidelines for clinical application of 5-aminolevulinic acid photodynamic therapy dermatology (2021 version). Chin J Dermatol. 2021;54(1):1–9.
89. Shi L, Wang H, Chen K, Yan J, Yu B, Wang S, et al. Chinese guidelines on the clinical application of 5-aminolevulinic acid-based photodynamic therapy in dermatology (2021 edition). Photodiagn Photodyn Ther. 2021;35:102340. https://doi.org/10.1016/j.pdpdt.2021.102340.
90. Ozog DM, Rkein AM, Fabi SG, Gold MH, Goldman MP, Lowe NJ, et al. Photodynamic therapy: a clinical consensus guide. Dermatologic Surg. 2016;42(7):804–27. https://doi.org/10.1097/DSS.0000000000000800.
91. Morton CA, Whitehurst C, McColl JH, Moore JV, MacKie RM. Photodynamic therapy for large or multiple patches of Bowen disease and basal cell carcinoma. Arch Dermatol. 2001;137(3):319–24.
92. Wu MF, Lv T, Wang HW. Successful treatment for multiple Bowen's disease using photodynamic therapy: a case report. Photodiagn Photodyn Ther. 2020;30:101783. https://doi.org/10.1016/j.pdpdt.2020.101783.
93. Lv T, Zhang JC, Miao F, Wang HW. Aminoleveulinate photodynamic therapy (ALA-PDT) for Bowen's disease in a SLE patient: case report and literature review. Photodiagn Photodyn Ther. 2017;18:20–3. https://doi.org/10.1016/j.pdpdt.2017.01.002.
94. Abramson AL, Alvi A, Mullooly VM. Clinical exacerbation of systemic lupus erythematosus after photodynamic therapy of laryngotracheal papillomatosis. Lasers Surg Med. 1993;13(6):677–9. https://doi.org/10.1002/lsm.1900130613.
95. Zhao Z, Wu Y, Zhou Z, Zhao Y, Sun X, Hu C, et al. ALA-PDT successfully treated multiple cSCC in situ and AK in a patient with epidermodysplasia verruciformis. Photodiagn Photodyn Ther. 2021;35:102395. https://doi.org/10.1016/j.pdpdt.2021.102395.
96. Wu Y, Wang P, Zhang L, Wang B, Wang X. Enhancement of photodynamic therapy for Bowen's disease using plum-blossom needling to augment drug delivery. Dermatologic Surg. 2018;44(12):1516–24. https://doi.org/10.1097/DSS.0000000000001608.
97. Yang JQ. Cinical efficacy of dermabrasion combined with photodynamic therapy forth treatment of Bowen disease. J Clin Dermatol. 2014;43(12):743–5.
98. Salim A, Leman JA, McColl JH, Chapman R, Morton CA. Randomized comparison of photodynamic therapy with topical 5-fluorouracil in Bowen's disease. Br J Dermatol. 2003;148(3):539–43. https://doi.org/10.1046/j.1365-2133.2003.05033.x.
99. Roopashree MR, Gondhalekar RV, Shashikanth MC, George J, Thippeswamy SH, Shukla A. Pathogenesis of oral lichen planus–a review. J Oral Pathol Med. 2010;39(10):729–34. https://doi.org/10.1111/j.1600-0714.2010.00946.x.
100. Zhong S, Zhang R, Mei X, Wang L. Efficacy of photodynamic therapy for the treatment of Bowen's disease: an updated systematic review and meta-analysis of randomized controlled trials. Photodiagn Photodyn Ther. 2020;32:102037. https://doi.org/10.1016/j.pdpdt.2020.102037.
101. Cervantes JA, Zeitouni NC. Photodynamic therapy utilizing 10% ALA nano-emulsion gel and red-light for the treatment of squamous cell carcinoma in-situ on the trunk and extremities: pilot study and literature update. Photodiagn Photodyn Ther. 2021;35:102358. https://doi.org/10.1016/j.pdpdt.2021.102358.
102. Kibbi N, Zhang Y, Leffell DJ, Christensen SR. Photodynamic therapy for cutaneous squamous cell carcinoma in situ: impact of anatomic location, tumor diameter, and incubation time on effectiveness. J Am Acad Dermatol. 2020;82(5):1124–30. https://doi.org/10.1016/j.jaad.2019.10.079.
103. Gomez C, Cobos M, Alberdi E. Methyl aminolevulinate-based photodynamic therapy of Bowen's disease: observational study of 21 lesions. Photodiagn Photodyn Ther. 2019;26:295–9. https://doi.org/10.1016/j.pdpdt.2019.04.011.
104. Alique-Garcia S, Alique D, Company-Quiroga J, Sanchez A, Nunez AH, Borbujo J. Treatment of Bowen's disease with photodynamic therapy. Observational study in 171 patients with 5-aminolaevulinic acid (BF-200 ALA) and methyl aminolaevulinate (MAL). Photodiagn Photodyn Ther. 2019;28:192–4. https://doi.org/10.1016/j.pdpdt.2019.08.011.
105. Aguilar-Bernier M, Rodriguez-Baron D, Rivas-Ruiz F, Segura-Palacios JM, de Troya Martin M. Long-

term efficacy of photodynamic therapy with methyl aminolevulinate in treating Bowen's disease in clinical practice: a retrospective cohort study (2006-2017). Photodermatol Photoimmunol Photomed. 2019;35(4):208–13. https://doi.org/10.1111/phpp.12453.
106. Zaar O, Fougelberg J, Hermansson A, Gillstedt M, Wennberg-Larko AM, Paoli J. Effectiveness of photodynamic therapy in Bowen's disease: a retrospective observational study in 423 lesions. J Eur Acad Dermatol Venereol. 2017;31(8):1289–94. https://doi.org/10.1111/jdv.14164.
107. Gracia-Cazana T, Mascaraque M, Salazar N, Vera-Alvarez J, Frias MP, Gonzalez S, et al. Photodynamic therapy: influence of clinical and procedure variables on treatment response in basal cell carcinoma and Bowen disease. Acta Derm Venereol. 2018;98(1):116–8. https://doi.org/10.2340/00015555-2756.
108. Jansen MH, Appelen D, Nelemans PJ, Winnepenninckx VJ, Kelleners-Smeets NWJ, Mosterd K. Bowen's disease: long-term results of treatment with 5-fluorouracil cream, photodynamic therapy or surgical excision. Acta Derm Venereol. 2018;98(1):114–5. https://doi.org/10.2340/00015555-2777.
109. Hambly R, Mansoor N, Quinlan C, Shah Z, Lenane P, Ralph N, et al. Topical photodynamic therapy for primary Bowen disease and basal cell carcinoma: optimizing patient selection. Br J Dermatol. 2017;177(3):e55–7. https://doi.org/10.1111/bjd.15281.
110. Stables GI, Stringer MR, Robinson DJ, Ash DV. Erythroplasia of Queyrat treated by topical aminolaevulinic acid photodynamic therapy. Br J Dermatol. 1999;140(3):514–7. https://doi.org/10.1046/j.1365-2133.1999.02720.x.
111. Feng G, Wang Y, Fang F. Current status and progress in the treatment of erythema proliferatum. Int J Dermatol Venereol. 2015;41(5):294–7.
112. Deen K, Burdon-Jones D. Imiquimod in the treatment of penile intraepithelial neoplasia: an update. Australas J Dermatol. 2017;58(2):86–92. https://doi.org/10.1111/ajd.12466.
113. Patrascoiu ST, Gingu C, Dick A, Cretu O, Surcel C, Vlaicu N, et al. Erythroplasia of Queirat, an unrecognized and undertreated disease. Eur Urol Suppl. 2013;12(4):e1184. https://doi.org/10.1016/s1569-9056(13)61924-7.
114. van Bezooijen BP, Horenblas S, Meinhardt W, Newling DW. Laser therapy for carcinoma in situ of the penis. J Urol. 2001;166(5):1670–1. https://doi.org/10.1097/00005392-200111000-00013.
115. Paoli J, Ternesten Bratel A, Lowhagen GB, Stenquist B, Forslund O, Wennberg AM. Penile intraepithelial neoplasia: results of photodynamic therapy. Acta Derm Venereol. 2006;86(5):418–21. https://doi.org/10.2340/00015555-0130.
116. Hanjun L, Xiaohua Z, Wei Q. Clinical observation of 8 cases of proliferative erythema treated with 5-aminolevulinic acid photodynamic therapy. Clin Med Res Pract. 2019;4(16):157–8. https://doi.org/10.19347/j.cnki.2096-1413.201916065.
117. Chen N, Lei X, Cheng Q. A successful treatment with ALA-PDT: a case-report on erythroplasia of Queyrat misdiagnosed as urethritis. Photodiagn Photodyn Ther. 2023;42:103506. https://doi.org/10.1016/j.pdpdt.2023.103506.
118. Kaprin AD, Ivanova-Radkevich VI, Urlova AN, Asratov AT, Gushchina YS, Libo L, et al. Successes of photodynamic therapy in treatment of erythroplasia of Queyrat. Biomed Photon. 2020;9(1):34–41. https://doi.org/10.24931/2413-9432-2020-9-1-34-41.
119. Park JY, Kim SJ, Kim YC. Erythroplasia of Queyrat refractory to photodynamic therapy. Clin Exp Dermatol. 2012;37(7):795–7. https://doi.org/10.1111/j.1365-2230.2012.04361.x.
120. Fai D, Romano I, Cassano N, Vena GA. Methylaminolevulinate photodynamic therapy for the treatment of erythroplasia of Queyrat in 23 patients. J Dermatolog Treat. 2012;23(5):330–2. https://doi.org/10.3109/09546634.2011.577405.
121. Maranda EL, Nguyen AH, Lim VM, Shah VV, Jimenez JJ. Erythroplasia of Queyrat treated by laser and light modalities: a systematic review. Lasers Med Sci. 2016;31(9):1971–6. https://doi.org/10.1007/s10103-016-2005-9.
122. Feldmeyer L, Krausz-Enderlin V, Tondury B, Hafner J, French LE, Hofbauer GF. Methylaminolaevulinic acid photodynamic therapy in the treatment of erythroplasia of Queyrat. Dermatology. 2011;223(1):52–6. https://doi.org/10.1159/000330328.
123. Iafrate M, Mancini M, Prayer Galetti T, Szekely S, Zattra E, Vaccari D, et al. Efficacy of topical photodynamic therapy in the treatment of Erythroplasia of Queyrat. Dermatol Reports. 2020;12(1):8566. https://doi.org/10.4081/dr.2020.8566.
124. Skroza N, La Viola G, Pampena R, Proietti I, Bernardini N, Tolino E, et al. Erythroplasia of Queyrat treated with methyl aminolevulinate-photodynamic therapy. G Ital Dermatol Venereol. 2020;155(1):103–6. https://doi.org/10.23736/S0392-0488.16.05163-4.
125. Peris K, Fargnoli MC, Garbe C, Kaufmann R, Bastholt L, Seguin NB, et al. Diagnosis and treatment of basal cell carcinoma: European consensus-based interdisciplinary guidelines. Eur J Cancer. 2019;118:10–34. https://doi.org/10.1016/j.ejca.2019.06.003.
126. Work G, Invited R, Kim JYS, Kozlow JH, Mittal B, Moyer J, et al. Guidelines of care for the management of basal cell carcinoma. J Am Acad Dermatol. 2018;78(3):540–59. https://doi.org/10.1016/j.jaad.2017.10.006.
127. Bartos V, Pokorny D, Zacharova O, Haluska P, Doboszova J, Kullova M, et al. Recurrent basal cell carcinoma: a clinicopathological study and evaluation of histomorphological findings in primary

and recurrent lesions. Acta Dermatovenerol Alp Pannonica Adriat. 2011;20(2):67–75.
128. Bichakjian CK, Olencki T, Aasi SZ, Alam M, Andersen JS, Berg D, et al. Basal cell skin cancer, version 1.2016, NCCN clinical practice guidelines in oncology. J Natl Compr Cancer Netw. 2016;14(5):574–97. https://doi.org/10.6004/jnccn.2016.0065.
129. Nahhas AF, Scarbrough CA, Trotter S. A review of the global guidelines on surgical margins for nonmelanoma skin cancers. J Clin Aesthet Dermatol. 2017;10(4):37–46.
130. Sin CW, Barua A, Cook A. Recurrence rates of periocular basal cell carcinoma following Mohs micrographic surgery: a retrospective study. Int J Dermatol. 2016;55(9):1044–7. https://doi.org/10.1111/ijd.13326.
131. Basset-Seguin N, Hauschild A, Kunstfeld R, Grob J, Dreno B, Mortier L, et al. Vismodegib in patients with advanced basal cell carcinoma: primary analysis of STEVIE, an international, open-label trial. Eur J Cancer. 2017;86:334–48. https://doi.org/10.1016/j.ejca.2017.08.022.
132. Migden MR, Guminski A, Gutzmer R, Dirix L, Lewis KD, Combemale P, et al. Treatment with two different doses of sonidegib in patients with locally advanced or metastatic basal cell carcinoma (BOLT): a multicentre, randomised, double-blind phase 2 trial. Lancet Oncol. 2015;16(6):716–28. https://doi.org/10.1016/S1470-2045(15)70100-2.
133. Bu W, Zhang M, Zhang Q, Yuan C, Chen X, Fang F. Preliminary results of comparative study for subsequent photodynamic therapy versus secondary excision after primary excision for treating basal cell carcinoma. Photodiagn Photodyn Ther. 2017;17:134–7. https://doi.org/10.1016/j.pdpdt.2016.11.003.
134. Li X, Tan L, Kou H, Zhang J, Wang Y, Li G, et al. Ocular preservation through limited tumor excision combined with ALA-PDT in patients with periocular basal cell carcinoma. Photodiagn Photodyn Ther. 2019;27:291–4. https://doi.org/10.1016/j.pdpdt.2019.06.016.
135. Cao D, Zhu W, Kuang Y, Zhao S. A safe and effective treatment: surgery combined with photodynamic therapy for multiple basal cell carcinomas. Photodiagn Photodyn Ther. 2019;28:133–5. https://doi.org/10.1016/j.pdpdt.2019.09.001.
136. Morton CA, Dominicus R, Radny P, Dirschka T, Hauschild A, Reinhold U, et al. A randomized, multinational, noninferiority, phase III trial to evaluate the safety and efficacy of BF-200 aminolaevulinic acid gel vs. methyl aminolaevulinate cream in the treatment of nonaggressive basal cell carcinoma with photodynamic therapy. Br J Dermatol. 2018;179(2):309–19. https://doi.org/10.1111/bjd.16441.
137. Wiegell SR, Skodt V, Wulf HC. Daylight-mediated photodynamic therapy of basal cell carcinomas - an explorative study. J Eur Acad Dermatol Venereol. 2014;28(2):169–75. https://doi.org/10.1111/jdv.12076.
138. Wang P, Zhou Z, Wei M, Shi L, Ji J, Yang D, et al. Plum-blossom needle tapping enhances the efficacy of aminolevulinic acid-based photodynamic therapy for actinic keratosis, basal cell carcinoma and squamous cell carcinoma. Chin J Dermatol. 2015;48(2):80–4.
139. Wolf P, Rieger E, Kerl H. Topical photodynamic therapy with endogenous porphyrins after application of 5-aminolevulinic acid. An alternative treatment modality for solar keratoses, superficial squamous cell carcinomas, and basal cell carcinomas? J Am Acad Dermatol. 1993;28(1):17–21. https://doi.org/10.1016/0190-9622(93)70002-b.
140. Christensen E, Mork C, Skogvoll E. High and sustained efficacy after two sessions of topical 5-aminolaevulinic acid photodynamic therapy for basal cell carcinoma: a prospective, clinical and histological 10-year follow-up study. Br J Dermatol. 2012;166(6):1342–8. https://doi.org/10.1111/j.1365-2133.2012.10878.x.
141. Cosgarea R, Susan M, Crisan M, Senila S. Photodynamic therapy using topical 5-aminolaevulinic acid vs. surgery for basal cell carcinoma. J Eur Acad Dermatol Venereol. 2013;27(8):980–4.
142. Zhang Y, Zhang H, Zhang L, Wang P, Shi L, Zhang G, et al. Modified 5-aminolevulinic acid photodynamic therapy to reduce pain in the treatment of moderate to severe acne vulgaris: a prospective, randomized, split-face study. J Am Acad Dermatol. 2021;84(1):218–20. https://doi.org/10.1016/j.jaad.2020.04.146.
143. Liao C, Zhang G, Wang P, Sun X, Wang X. Combination curettage and modified ALA-PDT for multiple basal cell carcinomas of the face and head. Photodiagn Photodyn Ther. 2021;35:102393. https://doi.org/10.1016/j.pdpdt.2021.102393.
144. Liao C, Shi L, Wang D, Wang X. Bimodal photodynamic therapy for treatment of a 91-year-old patient with locally advanced cutaneous basal cell carcinoma and postoperative scar management. Photodiagn Photodyn Ther. 2021;36:102553. https://doi.org/10.1016/j.pdpdt.2021.102553.
145. Kallini JR, Hamed N, Khachemoune A. Squamous cell carcinoma of the skin: epidemiology, classification, management, and novel trends. Int J Dermatol. 2015;54(2):130–40. https://doi.org/10.1111/ijd.12553.
146. Venables ZC, Autier P, Nijsten T, Wong KF, Langan SM, Rous B, et al. Nationwide incidence of metastatic cutaneous squamous cell carcinoma in England. JAMA Dermatol. 2019;155(3):298–306. https://doi.org/10.1001/jamadermatol.2018.4219.
147. Stratigos AJ, Garbe C, Dessinioti C, Lebbe C, Bataille V, Bastholt L, et al. European interdisciplinary guideline on invasive squamous cell carcinoma of the skin: part 1. Epidemiology, diagnostics and

prevention. Eur J Cancer. 2020;128:60–82. https://doi.org/10.1016/j.ejca.2020.01.007.
148. Muzic JG, Schmitt AR, Wright AC, Alniemi DT, Zubair AS, Olazagasti Lourido JM, et al. Incidence and trends of basal cell carcinoma and cutaneous squamous cell carcinoma: a population-based study in Olmsted County, Minnesota, 2000 to 2010. Mayo Clin Proc. 2017;92(6):890–8. https://doi.org/10.1016/j.mayocp.2017.02.015.
149. Gao T-W, Sun D-J, Li C-Y, He H, Li Q, Liu Y-S, et al. Retrospective analysis of 1905 patients with skin cancer from two general hospitals in western China from 1981 to 2000. J Peking Univ Health Sci. 2004;36(5):469–72.
150. Tu Q, Lv T, Lai Y, Zhang L, Shi L, Li J, et al. Epidemiological study of elderly skin tumors in a community in Shanghai. Geriatr Health Care. 2013;19:142–5.
151. de Gruijl FR, Rebel H. Early events in UV carcinogenesis–DNA damage, target cells and mutant p53 foci. Photochem Photobiol. 2008;84(2):382–7. https://doi.org/10.1111/j.1751-1097.2007.00275.x.
152. Que SKT, Zwald FO, Schmults CD. Cutaneous squamous cell carcinoma: incidence, risk factors, diagnosis, and staging. J Am Acad Dermatol. 2018;78(2):237–47. https://doi.org/10.1016/j.jaad.2017.08.059.
153. Brown VL, Harwood CA, Crook T, Cronin JG, Kelsell DP, Proby CM. p16INK4a and p14ARF tumor suppressor genes are commonly inactivated in cutaneous squamous cell carcinoma. J Invest Dermatol. 2004;122(5):1284–92. https://doi.org/10.1111/j.0022-202X.2004.22501.x.
154. Yan G, Li L, Zhu S, Wu Y, Liu Y, Zhu L, et al. Single-cell transcriptomic analysis reveals the critical molecular pattern of UV-induced cutaneous squamous cell carcinoma. Cell Death Dis. 2021;13(1):23. https://doi.org/10.1038/s41419-021-04477-y.
155. Zhang G, Yan G, Fu Z, Wu Y, Wu F, Zheng Z, et al. Loss of retinoic acid receptor-related receptor alpha (Rorα) promotes the progression of UV-induced cSCC. Cell Death Dis. 2021;12(3):247. https://doi.org/10.1038/s41419-021-03525-x.
156. Skin Tumor Research Center, Subcommittee on Skin Tumor, China Dermatologist Association. Consensus on diagnosis and treatment of cutaneous squamous cell carcinoma. Chin J Dermatol. 2021;54(8):653–64.
157. Work G, Invited R, Kim JYS, Kozlow JH, Mittal B, Moyer J, et al. Guidelines of care for the management of cutaneous squamous cell carcinoma. J Am Acad Dermatol. 2018;78(3):560–78. https://doi.org/10.1016/j.jaad.2017.10.007.
158. Leibovitch I, Huilgol SC, Selva D, Hill D, Richards S, Paver R. Cutaneous squamous cell carcinoma treated with Mohs micrographic surgery in Australia I. Experience over 10 years. J Am Acad Dermatol. 2005;53(2):253–60. https://doi.org/10.1016/j.jaad.2005.02.059.
159. Humphreys TR, Malhotra R, Scharf MJ, Marcus SM, Starkus L, Calegari K. Treatment of superficial basal cell carcinoma and squamous cell carcinoma in situ with a high-energy pulsed carbon dioxide laser. Arch Dermatol. 1998;134(10):1247–52. https://doi.org/10.1001/archderm.134.10.1247.
160. Peris K, Micantonio T, Fargnoli MC, Lozzi GP, Chimenti S. Imiquimod 5% cream in the treatment of Bowen's disease and invasive squamous cell carcinoma. J Am Acad Dermatol. 2006;55(2):324–7. https://doi.org/10.1016/j.jaad.2006.04.004.
161. Migden MR, Rischin D, Schmults CD, Guminski A, Hauschild A, Lewis KD, et al. PD-1 blockade with cemiplimab in advanced cutaneous squamous-cell carcinoma. N Engl J Med. 2018;379(4):341–51. https://doi.org/10.1056/NEJMoa1805131.
162. Preneau S, Rio E, Brocard A, Peuvrel L, Nguyen JM, Quereux G, et al. Efficacy of cetuximab in the treatment of squamous cell carcinoma. J Dermatolog Treat. 2014;25(5):424–7. https://doi.org/10.3109/09546634.2012.751481.
163. Wang X, Xu S, Zhang C, Zheng W. Photodynamic therapy of Bowen's disease using 5-aminolevulinic acid. Chin J Laser Med Surg. 1999;8(1):9–11.
164. Wang H, Wang X, Guo M, Yu Y. Topical 5-aminolaevulinic acid-photodynamic therapy in the treatment of precancerous changes and carcinoma of the skin in situ. Chin J Dermatol. 1995;35:102438.
165. Reginato E, Wolf P, Hamblin MR. Immune response after photodynamic therapy increases anti-cancer and anti-bacterial effects. World J Immunol. 2014;4(1):1–11. https://doi.org/10.5411/wji.v4.i1.1.
166. Lü T, Wang X, Zhou W, Wang H, Miao F, Li J. Establishment of mouse model for cutaneous squamous cell carcinoma induced by ultraviolet. Chin J Dermatol. 2011;3:174–7.
167. Wang H, Li J, Lv T, Tu Q, Huang Z, Wang X. Therapeutic and immune effects of 5-aminolevulinic acid photodynamic therapy on UVB-induced squamous cell carcinomas in hairless mice. Exp Dermatol. 2013;22(5):362–3. https://doi.org/10.1111/exd.12132.
168. Ji J, Fan Z, Zhou F, Wang X, Shi L, Zhang H, et al. Improvement of DC vaccine with ALA-PDT induced immunogenic apoptotic cells for skin squamous cell carcinoma. Oncotarget. 2015;6(19):17135–46. https://doi.org/10.18632/oncotarget.3529.
169. Zhang H, Wang P, Wang X, Shi L, Fan Z, Zhang G, et al. Antitumor effects of DC vaccine with ALA-PDT-induced immunogenic apoptotic cells for skin squamous cell carcinoma in mice. Technol Cancer Res Treat. 2018;17:1533033818785275. https://doi.org/10.1177/1533033818785275.
170. Ji J, Wang P, Zhou Q, Zhu L, Zhang H, Zhang Y, et al. CCL8 enhances sensitivity of cutaneous squamous cell carcinoma to photodynamic therapy by recruiting M1 macrophages. Photodiagn Photodyn Ther. 2019;26:235–43. https://doi.org/10.1016/j.pdpdt.2019.03.014.

171. Zhu L, Zhang G, Wang P, Zhang L, Ji J, Liu X, et al. The effect of C-X-C motif chemokine ligand 13 in cutaneous squamous cell carcinoma treated with aminolevulinic acid-photodynamic therapy. Photodiagn Photodyn Ther. 2019;26:389–94. https://doi.org/10.1016/j.pdpdt.2019.04.018.
172. Li S, Wang P, Zhang G, Ji J, Lv T, Wang X, et al. The effect of ALA-PDT on reversing the activation of cancer-associated fibroblasts in cutaneous squamous cell carcinoma. Photodiagn Photodyn Ther. 2019;27:234–40. https://doi.org/10.1016/j.pdpdt.2019.05.043.
173. Zhao Z, Zhang H, Zeng Q, Wang P, Zhang G, Ji J, et al. Exosomes from 5-aminolevulinic acid photodynamic therapy-treated squamous carcinoma cells promote dendritic cell maturation. Photodiagn Photodyn Ther. 2020;30:101746. https://doi.org/10.1016/j.pdpdt.2020.101746.
174. Copper MP, Triesscheijn M, Tan IB, Ruevekamp MC, Stewart FA. Photodynamic therapy in the treatment of multiple primary tumours in the head and neck, located to the oral cavity and oropharynx. Clin Otolaryngol. 2007;32(3):185–9. https://doi.org/10.1111/j.1365-2273.2007.01441.x.
175. Li Q, Gao T, Long HA, Ujiie H. Clearance of a thick invasive squamous cell carcinoma after multiple treatments with topical photodynamic therapy. Photomed Laser Surg. 2010;28(5):703–6. https://doi.org/10.1089/pho.2009.2610.
176. Wang P, Zhang G, Zhang L, Zhou Z, Shi L, Zeng Q, et al. 5-Aminolevulinic acid photodynamic therapy for early-stage lip squamous cell carcinoma. Photodiagn Photodyn Ther. 2021;35:102321. https://doi.org/10.1016/j.pdpdt.2021.102321.
177. Fargnoli MC, Kostaki D, Piccioni A, Di Stefani A, Peris K. Photodynamic therapy for the treatment of microinvasive squamous cell carcinoma of the lower lip: a case report. G Ital Dermatol Venereol. 2015;150(3):331–5.
178. Tarstedt M, Gillstedt M, Wennberg Larko AM, Paoli J. Aminolevulinic acid and methyl aminolevulinate equally effective in topical photodynamic therapy for non-melanoma skin cancers. J Eur Acad Dermatol Venereol. 2016;30(3):420–3. https://doi.org/10.1111/jdv.13558.
179. Yongpisarn T, Rigo R, Minkis K. Durable clearance rate of photodynamic therapy for Bowen disease and cutaneous squamous cell carcinoma: a systematic review and meta-analysis. Dermatologic Surg. 2022;48(4):395–400. https://doi.org/10.1097/DSS.0000000000003401.
180. Wang P, Zhang L, Zhang G, Zhou Z, Zhang H, Zhao Z, et al. Successful treatment of giant invasive cutaneous squamous cell carcinoma by plum-blossom needle assisted photodynamic therapy sequential with imiquimod: case experience. Photodiagn Photodyn Ther. 2018;21:393–5. https://doi.org/10.1016/j.pdpdt.2017.12.010.
181. Bhatta AK, Wang P, Keyal U, Zhao Z, Ji J, Zhu L, et al. Therapeutic effect of imiquimod enhanced ALA-PDT on cutaneous squamous cell carcinoma. Photodiagn Photodyn Ther. 2018;23:273–80. https://doi.org/10.1016/j.pdpdt.2018.07.010.
182. Ulrich M, Reinhold U, Dominicus R, Aschoff R, Szeimies RM, Dirschka T. Red light photodynamic therapy with BF-200 ALA showed superior efficacy in the treatment of actinic keratosis on the extremities, trunk, and neck in a vehicle-controlled phase III study. J Am Acad Dermatol. 2021;85(6):1510–9. https://doi.org/10.1016/j.jaad.2021.03.031.
183. Schmitz L, Novak B, Hoeh AK, Luebbert H, Dirschka T. Epidermal penetration and protoporphyrin IX formation of two different 5-aminolevulinic acid formulations in ex vivo human skin. Photodiagn Photodyn Ther. 2016;14:40–6. https://doi.org/10.1016/j.pdpdt.2015.11.004.
184. Morton CA, Brown SB, Collins S, Ibbotson S, Jenkinson H, Kurwa H, et al. Guidelines for topical photodynamic therapy: report of a workshop of the British Photodermatology Group. Br J Dermatol. 2002;146(4):552–67. https://doi.org/10.1046/j.1365-2133.2002.04719.x.
185. Barolet D. Light-emitting diodes (LEDs) in dermatology. Semin Cutan Med Surg. 2008;27(4):227–38. https://doi.org/10.1016/j.sder.2008.08.003.
186. Peter K, Lee BK. Current methods for photodynamic therapy in the US comparison of MAL PDT and ALA PDT. J Drugs Dermatol. 2013;12(8):925–30.
187. Maytin EV, Kaw U, Ilyas M, Mack JA, Hu B. Blue light versus red light for photodynamic therapy of basal cell carcinoma in patients with Gorlin syndrome: a bilaterally controlled comparison study. Photodiagn Photodyn Ther. 2018;22:7–13. https://doi.org/10.1016/j.pdpdt.2018.02.009.
188. Gholam P, Bosselmann I, Enk A, Fink C. Impact of red versus blue light on tolerability and efficacy of PDT: a randomized controlled trial. J Dtsch Dermatol Ges. 2018;16(6):711–7. https://doi.org/10.1111/ddg.13545.
189. Haedersdal M, Sakamoto FH, Farinelli WA, Doukas AG, Tam J, Anderson RR. Fractional CO(2) laser-assisted drug delivery. Lasers Surg Med. 2010;42(2):113–22. https://doi.org/10.1002/lsm.20860.
190. Zhi D, Yang T, O'Hagan J, Zhang S, Donnelly RF. Photothermal therapy. J Control Release. 2020;325:52–71. https://doi.org/10.1016/j.jconrel.2020.06.032.
191. Zhang GL, Keyal U, Shi L, Wang PR, Zhang LL, Bhatta AK, et al. Photodynamic therapy as an alternative treatment in patients with invasive cutaneous SCC where surgery is not feasible: single center experience. Photodiagn Photodyn Ther. 2020;32:101980. https://doi.org/10.1016/j.pdpdt.2020.101980.
192. Anand S, Rollakanti KR, Brankov N, Brash DE, Hasan T, Maytin EV. Fluorouracil enhances photodynamic therapy of squamous cell carcinoma via

a p53-independent mechanism that increases protoporphyrin IX levels and tumor cell death. Mol Cancer Ther. 2017;16(6):1092–101. https://doi.org/10.1158/1535-7163.MCT-16-0608.
193. Yang DF, Lee JW, Chen HM, Huang Z, Hsu YC. Methotrexate enhances 5-aminolevulinic acid-mediated photodynamic therapy-induced killing of human SCC4 cells by upregulation of coproporphyrinogen oxidase. J Formos Med Assoc. 2014;113(2):88–93. https://doi.org/10.1016/j.jfma.2013.12.005.
194. Zeng Q, Yang J, Ji J, Wang P, Zhang L, Yan G, et al. PD-L1 blockade potentiates the antitumor effects of ALA-PDT and optimizes the tumor microenvironment in cutaneous squamous cell carcinoma. Onco Targets Ther. 2022;11(1):2061396. https://doi.org/10.1080/2162402X.2022.2061396.
195. Bu W, Wang Y, Chen X, Fang F. Novel strategy in giant cutaneous squamous cell carcinoma treatment: the case experience with a combination of photodynamic therapy and surgery. Photodiagn Photodyn Ther. 2017;19:116–8. https://doi.org/10.1016/j.pdpdt.2017.05.006.
196. Yan J, Wang P, Li L, Zhang L, Zhang G, Tang Y, et al. Surgery sequential with 5-Aminolevulinic acid photodynamic therapy for lip squamous cell carcinoma: two cases reports. Photodiagn Photodyn Ther. 2020;32:102043. https://doi.org/10.1016/j.pdpdt.2020.102043.
197. Wang Y, Yang Y, Yang Y, Lu Y. Surgery combined with topical photodynamic therapy for the treatment of squamous cell carcinoma of the lip. Photodiagn Photodyn Ther. 2016;14:170–2. https://doi.org/10.1016/j.pdpdt.2016.04.008.
198. Fang S, Zhou Z, Wu Y, Zheng Z, Zhao Y, Sun X, et al. Photodynamic therapy combined with carbon dioxide laser for successful treatment of cutaneous squamous cell carcinoma within a long-standing and huge seborrheic keratosis. Photodiagn Photodyn Ther. 2021;36:102536. https://doi.org/10.1016/j.pdpdt.2021.102536.
199. Ang JM, Riaz IB, Kamal MU, Paragh G, Zeitouni NC. Photodynamic therapy and pain: a systematic review. Photodiagn Photodyn Ther. 2017;19:308–44. https://doi.org/10.1016/j.pdpdt.2017.07.002.
200. Wang B, Shi L, Zhang YF, Zhou Q, Zheng J, Szeimies RM, et al. Gain with no pain? Pain management in dermatological photodynamic therapy. Br J Dermatol. 2017;177(3):656–65. https://doi.org/10.1111/bjd.15344.
201. Cottrell WJ, Paquette AD, Keymel KR, Foster TH, Oseroff AR. Irradiance-dependent photobleaching and pain in delta-aminolevulinic acid-photodynamic therapy of superficial basal cell carcinomas. Clin Cancer Res. 2008;14(14):4475–83. https://doi.org/10.1158/1078-0432.CCR-07-5199.
202. Lam C, Funaro D. Extramammary Paget's disease: summary of current knowledge. Dermatol Clin. 2010;28(4):807–26. https://doi.org/10.1016/j.det.2010.08.002.
203. Weng S, Zhu N, Li D, Chen Y, Tan Y, Chen J, et al. Clinical characteristics, treatment, and prognostic factors of patients with primary extramammary Paget's disease (EMPD): a retrospective analysis of 44 patients from a single center and an analysis of data from the surveillance, epidemiology, and end results (SEER) database. Front Oncol. 2020;10:1114. https://doi.org/10.3389/fonc.2020.01114.
204. Siesling S, Elferink MAG, van Dijck JAAM, Pierie JPEN, Blokx WAM. Epidemiology and treatment of extramammary Paget disease in The Netherlands. Eur J Surg Oncol. 2007;33(8):951–5.
205. Ishizuki S, Nakamura Y. Extramammary Paget's disease: diagnosis, pathogenesis, and treatment with focus on recent developments. Curr Oncol. 2021;28(4):2969–86. https://doi.org/10.3390/curroncol28040260.
206. McCarter MD, Quan SHQ, Busam K, Paty PP, Wong D, Guillem JG. Long-term outcome of perianal Paget's disease. Dis Colon Rectum. 2003;46(5):612–6.
207. Guo L, Liu X, Li H, Tu P, Yang S, Li X, et al. Clinicopathological features of extramammary Paget's disease: a report of 75 cases. Chin Med J. 2015;95(22):1751–4. https://doi.org/10.3760/cma.j.issn.0376-2491.2015.22.010.
208. Pierie JPEN, Choudry U, Muzikansky A, Finkelstein DM, Ott MJ. Prognosis and management of extramammary Paget's disease and the association with secondary malignancies. J Am Coll Surg. 2003;196(1):45–50.
209. Cohen PR, Schulze KE, Tschen JA, Hetherington GW, Nelson BR. Treatment of extramammary Paget disease with topical imiquimod cream: case report and literature review. South Med J. 2006;99(4):396–402.
210. Miller RL, Gerster JF, Owens ML, Slade HB, Tomai MA. Imiquimod applied topically: a novel immune response modifier and new class of drug. Int J Immunopharmacol. 1999;21(1):1–14.
211. Henta T, Itoh Y, Kobayashi M, Ninomiya Y, Ishibashi A. Photodynamic therapy for inoperable vulval Paget's disease using delta-aminolaevulinic acid: successful management of a large skin lesion. Br J Dermatol. 1999;141(2):347–9.
212. Morris CR, Hurst EA. Extramammary Paget disease: a review of the literature-part I: history, epidemiology, pathogenesis, presentation, histopathology, and diagnostic work-up. Dermatologic Surg. 2020;46(2):151–8. https://doi.org/10.1097/DSS.0000000000002064.
213. Shim PJ, Zeitouni NC. Photodynamic therapy for extramammary Paget's disease: a systematic review of the literature. Photodiagn Photodyn Ther. 2020;31:101911. https://doi.org/10.1016/j.pdpdt.2020.101911.
214. Hu H, Cheng H. Clinical features and follow up analysis of 19 patients with extramammary Paget disease. Chin J Dermatovenereol. 2011;25(8):4.

215. Shieh S, Dee AS, Cheney RT, Frawley NP, Zeitouni NC, Oseroff AR. Photodynamic therapy for the treatment of extramammary Paget's disease. Br J Dermatol. 2002;146(6):1000–5.
216. Fontanelli R, Papadia A, Martinelli F, Lorusso D, Grijuela B, Merola M, et al. Photodynamic therapy with M-ALA as non surgical treatment option in patients with primary extramammary Paget's disease. Gynecol Oncol. 2013;130(1):90–4. https://doi.org/10.1016/j.ygyno.2013.04.008.
217. Shen S, Zhang G, Wang P, Zhang Y, Keyal U, Ji J, et al. ALA-PDT as palliative care in a patient with secondary perineum EMPD. Photodiagn Photodyn Ther. 2018;22:166–8. https://doi.org/10.1016/j.pdpdt.2018.04.002.
218. Wang H-W, Lv T, Zhang L-L, Lai Y-X, Tang L, Tang Y-C, et al. A prospective pilot study to evaluate combined topical photodynamic therapy and surgery for extramammary Paget's disease. Lasers Surg Med. 2013;45(5):296–301. https://doi.org/10.1002/lsm.22142.
219. Gao Y, Zhang XC, Wang WS, Yang Y, Wang HL, Lu YG, et al. Efficacy and safety of topical ALA-PDT in the treatment of EMPD. Photodiagn Photodyn Ther. 2015;12(1):92–7. https://doi.org/10.1016/j.pdpdt.2014.11.004.
220. Li C, Guo L, Wang P, Shi L, Sun X, Hu C, et al. ALA-PDT combined with holmium laser therapy of postoperative recurrent extramammary Paget's disease. Photodiagn Photodyn Ther. 2019;27:92–4. https://doi.org/10.1016/j.pdpdt.2019.05.011.
221. Dogan A, Hilal Z, Krentel H, Cetin C, Hefler LA, Grimm C, et al. Paget's disease of the vulva treated with imiquimod: case report and systematic review of the literature. Gynecol Obstet Investig. 2017;82(1):1–7. https://doi.org/10.1159/000449158.
222. Jing W, Juan X, Li X, Jiayuan C, Qin H, Qing L, et al. Complete remission of two patients with recurrent and wide spread extramammary Paget disease obtained from 5-aminolevulinic acid-based photodynamic therapy and imiquimod combination treatment. Photodiagn Photodyn Ther. 2014;11(3):434–40. https://doi.org/10.1016/j.pdpdt.2014.03.006.
223. Bauman TM, Rosman IS, Sheinbein DM. Extramammary Paget's disease of the scrotum with complete response to imiquimod and photodynamic therapy. BMJ Case Rep. 2018;2018:bcr2017221696. https://doi.org/10.1136/bcr-2017-221696.

6 HpD-PDT in the Treatment of Nonmelanoma Skin Cancer

Dixin Wang, Peiru Wang, Bo Wang, and Xiuli Wang

6.1 Introduction

Hematoporphyrin injection, which is primarily composed of hematoporphyrin derivatives (HpDs), is widely used as an intravenous photosensitizer. HpD enables the localization, diagnosis, and treatment of superficial cancers and precancerous lesions, including leukoplakia in the oral cavity, as well as lesions in the bladder, bronchus, lung, and digestive tract; it can also treat conditions such as port wine stain. Hematoporphyrin photodynamic therapy (HpD-PDT) is a noninvasive, simple, practical, and repeatable approach that has shown significant efficacy in treating nonmelanoma skin cancer (NMSC). In 1981, Chinese researchers first isolated HpD and successfully treated a patient with basal cell carcinoma via HpD-PDT. With over 40 years of clinical application, HpD-PDT continues to play a vital role in the treatment of NMSC.

D. Wang · P. Wang (✉) · X. Wang
Institute of Photomedicine, Shanghai Skin Disease Hospital, School of Medicine, Tongji University, Shanghai, China
e-mail: wangxiuli_1400023@tongji.edu.cn

B. Wang
Avera Medical Group Dermatology, Aberdeen, SD, USA

University of South Dakota, Vermillion, SD, USA
e-mail: makiwang@med.umich.edu

6.2 HpD-PDT in the Treatment of Extramammary Paget's Disease

6.2.1 Overview of Extramammary Paget's Disease

Extramammary Paget's disease (EMPD) is a relatively rare skin malignancy with a global incidence ranging from 0.1 to 2.4 cases per million annually. In Asian populations, the annual incidence is approximately four times greater than the global average, and the 5-year survival rate ranges from 72% to 87% [1–3]. It affects areas such as the scrotum, penis, labia, vagina, perianal region, groin, and armpits. Skin lesions often appear as eczematoid patches, progressing to ulcers, bleeding, nodules, and sclerosis in advanced stages [1].

6.2.2 Treatment

Currently, surgery is the first-line treatment for EMPD, with Mohs micrographic surgery (MMS) providing advantages over traditional excision, despite recurrence rates between 30% and 60% [2, 6]. The large lesion, multifocal presentation, and poorly defined margins of EMPD make surgery complex, invasive, and prone to recurrence. Additionally, owing to the EMPD location, large lesion areas, advanced patient age, and

X. Wang, B. Wang (eds.), *Photodynamic Therapy in Dermatology*,
https://doi.org/10.1007/978-981-96-8915-6_6

comorbidities, some patients are unsuitable candidates for surgery. Other treatment options, such as electrocautery and curettage, laser surgery, topical 5% imiquimod cream, radiotherapy, and local chemotherapy, are sometimes used, but they often have limited efficacy and high recurrence rates, making them secondary choices for EMPD [7, 8]. Therefore, optimizing and improving EMPD treatment remains a priority.

6.2.3 HpD-PDT

Owing to its strong tumor-targeting capabilities, photodynamic therapy (PDT) has gained attention as a treatment for EMPD. The photosensitizers used for EMPD include 5-aminolevulinic acid (ALA), methyl-aminolevulinate (MAL), hematoporphyrin derivative (HpD), and sodium porphyrin [1, 2]. The authors' group employed ALA-PDT for EMPD, achieving favorable clinical results while preserving the structure and function of surrounding healthy tissues. Combined approaches, such as ALA-PDT with surgery or holmium lasers, have further improved outcomes, establishing safe, effective treatment options after surgery, radiotherapy, or chemotherapy [3]. However, ALA-PDT faces limitations in EMPD treatment, including limited penetration depth, suboptimal efficacy as a monotherapy, and challenges with metastatic lesions. Intravenous photosensitizer-based PDT offers enhanced tissue penetration and improved clinical efficacy, addressing these limitations. In 1976, HpD-PDT was first used to treat skin cancer, lung cancer, head and neck cancer, breast cancer, and gastrointestinal cancer [4]. In 2002, HpD-PDT was first applied to EMPD in 2002, with promising results [5] A 2010 report on nine EMPD patients treated with HpD-PDT reported a complete remission rate of 78%, with no recurrence during a follow-up period of up to 68 months [6].

6.2.3.1 Treatment Mechanism

In HPD-PDT therapy, HpD targets tumor cells primarily via the lipid pathway, binding to low-density lipoprotein (LDL) and albumin to reach tumor sites and form concentrated deposits. In plasma, HpD binds mainly to high-density lipoprotein (HDL), allowing for extended plasma accumulation. After intravenous administration of 3H-labeled HpD in healthy mice, the tissue distribution peaked within 1 h, with the highest concentrations in the lung > liver > kidney > blood > stomach > intestine > spleen > heart > muscle > thymus > brain > bone. The tumor tissue initially ranked 8th–ninth among these tissues but rose to the fifth rank by 72 h. Five hours postinjection, 73.29% of the HpD dose had been excreted, reaching 91% by day 11. The HpD distribution within tumor tissues varies on the basis of cell density, size, cytoplasmic abundance, DNA/RNA content, and vascular supply, with higher HpD concentrations in well-supplied areas. The authors' group conducted fluorescence diagnostics on patients with malignant skin tumors treated with HpD-PDT, assessing drug accumulation within the lesion, margin, and distant sites. Fluorescence was detectable 24 h post-HpD injection, marking the lesion sites. The fluorescence intensity further increased at 48 h and then increased after PDT. The lesion fluorescence intensity was increased to the peak value at 72 h, indicating HpD re-enrichment. The fluorescence intensity decreased within 1 week after PDT and returned to baseline at approximately 4 weeks.

6.2.3.2 Clinical Efficacy and Parameter Selection

Light Source Selection and Illumination Parameters

HpD-PDT therapy commonly employs laser and light-emitting diode (LED) sources, with red LEDs and semiconductor lasers being the most frequently used for treating EMPD. No current studies have directly compared light sources for EMPD; however, when combined with other therapies, CO_2 or holmium lasers may also be utilized. In 2022, the authors' group treated 11 EMPD patients via HpD-PDT (630 nm red light semiconductor laser, output power of 1000–2000 mW, power density of 80–150 mW/cm^2, and energy density of 150–200 J/cm^2). Following a single HpD injection, red light irradiation was applied at 48 and 72 h without significant adverse effects. For patients with residual lesions, combination therapy with a holmium laser and ALA-PDT has proven effective in clearing the lesion [7]. Holmium laser treatment allows controlled operating depth by adjustable energy, offering advantages in precision, tissue cutting, and coagulation, with real-time lesion depth monitoring via ultrasound to guide treatment (settings: energy 0.5–0.9 J, rate 10 Hz, and fiber diameter 550 μm) [3].

Clinical Efficacy of HpD-PDT in Treating EMPD

The authors' group conducted a pioneering single-arm, prospective study treating 11 EMPD patients with HpD-PDT (averaging 73.4 years of age with a disease duration of 5.9 years). At 1 month, 90.1% (10/11) of patients achieved a complete response (CR), and 9.1% (1/11) achieved a partial response (PR). After 1 year, 81.8% (9/11) maintained CR, but at 2 years, this rate had decreased to 36.4% (4/11). The main adverse reactions included pain, urinary infection, scarring, photosensitivity, and urinary retention, with no liver dysfunction or significant changes in local tissue structure [7].

Currently, treatment consensus for EMPD, including surgery, laser, PDT, and radiotherapy, remains elusive, and there is a lack of multicenter, large-scale, randomized studies, leading to variability in CR rates. Surgical excision, which often requires extensive excision and reconstruction, remains the standard treatment but can result in anatomical and functional limitations. HpD-PDT offers an alternative, particularly for elderly or anatomically challenging patients, preserving tissue structure and function. Compared with surgical scars, those resulting from HpD-PDT are less severe [5]. The authors' group suggested that combined surgery and HpD-PDT may be suitable for patients with refractory EMPD with deep infiltration (Figs. 6.1, 6.2, 6.3, and 6.4).

PDT shows promising efficacy and safety for treating EMPD and holds significant potential for broader application. However, large-scale, multicenter, controlled studies comparing HpD-PDT to surgical treatments for EMPD are currently lacking. Further extensive, high-quality studies are needed to better assess and compare the effectiveness of HpD-PDT in managing EMPD.

Scope of Application

HpD-PDT is suitable for treating EMPD across various patient types, especially for those with lesions in complex anatomical areas, elderly patients, individuals unsuitable for surgery, or those experiencing recurrent EMPD postsurgery or with ineffective outcomes from other treatments. However, it is important to exclude patients with allergies, cicatricial predispositions, and allergic conditions (such as skin photoallergy or porphyria), as well as those who are pregnant, breastfeeding, or planning pregnancy during treatment [8].

Treatment Procedures

1. Skin test After necessary examinations and excluding contraindications, a skin test should be conducted via HpD injection. 0.5 mL of HpD was extracted, mixed with 250 mL of normal saline, and thoroughly mixed. All lights in the treatment room were turned off, and the switches were marked with anti-light tape. A 0.1 mL skin test dose was applied while avoiding light. A saline control was used on the opposite side, the time was recorded, and the samples were observed after 20 min. Drug administration was continued if the skin test was negative.
2. Drug formulation and intravenous infusion were used to calculate the dosage on the basis of body weight (3–5 mg/kg), and 250 mL of HpD in saline was prepared. The photosensitizer infusion was allowed to slow over 1–1.5 h, after which the mixture was rinsed with saline to ensure complete entry into the bloodstream. Direct light was avoided throughout the procedure.
3. The treatment area was identified, the fluorescence intensity and skin lesions were observed under Wood's lamp, and a treatment range 1–2 cm beyond the lesion was marked. Only the skin area intended for irradiation was exposed, shielding other areas, especially orifices.

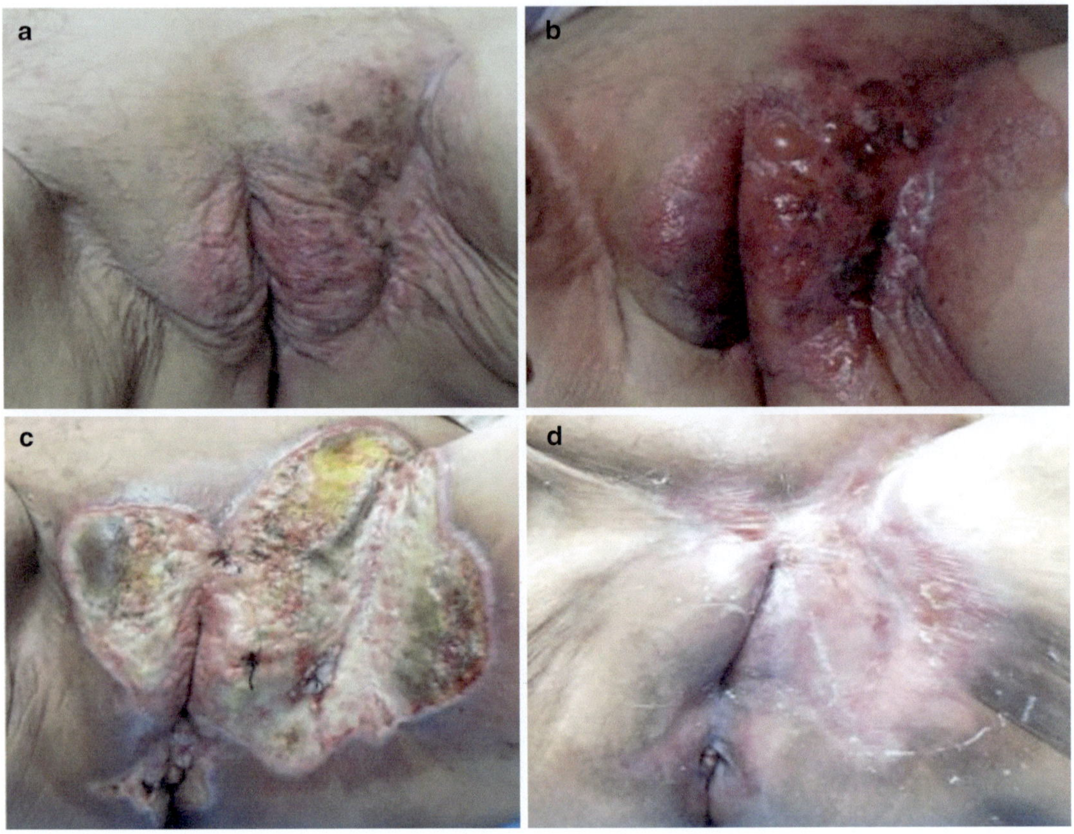

Fig. 6.1 HpD-PDT treatment of EMPD. (**a**) Extensive irregular vulva erythema before treatment, involving urethral opening and perineal skin. (**b**) Local erythema, swelling with blisters, and exudation immediately after treatment. (**c**) Dry wound surface 4 weeks after treatment, granulation tissue at the base. (**d**) Carring with intact structure and function 12 weeks after treatment

4. Light treatment was performed 48 and 72 h after infusion, and a red light therapy device with a 630 nm wavelength was used. The power density was set to 80–150 mW/cm^2, and the energy density was set to 150–200 J/cm^2. Each lesion was individually illuminated on the basis of its size.
5. Pain management Decided by general anesthesia on the basis of the patient's condition. For nongeneral anesthesia, a fentanyl patch was applied 6–8 h before light therapy, and lidocaine/artecaine was injected immediately before irradiation. Patient-reported pain scores were recorded, and cold air intervention was considered if needed. For severe cases, an anesthesiologist may evaluate intravenous general anesthesia or an analgesic pump.

Precautions

1. During drug administration, local extravasation is avoided; if it occurs, the infusion is stopped, a cold compress is applied, and the area is shielded from light until swelling subsides.
2. Postoperative care.
   (a) Wet compress and wound care immediately after surgery: Clean wound exudates, necrosis, and crusts with saline or boric acid solution. Ethacridine lactate solution was applied for 20 min, after which the mixture was covered with antibiotic ointment and a dressing. Blisters may be removed if necessary.
   (b) The temperature and urine output should be closely monitored, and regular blood

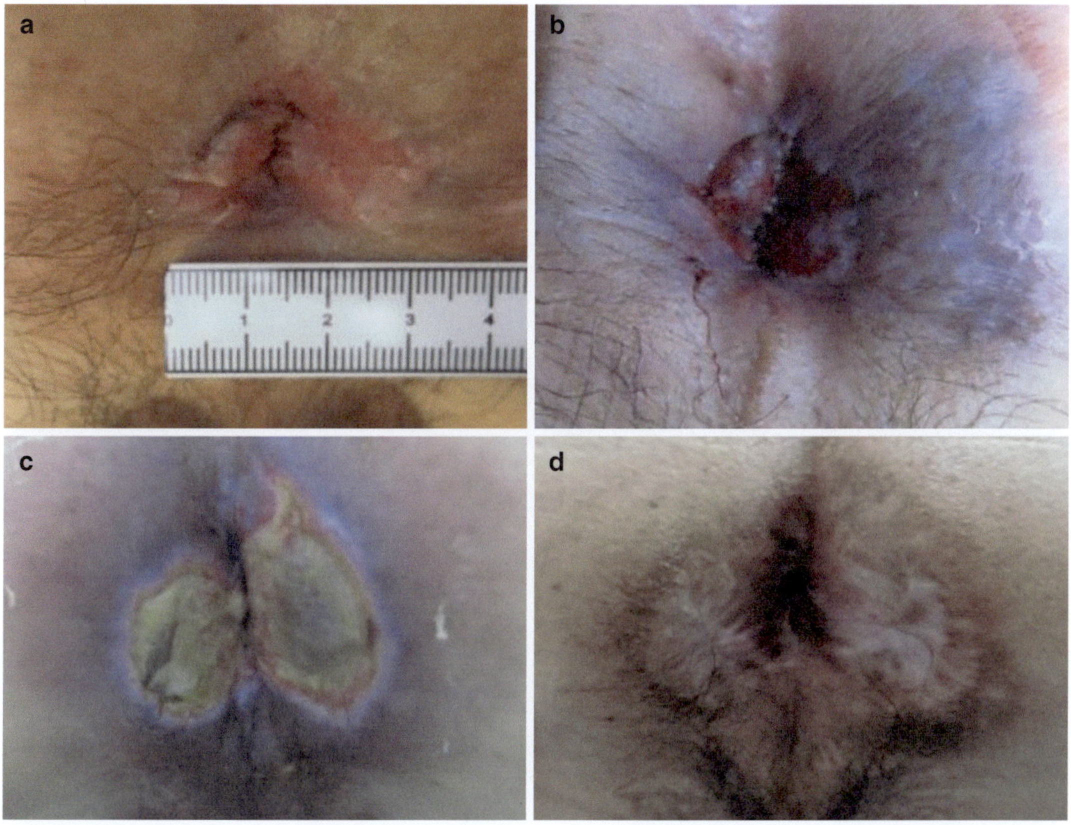

Fig. 6.2 HpD-PDT treatment of EMPD. (**a**) Continuous infiltrating erythema on the bilateral anal skin, measuring 3 × 3 cm in size, before treatment. (**b**) Local erythema, swelling, and necrosis immediately after treatment. (**c**) Yellow velvety plaque on the wound surface 4 weeks after treatment. (**d**) Scarring with mild contracture and intact structure and function 48 weeks after treatment

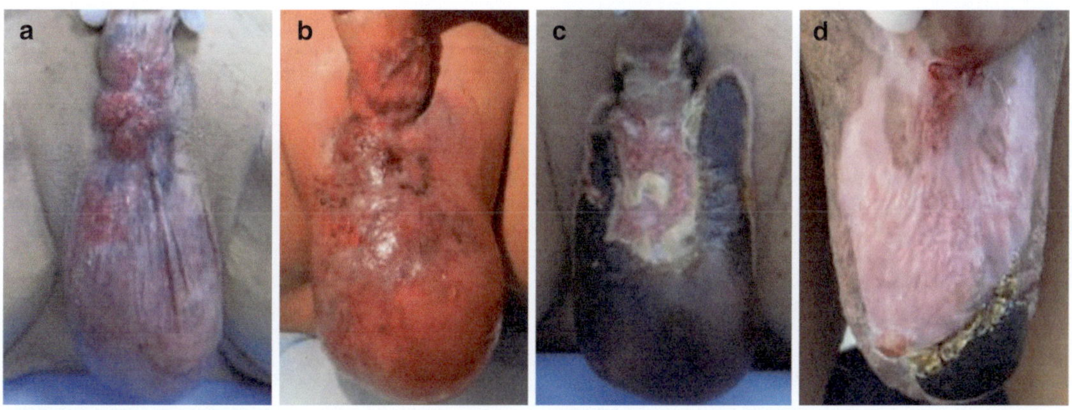

Fig. 6.3 HpD-PDT treatment of EMPD. (**a**) Irregular infiltrating erythema of the scrotum and ventral penis before treatment; a nodule measuring 3 × 2.5 cm was observed on the penile root. (**b**) Local erythema, swelling with blisters, and obvious exudation immediately after treatment. (**c**) Wound scabbed 4 weeks after treatment, and granuloma tissue at the base. (**d**) Scarring with mild contracture and intact structure and function 20 weeks after treatment

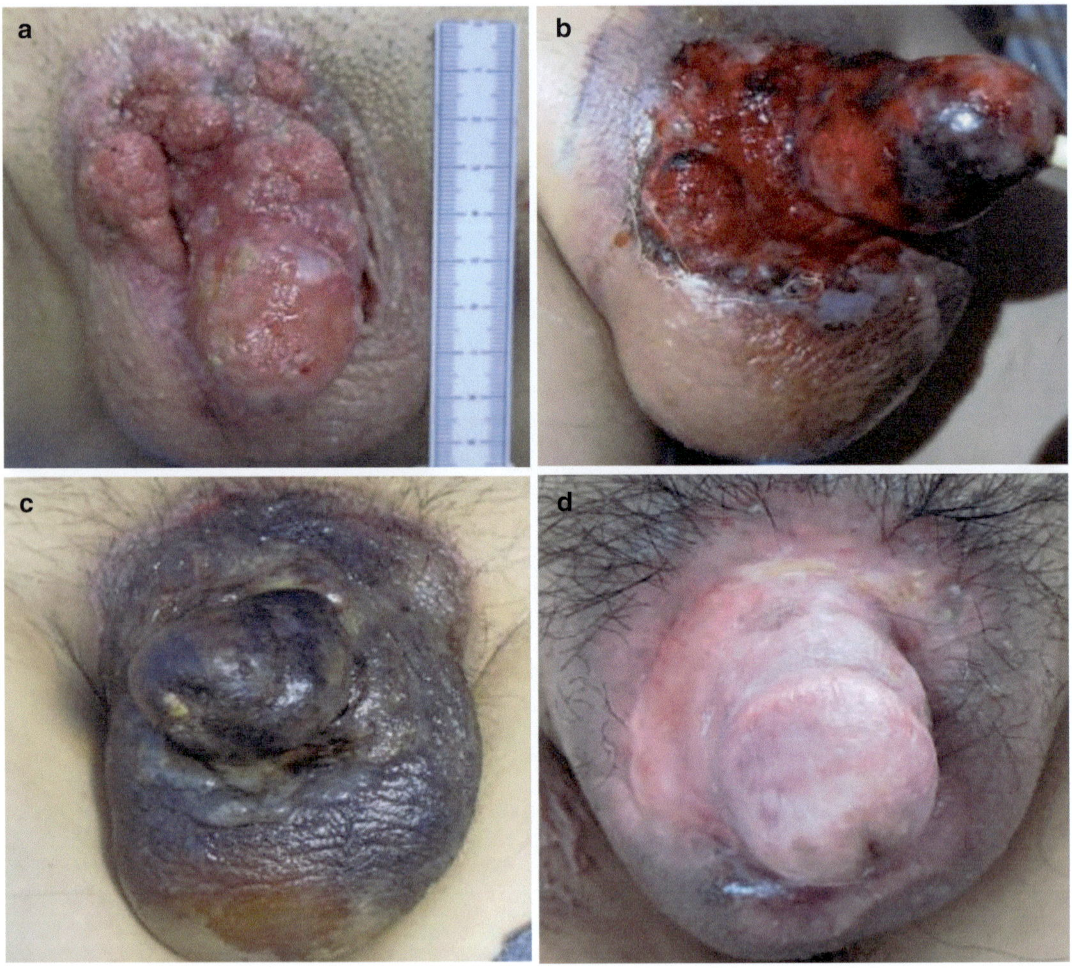

Fig. 6.4 HpD-PDT treatment of EMPD. (**a**) Before treatment, irregular infiltrating erythema and erosion of the scrotum and penis involving the glans head and urethral opening. Several 1–3 cm nodules were found at the penile base, with partial confluence. (**b**) Local erythema, swelling with exudation, and necrosis after treatment. (**c**) Scabbing at 4 weeks after treatment. (**d**) Scarring with intact structure and function at 24 weeks after treatment

tests and wound cultures should be conducted. Antibiotics should be administered if areas involving the anus or urethra are treated. Standard infection control principles should be followed, and treatment should be adjusted on the basis of laboratory results. Manage any chronic diseases such as diabetes or hypertension.

(c) For nongeneral anesthesia, cold compresses should be provided, and analgesics (e.g., fentanyl patches, NSAIDs) should be continued as needed. An analgesic pump was used postanesthesia if needed.

3. Light avoidance procedure after treatment.
   Strict light avoidance is essential post-HpD-PDT: (1) day of administration: staying in a dim room with curtains closed, max 100 lux; (2) days 1–7: remaining in a dark ward, with a maximum 40 W bulb; (3) days 7–30: patient can be discharged but recommend continuing to stay indoors, with a maximum 40 W bulb; (4) days 30–90: gradually increasing outdoor time in early morning or late evening, starting with 30 min and increasing 20 min daily, avoiding direct sunlight with UPF clothing and sunglasses; (5) months 3–6: if no skin pigmentation is observed 3 months after

administration, the patient can begin gradually resuming outdoor activities. If pigmentation is present, the patient should continue following light avoidance recommendations until the skin recovers. Fundus examination should not be conducted within the first 3 months. (6) After 6 months, the patient should be monitored for skin changes related to light exposure. Outdoor activity should follow a gradual, protected approach to prevent photosensitivity. If a photosensitive reaction occurs, appropriate symptomatic treatment should be administered.

The light intensity reference (on average) is as follows: 100,000 lux in summer sunshine; 10,000 lux outdoors on a cloudy day; the indoor fluorescent lamp is 100 lux; the 60 W desk lamp (measured 60 cm from the tabletop) is 300 lux; the television studio is 1000 lux; the evening room is 10 lux; the night street light is 0.1 lux; and the Candlelight (20 cm away) is 10–15 lux. This guide provides context for light exposure levels during HpD-PDT recovery, emphasizing the need to minimize light exposure for effective post-treatment care.

Adverse Reactions and Treatment

Owing to the systemic intravenous application and prolonged metabolic duration of the photosensitizer HpD, adverse reactions such as pain, skin ulceration, infection, scar formation, photosensitivity, and phototoxicity are more pronounced than those associated with local topical ALA-PDT. Proper management of these reactions is critical to achieving clinical efficacy and enhancing patient compliance.

Recommended Treatment Plan

The HpD-PDT is gaining acceptance as an effective treatment for EMPD. On the basis of a review of the relevant literature, alongside the research data and clinical experience from the authors' group, the following treatment protocol for HpD-PDT is recommended (Table 6.1).

Follow-up: daily follow-up within 1 week, weekly follow-up after 1 week, and monthly follow-up after 1 month.

Prognosis and Follow-Up

Following HpD-PDT treatment, wound healing typically occurs within 1–3 months. Patients should undergo evaluations at 1 month and 3 months post-treatment, including gross photography, dermoscopy, skin ultrasound, and RCM, to assess treatment efficacy. On the basis of the lesion type and characteristics, further evaluations at different intervals may be necessary to determine whether additional HpD-PDT or combination therapies are needed. In cases where recurrence or a suboptimal response is suspected, a biopsy may be warranted. Lifelong follow-up is recommended for these patients.

HpD-PDT offers a promising new approach for treating EMPD, with hope for patients with this condition. However, the treatment protocols and choice of light source require further optimization. Additionally, the potential benefits of combining HpD-PDT with other therapies to enhance efficacy remain areas for future research.

Table 6.1 Recommended HpD-PDT treatment for EMPD

	Preparation of photosensitizer				Illumination dose	
Preconditioning	HpD form	HpD dose	Duration of medication	Light source	Power density	Energy density
Expose skin lesions and protect surrounding normal skin	Solution	3–5 mg/kg	Light treatment 48 h, 72 h after drug injection	630 nm Semiconductor laser	80–100 mW/cm^2	150–200 J/cm^2

6.3 HpD-PDT in the Treatment of Other Nonmelanoma Skin Cancers

Basal cell carcinoma (BCC) accounts for approximately 75% of common nonmelanoma skin cancers (NMSCs), and squamous cell carcinoma of the skin (cSCC) accounts for approximately 20% [9]. The traditional treatments for NMSC include surgical excision, cryotherapy, and local chemotherapy. ALA-PDT was successfully applied to treat NMSCs. HpD-PDT provides another effective PDT option for patients with BCC and cSCC.

6.3.1 Basal Cell Carcinoma

BCC, the most common skin cancer worldwide, particularly among Caucasians, is a slow-growing malignant tumor with low risk of metastasis but high potential for local invasion. Its increasing incidence imposes a growing burden on healthcare systems worldwide. The primary goal in BCC treatment is complete tumor removal or destruction to achieve a clinical cure and minimize the risk of recurrence. Typically, BCCs are managed surgically via the first-line approach. Nonsurgical treatments, including PDT, are mainly considered for low-risk BCC subtypes [10]. According to the "Expert consensus on the diagnosis and treatment of cutaneous basal cell carcinoma (2021)" and National Comprehensive Cancer Network (NCCN) guidelines, BCC can be classified as high risk or low risk on the basis of recurrence risk. High-risk patients may receive PDT as a second-line option [11]. For diffuse BCC, surgical resection remains the primary treatment, although repeat surgeries may cause tissue damage. Studies have demonstrated that ALA-PDT is effective for superficial nodular BCCs less than 2 mm thick, with minimal impact on surrounding healthy skin, although ALA-PDT is less effective for larger or thicker lesions.

In 2006, two patients with neviform basal cell carcinoma syndrome (nBCC) were treated with porfimer sodium PDT. They received 1 mg/kg porfimer sodium intravenously, followed by irradiation with a 630 nm Diomed semiconductor laser at 373 mW/cm^2 48 h later. After 1 month, the tumor thickness was reduced by 86% and 88.5%, respectively, with significant clinical improvement and minimal impact on skin appearance [12]. Locally advanced basal cell carcinoma (laBCC) poses a challenge because of its invasive nature, especially in older patients. In 2021, the authors' group treated a 91-year-old woman with scalp laBCC via a combination of ALA-PDT and HpD-PDT. With a long history of diabetes and hypertension, the patient opted for a nonsurgical approach. The examination revealed a 5 × 4 × 1.5 cm tumor with ulceration and a crusted surface. Ultrasound indicated that the lesion extended to the galea aponeurotica, with a depth of 8.3–15 mm, and CT confirmed that there was no metastasis. On the basis of the 2019 European Consensus on Basal Cell Carcinoma, a laBCC diagnosis was made. The treatment included ALA-PDT administered biweekly for six sessions. After ultrasound confirmed lesion reduction, the patient received an intravenous HpD dose (5 mg/kg), followed 48 h later by 630 nm diode laser irradiation at 100 J/cm^2 and 33 mW/cm^2. A follow-up at 1.5 months revealed marked improvement. To reduce scarring, glucocorticoid injections were applied locally, along with 980 nm and 595 nm lasers, to close capillaries and limit angiogenesis [13].

6.3.2 Skin Squamous Cell Carcinoma

Surgical excision or Mohs microsurgery remains the primary treatment for cutaneous squamous cell carcinoma (cSCC). PDT offers an effective alternative, particularly given its excellent cosmetic outcomes. In the United States, ALA-PDT is FDA-approved solely for treating actinic keratosis (AK), whereas in the European Union and other regions, PDT is approved for treating superficial basal cell carcinoma (BCC) and cSCC [14]. According to the "Chinese guidelines on the clinical application of 5-aminolevulinic acid-based photodynamic therapy in dermatology (2021 edition)," the evidence for ALA-PDT in treating cSCC is grade II, with a clinical recommendation grade B [15]. However, ALA-PDT's limited tissue penetration can reduce its effectiveness on thicker lesions, whereas HpD-PDT, with its greater penetration depth, may offer advantages.

Owing to the strong tissue absorption of HpD, HpD-PDT has been explored for treating cSCC, although no standard clinical recommendation exists. The authors reported that after the administration of 5 mg/kg HpD, fluorescence in the tumor tissue intensified at 24 h, peaked between 48 and 72 h, and began to decrease after 72 h. On the basis of these findings, they recommend two irradiation sessions, at 48 and 72 h postinjection, to optimize efficacy [16]. In 1988, HpD-PDT was applied to treat cSCC via a 5 mg/kg dose of HpD, which was subsequently irradiated on days 3 and 5 with a 630 nm light source at a 30 J/cm^2 dose. Among 32 patients, the initial remission rate was 81%, although it decreased to under 50% after 6 months of follow-up [17]. In 2004, 34 SCCs in situ were treated with HpD-PDT (14 mg/m^2) with red light irradiation at different energy densities (60 J/cm^2, 120 J/cm^2, and 180 J/cm^2 at approximately 688 nm; power density, 200 ± 40 mW/cm^2) 1–3 h later. The complete response rates (CCRs) at 6 months were 78%, 88%, and 98%, with 24-months CCRs of 51%, 79%, and 95%, respectively [18]. The combination of local ALA-PDT and intravenous HpD-PDT was used in 16 patients with scalp and facial cSCC, whereas it was used in 10 patients treated with HpD-PDT alone and 14 treated with CO_2 laser ablation and ALA-PDT. The complete remission rates were 100% at 2 months post-PDT and 97.6% from 6 months to 6 years. The remission rates for HpD-PDT and ALA-PDT alone were 92.9% and 95.1%, respectively, indicating high efficacy with a reduced HpD dosage and shorter photosensitivity [19]. After HpD-PDT, protection of the skin wound from secondary infection is critical. The protocol involves washing with 3% boric acid, applying topical antibiotic ointment, and using wet dressings for healing [19]. The authors' group used HpD-PDT to treat a 93-year-old inoperable cSCC patient with a lesion in the right temporal region. After the administration of 5 mg/kg HpD and Wood lamp-guided illumination, the lesion was irradiated at 200 J/m^2 with a 630 nm semiconductor laser at 48 and 72 h postinjection. At follow-up (1 day to 8 weeks), clinical remission was achieved, with no recurrence and only mild scarring at the 6-week biopsy [20] (Fig. 6.5).

In summary, PDT has a good therapeutic effect on some NMSCs, with many advantages, such as repeatability, noninvasiveness, high selectivity, and few side effects, which provides a new option for clinical treatment, especially in addition to surgical treatment. In the treatment of EMPD, the HpD-PDT has broad applicability, especially for older patients or those who cannot undergo surgery. The HPD-PDT typically requires fewer treatment sessions, and the recurrence rates after a cure are low. If recurrence occurs, PDT can be repeated. However, few studies have focused on HpD-PDT for BCC, cSCC, and other NMSC, indicating a need for further research to optimize treatment plans, including parameters such as the light source, photosensitizer, and illumination dose. Clinical studies have confirmed that HpD-PDT effectively treats NMSCs, especially when conventional therapies such as drugs or surgical treatment are unsuitable or ineffective. To establish a strong theoretical foundation for the efficacy of HpD-PDT in treating EMPD, BCC, and cSCC, further extensive clinical studies and long-term practice are necessary.

This would help in the development of individualized treatment protocols and refine photosensitizer and light source selection, along with improving treatment methods. In addition, while encouraging, HpD-PDT lacks consensus on key treatment parameters, such as the application concentration, time, dose, and cycle, which needs further clinical study. Current parameters are based on prior literature and can guide clinical practice, but actual treatment settings should be tailored to each patient's condition. HpD-PDT preserves the tumor site structure, provides good cosmetic outcomes, and is well tolerated. It is expected to become a significant treatment option for NMSC over time.

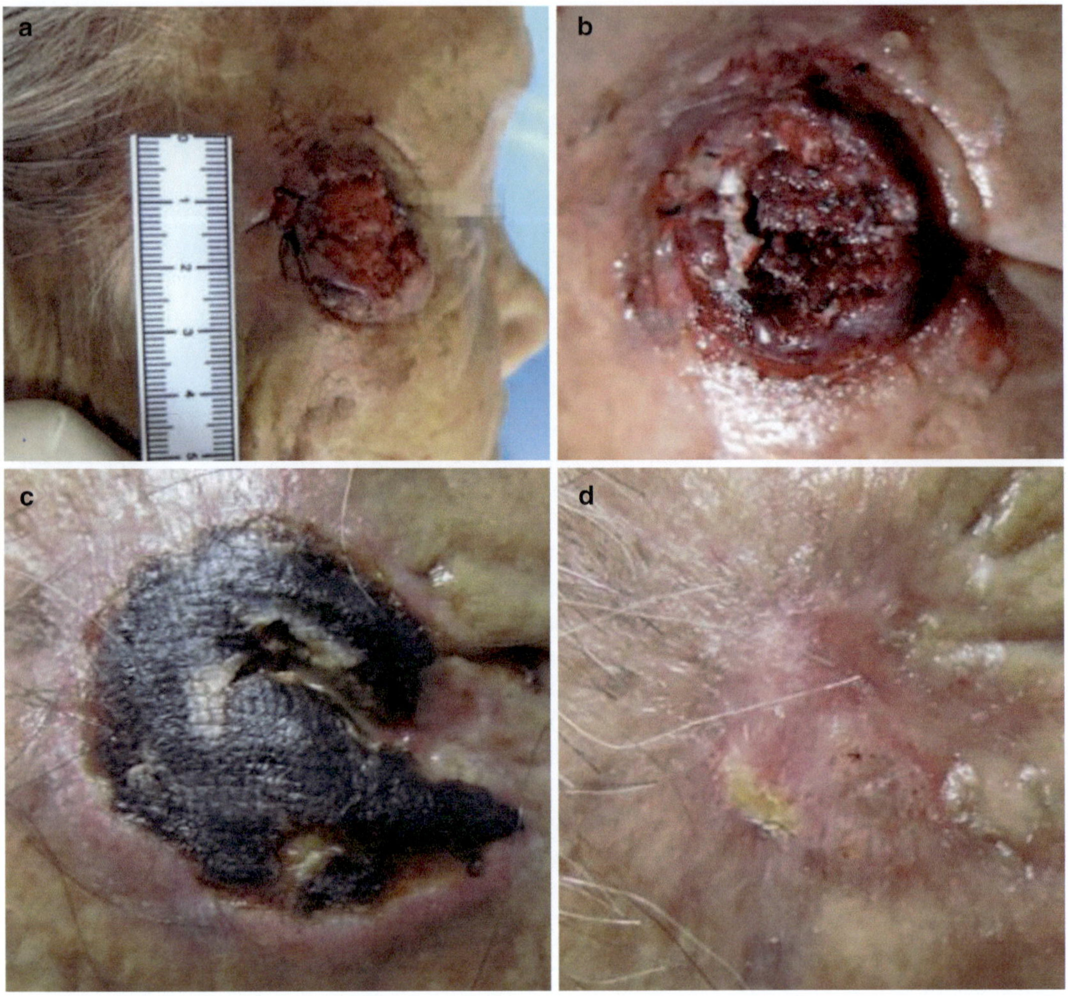

Fig. 6.5 HpD-PDT treatment for cSCC. (**a**) Dark red mass measuring 3 × 2.6 cm in the right temple skin before treatment. Ultrasound revealed depth of 5–7 mm. (**b**) Local erythema, swelling with exudation, and necrosis after treatment. (**c**) Wound scabbing at 4 weeks after treatment. (**d**) Scarcing with intact structure and function at 8 weeks after treatment

References

1. Shim PJ, Zeitouni NC. Photodynamic therapy for extramammary Paget's disease: a systematic review of the literature. Photodiagn Photodyn Ther. 2020;31:101911. https://doi.org/10.1016/j.pdpdt.2020.101911.
2. Gao Y, Zhang X-C, Wang W-S, Yang Y, Wang H-L, Lu Y-G, et al. Efficacy and safety of topical ALA-PDT in the treatment of EMPD. Photodiagn Photodyn Ther. 2015;12(1):92–7. https://doi.org/10.1016/j.pdpdt.2014.11.004.
3. Li C, Guo L, Wang P, Shi L, Sun X, Hu C, et al. ALA-PDT combined with holmium laser therapy of postoperative recurrent extramammary Paget's disease. Photodiagn Photodyn Ther. 2019;27:92–4. https://doi.org/10.1016/j.pdpdt.2019.05.011.
4. van Hillegersberg R, Kort WJ, Wilson JH. Current status of photodynamic therapy in oncology. Drugs. 1994;48(4):510–27.
5. Shieh S, Dee AS, Cheney RT, Frawley NP, Zeitouni NC, Oseroff AR. Photodynamic therapy for the treatment of extramammary Paget's disease. Br J Dermatol. 2002;146(6):1000–5.
6. Housel JP, Izikson L, Zeitouni NC. Noninvasive extramammary Paget's disease treated with photodynamic therapy: case series from the Roswell Park Cancer Institute. Dermatol Surg. 2010;36(11):1718–24. https://doi.org/10.1111/j.1524-4725.2010.01734.x.

7. Wang D, Wang P, Li C, Zhou Z, Zhang L, Zhang G, et al. Efficacy and safety of HpD-PDT for extramammary Paget's disease refractory to conventional therapy: a prospective, open-label and single arm pilot study. Photodiagn Photodyn Ther. 2021;37:102670. https://doi.org/10.1016/j.pdpdt.2021.102670.
8. Lu Z. Skin laser medicine and cosmetology. Shanghai: Fudan University Press; 2008.
9. Friedman R, Rigel D, Nossa R, Dorf R, Murphy G, Lawrence W, et al. Basal cell and squamous cell carcinoma of the skin. In: American Cancer Society textbook of clinical oncology. 2nd ed. Washington: American Cancer Society; 1995. p. 330–41.
10. Burns T, Breathnach SM, Cox N, Griffiths C. Rook's textbook of dermatology. Hoboken: Wiley; 2008.
11. Chinese Medical Association, Dermatologic Oncology Group, Branch of Dermatologists, Chinese Medical Doctor Association. Expert consensus on diagnosis and treatment of cutaneous basal cell carcinoma. Chin J Dermatol. 2021;54(9):757–64. https://doi.org/10.35541/cjd.20201139.
12. Madan V, Loncaster JA, Allan D, Lear JT, Sheridan L, Leach C, et al. Nodular basal cell carcinoma in Gorlin's syndrome treated with systemic photodynamic therapy and interstitial optical fiber diffuser laser. J Am Acad Dermatol. 2006;55(5):S86–9.
13. Liao C, Shi L, Wang D, Wang X. Bimodal photodynamic therapy for treatment of a 91-year-old patient with locally advanced cutaneous basal cell carcinoma and postoperative scar management. Photodiagn Photodyn Ther. 2021;36:102553. https://doi.org/10.1016/j.pdpdt.2021.102553.
14. Cohen DK, Lee PK. Photodynamic therapy for nonmelanoma skin cancers. Cancer. 2016;8(10):90.
15. Shi L, Wang H, Chen K, Yan J, Yu B, Wang S, et al. Chinese guidelines on the clinical application of 5-aminolevulinic acid-based photodynamic therapy in dermatology (2021 edition). Photodiagn Photodyn Ther. 2021;35:102340. https://doi.org/10.1016/j.pdpdt.2021.102340.
16. Li C, Wang P, Wang D, Shi L, Zhou Z, Zhang L, et al. Fluorescence kinetics study of twice laser irradiation based HpD-PDT for nonmelanoma skin cancer. Lasers Surg Med. 2022;54(7):945–54. https://doi.org/10.1002/lsm.23538.
17. Pennington DG, Waner M, Knox A. Photodynamic therapy for multiple skin cancers. Plast Reconstr Surg. 1988;82(6):1067–71.
18. Lui H, Hobbs L, Tope WD, Lee PK, Elmets C, Provost N, et al. Photodynamic therapy of multiple nonmelanoma skin cancers with verteporfin and red light-emitting diodes: two-year results evaluating tumor response and cosmetic outcomes. Arch Dermatol. 2004;140(1):26–32.
19. Wang Y, Lin Y, Zhang H-G, Zhu J. A photodynamic therapy combined with topical 5-aminolevulinic acid and systemic hematoporphyrin derivative is more efficient but less phototoxic for cancer. J Cancer Res Clin Oncol. 2016;142(4):813–21. https://doi.org/10.1007/s00432-015-2066-3.
20. Wang D, Li C, Zhou Z, Zhang Y, Zhang G, Wang P, et al. Photodynamic therapy of intravenous injection combined with intratumoral administration of photosensitizer in squamous cell carcinoma. Photodiagn Photodyn Ther. 2022;38:102857. https://doi.org/10.1016/j.pdpdt.2022.102857.

7 Photodynamic Therapy for Cutaneous Melanoma

Jiawen Gao, Lei Shi, Bo Wang, and Xiuli Wang

7.1 Overview of Cutaneous Melanoma

Cutaneous melanoma is a malignant tumor derived from melanocytes, and its etiology is not yet fully understood. Most people agree that race, heredity, trauma, stimulation, sunshine, and immunity are connected to it. Early on, it might present as black lesions on healthy skin, or the first melanocytic nevi can quickly enlarge and become darker. The rash might take on the appearance of a mushroom or cauliflower, with a surface that is prone to rupturing and bleeding, as the disease worsens and the lesion grows. The risk to human health is significant, and the death rate is high in the event of distant metastases. The incidence of cutaneous melanoma has been increasing annually in recent years. Early cutaneous melanoma identification is becoming more common as diagnostic technology advances. Doctors are presently faced with the problem of improving therapeutic efficacy and patient prognosis for patients with different stages of melanoma.

7.1.1 Classification of Primary Cutaneous Melanoma

From a histological standpoint, lentigo maligna melanoma, acral lentiginous melanoma, nodular melanoma, and superficial spreading melanoma are the most prevalent pathological types of melanoma. Epithelioid, fibroproliferative, and balloon-like cells; spindle cells; malignant amelanotic nevi; and gigantic nevus melanomas are rare types.

7.1.1.1 Superficial Spreading Melanoma (SSM)

The most common type among fair-skinned individuals frequently affects the lower limbs and backs of younger individuals and females. SSM typically develops horizontally before moving into a vertical growth phase and is generally associated with a favorable prognosis.

7.1.1.2 Nodular Melanoma (NM)

NM often appears as quickly growing, pigmented nodules, sometimes amelanotic, which may bleed

J. Gao · X. Wang
Institute of Photomedicine, Shanghai Skin Disease Hospital, School of Medicine, Tongji University, Shanghai, China
e-mail: wangxiuli_1400023@tongji.edu.cn

L. Shi
Department of Dermatology, Huadong Hospital, Fudan University, Shanghai, People's Republic of China

B. Wang (✉)
Avera Medical Group Dermatology, Aberdeen, SD, USA

University of South Dakota, Vermillion, SD, USA
e-mail: makiwang@med.umich.edu

X. Wang, B. Wang (eds.), *Photodynamic Therapy in Dermatology*,
https://doi.org/10.1007/978-981-96-8915-6_7

or ulcerate. NM is common in older males and is often found in areas with sporadic sun exposure. NM is highly malignant and frequently thick upon diagnosis, resulting in a poorer prognosis.

7.1.1.3 Lentigo Maligna Melanoma (LMM)

LMM is a high-grade chronic sun-damaged melanoma. It is characterized by linear or nested hyperplasia of atypical melanoma cells along the dermal–epidermal junction, extends to the hair follicle epithelium and sweat gland ducts, and is accompanied by severe sun damage. Atypical melanocytes can infiltrate the dermis. Accounting for only 10% of melanomas, it is less common than the previous two types. It commonly affects middle-aged and older individuals, especially those in frequently sun-exposed areas such as the face. LMM generally develops after years of sun exposure and is not derived from preexisting nevi. Early presentations include dark, irregular brown macules or patches, which can frequently be misdiagnosed as lentigo or seborrheic keratosis.

7.1.1.4 Acral Lentiginous Melanoma (ALM)

ALM is rare in white populations but more prevalent in Asian and African populations. ALM often affects areas such as nail beds, fingers, toes, and palms. Owing to its location, it is frequently overlooked in the early stages, which contributes to delayed diagnosis.

7.1.2 Treatment Methods

7.1.2.1 Surgical Excision

Surgical excision is the primary treatment for cutaneous melanoma. If melanoma is suspected, an initial incisional biopsy is recommended. According to the American Academy of Dermatology guidelines, melanomas less than 2 mm Breslow depth should be excised with a 1 cm margin [1].

7.1.2.2 Chemotherapy

Patients with metastases may receive chemotherapy alone or in combination with other therapies. Common medications include dacarbazine (DTIC), temozolomide, cisplatin/carboplatin, fotemustine, vinblastine, and paclitaxel. Combined regimens, including CVD (cisplatin, vinblastine, DITC) and BOLD (bleomycin, vincristine, fotemustine, DITC), are also used.

7.1.2.3 Targeted Therapy

Currently, most targeted therapies for melanoma focus on the MAPK pathway and the PI3K-AKT signaling pathway, especially in patients with BRAF V600 mutation. These therapies include BRAF inhibitors such as vemurafenib and dual-target combinations of BRAF and MEK inhibitors such as dabrafenib and trametinib. The COMBI-AD trial confirmed the superiority of dual-target therapy for stage III melanoma, with the tumor mutational burden (TMB) being an independent prognostic factor in the placebo group but not in the treatment group. IFNγ expression was associated with longer recurrence-free survival (RFS) in the treatment group, whereas treatment efficacy and prognosis were unaffected by the baseline mutation rate in the MAPK pathway [2]. The 2022 Chinese Society of Clinical Oncology (CSCO) melanoma guidelines recommend dual-target therapy with dabrafenib and trametinib for stage III melanoma with a grade I recommendation. For patients with KIT mutations, tyrosine kinase inhibitors such as imatinib and nilotinib are available in China. However, the effectiveness of targeted therapies for advanced melanoma is limited in China because of the lower prevalence of BRAF mutations than in the Caucasian population.

7.1.2.4 Immunotherapy

Immunotherapy activates the patient's immune system via vaccines derived from their own tumor cells. As an immunogenic tumor, melanoma can be treated by injecting cytokines such as IFN-α and IL-2. Immune checkpoint inhibitors, particularly PD-1, PD-L1, and CTLA-4 inhibitors, have become essential for treating metastatic melanoma. Commonly used immune checkpoint inhibitors include PD-1 monoclonal antibodies such as pembrolizumab and nivolumab and the CTLA-4 monoclonal antibody ipilimumab, which are used alone or in combination. Clinical trials have shown that patients treated with pembrolizumab have a 2-year survival rate of 53.6%, whereas those treated with both PD-1 and CTLA-4 inhibitors have a 2-year survival rate of 63.8% [3]. However, combining CTLA-4 and PD-1 inhibitors is associated with high toxicity and should be used with caution. Most trials have focused on advanced chronic sun-damaged melanoma, but immunotherapy is less effective in advanced acral melanoma, the most common melanoma type in China, underscoring the need for more research on melanoma immunotherapy.

Cutaneous melanoma is highly malignant and has a poor prognosis, particularly when metastasis occurs. Surgery remains the most effective treatment for early-stage melanoma without metastasis, with high success rates. Key treatments include surgery, immunotherapy, chemotherapy, and targeted therapy [4]. However, current therapies are not always sufficient, highlighting the importance of developing innovative treatment approaches for comprehensive melanoma management.

7.2 Photodynamic Therapy and Cutaneous Melanoma

Photodynamic therapy (PDT), which offers the benefits of a minimally invasive nature, reproducibility, and tissue-preserving qualities, is widely used in dermatology for nonmelanoma skin cancers. However, its application in treating cutaneous melanoma is still emerging.

7.2.1 Overview of Research on PDT for Melanoma Treatment

The use of PDT for cutaneous melanoma remains mostly in the experimental stage, with studies focusing on cell cultures and animal models.

In cellular experiments, Lang et al. investigated porphyrin synthesis in HaCaT cells, fibroblasts, and melanoma cells (Bro, SKMel-23, SKMel-28) via in vitro ALA-PDT [5]. All melanoma cells showed peak induction of porphyrin synthesis after 16–36 h of incubation with ALA (1 mM), with higher production of protoporphyrin and fecal porphyrin than keratinocytes did. Moreover, compared with primary melanoma cells, metastatic melanoma cells can accumulate higher levels of porphyrin. Using A375 cells with ALA-PDT, Yuangang Lu's team demonstrated that ALA-PDT increased E-cadherin expression, potentially reducing the invasive capacity of melanoma cells [6]. Additionally, research by Tahmasebi et al. indicated that coincubation with 5-fluorouracil (5-FU) enhanced the cytotoxic effect of ALA-PDT on melanoma cells (the MeL-Rm cell line) [7].

Haddad et al. investigated the effects of systemic ALA-PDT in animal models of melanoma and reported significantly improved survival rates in treated mice ($p < 0.05$). In cellular experiments, PDT was more effective at reducing melanoma cell viability than both untreated melanoma cells and treated normal splenic tissue cells were ($p < 0.001$), suggesting the potential of ALA as a photosensitizer for melanoma treatment [8]. In related research, Pahernik et al. used topical ALA on Syrian golden hamsters with the amelanotic melanoma cell line A-Mel-3 and observed the selective accumulation of porphyrin within tumor tissues [9]. Additionally, Hao Fei's team applied a combination of 10% 5-ALA and Ce6 via topical and intraperitoneal routes, along with 652 nm semiconductor laser irradiation, in melanoma-bearing mice. These results demonstrated effective melanoma cell destruction with the Ce6 and 5-ALA PDT approach [10].

Melanin produced by melanoma cells can limit light penetration, potentially reducing the effectiveness of photodynamic therapy (PDT) for melanoma. This challenge has led to ongoing debate among researchers about the suitability of PDT for treating cutaneous melanoma. Some suggest that animal models, in which melanoma cell lines are introduced into animals, show enhanced sensitivity to PDT, supporting the translation of results to human applications; however, other researchers have argued against this.

Von Felbert et al. examined the impact of ALA-PDT on melanoma via MT-Ret transgenic mice, a model closely resembling human melanoma. Their studies revealed that while ALA-PDT showed sensitivity in melanoma cells in vitro, it failed to significantly inhibit tumor growth in vivo and caused minimal increases in fibrosis and bleeding at tumor sites, indicating resistance to PDT in malignant MT-Ret melanomas [11]. These findings suggest that malignant MT-Ret melanomas are resistant to PDT in vivo despite their sensitivity in vitro. In earlier work, Nelson et al. reported in nude mice that hematoporphyrin derivatives (HpD) used in PDT were effective against amelanotic melanomas but not melanotic melanomas. They attributed this to melanin's interference with PDT, where melanin competes for photons or redirects energy from excited photosensitizers. The broad absorption range of stabilized protein complexes is limited by the presence of melanin, leading to an inefficient phototoxic response [12]. Busetti et al. later proposed a solution using pulsed laser preirradiation at 1064 nm along with the benzoporphyrin derivative cyclic A monoacid (verteporfin, BPD-MA) as a photosensitizer. This combination enhances the therapeutic effect of PDT on B16 pigmented melanoma cells, offering a potential way to overcome the limiting effects of melanin on PDT efficacy [13].

Improving the effectiveness of PDT for treating melanoma involves increasing photosensitizer bioavailability, enhancing light penetration, and optimizing tumor light absorption. Recently, nanoparticles have gained interest in skin tumor treatments because of their biocompatibility, which allows them to cross biological barriers such as blood vessels, dense interstitial spaces in tumors, and cellular membranes. This capability also enhances the bioavailability of drugs carried by nanoparticles [14]. An increasing number of nanoparticles, including second-generation polyamide dendrimer (PAMAM-G2), gold, organosilicon, and poly-N-phenylglycine, are being explored for their potential in PDT, although most studies are still in preclinical stages, including studies with cellular and animal models. The use of nanoparticles to combine PDT with immunotherapy is also under investigation. Zhenxi Zhang's research team constructed a tumor microenvironment/light multiresponsive lipid nanomedicine control system (MRPL-SC), which demonstrated the synergistic antimelanoma effect of natural killer (NK) cell immunotherapy and PDT via the MRPL-SC in cellular and nude mouse xenograft models. This system enables the programmed release of antitumor drugs, suggesting an integrated approach for PDT and immunotherapy against melanoma [15].

7.2.2 The Mechanism of PDT in the Treatment of Melanoma

Research on the mechanism of action of PDT for treating cutaneous melanoma is currently ongoing; however, it has focused primarily on the signaling pathways associated with melanoma cell survival, proliferation, autophagy, and apoptosis.

7.2.2.1 PDT Induces Apoptosis in Melanoma Cells

Apoptotic processes include the activation of cysteine proteases (caspases), cytochrome C-dependent mitochondrial pathways, and other mechanisms [16]. Apoptosis can be initiated through an intrinsic mechanism (mitochondrial outer membrane permeabilization), or the extrinsic pathway (death receptor activation) can initiate the cysteine protease cascade, both of which PDT can activate. PDT has been reported to activate mitochondria-mediated caspase pathways with photosensitizers such as chrysin [17, 18]. Certain photosensitizers directly target mitochondria, which play a key role in apoptosis. For example, Barge et al. studied the photocidal effects of the photosensitizer silicone phthalocyanine in human melanoma and reported that its cholesterol derivatives enhance mitochondrial permeability and generate substrates resembling caspases, inhibiting cystatinase activity and leading to apoptotic cell death [19].

7.2.2.2 PDT Induces Autophagy in Melanoma Cells

Autophagy, a self-degradative process found in most eukaryotic cells, is tightly regulated by various intracellular genes and signaling pathways. In melanoma cells, PDT-induced oxidative stress has been linked to triggering autophagy, which breaks down organelles and depletes intracellular nutrients [20]. Although research specific to melanoma cells is limited, studies in other tumor cells indicate that PDT-induced disruption of the lysosomal system, which is crucial for processing ROS-damaged organelles, can initiate autophagy [8]. Furthermore, autophagy may be influenced by PDT-induced loss of the antiapoptotic protein Bcl-2 in mitochondria [21].

7.2.2.3 Effects of PDT on Melanoma Cell Proliferation and Survival Pathways

Cell proliferation, a primary driver of carcinogenesis, is regulated by the Ras/Raf/MEK/ERK signaling pathway, a major mechanism controlling melanoma cell growth, differentiation, and proliferation. Approximately 90% of melanoma patients exhibit high ERK expression [22], with the common BRAF mutation V600E causing excessive ERK signaling. Research by Zhimin Tong et al. demonstrated that prolonged ERK1/2 activation can protect tumor cells from PDT-induced death, as shown by ERK1/2 activity in both PDT-sensitive (GM38A) and PDT-resistant (LFS087) cell lines post-PDT [23]. Nuclear factors, such as NF-κB, are critical regulators of cell proliferation, metastasis, and survival, making them key targets in the antiproliferative effects of PDT. The primary mechanisms of PDT-induced oxidative stress include ROS-induced activation of NF-kß and I-kß inhibition [24]. Thus, targeting NF-κB inhibition in PDT could be pivotal in controlling the growth of malignant cells.

7.2.3 Photothermal Therapy and Cutaneous Melanoma

In photothermal therapy (PTT), a substance with high photothermal conversion efficiency is administered to target and accumulate near tumor tissue. Upon irradiation with an external light source, this substance converts light energy into heat, killing cancer cells. Melanin particles in melanoma are adept at absorbing photons for photothermal conversion, an ability not present in surrounding normal tissues. Therefore, PTT can theoretically provide precise melanoma treatment with minimal impact on healthy tissues. The benefits of this approach include reduced side effects, high specificity, and suitability for outpatient care. The authors' group reported that PTT primarily affects melanoma cells, ablating and destroying melanoma cells via photothermal impact, further releasing significant tumor-associated antigens and activating immune responses. Animal studies with transcriptome sequencing confirmed the dual effects of PTT in "ablation" and "immune activation."

After laser irradiation of the tissue surface, the treated area is divided into five temperature-based zones: (1) the evaporative charring region (>105 °C), which causes tissue charring and evaporation, eliminating tumor cells and associated immune suppression related to tumor cells (Fig. 7.1); (2) the cytotoxic region (46–100 °C); (3) the heat shock region (41–43 °C); (4) the hypothermia region (39–41 °C); and (5) the photobiological region (normal body temperature), which has a photobiological modulatory effect and enhances immune and antitumor activities through photobiological modulation, promoting photochemical and photophysical reactions.

These regions work together to activate the immune response. For example, the evaporative charring region eliminates many tumor cells, alleviating immune suppression. Other regions enhance cellular immunity by promoting DC maturation, antigen uptake, and phagocytosis capacity through the expression of DAMPs (HSP70 and HSP90) in tumor cells. Additionally, the migration of mature and activated DCs to draining lymph nodes further activates T cells, which in turn induce antitumor cellular immunity [25, 26]. PTT establishes a photothermal gradient within tumor tissue, either by inhibiting tumor growth through immune responses induced by tumor-specific antigens or controlling apoptosis and necrosis by influencing heat shock proteins (HSPs) in tumor cells, thereby increasing cellular immunity.

An iHRANP molecular probe with ultrasensitive H_2O_2 responsiveness was developed by Professor Bingbo Zhang's research team at Tongji University School of Medicine via

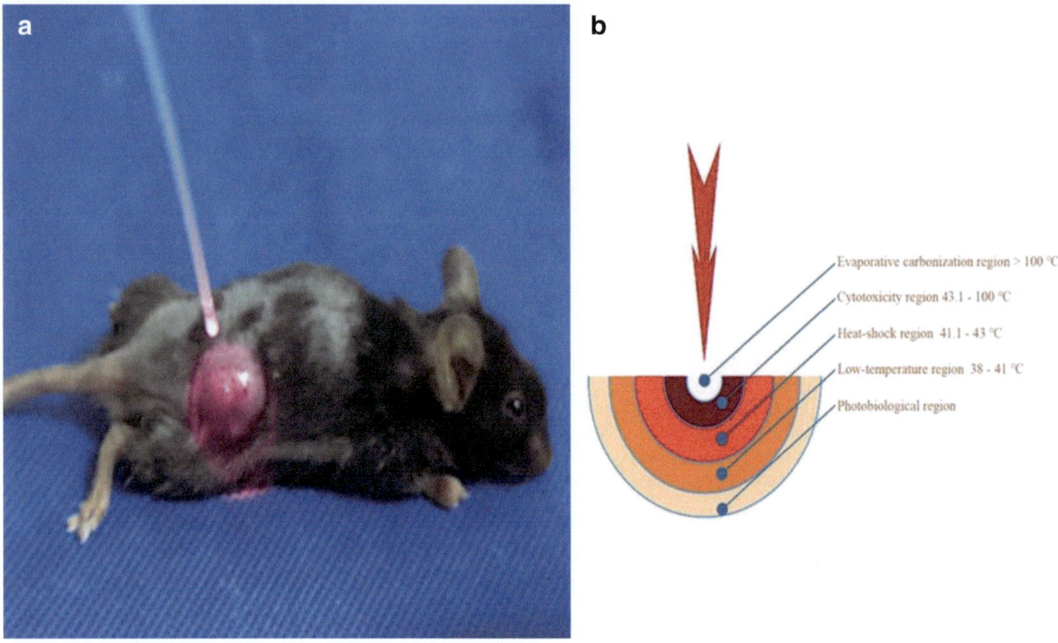

Fig. 7.1 Photothermal treatment of mouse melanoma produces a photothermal gradient that activates immunity to inhibit tumor growth

enzyme–protein-mediated simulation and biomimicry. Under 808 nm laser irradiation, this probe demonstrated strong photoacoustic imaging and effective photothermal conversion. The authors' group, in collaboration with Prof. Zhang's team, conducted a comparative study on mice with squamous carcinoma and melanoma. After iHRANP injection into the mouse tail vein, both tumor models presented strong and comparable MRI signals, yet the photoacoustic signals differed significantly: melanoma tissues presented weaker signals than squamous carcinoma tissues did, suggesting higher H_2O_2 levels in melanoma. This distinction was confirmed through in vitro and ex vivo studies, which successfully identified and differentiated the two types of tumors via photoacoustic imaging. Further photothermal treatment experiments revealed that the tumor-suppressive effect was stronger in melanoma than in squamous carcinoma under the same iHRANP dose and 808 nm light exposure. In squamous carcinoma tissues, locally injected H_2O_2 enhanced the photothermal effect of iHRANPs, increasing their antitumor efficacy. This method achieves precise treatment for squamous carcinoma and melanoma, with MRI guiding the process. This research laid the foundation for clinical advancements in noninvasive, precise diagnostic and therapeutic integration in animal research [27] (Fig. 7.2).

After PTT treatment, the authors' group analyzed gene expression and immune cell composition in mouse melanoma via microarray analysis. A total of 256 DEGs were identified, 215 of which were downregulated and 41 of which were upregulated. Gene function annotations indicated that most of these genes were associated with inflammatory and immune responses. Analysis of immune cell composition revealed shifts in several immune cell ratios, including M2 macrophages, dendritic cells (DCs), natural killer (NK) cells, and regulatory T cells (Tregs) (Fig. 7.3). Specifically, M2 macrophages tended to polarize toward the M1 type and significantly decreased following PTT, enhancing antitumor immunity. Additionally, the increase in activated DCs and NK cells after PTT further promoted antitumor-specific and innate immune responses. Treg cells are known to facilitate tumor growth and express CTLA-4, a cytotoxic T-lymphocyte-

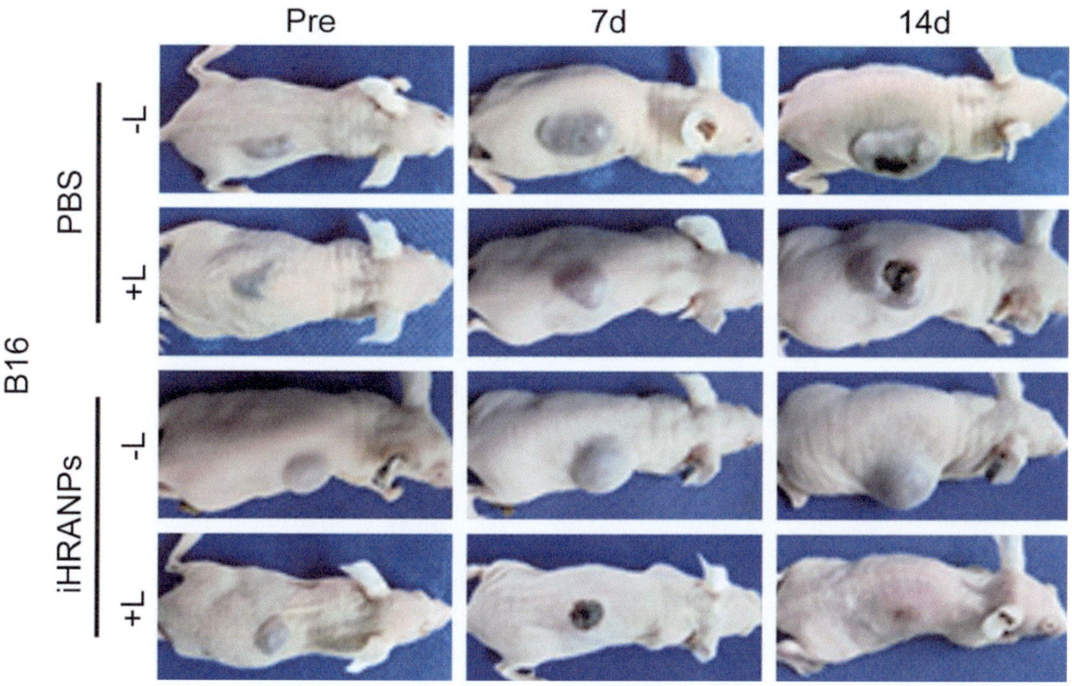

Fig. 7.2 Before and after iHRANP nanoprobe-mediated PTT treatment of melanoma in mice

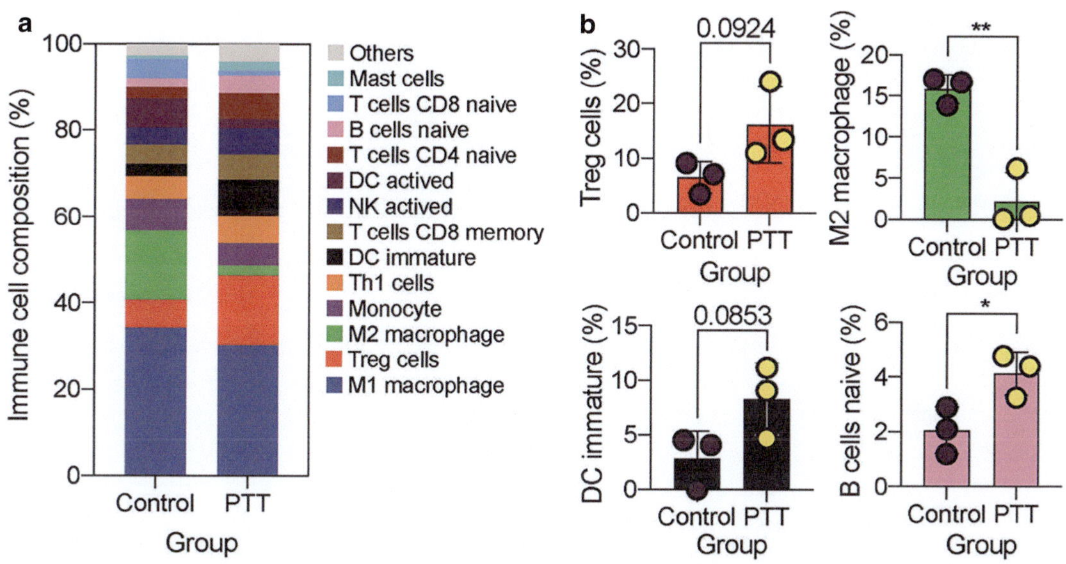

Fig. 7.3 (**a**) Analysis of changes in immune cell composition before and after PTT treatment on the basis of gene expression profiles. (**b**) Significantly changed immune cells before and after PTT treatment on the basis of gene expression profiles

associated antigen. Treg cells significantly increase following PTT, possibly as a defense mechanism against excessive immune responses. These findings suggest that combining PTT with checkpoint inhibitors such as anti-CTLA-4 could further enhance PTT efficacy in melanoma treatment [28].

Currently, the clinical effect of using melanin particles in melanoma to absorb photons and generate a thermal effect is limited; however, exogenously administered photothermal agents concentrated in melanoma tissues may enhance the effectiveness of PTT. The authors' group successfully developed Prussian blue nanoparticles with high photothermal conversion efficiency and good biocompatibility to mediate PTT for melanoma treatment. These nanoparticles inhibited melanoma cell proliferation in a concentration-dependent manner. Through animal models, they demonstrated the high photothermal conversion effectiveness of Prussian blue nanoparticles. After 10 min of illumination, tumor-adjacent temperatures reached 62.9 °C, and tumors either significantly reduced or disappeared after treatment compared with those of the controls. H&E staining further suggested that Prussian blue nanoparticles had no notable toxic effects on the organs of the mice [29]. These results imply that Prussian blue nanoparticle-mediated PTT could represent a promising strategy for melanoma treatment.

PTT and PDT are viable treatments for melanoma, either alone or in combination. The authors discovered that bionanoparticle-mediated PTT in conjunction with PDT can effectively slow tumor progression in melanoma models. This study used indocyanine green loaded into a bovine serum albumin–manganese dioxide complex to form biomimetic nanoparticles called MnO2-ICG@BSA. These nanoparticles can absorb near-infrared light, maintain stable photothermal conversion, and improve the local hypoxic environment of the tumor, increasing the effectiveness of PDT. As a result, they significantly reduced proliferation in melanoma cell lines and murine melanoma models [30]. MnO_2-ICG@BSA nanoparticle-mediated PTT combined with PDT thus appears to be a promising melanoma treatment approach (Fig. 7.4).

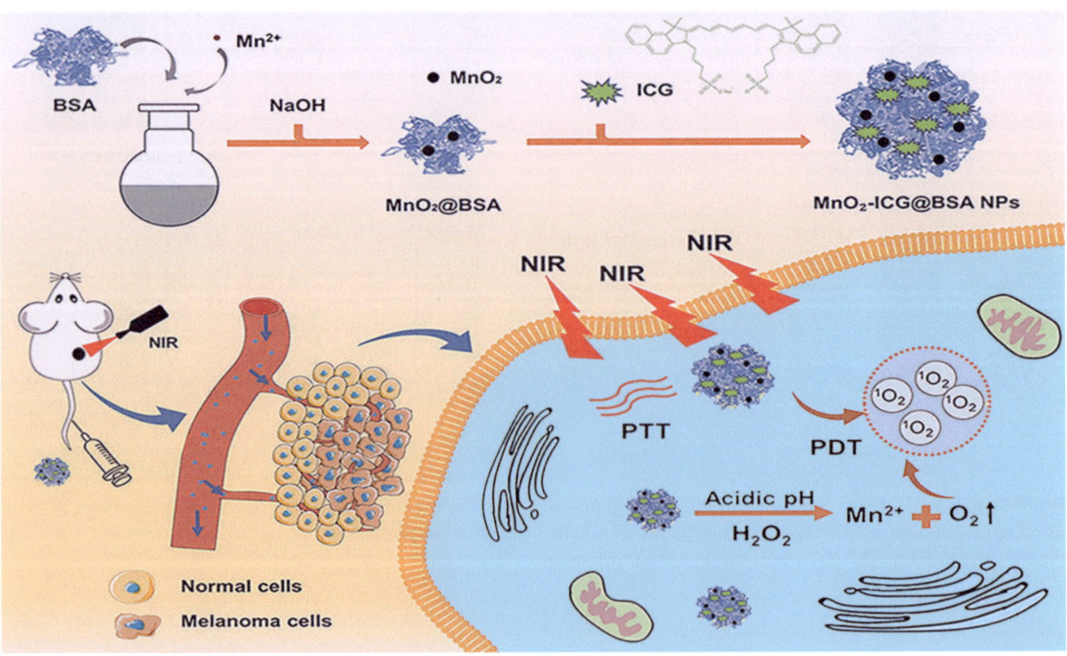

Fig. 7.4 Mechanism of MnO2-ICG@BSA nanoparticle-mediated PTT combined with PDT for the treatment of melanoma in mice

Although PDT and PTT for cutaneous melanoma are still under investigation, their efficacy currently falls short of clinical application. However, various new photosensitizers, photothermal agents, and light source devices for treating melanoma are being researched and developed, which are expected to improve the effectiveness of PDT and PTT for the treatment of cutaneous melanoma. These advancements are anticipated to gradually become part of treatment or adjuvant therapy for this condition [31].

References

1. Swetter SM, Tsao H, Bichakjian CK, Curiel-Lewandrowski C, Elder DE, Gershenwald JE, et al. Guidelines of care for the management of primary cutaneous melanoma. J Am Acad Dermatol. 2019;80(1):208–50. https://doi.org/10.1016/j.jaad.2018.08.055.
2. Dummer R, Brase JC, Garrett J, Campbell CD, Gasal E, Squires M, et al. Adjuvant dabrafenib plus trametinib versus placebo in patients with resected, BRAF(V600)-mutant, stage III melanoma (COMBI-AD): exploratory biomarker analyses from a randomised, phase 3 trial. Lancet Oncol. 2020;21(3):358–72. https://doi.org/10.1016/S1470-2045(20)30062-0.
3. Hodi FS, Chesney J, Pavlick AC, Robert C, Grossmann KF, McDermott DF, et al. Combined nivolumab and ipilimumab versus ipilimumab alone in patients with advanced melanoma: 2-year overall survival outcomes in a multicenter, randomized, controlled, phase 2 trial. Lancet Oncol. 2016;17(11):1558–68. https://doi.org/10.1016/s1470-2045(16)30366-7.
4. Luke JJ, Schwartz GK. Chemotherapy in the management of advanced cutaneous malignant melanoma. Clin Dermatol. 2013;31(3):290–7. https://doi.org/10.1016/j.clindermatol.2012.08.016.
5. Lang K, Bolsen K, Stahl W, Ruzicka T, Sies H, Lehmann P, et al. The 5-aminolevulinic acid-induced porphyrin biosynthesis in benign and malignant cells of the skin. J Photochem Photobiol B. 2001;65(1):29–34.
6. Dong L, Shen X, Zhang W, Lu Y. Photodynamic therapy inhibits migration, invasion and epithelial mesenchymal transition in melanoma. Immunol J. 2020;36(6):516–20. https://doi.org/10.13431/j.cnki.immunol.j.20200082.
7. Tahmasebi H, Khoshgard K, Sazgarnia A, Mostafaie A, Eivazi MT. Enhancing the efficiency of 5-aminolevulinic acid-mediated photodynamic therapy using 5-fluorouracil on human melanoma cells. Photodiagn Photodyn Ther. 2016;13:297–302. https://doi.org/10.1016/j.pdpdt.2015.08.011.
8. Haddad R, Kaplan O, Greenberg R, Siegal A, Skornick Y, Kashtan H. Photodynamic therapy of murine colon cancer and melanoma using systemic aminolevulinic acid as a photosensitizer. Int J Surg Investig. 2000;2(3):171–8.
9. Pahernik S, Langer S, Botzlar A, Dellian M, Goetz AE. Tissue distribution and penetration of 5-ALA induced fluorescence in an amelanotic melanoma after topical application. Anticancer Res. 2001;21(1A):59–63.
10. Deng J, Hao F. Therapeutic effect of photodynamic therapy with chlorin e6 and 5-aminolevulinic acid on malignant melanoma in mice. Acta Acad Med Militaris Tertiae. 2006;28(16):1675–8.
11. Cordoba F, Braathen LR, Weissenberger J, Vallan C, Kato M, Nakashima I, et al. 5-aminolaevulinic acid photodynamic therapy in a transgenic mouse model of skin melanoma. Exp Dermatol. 2005;14(6):429–37. https://doi.org/10.1111/j.0906-6705.2005.00303.x.
12. Nelson JS, McCullough JL, Berns MW. Photodynamic therapy of human malignant melanoma xenografts in athymic nude mice. J Natl Cancer Inst. 1988;80(1):56–60.
13. Busetti A, Soncin M, Reddi E, Rodgers MA, Kenney ME, Jori G. Photothermal sensitization of amelanotic melanoma cells by Ni(II)-octabutoxy-naphthalocyanine. J Photochem Photobiol B. 1999;53(1-3):103–9.
14. Borgheti-Cardoso LN, Viegas JSR, Silvestrini AVP, Caron AL, Praca FG, Kravicz M, et al. Nanotechnology approaches in the current therapy of skin cancer. Adv Drug Deliv Rev. 2020;153:109–36. https://doi.org/10.1016/j.addr.2020.02.005.
15. Liu H, Qin F, Wang S, Zhang Z. Multi-responsive liposomal nanocomplex encapsulating Ce6 & MMP-2 inhibitors for photodynamic-immune synergistic treatment of melanoma. Chin J Lasers. 2023;50(3):14. https://doi.org/10.3788/CJL221212.
16. Danial NN, Korsmeyer SJ. Cell death: critical control points. Cell. 2004;116(2):205–19.
17. Agostinis P, Buytaert E, Breyssens H, Hendrickx N. Regulatory pathways in photodynamic therapy induced apoptosis. Photochem Photobiol Sci. 2004;3(8):721–9. https://doi.org/10.1039/b315237e.
18. Oleinick NL, Morris RL, Belichenko I. The role of apoptosis in response to photodynamic therapy: what, where why, and how. Photochem Photobiol Sci. 2002;1(1):1–21.
19. Barge J, Decreau R, Julliard M, Hubaud JC, Sabatier AS, Grob JJ, et al. Killing efficacy of a new silicon phthalocyanine in human melanoma cells treated with photodynamic therapy by early activation of mitochondrion-mediated apoptosis. Exp Dermatol. 2004;13(1):33–44. https://doi.org/10.1111/j.0906-6705.2004.00147.x.
20. Davids LM, Kleemann B, Cooper S, Kidson SH. Melanomas display increased cytoprotection to hypericin-mediated cytotoxicity through the induction of autophagy. Cell Biol Int. 2009;33(10):1065–72. https://doi.org/10.1016/j.cellbi.2009.06.026.

21. Pattingre S, Tassa A, Qu X, Garuti R, Liang XH, Mizushima N, et al. Bcl-2 antiapoptotic proteins inhibit Beclin 1-dependent autophagy. Cell. 2005;122(6):927–39. https://doi.org/10.1016/j.cell.2005.07.002.
22. Cohen C, Zavala-Pompa A, Sequeira JH, Shoji M, Sexton DG, Cotsonis G, et al. Mitogen-actived protein kinase activation is an early event in melanoma progression. Clin Cancer Res. 2002;8(12):3728–33.
23. Tong Z, Singh G, Rainbow AJ. Sustained activation of the extracellular signal-regulated kinase pathway protects cells from photofrin-mediated photodynamic therapy. Cancer Res. 2002;62(19):5528–35.
24. Mercurio F, Manning AM. NF-kappaB as a primary regulator of the stress response. Oncogene. 1999;18(45):6163–71. https://doi.org/10.1038/sj.onc.1203174.
25. Luo M, Shi L, Zhang F, Zhou F, Zhang L, Wang B, et al. Laser immunotherapy for cutaneous squamous cell carcinoma with optimal thermal effects to enhance tumor immunogenicity. Int J Hyperth. 2018;34(8):1337–50. https://doi.org/10.1080/02656736.2018.1446221.
26. Zhou F, Li X, Naylor MF, Hode T, Nordquist RE, Alleruzzo L, et al. InCVAX–a novel strategy for treatment of late-stage, metastatic cancers through photoimmunotherapy induced tumor-specific immunity. Cancer Lett. 2015;359(2):169–77. https://doi.org/10.1016/j.canlet.2015.01.029.
27. Wang P, Yang W, Shen S, Wu C, Wen L, Cheng Q, et al. Differential diagnosis and precision therapy of two typical malignant cutaneous tumors leveraging their tumor microenvironment: a photomedicine strategy. ACS Nano. 2019;13(10):11168–80. https://doi.org/10.1021/acsnano.9b04070.
28. Yan G, Shi L, Zhang F, Luo M, Zhang G, Liu P, et al. Transcriptomic analysis of mechanism of melanoma cell death induced by photothermal therapy. J Biophotonics. 2021;14(8):e202100034. https://doi.org/10.1002/jbio.202100034.
29. Li M, Wang X, Wei Z. The study of Prussian blue nanoparticles photothermal therapy on skin melanoma. Chin J Dermatovenereol. 2017;31(9):941–5. https://doi.org/10.13735/j.cjdv.1001-7089.201701055.
30. Wen L, Hyoju R, Wang P, Shi L, Li C, Li M, et al. Hydrogen-peroxide-responsive protein biomimetic nanoparticles for photothermal-photodynamic combination therapy of melanoma. Lasers Surg Med. 2021;53(3):390–9. https://doi.org/10.1002/lsm.23292.
31. Davids LM, Kleemann B. Combating melanoma: the use of photodynamic therapy as a novel, adjuvant therapeutic tool. Cancer Treat Rev. 2011;37(6):465–75. https://doi.org/10.1016/j.ctrv.2010.11.007.

8 ALA-PDT in the Treatment of HPV-Related Diseases

Haiyan Zhang, Yutong Yang, Jia Yan, Jingjuan Shi, Lei Shi, Hongwei Wang, Bo Wang, and Xiuli Wang

8.1 ALA-PDT for the Treatment of Condyloma Acuminata

8.1.1 Introduction

Condyloma acuminata, commonly referred to as genital or venereal warts, are skin conditions caused by HPV infection affecting the external genital and perianal skin and mucosa. HPV is a double-stranded circular DNA virus with more than 200 subtypes identified. In China, common HPV types include HPV6, HPV11, HPV16, HPV52, HPV58, HPV18, HPV33, etc. [1, 2]. HPV types are categorized as low-risk (e.g., HPV6, HPV11) or high-risk (e.g., HPV16, HPV18, HPV52, HPV58, HPV33) [3].

High-risk HPV types are prone to integrate into host cell DNA, leading to squamous intraepithelial lesions in cervical epithelial cells and potentially cervical cancer [4, 5]. Previously, genital warts were thought to result primarily from low-risk HPV infections. However, in 2009, the authors' group investigated cervical HPV infection and the HPV subtype distribution in female patients with vulvar condyloma acuminata in Shanghai. Their findings revealed that 22.2% of patients had coinfections of low- and high-risk HPV types, with 85.6% of these patients also experiencing cervical HPV infection. Vulvar and cervical HPV infections were consistent in 95.8% of cases, with high-risk HPV infections significantly increasing the risk of genital squamous intraepithelial lesions, squamous cell carcinoma, and cervical cancer [6].

8.1.1.1 Clinical Manifestations

Condyloma acuminata typically present in men on the glans penis, coronal sulcus, inner foreskin, and frenulum, whereas in women, they generally affect the vulva, vagina, and cervix. In both sexes, lesions may also occur in other areas, such as the urethra and anal canal. Lesions often appear as red, skin-colored, or brown papules with a papillomatous or cauliflower-like appearance, and some may develop into keratinizing papules or plaques. Lesions can progressively enlarge and may ulcerate, ooze, bleed, or become infected. Although generally asymptomatic, some patients report mild

H. Zhang · Y. Yang · J. Yan · J. Shi · X. Wang
Institute of Photomedicine, Shanghai Skin Disease Hospital, School of Medicine, Tongji University, Shanghai, China
e-mail: wangxiuli_1400023@tongji.edu.cn

L. Shi · H. Wang (✉)
Department of Dermatology, Huadong Hospital, Fudan University, Shanghai, People's Republic of China

B. Wang
Avera Medical Group Dermatology, Aberdeen, SD, USA

University of South Dakota, Vermillion, SD, USA
e-mail: makiwang@med.umich.edu

X. Wang, B. Wang (eds.), *Photodynamic Therapy in Dermatology*,
https://doi.org/10.1007/978-981-96-8915-6_8

itching, a sensation of a foreign body, or dyspareunia. Genital warts are categorized on the basis of their location, with external genital warts affecting areas such as the vulva or penis and intracavitary warts affecting areas such as the urethra, vagina, cervix, and anal canal (Fig. 8.1). In 2008, the authors' group reported that male patients with genital warts and diabetes presented unique clinical characteristics, with warts forming a "wreath-like" pattern around the foreskin (Fig. 8.2) and often accompanied by redundant foreskin, maceration, cracks, phimosis, and candidal balanitis [7].

8.1.1.2 Histopathology

The primary histological features include hyperkeratosis with parakeratosis, acanthosis, and papillomatous hyperplasia of the epidermis. In the middle and upper portions of the granular and spinous layers, numerous vacuolated cells are present, with large cell bodies and round, deeply stained nuclei. The dermal papillae exhibit vasodilation along with perivascular inflammatory infiltrates.

8.1.2 Treatment

8.1.2.1 Pharmacological Treatment

The primary treatment for condyloma acuminata involves topical medications aimed at removing warts and addressing surrounding subclinical infection, which are primarily suited for small, visible warts on the body surface [8]. The most commonly used topical agents in clinical settings include 0.5% Podophyllum emodin tincture, 5% imiquimod cream, and 33.3% trichloroacetic acid solution. However, these treatments often have low cure rates, a high likelihood of recurrence, and may require repeated applications. Treatment sites may also experience localized irritation, including redness, swelling, erosion, and, occasionally, secondary infections (Table 8.1). Intracavitary genital warts present additional challenges due to their concealed locations, making it harder for topical agents to reach the affected areas (Table 8.1). In 2013, a study by the authors' group noted adverse reactions in a couple using imiquimod cream for genital warts. The woman developed vitiligo-like depigmentation at

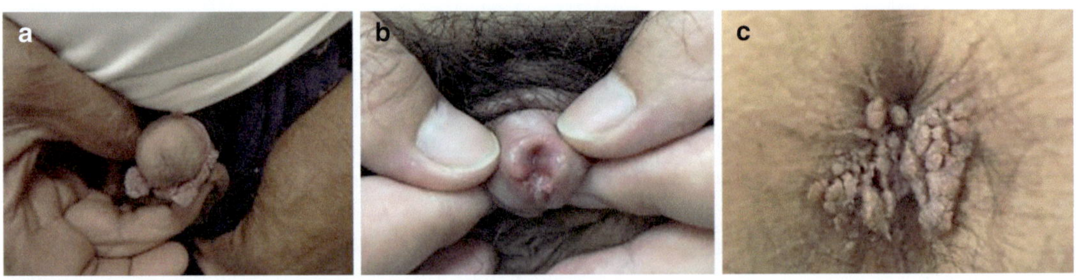

Fig. 8.1 Clinical manifestations of condyloma acuminata: (**a**) condyloma acuminata in the coronary sulcus, (**b**) condyloma acuminata at the urethral orifice, and (**c**) perianal condyloma acuminata

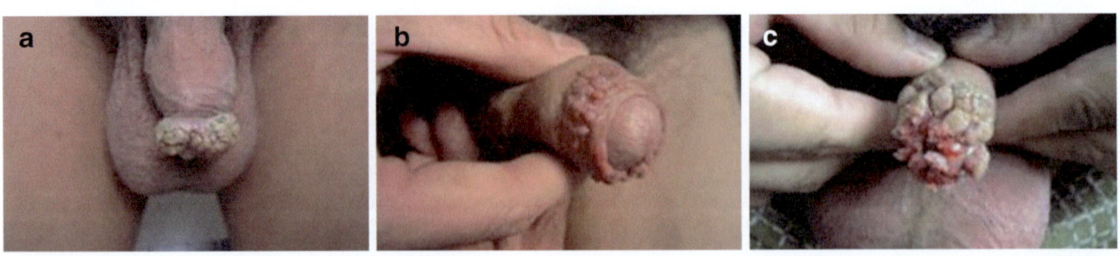

Fig. 8.2 Special clinical manifestations of genital warts in diabetic men: (**a**) warts grow exophytically around the foreskin, with visible phimosis and candidal balanitis, (**b**) warts present in a "wreath-like" pattern around the foreskin ring, with visible phimosis, and (**c**) many warts grow exophytically covering the foreskin, accompanied by maceration, fissures, bleeding of the foreskin, and candidal balanitis

Table 8.1 The main traditional treatments for condyloma acuminata

Treatment	Treatment options	advantage	disadvantage
0.5% podophyllum emodin tincture	After cleaning the warts, apply the tincture to the warts and surroundings, twice daily for 3 days, stop for 4 days (repeat as needed)	Can be treated at home	Local irritation: redness, swelling, erosion, and secondary infection
5% imiquimod cream	After cleaning the warts, apply the cream to the warts and surroundings, once every other day at night, rinse off in the next morning, course of treatment can be up to 16 weeks	Can be treated at home and can activate antiviral immunity to reduce recurrence	Local irritation, risk of secondary vitiligo
33.3% trichloroacetic acid solution	Apply to the wart with a cotton swab or bamboo stick, protect the surrounding normal skin and mucous membranes, retreat with 1–2-week intervals	Easy to operate and low cost	Local irritation, low cure rate, high recurrence rate
CO_2 laser, electrocautery, microwave, surgery	After local anesthesia, cautery or incision are used to remove visible warts, with 1–2-week intervals	Fast onset, high cure rate	Significant local trauma, risk for scarring, and high recurrence rate
Thermotherapy	Mainly through irradiation of the warts and surrounding areas with heat-generating light sources such as 808 nm or infrared, the temperature within the wart tissue is increased to exert thermal damage and immune effects	Mild side effects	Low cure rate
Liquid nitrogen cryotherapy	After local anesthesia, liquid nitrogen is placed in and around the wart with a liquid nitrogen treatment instrument or cotton swab and repeatedly freeze–thaw until a pale edema band appears around the wart, with 1–2-week intervals	Easy to operate and low cost	Low cure rate, with local pain, tissue edema, necrosis, and a high recurrence rate

the site of her vulvar lesion after 6 weeks of treatment with 5% imiquimod cream. Discontinuing imiquimod and switching to 0.1% tacrolimus ointment resulted in repigmentation after 4 months. Her husband developed localized lichen planus after 3 months of imiquimod cream use, which resolved after five sessions of ALA-PDT (Fig. 8.3) [9].

8.1.2.2 Nonpharmacological Treatment

Nonpharmacological treatments mainly include CO_2 lasers, liquid nitrogen cryotherapy, electrocautery, microwave therapy, thermotherapy, and surgery. Among these methods, CO_2 laser therapy is the most widely used traditional treatment method in China. The CO_2 laser allows for the direct removal of visible warts and is relatively easy to perform. However, it is highly invasive and often associated with serious adverse reactions, such as skin ulcers, scarring, and narrowing or adhesion of cavities (Fig. 8.4). Additionally, the recurrence rate following treatment is high. Cryotherapy with liquid nitrogen has a low cure rate and is commonly accompanied by significant local edema and necrosis, which can lead to discomfort and complications. Thermotherapy is a physical therapy method that works by activating the body's antiviral immune response. While it has the advantage of causing fewer adverse reactions, its effectiveness is limited, as the cure rate remains low (Table 8.1).

8.1.3 ALA-PDT in the Treatment of Condyloma Acuminata

8.1.3.1 ALA-PDT

In 1997, Professor Xiuli Wang pioneered the application of ALA-PDT for the treatment of condyloma acuminata in the urethra, initiating a series of clinical and foundational studies. In 2000, the authors' group became the first to systematically

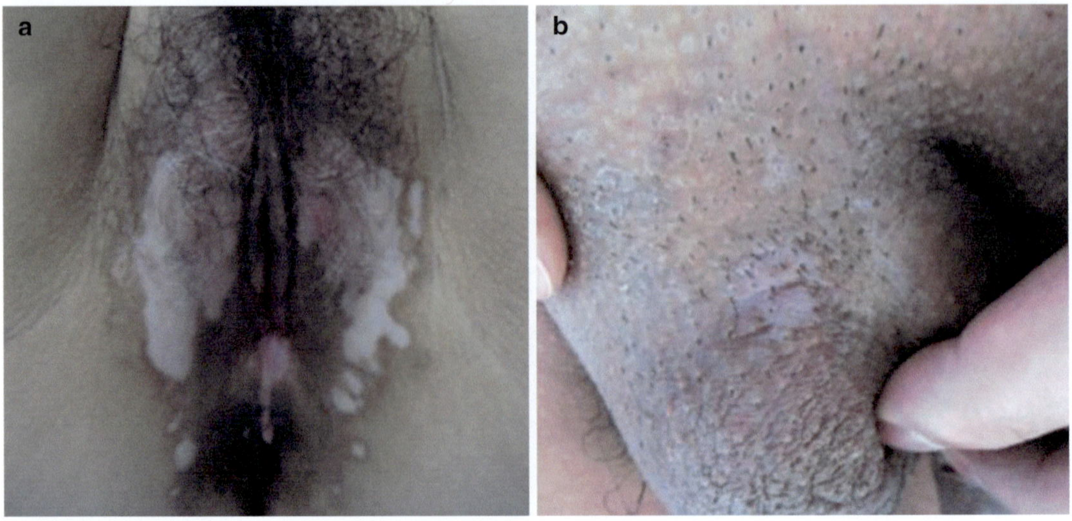

Fig. 8.3 Adverse reactions of a couple with condyloma acuminata after topical treatment with 5% imiquimod cream: (**a** vulvar vitiligo (wife) and (**b** lichen planus over the scrotum (husband)

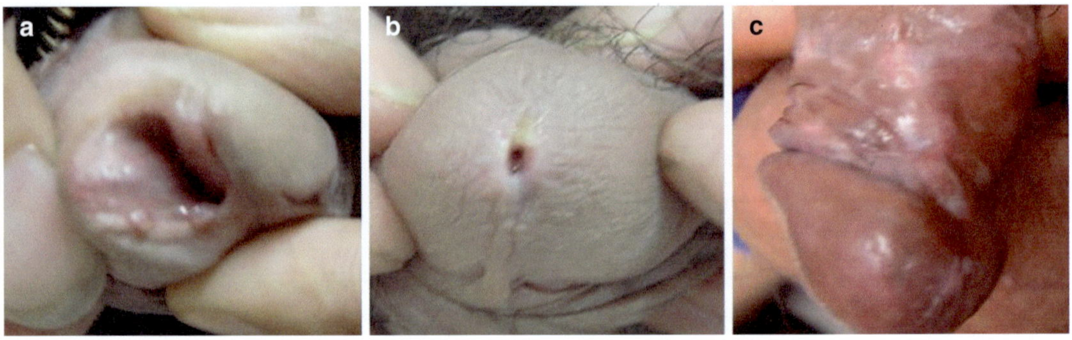

Fig. 8.4 Adverse reactions of traditional physical therapies in the treatment of condyloma acuminata: (**a**) recurrence of warts after surgical incision of the urethral orifice, (**b**) adhesion stricture of the urethral orifice caused by CO_2 laser treatment, and (**c**) scarring of the penis and foreskin after CO_2 laser and cryotherapy

report the safety and efficacy of ALA-PDT for genital urethral warts. In a study involving 18 patients with urethral condyloma acuminata, all achieved complete lesion resolution after four treatments. The cure rate was 100%, with no adverse reactions, such as scarring, urethral adhesion, or stricture [10]. Later studies from the authors' group involving 164 patients with condyloma acuminata confirmed a cure rate of 95% and a recurrence rate of only 5%. These studies reiterated the safety of ALA-PDT, with no reports of scarring, urethral adhesion, or stricture. The team also revealed two primary mechanisms by which ALA-PDT treats condyloma acuminata: (1) Direct effects: ALA-PDT causes the apoptosis and necrosis of HPV-infected keratinocytes. (2) Immune activation: This process stimulates immune cells such as neutrophils and lymphocytes, enhancing the immune response. These findings were published in the *British Journal of Dermatology* in 2004 and received widespread international recognition, with 361 citations. These contributions have significantly bolstered the academic influence of Chinese researchers in the field [11].

In 2006, the authors compared the efficacy of ALA-PDT and CO_2 laser therapy for treating condyloma acuminata of the external genitalia and reported that ALA-PDT offers significant advantages over CO_2 laser. ALA-PDT demonstrated a "field therapy" effect, effectively targeting subclinical and latent infections around warts, resulting in a higher cure rate, lower recurrence rate, mild trauma, no scarring, and preservation of local tissue structure and function (Fig. 8.5) [12]. In contrast, CO_2 laser therapy provided only a "focal ablation" effect. This study introduced the concept of ALA-PDT's "field therapy" effect, which has since been applied to "field therapy" for field cancerization of AK.

In 2007, a phase III clinical study of ALA-PDT for treating small condyloma acuminata, led by Professor Xuejun Zhu and designed by Professor Xiuli Wang, was conducted across five academic centers in China. A total of 453 patients were enrolled and divided into an ALA-PDT experimental group and a CO_2 laser control group, with up to three treatments and 12 weeks of follow-up. While the wart clearance rate 1 week after the final treatment was similar in both groups, the recurrence rate in the ALA-PDT group was significantly lower (10.77%) than that in the CO_2 laser group (33.33%, $P < 0.0001$). Additionally, the incidence of local adverse reactions in the ALA-PDT group was only 7.67%, primarily mild erosion, whereas it was 53.57% in the CO_2 laser group, where ulcers, pain, and scarring were common ($P < 0.0001$). These results demonstrate that ALA-PDT offers a lower recurrence rate, greater safety, and better tolerability than CO_2 laser therapy does, making it especially suitable for treating small condyloma acuminata [13, 14].

The authors' group has made significant contributions to the field of HPV-related diseases [15, 16]. In 2008, Professor Xiuli Wang first introduced the concept of HPV-related diseases in the *Chinese Journal of Dermatology* and initiated a series of studies on ALA-PDT [17]. In 2015, she led the development of China's first "*Expert Consensus on the Clinical Application of Aminolevulinic Acid Photodynamic Therapy*," officially recommending ALA-PDT as a first-line treatment for intralesional condyloma acuminata [18]. These findings were later incorporated into the 2014 *Chinese Guidelines for the Diagnosis and Treatment of Condyloma Acuminata* and the 2019 *European Guidelines for Photodynamic Therapy* [8, 19]. In 2021, Professor Xiuli Wang spearheaded the creation of the *Guidelines for the Clinical Application of Aminolevulinic Acid Photodynamic Therapy in Dermatology (2021 Edition)* [20], elevating the recommendation level of ALA-PDT for condyloma acuminata to

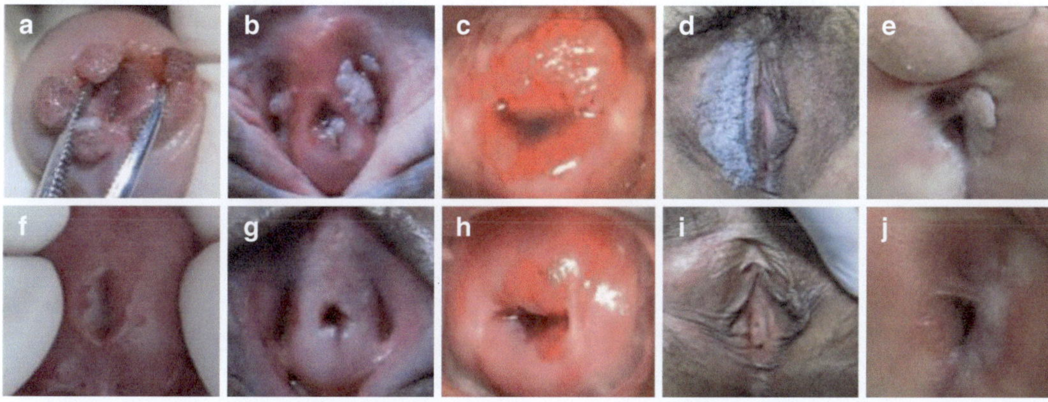

Fig. 8.5 ALA-PDT for the treatment of refractory condyloma acuminata. ALA-PDT is highly effective in removing skin lesions, with few adverse reactions, high safety, a low recurrence rate, minimal scarring, preservation of organ structure and function, and promotion of physical and psychological recovery in patients. (**a**, **f**) Before and after ALA-PDT treatment of condyloma acuminata of the urethral orifice, (**b**, **g**) before and after ALA-PDT treatment of condyloma acuminata of the urethral orifice, (**c**, **h**) before and after ALA-PDT treatment for female cervical condyloma acuminata, (**d**, **i**) before and after ALA-PDT treatment for female condyloma acuminata of the vulva, and (**e**, **j**) before and after ALA-PDT treatment for perianal condyloma acuminata in the toddler

Grade A with Grade I evidence, as published in *Photodiagnosis and Photodynamic Therapy* [21].

8.1.3.2 Treatment Mechanism

HPV-infected keratinocytes exhibit hyperplasia and heightened metabolic activity, allowing them to absorb significant amounts of ALA during ALA-PDT treatment for condyloma acuminata. These cells synthesize and convert ALA into protoporphyrin IX (PpIX), which, under specific wavelengths of light irradiation, undergoes a photodynamic reaction to produce reactive oxygen species, effectively targeting and killing HPV-infected keratinocytes [22]. In 2001, the authors' group treated 15 patients with condyloma acuminata via ALA-PDT and observed rapid neutrophil chemotaxis to the affected tissues within 1 h, which induced keratinocyte apoptosis and necrosis while preserving adjacent normal cells (Fig. 8.6), thereby clearing lesional, subclinical, and latent infections [23]. In 2011, the group established an HPV16-E7-HaCaT keratinocyte model stably expressing the HPV16E7 protein and demonstrated that ALA-PDT induces mitochondrial membrane potential collapse, activates the apoptotic cascade, and triggers apoptosis via cysteine protease-3 activators, confirming the pivotal role of the mitochondrial pathway in killing HPV-infected cells [24, 25]. In 2013, histopathological studies revealed that ALA-PDT mobilizes local immune responses, with an early Th1 response dominated by CD4+ T cells and a subsequent cytotoxic response driven by activated CD8+ T cells, effectively clearing HPV-infected cells [26]. Collectively, these findings demonstrate that ALA-PDT targets HPV-infected keratinocytes through apoptosis and necrosis, enhances neutrophil-dominated innate immunity and T lymphocyte-mediated acquired immunity, and provides robust theoretical support for eliminating condyloma acuminata, subclinical lesions, and latent HPV infections.

8.1.3.3 Clinical Application and Parameter Optimization

Since 1997, when Professor Xiuli Wang first successfully applied ALA-PDT to treat urethral condyloma acuminata, its use has expanded to other forms. Progressing from initial case series reports to randomized controlled trials, multicenter clinical studies, and meta-analyses, the evidence base for ALA-PDT has steadily advanced, consistently demonstrating its safety, efficacy, high cure rates, and low recurrence rates in treating condyloma acuminata. To promote and standardize its clinical application, the authors' group optimized treatment parameters and operational protocols, ensuring consistent efficacy and minimizing adverse reactions. ALA-PDT is now recognized as a first-line treatment for condyloma acuminata and is supported by grade I evidence-based medicine and a grade A recommendation [19, 27].

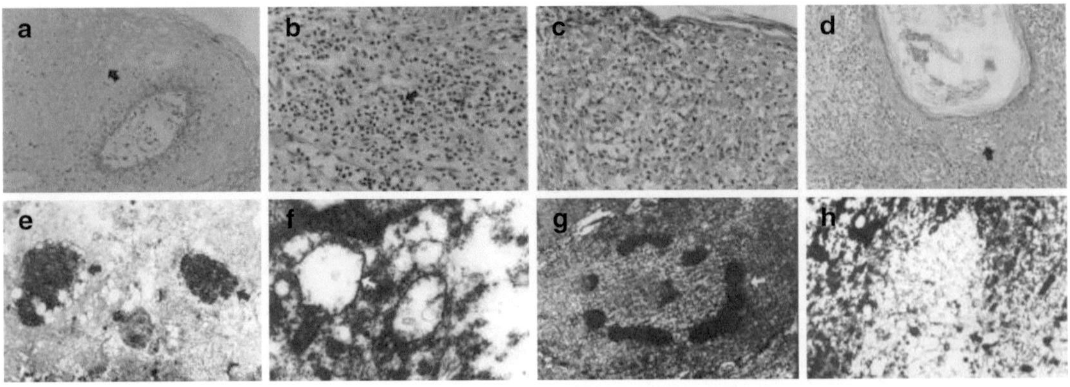

Fig. 8.6 H&E staining and electron microscopy revealed rapid neutrophil chemotaxis to wart and dermis tissues and gradual necrosis and apoptosis of keratinocytes. (**a**, **e**) Before treatment, (**b**, **f**) 1 h after treatment, (**c**, **g**) 3 h after treatment, and (**d**, **h**) 5 h after treatment

ALA-PDT for the Treatment of Condyloma Acuminata in Cavities

In 1997, Professor Xiuli Wang treated 18 male patients with urethral condyloma acuminata via a 10% ALA solution for wet compression for 3 h, followed by irradiation of the urethral lesion area with a specially designed laser probe emitting a 632.8nm HeNe laser at 100 J/cm^2. The treatment intervals were 7–10 days, with follow-ups every 2 weeks posttreatment. Complete remission, defined as the complete disappearance of lesions with a normal mucosal appearance, was achieved in all patients, with smaller lesions (≤3 mm) resolving after one to two sessions and larger lesions (>3 mm) resolving after three to four sessions. To prevent subclinical recurrence, patients received 2–3 additional consolidative treatments postremission. Mild local burning or stinging sensations and transient edema were observed but resolved without complications, and no ulceration, infection, or significant discomfort occurred. Two patients with diabetes and lymphoma experienced recurrence at 4 weeks posttreatment but achieved remission with retreatment, while the remaining 16 patients remained recurrence-free during 13 months of follow-up. The recurrent patients were retreated with ALA-PDT and achieved complete remission again, with weekly follow-up visits showing no recurrence for 8 weeks [10]. Subsequent studies by the authors' group in 2003 further demonstrated the efficacy of ALA-PDT, with 101 cases of genital urethral warts achieving complete remission after one to six treatments and no infections, ulcers, or urethral strictures [28]. A 2004 study involving 164 patients reported a cure rate of 95% and a recurrence rate of only 5% after 24 months of follow-up [11]. The treatment of deep urethral condyloma acuminata in males is challenging and prone to recurrence. In 2022, authors' group treated 16 cases of refractory and recurrent male urethral condyloma acuminata with a 20% ALA solution in a thermosensitive gel and irradiated the deep urethra with a 630-nm cylindrical optical fiber at a power density of 100 mW/cm^2 and an energy density of 120 J/cm^2. All lesions were cleared after three to six sessions, with no recurrences during the 6 months of follow-up, highlighting the high efficacy and low recurrence rate of ALA-PDT for challenging urethral lesions.

In 2008, a prospective study by the authors evaluated the efficacy and safety of ALA-PDT compared with CO_2 laser treatment for the treatment of cervical condyloma acuminata. The study involved 45 patients treated with ALA-PDT, in which a 10% ALA temperature-sensitive gel was applied to the cervix for 4 h, followed by red-light irradiation at an energy density of 80–100 J/cm^2, and 35 patients treated with a CO_2 laser. After one to four treatments and 3 months of follow-up, the ALA-PDT group achieved a complete remission rate of 97.8% (44/45), with a recurrence rate of 6.8% (3/44), whereas the CO_2 laser group had a complete remission rate of 100% (35/35) but a significantly higher recurrence rate of 31.4% (11/35). Although both groups had similar remission rates ($P > 0.05$), ALA-PDT resulted in a significantly lower recurrence rate ($P < 0.05$). Patients treated with ALA-PDT experienced mild lower abdominal discomfort during red-light irradiation but experienced no bleeding, scarring, or other adverse effects, whereas those in the CO_2 laser group experienced bleeding, shallow ulcers, and scarring [29]. In 2011, the authors' group further compared the two treatments in 44 patients with cervical intraepithelial neoplasia grade I and reported that ALA-PDT achieved a significantly higher HPV clearance rate (90.5%) after 12 months of follow-up than did the CO_2 laser group (43.5%) ($P < 0.005$). These findings suggest that ALA-PDT is a safe, effective treatment for cervical condyloma acuminata and HPV infection, with low recurrence rates and no significant side effects, making it an essential tool for early intervention and cervical cancer prevention [30]. The *2021 Guidelines for the Clinical Application of Aminolevulinic Acid Photodynamic Therapy in Dermatology* and the *2022 Expert Consensus on the Clinical Application of Aminolevulinic Acid Photodynamic Therapy in Women with Lower Genital Tract Diseases* recommend ALA-PDT as the first-line treatment for cervical condyloma acuminata [27, 31].

In 2005, Professor Xiuli Wang conducted a study at the University of Munich in Germany to determine the optimal ALA concentration and duration for ALA-PDT for treating urethral condyloma acuminata by analyzing PpIX fluorescence kinetics in vivo [22]. A total of 60 patients were divided into five groups according to ALA concentrations of 0.5%, 1%, 3%, 5%, and 10%, with samples taken at 1, 3, 5, and 7 h after application for in situ PpIX quantification. The results revealed varying degrees of PpIX brick-red fluorescence in the local epidermis of the lesions, with the strongest fluorescence observed in the germinative layer (basal cell layer and the lower part of the spinous cell layer), whereas the dermis exhibited minimal fluorescence. This finding indicated that ALA absorption and conversion occurred only in the epidermis, providing a theoretical basis for the lack of ulcers, scars, or strictures in ALA-PDT. The fluorescence intensity increased with application time, becoming significant at 3 h, peaking at 5 h, and then declining by 7 h to the levels observed at 3 h (Figs. 8.7 and 8.8). Higher ALA concentrations also increased PpIX fluorescence, with 5% and 10% concentrations producing significantly stronger fluorescence than lower concentrations did ($P < 0.05$). Thus, the optimal ALA concentration for treating urethral condyloma acuminata was determined to be 5% or 10%, with an application duration of 3–5 h.

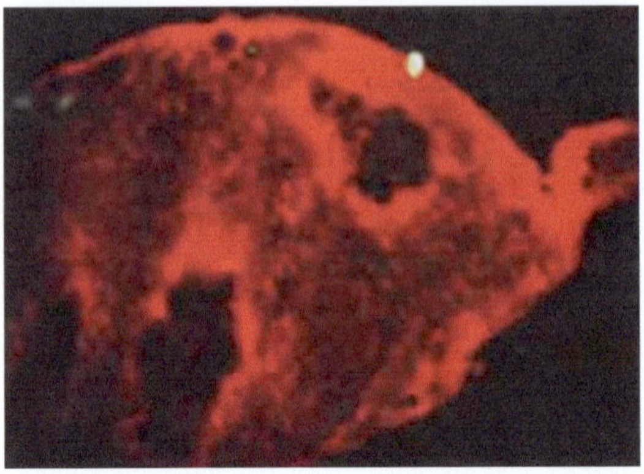

Fig. 8.7 PpIX fluorescence within condyloma acuminata lesions after 3 h of wet compression with 5% ALA (×200). The full-thickness epidermis showed PpIX brick-red fluorescence, and the fluorescence intensity of the germinal layer was significantly greater than that of the upper spinous layer

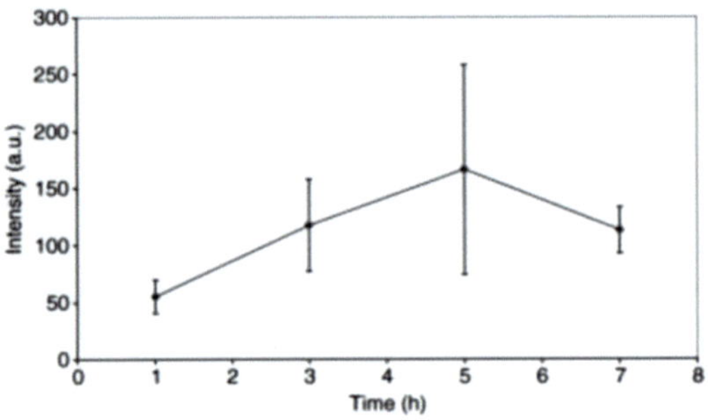

Fig. 8.8 Relationship between 10% ALA incubation time and epidermal fluorescence intensity

ALA-PDT for the Treatment of Condyloma Acuminata of the External Genitalia

Historically, CO_2 laser treatment has been the primary method for treating condyloma acuminata because of its high cure rate and rapid wart removal. However, a comparative study conducted in 2006 evaluated the efficacy of ALA-PDT vs a CO_2 laser. In this randomized controlled trial with 30 patients in each group, the CO_2 laser group had a higher cure rate (100.0% vs 63.3%) and superior one-time wart removal efficiency. Nevertheless, the ALA-PDT group presented significantly lower recurrence rates (15.8% vs 60.0%) and offered broader benefits by targeting visible warts, subclinical lesions, and latent infections simultaneously, achieving "field therapy" without structural damage [32]. ALA-PDT removes condyloma acuminata from external genitalia with minimal damage to anatomical structure and is beneficial to the physical and mental health of patients, as shown in Figs. 8.9 and 8.10. A 2018 study led by Kang Zeng further demonstrated the efficacy of ALA-PDT in treating latent and subclinical HPV infections. When a 20% ALA solution with a light dose of 100 J/cm^2 was used, active HPV infectors experienced a significant reduction in viral load after three treatments ($P < 0.001$). Among patients with latent or subclinical lesions, 80% (12/15) tested negative for HPV DNA after a single treatment. These findings support ALA-PDT as an effective, safe, and comprehensive treatment for condyloma acuminata and latent HPV infections,

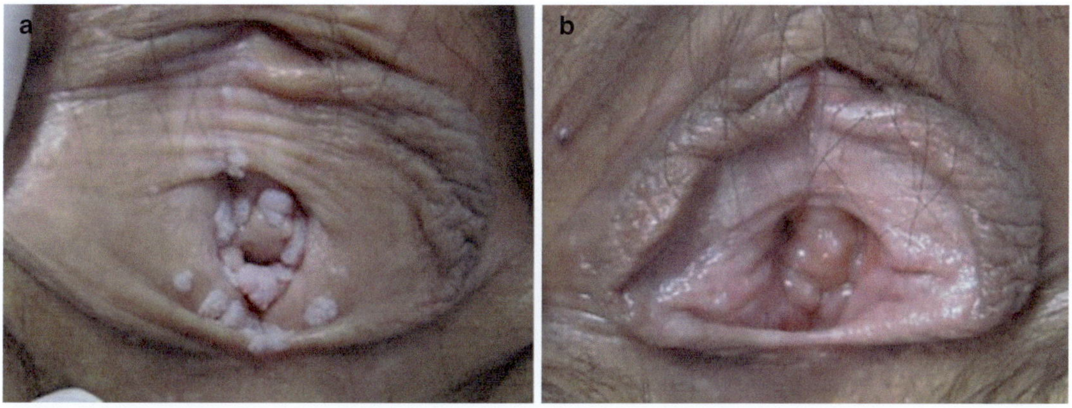

Fig. 8.9 Condyloma acuminata of the vulva in women cured after 3 ALA-PDT treatments: (**a**) before treatment and (**b**) after treatment

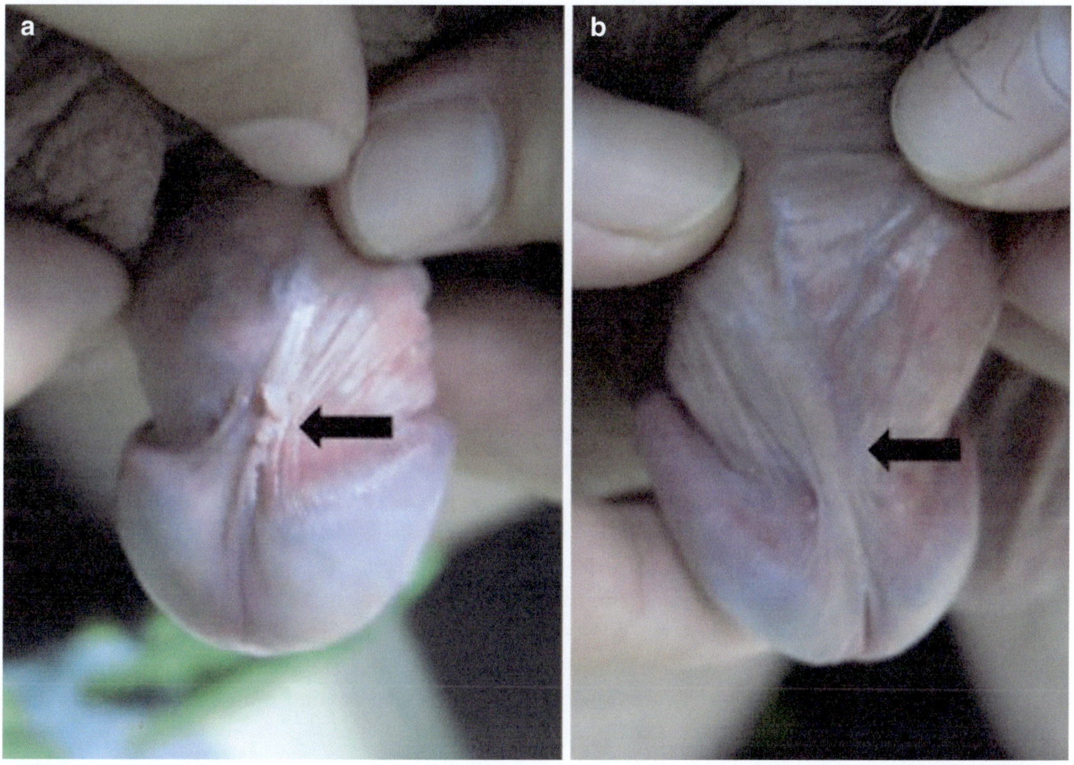

Fig. 8.10 Condyloma acuminata of the penile frenulum before and after ALA-PDT treatment: (**a**) before treatment and (**b**) after treatment, the wart disappeared without damage to the frenulum of the foreskin

emphasizing the importance of HPV DNA and viral load monitoring to guide therapy [33].

Professor Xiuli Wang guided a multicenter, randomized, controlled clinical study in China on ALA-PDT for small-volume urethral condyloma acuminata, enrolling 453 patients, with 442 completing follow-ups (331 in the ALA-PDT group and 111 in the CO_2 laser group). The study applied a 20% ALA solution for 3 h with a light dose of 100–150 J/cm^2, allowing up to three treatments, and monitored recurrence over 12 weeks. The wart clearance rates at the urethral orifice were 99.43% (ALA-PDT) and 100% (CO2 laser) ($P > 0.05$), but the recurrence rates were significantly lower in the ALA-PDT group (10.77%) than in the CO_2 laser group (33.33%) ($P < 0.0001$). Compared with the CO_2 laser group, the ALA-PDT group presented fewer local adverse reactions (7.67%, mainly mild erosion) (53.57%, including ulcers, pain, and 14 cases of scarring) ($P < 0.0001$). No systemic adverse reactions occurred in either group. ALA-PDT demonstrated comparable efficacy to the CO_2 laser but offered superior safety, tolerability, and a lower recurrence rate without urethral stricture or scarring. These findings, published in journals such as the *Journal of the American Academy of Dermatology*, support ALA-PDT as a first-line treatment for condyloma acuminata, with grade I evidence and an A-grade recommendation [13, 14].

ALA-PDT in the Treatment of Subclinical and Latent HPV Infection

The high recurrence rate of HPV-related diseases is linked to subclinical lesions and latent infections. In 2008, authors' group applied photodynamic diagnosis (PDD) to HPV-related diseases and conducted one of the few comprehensive studies on this method. In a study of 30 patients with condyloma acuminata, a 20% ALA cream was applied to lesions and a surrounding 2 cm area for 2 h, followed by fluorescence detection alongside acetowhitening tests, histopathology, and HPV DNA analysis. The results revealed PpIX brick-red fluorescence not only in warts and subclinical lesions but also in areas 0.5–2 cm beyond lesions, with matching HPV DNA. Some areas with negative acetowitening tests also showed fluorescence, highlighting the superiority of ALA-PDD over traditional methods for detecting latent HPV infections (Figs. 8.11 and 8.12). However, nonspecific fluorescence may occur in mucosal regions or areas with inflammation or ulcers, requiring careful differentiation [34]. On the basis of these findings, expanding ALA application to 2 cm beyond lesions for PDD diagnosis and at least 1 cm for ALA-PDT treatment to fully eliminate subclinical and latent HPV infections is recommended, thereby reducing recurrence [35]. Additionally, the team developed China's first urethroscopic PDD system to locate deep urethral lesions, addressing recurrence issues caused by residual warts in hard-to-reach areas [22].

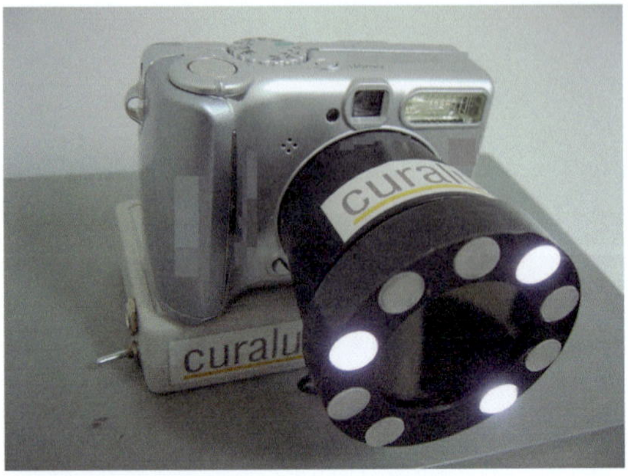

Fig. 8.11 Fluorescence camera for PDD

Modified Painless Photodynamic Therapy for Condyloma Acuminata

During ALA-PDT treatment for condyloma acuminata, many patients experience severe burning and stinging pain, which can significantly impact their therapeutic experience, with some interrupting or refusing further treatment out of fear, limiting the clinical application of ALA-PDT. To address this challenge, authors' group began exploring "modified ALA-PDT (M-PDT)" technology in 2017. They reported that treatment-associated pain is positively correlated with light irradiation power density, whereas therapeutic efficacy is correlated with energy density. By reducing the power density and extending the irradiation time, they effectively minimized pain without compromising clinical outcomes, overcoming a major obstacle in ALA-PDT applications [36].

In 2018, the authors' group conducted a prospective, randomized, self-controlled study on modified painless ALA-PDT for condyloma acuminata, enrolling 20 patients aged 18–65 years. The lesions were divided into a modified ALA-PDT group and a conventional ALA-PDT (C-PDT) group, both of which used 20% ALA cream. The modified group received LED red-light irradiation (630 nm, 300 J/cm^2) after 30 min of application, whereas the conventional group

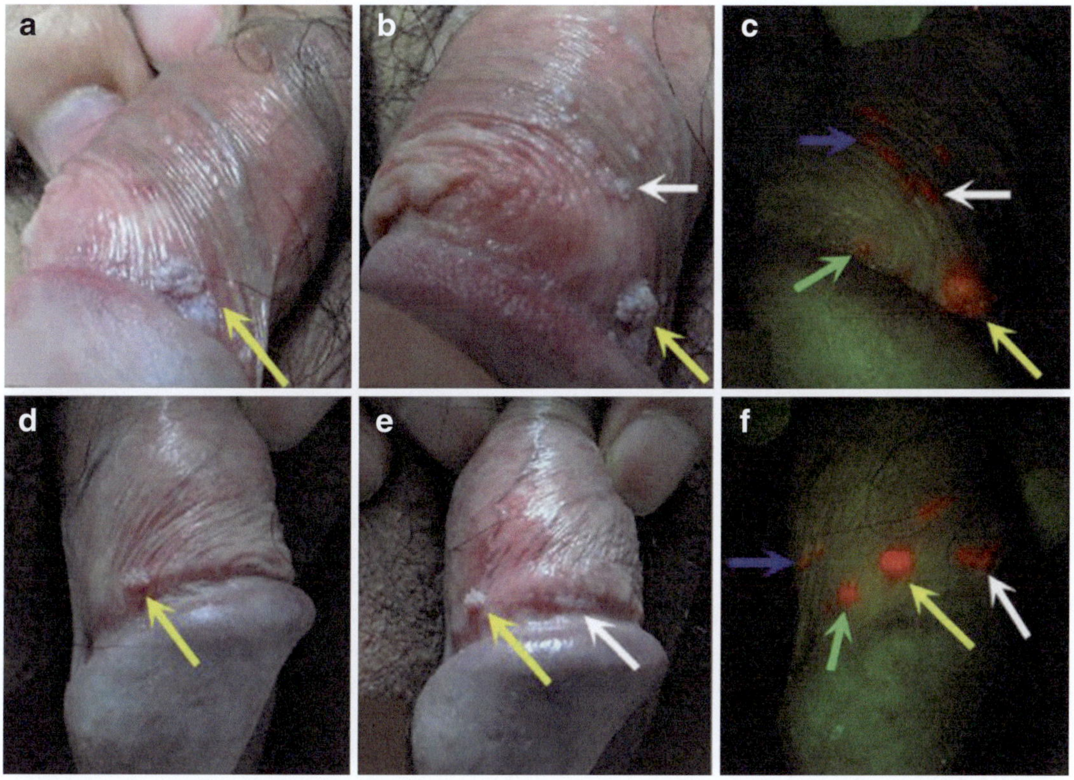

Fig. 8.12 Condyloma acuminata, subclinical lesions, and latent infection PDD showing brick-red fluorescence: (**a**, **d**) macroscopic observation, (**b**, **e**) acetate white test, and (**c**, **f**) PDD

underwent irradiation (100 J/cm^2) after 3 h of application. Treatments were administered weekly for up to three sessions if necessary. The lesion clearance rates were 98.17% in the modified group and 98.20% in the conventional group, with similar recurrence rates (11.11% vs 10.53%; $P > 0.05$). However, the average pain score in the modified group was significantly lower (0.3 ± 0.47, range 0–1) than that in the conventional group (3.6 ± 0.94, range 3–6; $P < 0.05$). These results demonstrate that modified ALA-PDT is as effective as conventional ALA-PDT but nearly eliminates treatment-associated pain, addressing a key limitation of this therapy [37].

ALA-PDT in Combination with Other Therapies for the Treatment of Condyloma Acuminata

For complex and refractory condyloma acuminata, combining ALA-PDT with other physical therapies is recommended. In 2002, the authors' group treated 86 refractory patients with ALA-PDT following microwave therapy, achieving a cure rate of 100%, with a 12-month recurrence rate of 31.4%, significantly extending the average recurrence cycle. Relapsed patients were cured with one to two additional treatments, with no further recurrences [38]. In 2014, Jinhua Huang's team combined a CO_2 laser and ALA-PDT for 119 patients with external genital warts (size >2 mm, 20% ALA, 3–5 h of incubation, energy density of 100–150 J/cm^2), achieving a 7.1% recurrence rate over 6 months. Half of the patients required only one ALA-PDT session for clearance, whereas the remaining patients needed two to six sessions [39]. In 2020, the authors' group demonstrated that a holmium laser combined with ALA-PDT was more effective for intracavitary anal canal condyloma acuminatum than was a CO_2 laser combined with ALA-PDT, resulting in greater clearance and lower recurrence rates without serious adverse effects (Fig. 8.13) [40]. These studies highlight the

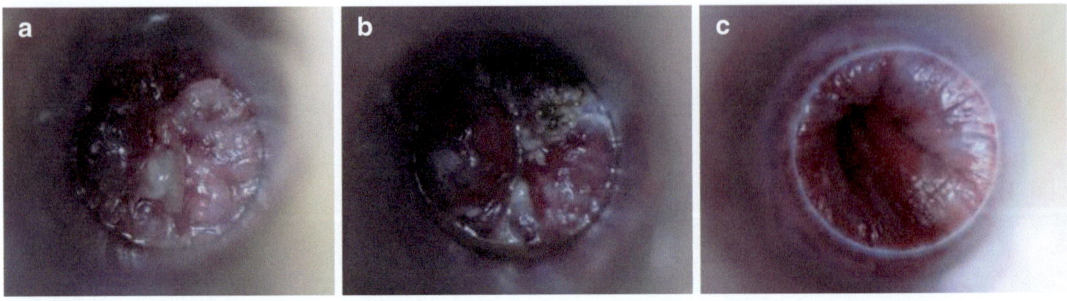

Fig. 8.13 Holmium laser combined with ALA-PDT for the treatment of condyloma acuminata in the anal canal: (**a**) wrinkled warts of the mucosa before treatment, (**b**) no bleeding on the surface after holmium laser treatment, and (**c**) complete removal of warts after two treatments

effectiveness of combining ALA-PDT with physical therapies to improve cure rates and reduce recurrences in complex cases.

8.1.3.4 Recommended Protocol

Condyloma acuminata in cavities include those located in the urethra, canal, vagina, and cervix. ALA-PDT can be used as a first-line treatment. For condyloma acuminata of the urethra and cervix, ALA-PDT is preferred.

Recommended protocol: (a) Urethroscopy, colposcopy, anoscopy, and other laparoscopes can be used to assist in the diagnosis and localization of lesions (Fig. 8.14). (b) A 10–20% ALA solution or gel is applied to the surface of the lesion and 1 cm periphery through a special urethral mucosal dressing device (Fig. 8.14, invented by the authors' group) or a cotton swab. If the lesion is located in the posterior urethra, a 20% ALA solution is injected directly through the catheter. (c) Red-light irradiation is performed by an optical fiber. The diode laser has an energy density of 100–150 J/cm^2 and a power density of 60–100 mW/cm^2. (d) Patients are re-evaluated at a 1-week posttreatment follow-up. Persisting lesions warrant re-administration of the initial therapy. Failure to achieve ≥50% clinical response after three sessions necessitates transition to either combination therapy or alternative regimens as per standard guidelines (Tables 8.2 and 8.3).

Key Points of Treatment

(a) Condyloma acuminata of the urethra: a) Patients should be educated to reduce psychological tension that may cause urinary difficulties, and elderly women should be monitored for acute urinary retention posttreatment. b) Advise drinking less water and emptying the bladder before applying medication. c) Recommend the use of a 630–635-nm semiconductor laser and a cylindrical diffusing optical fiber. d) Hydration and regular urination should be encouraged posttreatment to prevent infections.
(b) Condyloma acuminata of the cervix: a) Clear cervical mucus before treatment. b) If available, use a fiber optic cervical cap for phototherapy.
(c) Condyloma acuminata of the canal and vagina: a) Due to the wrinkled nature of the cavity, ALA may be applied insufficiently, and light may be irradiated at a lower dosage. It is recommended to first use other physical methods to remove visible warts before ALA-PDT. b) Regular soft bowel movements must be ensured posttreatment to prevent anal fissures. c) Monitoring for bleeding or exacerbated hemorrhoids.

Condyloma Acuminata on the External Genitalia and Perianal Area

Special areas such as the coronal sulcus of the penis and the inner side of the labia minora, where lesions appear in a carpet-like pattern, have a pinkish surface, or present as multiple smaller warts, ALA-PDT can be applied directly to address warts, subclinical warts, and latent infections, whereas for nonspecial areas with fewer lesions, warts larger than 0.5 cm, or those with increased keratinization and thickening, ini-

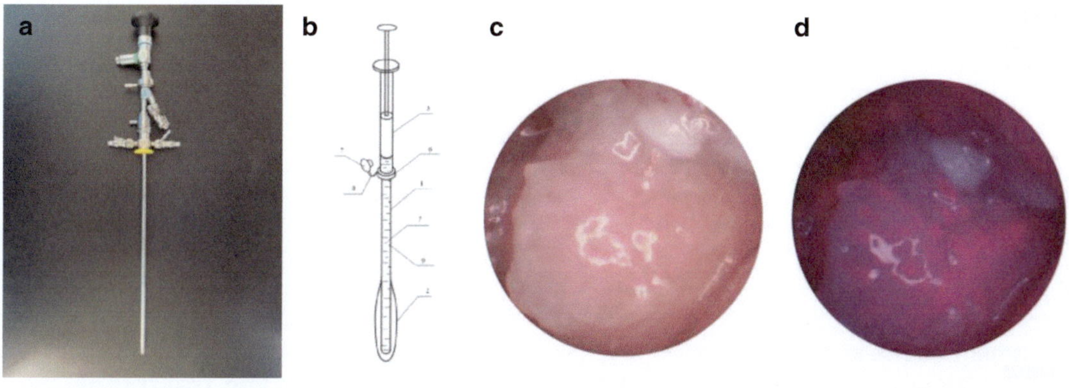

Fig. 8.14 (**a**) Urethroscope for ALA-PDT treatment of genital urethral warts. (**b**) The authors' group invented a controllable urethral mucosal dressing device (ZL201120194325. X) for intraurethral administration of ALA. (**c**) The wart between the external urethral orifice and the scaphoid fossa was observed under urethroscopy. (**d**) Specific red fluorescence was visible on the surface of the wart under blue light

Table 8.2 Recommended regimens of ALA-PDT for condyloma acuminata in cavities

	ALA distribution			Dose of light	
Pretreatment	ALA dosage form	ALA concentration (%)	Dressing time (h)	Energy density (J/cm^2)	Power density (mW/cm^2)
Cleaning and disinfection	Solution or gel	10–20	3	100–150	60–100

Table 8.3 Fiber optic options in ALA-PDT for the treatment of cavity condyloma acuminata

Location	Optical fiber
Urethra	Diode lasers approximately 630 nm and columnar diffuse fibers are recommended
Cervix	Semiconductor lasers of approximately 630 nm, bare fibers, and microlens fibers are recommended, and optical fibers with cervical caps can be used in hospitals with conditions
Anal canal	Specially designed LED light sources for cavities or semiconductor lasers approximately 630 nm and columnar diffuse fibers are recommended

tial removal of visible warts via other physical methods is recommended before proceeding with ALA-PDT treatment.

The recommended regimen for conventional ALA-PDT is as follows: (a) Pretreatment can be applied for hyperkeratotic warts, and physical methods, including CO_2 lasers, can be used to remove wart surfaces. (b) Apply 10–20% ALA cream, gel, or solution to the lesion surface with a 1 cm periphery, seal and avoid light exposure for 3–6 h. (c) Wipe off the drug and irradiate with red light. The use of a semiconductor laser or LED light source, with an energy density of 100–150 J/cm^2 and a power density range of 60–100 mW/cm^2, is recommended. (d) Follow-up 1 week after treatment; if the warts are not completely removed, the treatment can be repeated. If improvement is less than 50% after three treatments, combination therapy or switching to other treatments is recommended (Table 8.4).

The recommended regimen for modified ALA-PDT is as follows: (a) Apply 10–20% ALA cream, gel, or solution to the surface of the lesion and 1 cm periphery, and incubate in the dark for 30 min. (b) ALA is kept on the lesion surface and irradiated with red light. Diode lasers or LED light sources are recommended, with an energy density of 150–300 J/cm^2 and a power density range of 40–60 mW/cm^2. (c) The remaining treatment is the same as conventional ALA-PDT.

Table 8.4 Recommended regimens for the treatment of genital genitalia and perianal condyloma acuminata by ALA-PDT

	ALA formulation			Dose of light	
Pretreatment method	ALA dosage form	ALA concentration (%)	Dressing time	Energy density	Power density
CO_2 laser removes large warts or hyperkeratinization on the surface	Solution, gels, creams	10–20	3–6 h (C-PDT) 30 min (M-PDT)	100–150 J/cm^2 (C-PDT) 150–300 J/cm^2 (M-PDT)	60–100 mW/cm^2 (C-PDT) 40–60 mW/cm^2 (M-PDT)

Treatment Course and Follow-up

Regular follow-up is essential after ALA-PDT treatment, with routine assessments 1 week after each session and before the next, including photographic documentation for objective evaluation; subsequent treatments should be guided by therapeutic effects and adverse reactions, with significant reactions such as redness and swelling warranting a 2-week delay until they subside. Initial cases typically require three to four sessions per course, whereas recurrent or persistent cases often need four to six sessions, with additional courses as necessary. If the lesion volume decreases by less than 50% after three treatments, combining ALA-PDT with other therapies or switching methods is advised. During the first 3 months postcure, patients should follow-up every 2 weeks and seek prompt care for special concerns, transitioning to monthly follow-ups until 6 months.

Since 1997, the authors' group has pioneered the use of ALA-PDT for treating urethral condyloma acuminata, addressing clinical challenges and expanding its application to genital warts in various cavities; this approach has since been widely adopted nationwide, becoming a key criterion for dermatology departments in top Chinese hospitals and enriching dermatological treatment as a novel technology alongside cryotherapy, laser, and ultraviolet therapies, with its inclusion in professional dermatological texts and standardized medical textbooks for medical students.

8.2 ALA-PDT in the Treatment of Bowenoid Papulosis

8.2.1 Introduction

Bowenoid papulosis (BP) is a precancerous disease caused by HPV infection, and its incidence rate has increased in recent years. The typical clinical manifestation is multiple pigmented flat papules that occur in the external genitalia or perianal area, with histopathological presentation of low-grade malignant carcinoma in situ. In 1970, Lloyd first reported this disease [41], and Wade et al. officially named it Bowenoid papulosis in 1978 [42].

8.2.1.1 Clinical Features

BP predominantly affects sexually active individuals aged 21–30 years, presenting as single or multiple well-demarcated papules that can be skin-colored, flesh-colored, reddish-brown, or black, measuring 2–10 mm in diameter, with round, oval, or irregular shapes. The papules may have a bright, velvety surface or appear slightly keratinized and warty, commonly occurring in the groin, external genitalia, and perianal skin or mucosa, often without symptoms but occasionally causing itching or burning sensations; the condition is chronic, with rare progression to invasive cancer. Since 1997, the authors' group has studied BP, and in 2004, they analyzed 60 cases—36 males with lesions primarily on the glans penis, coronal sulcus, medial prepuce, penis, scrotum, and perianal region, 75% of which involved the coronal sulcus and medial prepuce—and 24 females with lesions mainly on the labia majora, labia minora, vaginal orifice, perineum, and perianal region, 87.5% of which were concentrated between the labia majora, labia minora, and perineum. All the patients had a history of sexual contact, with no lesions outside the genital or perianal areas. The lesions range from 2 to 12 mm in size and are generally larger and coalescing into larger patches in female labia and perineum; in male patients, BP lesions tend to align along the coronal sulcus and may coalesce into patches or linearly orient [43].

8.2.1.2 Histopathology

BP is often mistaken for keratinizing and verrucous lesions such as condyloma acuminata, Bowen's disease (BD), lichen planus, and seborrheic keratosis, making histopathological examination crucial for accurate diagnosis. While BP and condyloma acuminata are similar, they differ significantly in pathology; BP is characterized by epidermal hyperkeratosis, parakeratosis, acanthosis, widening and elongation of rete ridges, occasional papilloma-like hyperplasia, disordered and atypical keratinocytes, frequent mitotic figures, dyskeratotic cells, vacuolated cells, and intact basal layers (Fig. 8.15). Inflammatory infiltrates in the dermis consist mainly of lymphocytes, with occasional histiocytes and rare plasma cells, alongside melanin granules, melanophages, and dilated dermal vessels [43]. Through long-term research and case accumulation, the authors identified a correlation between the clinical and histopathological features of BP and proposed its first pathological classification on the basis of 60 BP cases, which were divided into three types. Type I lesions include (1) tightly packed atypical keratinocytes, (2) hyperchromatic nuclei and scant cytoplasmic content (increased N/C ratio), (3) acanthosis, which is present but less prominent than in type III lesions, and (4) extended rete ridges with minimal anastomosis. The frequency of type I lesions was 44 out of the 60 cases examined (73.3%). Clinically, most lesions have a maculopapular appearance with a diameter less than 1 cm. Most lesions are biopsied during the early course of disease and are responsive to treatment, such as cryotherapy and photodynamic therapy. The features of type III lesions include (1) larger atypical cells with increased cytoplasmic content and a decreased N/C ratio, (2) more prominent acanthosis, and (3) anastomotic rete ridges. These features were observed in 12 out of 60 patients (20%), with a female predominance. Clinically, type III lesions present as larger papules and plaques. These patients tend to respond poorly to canonical treatments (imiquimod or photodynamic therapy) and have a high recurrence rate. Type II lesions have features that overlap between type I and type II lesions. Of the 60 patients, 4 were categorized as type II, and the lesions appeared as large papules. Another pathological feature of BP is its unique parakeratosis pattern: parakeratotic nuclei are more basophilic and larger in size than are the nuclei of keratinocytes. They are frequently oval to round in shape. The distribution of retained nuclei is disorganized, rarely in a linear pattern. No parakeratosis was present in the surrounding nonlesional sites. Such distinct parakeratosis can be observed in 50 out of 60 (83.3%) BP patients. Other unique histological features of BP include distinctive cuticle structures, the compression of proliferative granular layers into flat, horizontal arrangements, and the absence of plasma cell infiltration. These findings were corroborated in 2006 during a national PDT education class, where histopathological classifications of female vulvar intraepithelial lesions in gynecology were found to align with the BP classifications described by the authors in 2004 [43].

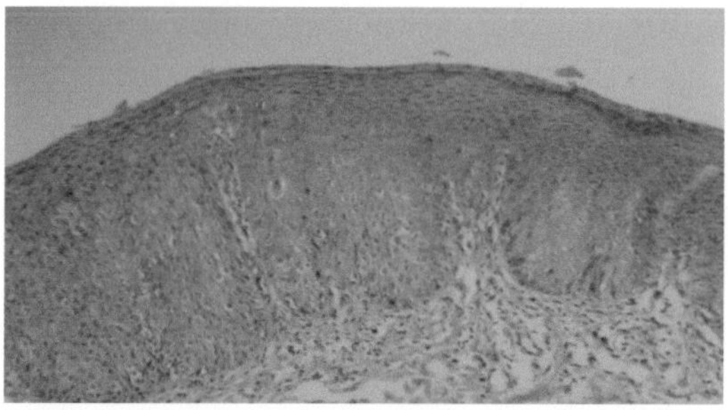

Fig. 8.15 Pathological manifestations of BP include disordered parakeratosis, acanthosis, and the presence of numerous mitotic figures and dyskeratotic cells

8.2.1.3 BP and HPV

Clinically, HPV is categorized into low-risk and high-risk types on the basis of its carcinogenic potential; low-risk types, mainly HPV6 and 11, cause benign tumors or warts, whereas high-risk types, primarily HPV16 and HPV18, are associated with precancerous lesions of the external genitalia, the female genital tract, and invasive cervical cancer [44]. Both condyloma acuminata and BP are linked to HPV infection and are sexually transmitted, with similar clinical manifestations and lesion locations, often leading to misdiagnosis, especially when they occur sequentially or coexist.

In 1985, Gross et al. identified HPV antigen structures and HPV6-related gene sequences in BP skin lesions, suggesting a link between BP and HPV infection, which has since been confirmed [45]. Studies have shown that HPV16 and HPV18, the most prevalent high-risk HPV types, account for 70% of all cervical cancers [44]. In 2006, the authors' group detected high-risk HPV16 and HPV18 in 77.8% of vulvar BP lesions in 18 female patients, aligning with cervical HPV infections and indicating a shared source. A 2008 study of 45 BP patients further confirmed that high-risk HPV, especially HPV16, is closely tied to BP development [46]. Persistent high-risk HPV infection in the vulva increases the risk of cervical cancer, highlighting the need for long-term follow-up of patients and their partners. Histopathologically, BP presents as atypical in situ carcinoma with full-thickness epidermal cell involvement, leading some patients to seek treatment in other specialties, resulting in invasive procedures such as vulvar resection and significant physical and psychological harm. The authors advocate for a proactive approach to HPV-related tumor prevention, emphasizing early detection and treatment of skin HPV-related diseases, reducing cavity infections, managing vulvar HPV infections, and addressing HPV infections at the entry point of the female reproductive tract to lower the risk of cervical cancer. This strategy aims to improve national health outcomes and enhance cervical cancer prevention.

8.2.1.4 BP and Squamous Intraepithelial Lesions (SILs)

The anus and genitalia, areas of overlap for dermatology, gynecology, urology, and pathology, have led to differing disease names and interpretations across disciplines. Since 1978, dermatology has identified BP on the basis of clinical papules with BD-like pathological changes, whereas obstetrics and urology have classified it as vulvar intraepithelial neoplasia (VIN) or penile intraepithelial neoplasia (PIN) [47, 48]. The definition of vulvar intraepithelial lesions varies internationally. The International Society for the Study of Vulvovaginal Disease (ISSVD) introduced a three-tier system in 1986 for intraepithelial neoplasia—VIN1 (mild atypia), VIN2 (moderate atypia), and VIN3 (severe atypia/carcinoma in situ)—to standardize the pathological diagnosis of HPV-related proliferative diseases [49]. The authors' group confirmed in 2005 that most VIN1 specimens were HPV16 positive and that HPV oncogene integration in VIN3 lesions correlates with progression to vulvar squamous cell carcinoma. In 2013, the College of American Pathologists (CAP) and American Society for colposcopy and cervical pathology (ASCCP) replaced this system with a two-tier classification: low-grade squamous intraepithelial lesion (LSIL, formerly VIN1) and high-grade squamous intraepithelial lesion (HSIL, formerly VIN2/3). This nomenclature distinguishes LSIL's low malignant potential from HSIL's high risk [50]. By 2015, the WHO further refined these categories into LSIL (HPV infection or condyloma acuminata), HSIL and differentiated VIN (dVIN), emphasizing the nonprecancerous nature of LSIL to prevent overtreatment [51]. As BP is associated with high-risk HPV, particularly HPV16, it is histologically considered an HSIL and is often surgically treated. However, histopathology must integrate clinical presentation, disease progression, and prognosis to guide appropriate management.

8.2.2 Treatment Methods

BP is an HPV-related disease, with some lesions spontaneously regressing while others persist for years; in untreated, older, or immunosuppressed patients, it can progress to Bowen disease (BD) or invasive cutaneous squamous cell carcinoma (cSCC) [51, 52]. Although histologically similar to BD, BP lesions in young individuals often follow a benign clinical course. The development of BP is closely linked to high-risk HPV, particularly HPV16, whose persistence in the vulva increases the risk of cervical HPV infection and subsequent cervical cancer [53]. An improved understanding and active management of BP, along with long-term follow-up of female patients and their partners, are essential due to its multicentric and discrete lesion distribution, which poses significant treatment challenges. Currently, there is no consensus on the optimal treatment for BP, which is similar to the situation with genital warts. Historically, treatments have included laser therapy, cryotherapy, and topical agents such as 5-fluorouracil, podophyllotoxin, interferon, and imiquimod, with clinicians often selecting approaches on the basis of their own clinical experience. The presence of subclinical skin lesions and latent HPV infection often means that the actual extent of BP lesions is greater than what is clinically visible. Traditional treatments such as CO_2 lasers and cryotherapy can quickly remove visible lesions and provide immediate clinical efficacy. However, these methods do not address subclinical lesions or latent infection, leading to frequent relapses, particularly in patients with extensive or longstanding disease. Repeated laser treatments can damage the normal structure of the vulva or external genitalia, resulting in scarring and significantly impacting patients' physical and mental well-being. Considering treatment safety, tissue trauma, and recurrence rates, individualized combination therapies such as CO_2 lasers with 5% imiquimod cream or ALA-PDT with 5% imiquimod cream are recommended. These approaches are less traumatic, typically avoid ulcers and scarring, and preserve vulvar structure and function, improving patients' quality of life and mental health. Clinical observations by the authors' group revealed that CO_2 laser treatment had an effective rate of 82.8%, but patients reported pain, slow wound healing, and a high recurrence rate of 62.1% within 3 months [54]. These data were confirmed by other studies, which reported a 10-year recurrence rate of 79% following CO_2 laser treatment [55]. Over 40 years ago, partial or total vulvar resection was a common treatment for female BP, but this approach often resulted in significant structural damage and functional impairment of the vulva (Fig. 8.16). In 2007, the authors' group conducted a retrospective study on 39 BP patients to evaluate the efficacy and recurrence of different

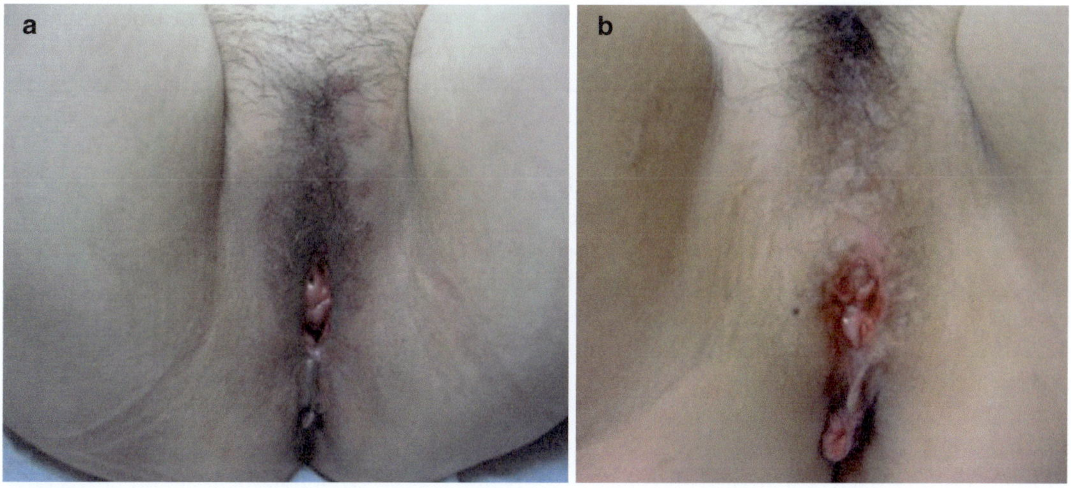

Fig. 8.16 Partial (**a**) or complete surgical (**b**) resection causing structural damage and functional impact on the external genitalia

treatments. The first group (15 patients) was treated with 5% imiquimod cream three times weekly for 8 weeks, achieving a 33.33% (5/15) cure rate with no recurrence, although adverse reactions such as erythema, edema, erosion, and pain were observed without systemic effects. The second group (12 patients) received CO_2 laser treatment, which cured all patients but had a high recurrence rate of 66.66% (8/12). The third group (12 patients) underwent combined CO_2 laser and 5% imiquimod cream treatment, achieving a 75% cure rate with only 25% (3/12) recurrence. The study concluded that 5% imiquimod cream offers good efficacy with a low recurrence rate for small lesions but may cause localized adverse effects. For hypertrophic or mild verrucous lesions, combining a CO_2 laser with 5% imiquimod cream effectively reduces recurrence [56].

8.2.3 ALA-PDT

In 1997, the authors' group pioneered the use of ALA-PDT for treating condyloma acuminata, demonstrating its ability to simultaneously target visible warts, subclinical lesions, and latent infections, effectively achieving "field therapy" while proving its safety and efficacy. This approach has also been extended to the treatment of BP lesions.

8.2.3.1 Mechanism

ALA, a precursor in hemoglobin production, is a commonly used topical photosensitizer. Upon application, ALA is selectively absorbed by hyperplastic tissues and converted into PpIX, which, when exposed to a specific red-light wavelength, produces singlet oxygen and free radicals. This process induces necrosis and apoptosis of HPV-infected cells while simultaneously clearing HPV by triggering robust local inflammation, cellular responses in surrounding tissues, and the activation of host immunity [57].

8.2.3.2 Clinical Efficacy

In 1998, Martin Hirsch et al. treated eight patients with high-grade VIN via 20% ALA applied locally for 4 h, followed by 100 J/cm^2 red-light irradiation, achieving a 37% resolution rate for VIN lesions after a single ALA-PDT session [58]. In 2001, Fehr et al. compared laser, surgery, and ALA-PDT for VIN3 lesions. In all, 15 patients received 10% ALA gel for 2–3 h and 635-nm laser irradiation at 120 J/cm^2 for one to four sessions. The results revealed that 73% of patients achieved complete lesion resolution 8 weeks posttreatment, with intact vulvar tissue and no ulcers or scarring. Long-term disease-free survival was comparable to that of laser therapy and surgery ($P < 0.67$), while ALA-PDT offered faster healing and preserved the vulvar appearance [59]. Later, Fehr et al. reported a 57% complete resolution rate in 22 VIN2/3 patients treated with 10% ALA and an 80–100 J/cm^2 635 nm laser for one to four sessions, although the outcomes were poorer for pigmented and hyperkeratotic VIN [60]. Additionally, Yang treated two penile BP cases with 20% ALA for 6–12 h followed by 634 ± 20-nm red-light irradiation at 90 mW/cm^2 at two 25-min intervals separated by 90 min. Both patients achieved complete resolution after one ALA-PDT session, with no recurrence observed during follow-up [61].

In 2006, Hillemans and the authors' group assessed the clinical efficacy of CO_2 lasers, ALA-PDT, and surgery for treating VIN3 lesions. The ALA-PDT group was treated with 20% ALA gel for 2–4 h in the dark, followed by 635-nm argon ion dye laser irradiation at 100 J/cm^2 energy density and 150 mW/cm^2 power density. After an average follow-up of 53.7 weeks, the recurrence rates for CO_2 laser, ALA-PDT, and surgery were 40.4%, 48.1%, and 41.7%, respectively, with no statistically significant difference. However, ALA-PDT had fewer side effects than the CO_2 laser or surgery. Paoli et al. treated ten patients with penile PIN3 (older than 40 years) via PDT, with seven showing effectiveness after two to eight treatments. Among these patients, four experienced no recurrence after an average 35-month follow-up, three experienced recurrence, and three experienced treatment failure. Importantly, no patients developed invasive penile cancer. Although there are no prospective randomized controlled trials, PDT represents a promising new treatment option for PIN [62].

In 2007, the authors' group reported that ALA-PDT and imiquimod share similar indications and immunomodulatory pathways for treating HPV-related diseases, both of which induce skin immune responses characterized by activated dendritic cells and increases in CD4+ and CD8+ T cells. This led to a clinical study exploring the feasibility of combining imiquimod with ALA-PDT for treating BP. The study included 27 patients, 15 of whom received imiquimod (5% applied three times a week) combined with ALA-PDT (once a week for a total of four sessions). The control group of 12 patients received CO_2 laser treatment. The results revealed that 60% (9/15) of the patients in the combined treatment group achieved complete remission, with only one patient (11.1%) experiencing recurrence, and mild local side effects, such as erythema, edema, and burning, were observed. In contrast, 83.3% (10/12) of the patients in the CO_2 laser group experienced complete remission, but 60% (6/12) experienced relapse, with more significant local side effects, including edema, ulceration, delayed healing, persistent pain, and scarring. This was the first study globally to propose the combination of imiquimod and ALA-PDT for BP treatment, showing that this combination is a safe, effective approach with a low recurrence rate and minimal side effects [63]. Additionally, Welbourn et al. treated 15 patients with perianal IN3 via ALA-PDT and achieved complete remission in six out of ten patients after one to four treatments, with an average follow-up of 19 months [64]. Furthermore, a study by Kang Zeng involving 200 BP patients compared ALA-PDT (100 patients) with other treatments, such as radiofrequency cauterization, microwave ablation, and surgical resection (control group). ALA-PDT involves the application of 20% ALA cream for 4 h followed by laser irradiation, with patients receiving an average of 5.53 sessions for multiple lesions and 3.63 for single lesions. The ALA-PDT group presented a 100% lesion clearance rate and no recurrence after 1 year, whereas 20 patients in the control group experienced recurrence [65].

8.2.3.3 Photodynamic Diagnosis (PDD)

Akoel et al. used photodynamic detection (PDD) to assess 107 patients with VIN. After 3% ALA was applied topically for 3–6 h, the lesions were irradiated with a 20 mW xenon lamp emitting light at wavelengths of 380–440 nm. Brick-red fluorescence was observed through a filter, and the results were compared with histopathological findings. The sensitivity, specificity, and predictive values of the PDD for diagnosing VIN were 85.7%, 81.2%, 80.0%, and 86.6% for VIN1; 93.3%, 93.7%, 93.3%, and 93.7% for VIN2; and 96.3%, 94.7%, 96.3%, and 94.7% for VIN3 and vulvar noninvasive squamous cell carcinoma, respectively [66]. These findings suggest that PDD, as a noninvasive diagnostic tool, has significant value in diagnosing VIN and vulvar noninvasive squamous cell carcinoma. In 2008, the authors' group applied 20% ALA cream to five clinically diagnosed BP lesions and the surrounding 2 cm area, followed by fluorescence PDD after 2 h. White acetate testing and histopathological examination were performed on the lesions, including subclinical areas and the surrounding 0.5 cm and 2 cm regions, along with HPV DNA detection via gene profiling. The results revealed PpIX brick-red fluorescence at BP lesions, indicating the potential of PDD for detecting both clinical and subclinical HPV-related lesions [67] (Fig. 8.17).

8.2.3.4 Recommended Protocols (Table 8.5)

In 2010, the authors' group summarized the treatment outcomes of 135 BP patients, comparing the clinical efficacy and adverse reactions of CO_2 lasers, ALA-PDT, 5% imiquimod topical treatment, and the combination of 5% imiquimod topical treatment with ALA-PDT. The results indicated that the combination of ALA-PDT with 5% imiquimod cream significantly improved the cure rate and reduced the recurrence rate. Additionally, PpIX fluorescence in the lesions of some patients treated with imiquimod cream was markedly enhanced, suggesting that the skin irritation caused by imiquimod improved the absorption and conversion efficiency of the photosensitizer. This may contribute to the supe-

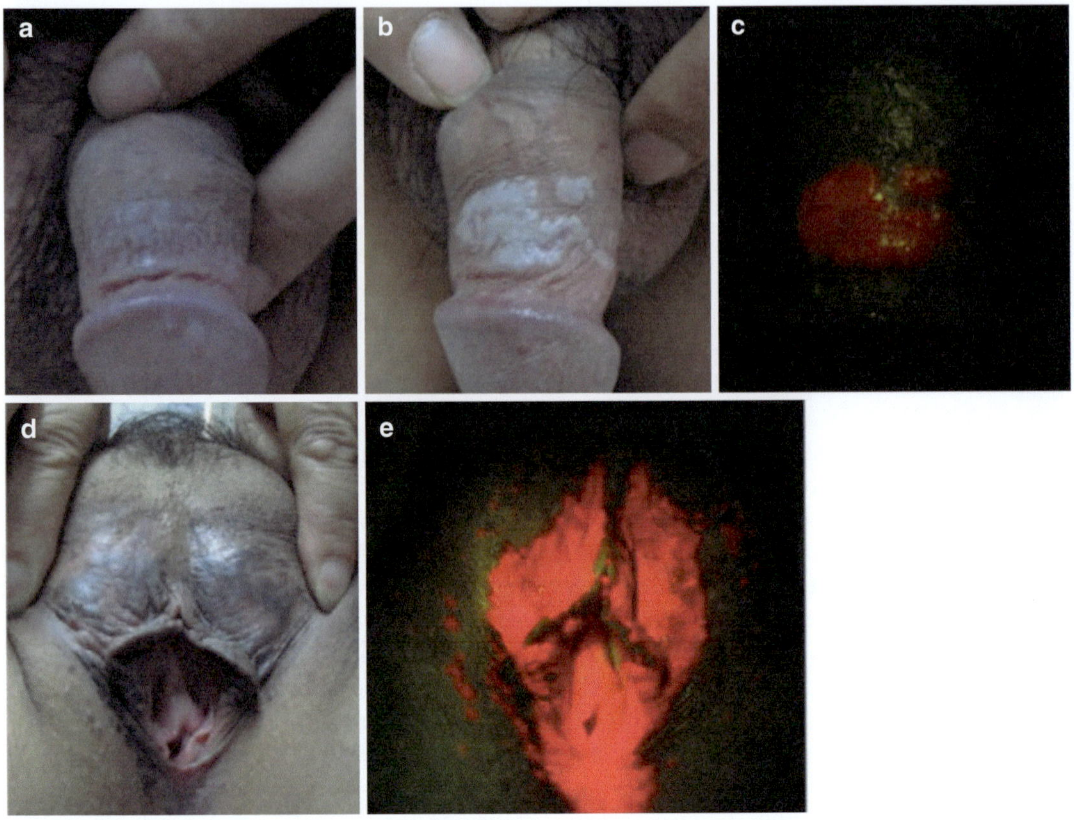

Fig. 8.17 PDD of BP: (**a**) male penile BP lesions, (**b**) acetic acid white test, (**c**) ALA PDD, (**d**) BP lesions on the female external genitalia, and (**e**) brick-red fluorescence appeared in skin lesions and subclinical lesions

Table 8.5 Recommended regimen of ALA-PDT for BP

Pretreatment	Recommend combination therapy	ALA preparation			Application time (h)	Illumination dose	
		ALA dosage form	PDT type	ALA concentration (%)		Energy density (J/cm^2)	Power density (mW/cm^2)
Cleaned the surface and removed the tumor on the surface by laser or scraper to increase the drug permeability	5% Imiquimod cream combined with ALA-PDT	Cream or gel	C-PDT	10–20	3–6	100–150	60–100
			M-PDT	10–20	0.5–1 No cleaning	300–400	60–100

rior efficacy of the combination therapy compared with ALA-PDT or imiquimod alone. On the basis of these findings, the authors' group suggested that BP patients with fewer skin lesions could be treated with a CO_2 laser or direct topical imiquimod cream, whereas those with more extensive or disseminated lesions would benefit more from combined ALA-PDT and imiquimod treatment (Fig. 8.18).

Combination therapy: five percent imiquimod cream is applied externally to the skin lesions, which are gently rubbed several times a week, typically three times. The cream should be washed off with water or neutral soap 6–10 h after application, and attention should be given to monitoring for adverse reactions. Imiquimod cream can cause mild to moderate erythema, pruritus, edema, and burning sensa-

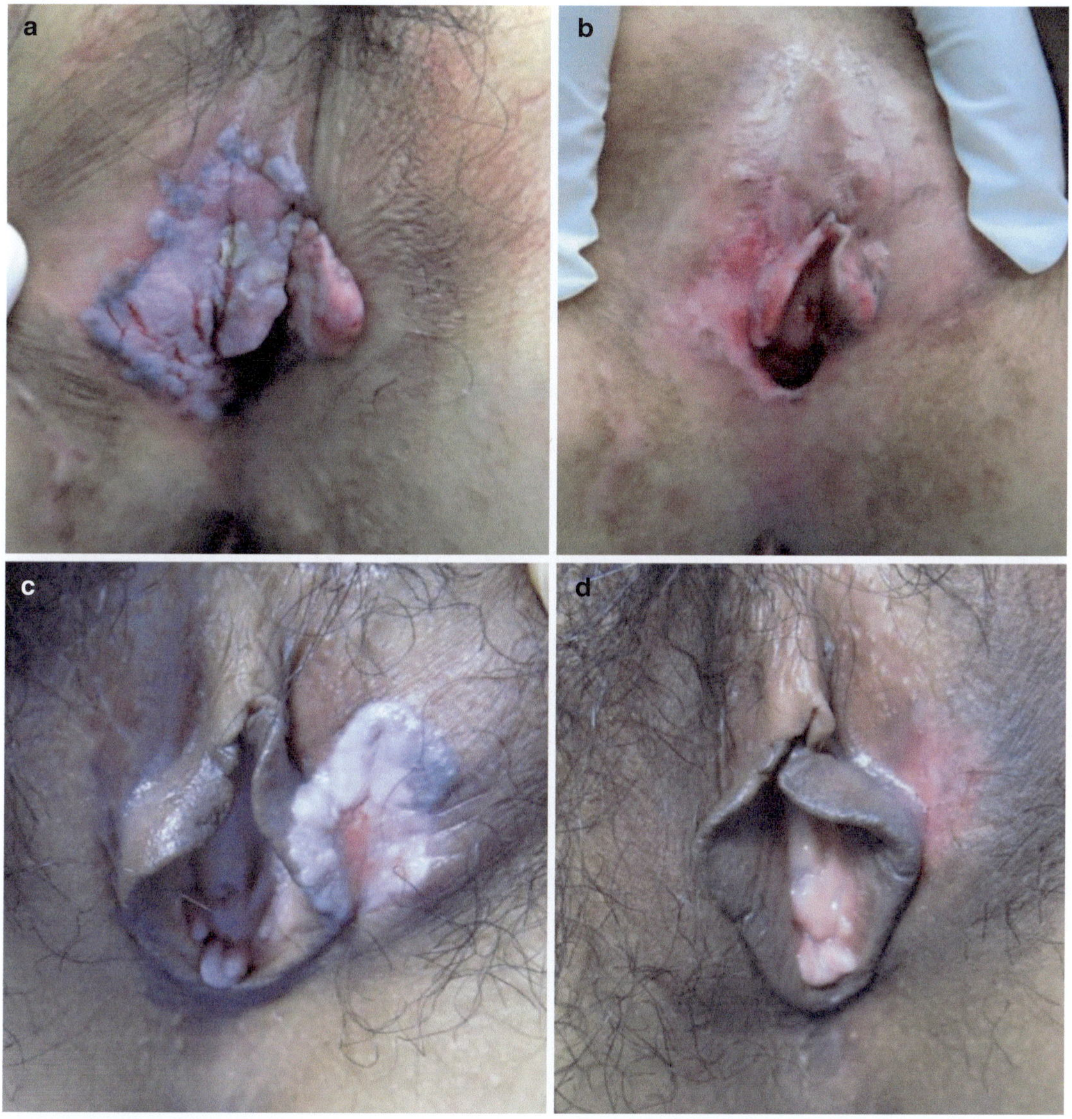

Fig. 8.18 ALA-PDT treatment for BP before treatment (**a**, **c**, **e**) and after treatment (**b**, **d**, **f**). There was minimal scarring after recovery, with preservation of structure and function

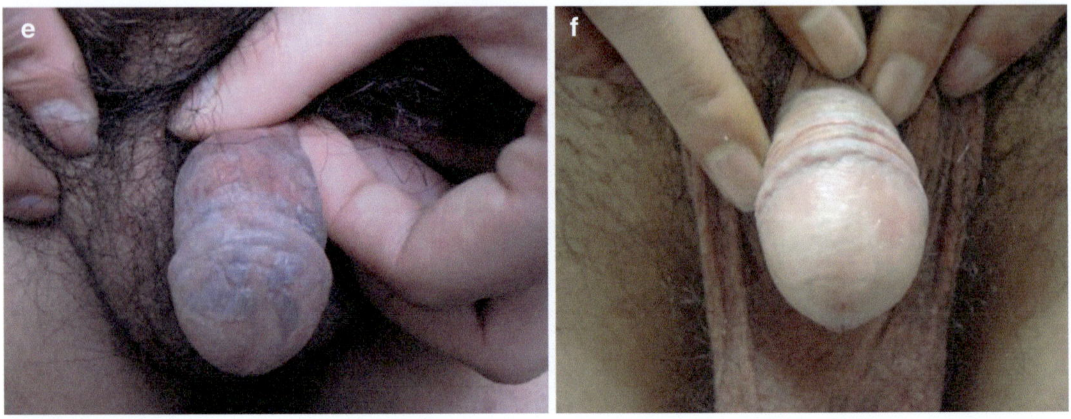

Fig. 8.18 (continued)

tions on the local skin, which are considered normal treatment responses. If pain or erosion occurs, treatment can be paused for 2–3 days. After 2 weeks of continuous application, ALA-PDT was then used sequentially.

The treatment interval was as follows: the treatment was repeated every 1–2 weeks, and the curative effect was evaluated before each session. Given that the persistence of BP in the anogenital region may increase the risk of cSCC formation, pathological examination is necessary if the treatment is ineffective or if the skin lesions continue to expand during therapy. Close attention should be given to the risk of malignant transformation.

Adverse reactions may include varying degrees of burning sensations or pain, which are generally tolerable. If symptoms are unbearable, symptomatic pain relief can be provided. Posttreatment erythema, edema, and mild erosion typically resolve without additional intervention. When combined with 5% imiquimod cream, the main adverse reactions are mild to moderate erythema, pruritus, edema, burning, pain, and erosion at the application site, which usually occur 1 week after application. In severe cases, the treatment can be temporarily discontinued, or the application interval can be extended.

8.3 ALA-PDT in the Treatment of Cervical HPV-Related Disease

8.3.1 Introduction of Cervical HPV-Related Disease

8.3.1.1 Introduction of HPV

In 1949, Strauss first observed HPV particles via electron microscopy, noting their spherical shape with icosahedral symmetry and measuring approximately 45–55 nm in diameter [68]. HPV consists of capsid proteins (L1) and secondary capsid proteins (L2), along with uncoated loop DNA in the form of small double strands. The virus contains approximately 8000 base pairs of double-stranded closed-loop DNA, which includes eight early open reading frames (E1–E8), two late reading frames, and a long noncoding control region [69]. With nearly 130 genotypes identified, HPV is classified on the basis of its genetic sequence. Among the early open reading frames, the E6 and E7 genes play crucial roles in stimulating cellular growth. The proteins encoded by these genes contribute to the immortalization of cervical epithelial cells. HPV is categorized into low-risk and high-risk types on the basis of its biological characteristics and potential for carcinogenesis.

8.3.1.2 Cervical HPV Infection

Cervical HPV infection is a prevalent sexually transmitted infection in women and is strongly associated with sexual behaviors. Its infection rate largely depends on the age and sexual behavior patterns of the population. HPV has high host specificity and can infect only humans. In most women, the immune system clears HPV naturally, but in individuals with impaired immune function, persistent infection can occur. Low-risk HPV (LR-HPV) infections are commonly linked to conditions such as condyloma acuminata, whereas persistent infection with high-risk HPV (HR-HPV) is a significant factor in the development of cervical cancer. In a study conducted by the authors' group in Shanghai involving HPV genotyping of lesions and exfoliated cervical cells from 194 female patients with genital condyloma acuminatum, the detection rate of HPV lesions was 100%. Among these, 74.2% (144 cases) were infected with LR-HPV, and 25.8% (50 cases) were infected with HR-HPV. Among the LR-HPV infections, 94.4% (136 cases) were monotypic infections, which were caused primarily by HPV6 or HPV11. Additionally, 43 patients had mixed infections of LR-HPV and HR-HPV. Among the 194 patients, 85.6% (166) were infected with cervical HPV, with 61.4% being infected with LR-HPV and 23.7% with HR-HPV. There was 95.8% consistency in HPV types between vulvar and cervical lesions. The most common LR-HPV types were HPV11, HPV6, and HPV53, whereas the HR-HPV types included HPV16, HPV18, HPV52, HPV31, HPV45, and HPV58. Although many individuals are infected with HPV, approximately 90% experience transient infections, whereas a small percentage of patients have persistent HR-HPV infections. This persistent infection can lead to the integration of HPV DNA into human DNA, potentially progressing to precancerous lesions or tumors. Persistent HR-HPV infection is considered a major cause of cervical cancer, with infection lasting 6–12 months referred to as "persistent infection." If HR-HPV infection persists for 8–12 years, it can develop into cervical cancer [70, 71]. In 2018, approximately 570,000 new cases of cervical cancer were reported to occur globally each year, with 311,000 related deaths [70, 72]. Therefore, appropriately managing persistent HR-HPV infections is critical for preventing the development of cervical squamous intraepithelial lesions and cervical cancer.

8.3.1.3 Cervical Squamous Intraepithelial Lesions

Cervical intraepithelial neoplasia (CIN) refers to a pathological diagnosis of cervical dysplasia and carcinoma in situ. CIN is categorized into three grades on the basis of the degree of cellular atypia observed in the cervix: CIN1 (mild), CIN2 (moderate), and CIN3 (severe or carcinoma in situ). These categories are determined by the proportion of abnormal, or heteromorphic, cells present in the upper third, middle two-thirds, and entire epithelial layer of the cervix. In 2012, the American Pathological Society (CAP) and the American Society for Colposcopy and Cervical Pathology (ASCCP) introduced a new standardized classification system for squamous intraepithelial lesions of the genital tract. The term squamous intraepithelial lesion (SIL) is now recommended for all squamous intraepithelial lesions associated with HPV infection. SILs can be further divided into low-grade squamous intraepithelial lesions (LSILs) and high-grade squamous intraepithelial lesions (HSILs). SIL can be further subclassified into intraepithelial neoplasia (IN) on the basis of the severity of the lesions. LSIL includes CIN1 and p16-negative CIN2, whereas HSIL encompasses p16-positive CIN2 and CIN3. The majority of LSIL lesions are associated with HPV infections, with approximately 83% of these cases testing positive for HR-HPV [73]. In LSIL lesions, HPV often remains in a free state, and the host cells do not undergo malignant transformation, making it easier for the immune system to clear the infection. In contrast, HSIL lesions are characterized by the integration of HPV DNA into the host genome. As the severity of the lesions increases, the degree of HPV integration also increases, making it more difficult for the immune system to recognize and clear the infection. This integration can lead to cervical precancerous lesions or even cervical cancer. The progression of cervical cancer follows a continuous evolutionary process, from a quantitative change (LSIL) to a qualitative change, progressing from early invasive cancer to invasive cancer. Thus, early screening and intervention are crucial for preventing the development of cervical cancer [74].

8.3.1.4 Management Principles of Cervical LSIL

Cervical LR-HPV infection is primarily associated with condyloma acuminata. According to the latest American Society for Colposcopy and Cervical Pathology risk-based guidelines for abnormal management of cervical cancer screening [75] and Chinese expert consensus [76], individuals with persistent HR-HPV infection for 1 year should undergo colposcopy to evaluate for potential cellular or tissue abnormalities. Management of CIN1, which is caused primarily by persistent HR-HPV, focuses on identifying and treating HSIL to prevent cervical cancer. While 60% of CIN1 lesions resolve naturally, 30% persist, and 10% progress to HSIL within 2 years. CIN1 with cytological HSIL carries a 3.9% risk of CIN3 within a year, warranting active treatment, including diagnostic conization if needed. In women under 25 years of age, CIN1 is often transient, with over 80% clearing naturally, favoring follow-up over immediate treatment. Persistent lesions for more than a year or LSIL with cytological HSIL indications should be treated proactively.

8.3.2 Physical and Surgical Treatment

Physical therapy includes microwaves, CO_2 lasers, cryotherapy, and electrocoagulation, whereas surgical options include loop electrosurgical excision procedure (LEEP) and cold knife conization (CKC). Comprehensive treatments may combine Chinese and Western medicine, integrate physical therapy with medication, or pair surgery with pharmacological interventions. However, medications alone are often ineffective, and physical or surgical treatments may cause complications such as damage to adjacent tissues and organs, bleeding, infection, cervical stenosis or adhesion, impaired cervical function, cervical endometriosis, and a high risk of recurrence posttreatment.

8.3.3 ALA-PDT

During her doctoral studies at the University of Munich in 2003, under the guidance of Professor Hillemanns, Professor Xiuli Wang investigated hexyl aminolevulinate (HAL)-mediated photodynamic therapy (PDT) for treating CIN, vaginal intraepithelial neoplasia (VaIN), and vulvar intraepithelial neoplasia (VIN). Upon returning to China in 2005, she introduced this therapeutic experience. In 2006, the first national continuing medical education course on PDT in dermatology was held, encompassing dermatology, gynecology, and urology. HAL-PDT for CIN, VaIN, and VIN was highlighted in collaboration between Dr. Wang's team and Professor Hillemanns, promoting academic exchanges and clinical collaborations with gynecologists, advancing the application of ALA-PDT in gynecology and paving the way for the recent development of the "Expert Consensus on Clinical Application of Aminolevulinic Acid Photodynamic Therapy in Female Lower Genital Tract Diseases in Gynecology".

8.3.3.1 Therapeutic Mechanism

The mechanism of ALA-PDT in treating HR-HPV infection or cervical LSIL leading to apoptosis and necrosis of diseased cells mirrors that described earlier in this chapter. The authors' group, along with Professor Hillemanns, reported that the cervical and urethral mucosa can specifically absorb ALA and convert it to PpIX throughout the cervical mucosal epidermis, with minimal impact on the dermis, making ALA-PDT both effective and safe for treating cervical HPV infections [77]. Research indicates that HR-HPV infection significantly reduces both the activity and number of natural killer (NK) cells and langhans cells involved in immune surveillance, whereas PDT enhances NK cell activity, promoting antiviral immune responses [78]. Furthermore,

ALA-PDT induces apoptosis in HR-HPV-infected cervical cancer cells (HeLa and SiHa) via caspase-dependent pathways, endoplasmic reticulum stress, and autophagy, effectively eliminating HR-HPV infection [79]. Additionally, ALA-PDT facilitates HeLa cell autophagy and death through the $Ca2^{+}$-CaMKK-β-AMPK pathway, suggesting that this pathway and autophagy are potential therapeutic targets for HR-HPV infection management [80].

8.3.3.2 Clinical Efficacy

Clinical studies have demonstrated that ALA-PDT is effective in treating cervical HPV infection. In 1998, Pahernik, Hillemanns, and colleagues observed peak porphyrin fluorescence 3–4 h after applying 3% ALA solution to cervical CIN lesions [81]. Although early studies revealed no significant differences in efficacy compared with placebo [82, 83], Bodner successfully treated CIN2 with ALA-PDT, achieving outcomes comparable to those of cold knife conical excision without severe tissue damage [84]. In 2003, Hillemann and the authors' group enhanced the efficacy of 10% ALA thermosensitive gel, which increased porphyrin levels at lesion sites [85]. This gel adhered effectively to cervical lesions, being liquid at 4 °C and viscous above 31 °C. Subsequently, ALA thermosensitive gels have been widely used for ALA-PDT in the cervix and other special sites. In 2011, the authors treated 44 chronic CIN1 patients with HR-HPV via ALA-PDT and 10% gel for 4 h. Brick-red fluorescence of PpIX in CIN1 was observed in the full-thickness epidermis (Fig. 8.19), followed by 635-nm laser irradiation at 80–100 J/cm^2 every 2 weeks for three sessions [86]. Follow-up revealed HR-HPV negative conversion rates of 81% at 6 months and 90.5% at 12 months, with CIN reversal rates of 85.7%. In 2012, 75 HR-HPV patients were treated, resulting in a significantly higher conversion rate in the ALA-PDT group (72.5%) than in the control group (37.4%) [87]. Further studies revealed histological remission rates above 90% at 3–12 months and recurrence rates of 3.7–13.9% at 12–37 months [88, 89], with ALA-PDT also showing promise for positive margins or recurrence afterLEEP/CKC [90, 91].

ALA-PDT is also effective for treating vaginal LSIL/VaIN (Fig. 8.20). A retrospective analysis by the authors' group compared ALA-PDT combined with one CO_2 laser with CO_2 laser alone. In the CO_2 laser group, the complete remission rate was 66.67% (10/15), and the HR-HPV remission rate was 33.33% (5/15) at 1 month posttreatment. In contrast, the ALA-PDT combined with CO_2 laser group achieved a complete remission rate of 86.67% (13/15) and an HR-HPV remission rate of 93.33% (14/15). Adverse events, including severe bleeding in one patient and tissue adhesion and vaginal stenosis in 12 patients, were more common in the CO_2 laser group. No serious adverse events or systemic side effects were reported in the ALA-PDT plus CO_2 laser combination group [92]. ALA-PDT is now widely used for treating cervical and vaginal HPV-related diseases.

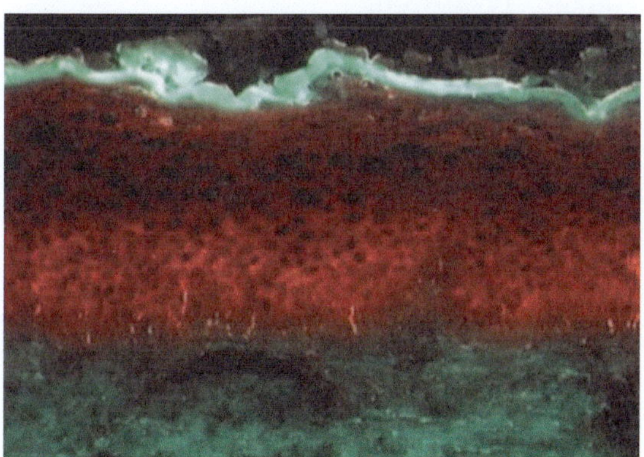

Fig. 8.19 Brick-red fluorescence of PpIX over the full-thickness epidermis with clear demarcation at the dermal–epidermal junction in CIN1 lesions

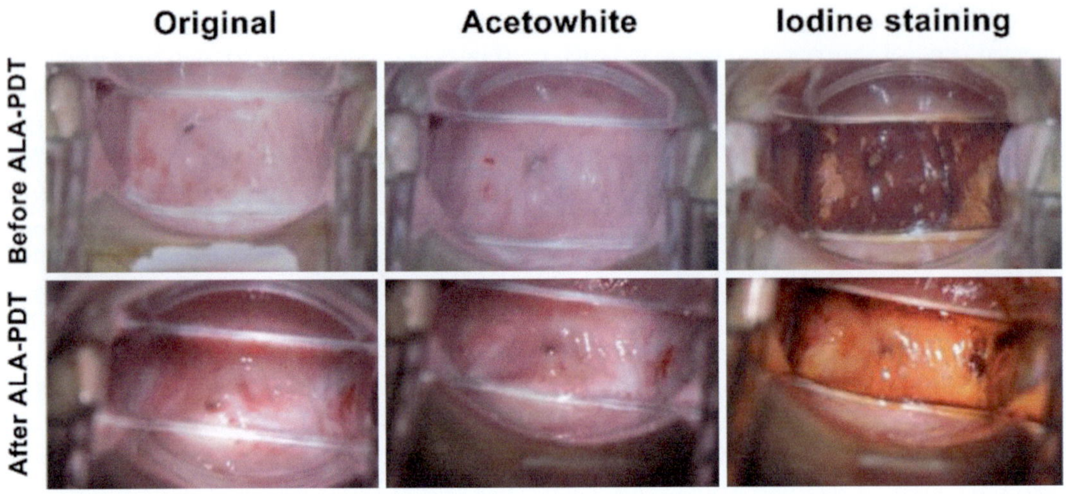

Fig. 8.20 Vaginal LSIL was treated with ALA-PDT. After treatment, there was no obvious abnormality under colposcopy, both in the acetowhite and iodine staining images

8.3.3.3 Recommended Protocol (Table 8.6)

According to the 2022 "Expert Consensus on the Clinical Application of Aminolevulinic Acid Photodynamic Therapy in Female Lower Genital Tract Diseases" the recommended protocol includes the following:

Indications: Histopathologically confirmed LSIL/CIN1, as well as histopathologically confirmed HSIL/CIN2, provided that the cervical squamo-columnar junction and lesion margins are visible during colposcopy.

Contraindication: Cytological and histological examinations showing atypical glandular cells (AGC), adenocarcinoma in situ (AIS), or suspected malignant lesions.

8.3.3.4 Precautions

During ALA-PDT for cervical HPV-related diseases, abdominal pain may occur but typically resolves within a few hours. However, in pregnant women, pain can potentially trigger uterine contractions and premature labor. After treatment, patients may experience increased vaginal discharge, which usually subsides naturally within 3–5 days without treatment. Prior to ALA-PDT, a thorough evaluation by a gynecologist should be conducted, with strict adherence to the indications and contraindications. Notably, due to the significant risk of high-grade squamous intraepithelial lesions (HSIL) progressing to invasive squamous cell carcinoma, extreme caution is warranted when considering ALA-PDT for HSIL management.

8.3.3.5 Other PDT Regimens

Currently, photosensitizers for treating cervical intraepithelial neoplasia are limited primarily to ALAs, although Photofrin is also used. Photofrin treatment involves intravenous injection at a dose of 2 mg/kg, followed by irradiation 48–60 h later with 630 nm light and an energy density of 100 J/cm^2 [94].

In all, 10 mm of 10 mM HAL thermosensitive gel was applied locally to CIN1, CIN2, and CIN3 lesions for 3–5 h and then irradiated with a 633-nm semiconductor laser. At 6 months posttreatment, 15 out of 24 patients (63%) demonstrated complete CIN remission and HPV clearance, with response rates of 71%, 50%, and 71% for CIN1, CIN2, and CIN3, respectively [95].

ALA-PDT offers distinct advantages, including simultaneous clearance of CIN1 and HR-HPV infection, ease of operation, lack of tissue damage, and minimal side effects compared with traditional therapies. These features highlight its importance in reducing the incidence of cervical cancer and underscore its potential for widespread application.

Table 8.6 Recommended protocol for the treatment of cervical HPV-associated disease with ALA-PDT [31, 93]

		Preparation of ALA				Illumination dosage	
Pretreatment	Recommended protocol	ALA dosage form	ALA concentration (%)	Incubation time (h)	Recommended light source	Energy density (J/cm^2)	Power density (mW/cm^2)
Sanitize treatment area (e.g., germanium) and remove mucus over cervix	Can be combined with CO_2 laser	Thermosensitive gel	10–20	3–5	Optical fiber with cervical cap is recommended	60–150	40–120

8.4 ALA-PDT in the Treatment of Cutaneous Warts

8.4.1 Overview of Cutaneous Warts

Cutaneous warts, a common benign proliferative skin disease caused by HPV infection, can occur at any age. On the basis of their location and clinical presentation, they are categorized into common warts, plantar warts, and flat warts.

8.4.1.1 Clinical Manifestations

Common warts (verrucae vulgares) demonstrate a predilection for the palms, soles, fingers, and periungual regions. While facial and scalp lesions may occur, subungual involvement is rare and warrants specialized management. They are caused primarily by HPV types 1, 2, 4, 27, and 57. The lesions are hard, grayish-yellow or dirty-brown papules with keratinized, rough surfaces. Initially, the size of a pinhead gradually increases to the size of a soybean, with numbers potentially increasing to several or dozens. They are generally asymptomatic but may occasionally cause tenderness.

Plantar warts are found on the soles of the feet and the bottoms of toes and often linked to trauma, friction, and excessive foot sweating. They are typically caused by HPV types 2, 27, and 57. The lesions are round, hard, well defined, and surrounded by a thickened keratinous ring. They may appear as isolated papules, coalesced plaques, or lesions secondary to calluses, with satellite foci. Tenderness with varying intensity is common.

Flat warts are common among adolescents and often occur on the face, dorsal hands, and other exposed skin. They are caused primarily by HPV types 3 and 10. The lesions are light brown or skin-colored, flat papules ranging in size from a corn kernel to a mung bean. They can coalesce into patches or form linear arrangements along scratch lines (Koebner phenomenon). Lesions are usually asymptomatic or mildly pruritic.

8.4.1.2 Histopathology

Cutaneous warts exhibit histological features such as hyperkeratosis, parakeratosis, acanthosis, and papillomatous hyperplasia. The overlying stratum corneum of the elevated papillary ridges shows tile-like parakeratosis with large, darkly stained nuclei, often accompanied by pinpoint hemorrhages. The granular layer and upper spinous layers contain multiple vacuolated cells and basophilic coarse hyaline granules. Dilated capillaries with mild inflammatory cell infiltration can be observed in the papillary dermis. Different wart types display distinctive pathological characteristics: common warts present papillomatous hyperplasia with inward bending of rete ridges at lesion edges (toeing in); plantar warts extend deeper into the dermis with a thickened stratum corneum; flat warts present a basket-weave stratum corneum with alternating hyperkeratosis and parakeratosis; and numerous vacuolated cells in the upper spinous and granular layers.

8.4.2 Treatment

The treatment of cutaneous warts primarily involves local therapies categorized by their mechanisms: destructive, cytotoxic, and immunomodulatory. Destructive therapies include cryotherapy, trichloroacetic acid (TCA), salicylic acid, electrocautery, laser treatment, and surgical excision. Cytotoxic treatments utilize agents such as topical fluorouracil, 0.5% podophyllotoxin, cantharidin, and bleomycin. Immunomodulatory therapies include 5% imiquimod. These treatments often lead to side effects such as pain, redness, swelling, erosion, infection, and scarring and are associated with low cure rates and high recurrence rates.

8.4.3 PDT

In 1975, Morison utilized proflavin photodynamic therapy (PDT) to treat five patients with cutaneous warts [96], applying a 1% aqueous solution of proflavin externally and irradiating them with a daylight-type fluorescent tube for 20 min daily over 4 weeks, with repeat treatment permitted for up to 3 months. Three patients experienced resolution of skin lesions after treatment. In 1979, Stahl treated 65 patients with palmoplantar warts via methylene blue PDT and compared the results to those of a control group treated with salicylic acid and creosote [97]. The PDT applied a 1% methylene blue solution for 0.5 h followed by irradiation with a mercury vapor lamp (500–600 nm, 30 mW/cm²) once weekly for 8 weeks. In the control group, a solution of 16% salicylic acid and 24% creosote was applied overnight daily for 8 weeks. Eight weeks posttreatment, the cure rate was 8% in the PDT group and 15% in the control group. In 1997, the authors' group pioneered the use of ALA-PDT for urethral condyloma acuminata and later extended its application to cutaneous warts.

8.4.3.1 Therapeutic Mechanisms

Cutaneous warts and condyloma acuminata are similar to HPV-infected skin diseases and have the same mechanism as discussed in Sect. 8.1.3.2.

8.4.3.2 Clinical Efficacy of PDT

Cutaneous warts exhibit papillomatous hyperplasia with prominent hyperkeratotic surfaces, which directly impairs the effectiveness of ALA-PDT. Therefore, proper pretreatment to address hyperkeratosis is crucial for enhancing therapeutic outcomes.

Common warts: In 1995, Ammann explored the use of ALA-PDT to treat six cases of intractable common warts on hands resistant to traditional therapies and with disease durations ranging from 2 to 10 years [98]. A 20% ALA cream was applied externally for 5–6 h, followed by visible light irradiation for 30 min. After 2 months of follow-up, acute skin inflammation was noted in the treated areas; five patients showed no improvement, whereas one experienced complete lesion clearance. In 2000, Stender conducted a randomized study involving 45 patients with 232 common warts on their hands and feet [99]. The lesions were divided into ALA-PDT and placebo-PDT groups, which received either 20% ALA cream or placebo cream under occlusion for 4 h, followed by irradiation with 590–700 nm red light at an energy density of 70 J/cm². Treatments were administered biweekly for three to six sessions. At the 14th week, wart areas were reduced by 98% in the ALA-PDT group compared with 52% in the placebo group; by the 18th week, the reductions were 100% and 71%, respectively. Pain was the primary adverse reaction and was more pronounced in the ALA-PDT group. Additionally, the authors' group treated a patient with subungual and periungual warts via a combination of an electric knife, curetting, and ALA-PDT [100]. The toenail was separated and removed with an electric knife to expose subungual warts, followed by surface removal with a curette. A 20% ALA cream was applied for 3 h under light protection, and a 635-nm diode laser was used for 20 min at 100 mW/cm². Complete lesion resolution occurred after two ALA-PDT sessions, with no recurrence observed during the 2-year follow-up, and the toenail plate returned to normal (Fig. 8.21).

Plantar warts: In 2001, Fabbrocini investigated the efficacy of ALA-PDT for refractory plantar warts in a study involving 67 patients who had not responded to conventional treatments [101]. A total of 121 lesions were randomized, with 64 lesions treated with ALA-PDT and 57 lesions treated with placebo-PDT. A 20% ALA cream or placebo cream was applied to the lesions for 5 h, followed by irradiation with 400–700-nm visible light at an energy density of 50 J/cm². Treatments were administered every 2 weeks for a total of three sessions, and patients were followed up for 22 months. At 2 months posttreatment, the cure rate was significantly greater in the ALA-PDT group (75%) than in the placebo-PDT group (22.8%).

Flat warts: In 2003, Mizuki described treating a patient with multiple flat warts on the face via ALA-PDT [102]. The patient had a 2-year history of this condition, with previous treatments such as cryotherapy and dinitrochlorobenzene proving ineffective. A 20% ALA cream was applied for 6 h, followed by irradiation with a metal halide lamp (with wave peaks at 630 nm and 700 nm) for 20 min at an energy density of 120 J/cm². After two treatments, the lesions were completely eradicated within 5 months, with no recurrence. In 2010, Lu conducted a study involving 18 patients with multiple flat warts on the face, all of whom had experienced prolonged disease (1–6 years) and resistance to traditional therapies [103]. The treatment involved applying

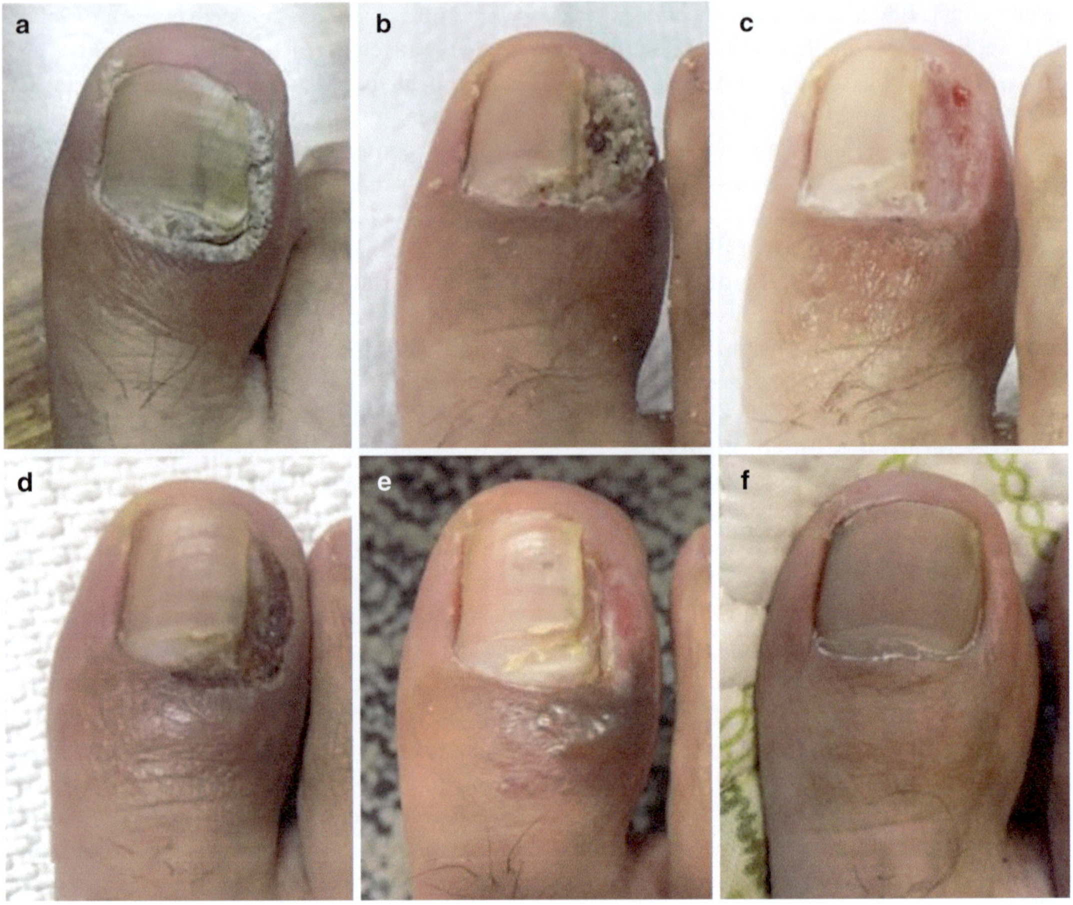

Fig. 8.21 Clinical pictures of ALA-PDT combined with curettage for the treatment of subungual and periungual warts. (**a**) Thickened keratinization of the lateral margin of the right great toenail, gray and yellow discoloration under the nail, and partial onycholysis. (**b**) Thickened and keratinized warts under the nail can be seen after partial nail avulsion. (**c**) An electric knife and curette were used to remove the surface hyperkeratotic lesions. (**d**) Localized dark red scabs, erythema and swelling of periungual tissues after the first ALA-PDT. (**e**) Warts are removed after the second ALA-PDT. (**f**) Two years after treatment, there was no wart recurrence and the nail plate appeared normal

10% ALA cream for 4 h, followed by 635-nm red-light irradiation with an energy density of 120 J/cm^2. Sessions were held every 15 days, with two to three treatments per patient. The results revealed that 17 patients were cured after two treatments, with one patient experiencing recurrence within 6 months. One patient withdrew from the study because of a lack of efficacy. In 2014, Li conducted a split-face-controlled study to evaluate the efficacy of ALA-PDT for treating multiple flat warts on the face [104]. The study included 55 patients divided into groups treated with 5%, 10%, or 20% ALA cream, all of which were incubated for 4 h. Red-light irradiation (633 nm) was applied at an energy density of 113 J/cm^2, with treatments every 2 weeks for a total of three sessions. The clearance rate of lesions was slightly lower in the 5% ALA group than in the 10% and 20% ALA groups, but the differences were not statistically significant. The highest incidence of adverse effects, including localized hyperpigmentation (61%), was observed in the 20% ALA group. The 10% ALA-PDT group showed the best balance of efficacy and tolerability, achieving a 33.3% clearance rate of lesions within 12 weeks.

8.4.3.3 Recommended Protocol

ALA-PDT is effective in treating cutaneous warts. Owing to the papillomatous hyperplasia and hyperkeratosis of these lesions, the limited penetration depth of the photosensitizer requires pretreatment with keratolytic agents or scraping to enhance drug absorption. A single session of ALA-PDT is often insufficient, necessitating multiple treatments for thorough lesion clearance. Additionally, ALA-PDT is more costly than topical medications and other traditional physical therapies. Therefore, ALA-PDT is recommended after pretreatment in cases where conventional treatments are ineffective, where lesions are in sensitive or challenging areas, or when preserving local tissue structure and function is a priority.

Common warts: The following ALA-PDT regimens are recommended for treating refractory common warts (Table 8.7) and may be adjusted accordingly.

Plantar warts: Same as common warts.

Flat warts: The following ALA-PDT regimens are recommended for treating flat warts (Table 8.8) and may be adjusted accordingly.

8.4.3.4 Optimization of the Protocol

Promoting the transdermal absorption of ALA is crucial for the success of ALA-PDT in treating cutaneous warts, as hyperkeratosis on the wart surface hinders absorption and limits efficacy. Various methods have been explored to increase ALA absorption, including curettage, electrodermabrasion, ultrasound, iontophoresis, microdermabrasion, laser ablation, fire needling, and salicylic acid under occlusion [100, 105, 106]. Yoo [107] treated 12 patients with refractory periungual warts via a carbon dioxide laser combined with methyl 5-aminolevulinic acid photodynamic therapy (MAPT), achieving a 90% clearance rate with no recurrence after 6 months and a significantly shorter treatment period than ALA-PDT alone.

Light source optimization: The choice of light source significantly impacts the therapeutic efficacy of ALA-PDT. While 410-nm blue light offers maximum PpIX absorption, its limited tissue penetration makes 630-nm red light the preferred option in clinical settings for treating warts. In 1999, Stender evaluated ALA-PDT for refractory hand and foot warts using various excitation light sources and reported that white light achieved a significantly higher cure rate than red light, blue light, or cryotherapy alone did, highlighting the potential of white light for enhanced treatment outcomes [108].

Combined treatment strategies can increase the efficacy and reduce the duration of ALA-PDT for the treatment of cutaneous warts. Options

Table 8.7 Recommended regimens for ALA-PDT for refractory common warts

	ALA formulation			Light doses		
Pretreatment	ALA dosage form	ALA concentration (%)	Application time (h)	Energy density (J/cm^2)	Power density (mW/cm^2)	Treatment interval (weeks)
Keratolytic agents, curette, etc., to remove hyperkeratotic lesions	Solution/cream	10–20	3–6	60–150	60–100	1–2

Table 8.8 Recommended regimens for ALA-PDT for the treatment of flat warts

	ALA formulation			Light doses		
Pretreatment	ALA dosage form	ALA concentration (%)	Application time (h)	Energy density (J/cm^2)	Power density (mW/cm^2)	Treatment interval (weeks)
Tape stripping	Solution/cream	10–20	3–6	60–150	60–100	1–2

include combining ALA-PDT with salicylic acid, photothermal therapy, imiquimod, or surgery. In 2018, a study combining photothermal therapy with imiquimod for 36 patients with refractory warts achieved a 61.1% complete remission rate, which was significantly higher than the 32.4% reported in the imiquimod-only group [109]. In 2019, Mo Xingfan reported a 100% clearance rate for refractory plantar warts treated with surgery combined with ALA-PDT, with no adverse reactions after 6 months [110]. Additionally, Zhao Shuang's team treated 23 patients with periungual warts via shallow scraping and ALA-PDT, resulting in over 50% clearance in 96% of the patients after three treatments within 3 months [111].

8.4.4 Photothermal Therapy for Cutaneous Warts

Photothermal therapy (PTT) is increasingly recognized as an effective modality for treating tumors and infectious diseases through the use of photothermal agents (PAs), such as carbon, gold, silver nanomaterials, and germanium nanocrystals, to convert light energy into heat, leading to localized tissue ablation [13, 112]. Upon light irradiation at specific wavelengths, these agents absorb photons, transition to an excited state, and release energy through vibrational relaxation, generating heat in the surrounding tissue. A heat shock response occurs when the tissue temperature reaches 41 °C, triggering changes in gene expression and heat shock protein production [113]. Irreversible damage begins at 42 °C, with necrosis occurring after 10 min at 42–46 °C. At 46–52 °C, cells die rapidly from microvascular thrombosis and ischemia, whereas temperatures above 60 °C cause immediate cell death due to protein denaturation and membrane disruption [114].

In 2018, the authors' group first applied intense pulsed light (IPL) as PTT for facial flat warts, treating 23 patients with a 590-nm filter at 12–16 J/cm^2, combined with intramuscular BCG-PSN injections twice weekly for 8 weeks and two IPL sessions per month [115]. A total of 17 patients (74%) achieved complete remission, with 548 of the 676 warts eradicated, resulting in an overall clearance rate of 81% and only four recurrences at the 20-week follow-up. In 2019, the group demonstrated that PTT enhanced the efficacy of 5% imiquimod cream for refractory cutaneous warts when combined with 808-nm laser irradiation, resulting in a significantly higher remission rate (61.1%) than imiquimod alone (32.4%). PTT also showed additional benefits in improving skin pigmentation, tone, and elasticity [109].

In summary, both ALA-PDT and PTT have proven to be effective treatments for common, flat, plantar, and other cutaneous warts, and their clinical application continues to expand.

References

1. Zhang J, Gao B, Kang Y, Ma ZJ, Li QM. Genotype distribution of human papillomavirus strains in cervix samples from Chinese women:a meta-analysis. Chin J Microbiol Immunol. 2014;34(12):913–20.
2. Zhao YQ, Zhao FH, Hu SY, Chen W, Chen F, Cui JF, et al. Multicenter cross-sectional study on type-specific human papillomavirus infection among Chinese women. Chin J Epidemiol. 2015;36(12):1351–6.
3. Branch CPMAV. Expert consensus on immunological prevention of human papillomavirus?Related diseases. Chin J Prevent Med. 2019;8:761–803.
4. Hillemanns P, Wang XL. Integration of HPV-16 and HPV-18 DNA in vulvar intraepithelial neoplasia. Gynecol Oncol. 2006;100(2):276.
5. Wang XL, Liao KH, Hillemanns P. Integration of HPV 16/18 DNA in vulvar intraepithelial neoplasia. Chin J Dermatol. 2005;38(10):615–8. https://doi.org/10.3760/j.issn:0412-4030.2005.10.006.
6. Wang XL, Wang HW, Yang LJ, Xiao Q, Lv T. Cervical human papillomavirus(HPV)infection and associated genotypes in female patients with vulvar condyloma acuminatum from Shanghai area. Chin J Dermatol. 2009;11:739–41.
7. Wang XL, Wang HW, Hillemanns P, Hamblin MR. Distinctive features of foreskin condylomata acuminata associated with diabetes mellitus. Acta Derm Venereol. 2008;88(6):578–83. https://doi.org/10.2340/00015555-0537.
8. Group CMADBV. Guidelines for the diagnosis and treatment of genital warts. Chin J Dermatol. 2014;47(8):598–9.
9. Wang HW, Miao F, Shi L, Lv T, Huang Z, Wang XL. Imiquimod-induced localized vitiligo in wife and lichen planus in husband. Chin Med J. 2013;126(13):2593.

10. Wang XL, Xu SZ, Zhang CR, Zhu XJ, Xia W. Δ-Aminolevulinic acid photodynamic therapy for male urethra Condyloma Acuminatum. Chin J Dermatovenereol. 2000;2:34–5.
11. Wang XL, Wang HW, Wang HS, Xu SZ, Liao KH, Hillemanns P. Topical 5-aminolaevulinic acid-photodynamic therapy for the treatment of urethral condylomata acuminata. Br J Dermatol. 2004;151(4):880–5. https://doi.org/10.1111/j.1365-2133.2004.06189.x.
12. Wang HW, Wang XL, Guo MX, Liu F. 5-aminolevulinic acid-photodynamic therapy and CO_2 laser for condylomata acuminatam. J Clin Dermatol. 2006;35(10):674–5.
13. Tu P, Zhang HY, Zheng HY, Gu H, Xu JH, Tao JN. 5-Aminolevulinic photodynamic therapy versus carbon dioxide laser therapy for small genital warts: a multicenter, randomized, open-label trial. J Am Acad Dermatol. 2021;84(3):779–81. https://doi.org/10.1016/j.jaad.2019.07.073.
14. Tu P, Zheng HY, Gu H, Xu JH, Wang XL, Chen W, et al. Topical 5-aminolevulinic acid photodynamic therapy for the treatment of condyloma acuminatum: a multicenter, randomized, CO_2 laser-controlled trial. Chin J Dermatol. 2007;40(2):67–70.
15. Hillemanns P, Wang XL, Staehle S, Michels W, Dannecker C. Evaluation of different treatment modalities for vulvar intraepithelial neoplasia (VIN): CO(2) laser vaporization, photodynamic therapy, excision and vulvectomy. Gynecol Oncol. 2006;100(2):271–5. https://doi.org/10.1016/j.ygyno.2005.08.012.
16. Wang HW, Wang XL, Guo MX, Yu YF. Topical 5-aminolaevulinic acid-photodynamic therapy in the treatment of precancerous changes and carcinoma of the skin in situ. Chin J Dermatol. 2006;3:137–9.
17. Wang XL, Wang HW, Le JY. Focus on the diagnosis and treatment of certain HPV-related skin diseases. Chin J Dermatol. 2008;41(05):279–81.
18. Association PTRC. Expert consensus on the clinical application of aminolevulinic acid photodynamic therapy. Chin J Dermatol. 2015;48(10):675–8.
19. Morton CA, Szeimies RM, Sidoroff A, Braathen LR. European guidelines for topical photodynamic therapy part 2: emerging indications field cancerization, photorejuvenation and inflammatory/infective dermatoses. J Eur Acad Dermatol Venereol. 2013;27(6):672–9.
20. Association PTRC. Chinese guidelines for clinical application of aminolevulinic acid-based photodynamic therapy in dermatology (2021 edition). Chin J Dermatol. 2021;54(1):1–9.
21. Shi L, Wang HW, Chen K, Yan J, Yu B, Wang SC, et al. Chinese guidelines on the clinical application of 5-aminolevulinic acid-based photodynamic therapy in dermatology (2021 edition). Photodiagn Photodyn Ther. 2021;35:102340. https://doi.org/10.1016/j.pdpdt.2021.102340.
22. Wang XL, Wang HW, Huang Z, Stepp H, Baumgartner R, Dannecker C, et al. Study of protoporphyrin IX (PpIX) pharmacokinetics after topical application of 5-aminolevulinic acid in urethral condylomata acuminata. Photochem Photobiol. 2007;83(5):1069–73. https://doi.org/10.1111/j.1751-1097.2007.00178.x.
23. Wang XL, Xu SZ, Zhang CR, Wang HW. Study of the mechanism of δ-aminolevulinic acid-induced photodynamic therapy on patients with condyloma accuminata. Chin J Dermatovenereol. 2001;15(4):234–7.
24. Liao F, Wang XL, Wang HW, Ding HL, Lv T, Zhang LL. Establishment of a human keratinocyte cell line (HaCaT) stably expressing human papillomavirus type 16 E7 (HPV16E7) protein. Chin J Dermatol. 2011;044(005):310–3.
25. Miao F, Lv T, Zhang YF, Huang Z, Wang XL, Wang H. Induction of apoptosis in HPV16 E7 transfected human keratinocyte by ALA-mediated photodynamic therapy. Photodiagn Photodyn Ther. 2016;13:205–10. https://doi.org/10.1016/j.pdpdt.2015.07.004.
26. Zhang YF, Miao F, Wang HW, Lv T, Li JJ, Wang XL. Local immune response in condyloma acuminatum treated with aminolevulinic acid-photodynamic therapy. Chin J Dermatol. 2013;46(5):309–12.
27. Center, C. M. A. D. B. P. T. R., Committee, C. A. & Group, C. M. E. A. D. Chinese guidelines for clinical application of aminolevulinic acid-based photodynamic therapy in dermatology (2021 edition). Chin J Dermatol. 2021;54(1):1–9.
28. Wang XL, Wang HW, Ding YF, Shao YL, Yang Q, Xu SZ. Clinical efficacy observation of δ-aminolevulinic acid photodynamic therapy in treating 101 cases of urethral condyloma acuminatum. J Clin Dermatol. 2003;8:479.
29. Wang XL, Miao F, Zhang LL, Guo MX, Zhang HQ, Wang HW. Topical photodynamic therapy with 5-aminolevulinic acid for cervical condyloma acuminatum. Chin J Dermatol. 2010;10:694–7.
30. Wang XL, Yao HX, Miao F, Wang L, Wang HW. Topical photodynamic therapy with 5-aminolevulinic acid for cervical intraepithelial neoplasia. Chin J Clin. 2011;5(16):4751–5.
31. Qiu LH, Li JR, Chen F, Huang Z, Sui L, Wei LH, et al. Expert consensus on the clinical application of aminolevulinic acid photodynamic therapy in diseases of the female lower reproductive tract. Chin J Clin Obstet Gynecol. 2022;23(4):446–8. https://doi.org/10.13390/j.issn.1672-1861.2022.04.037.
32. Wang HW, Wang XL, Guo MX, Liu F. 5-aminolevulinic acid-photodynamic therapy and CO_2 laser for condylomata acuminata. J Clin Dermatol. 2006;35(10):674–5.
33. Hu ZL, Li JP, Liu H, Liu LS, Jiang LF, Zeng K. Treatment of latent or subclinical genital HPV infection with 5-aminolevulinic acid-based photodynamic therapy. Photodiagn Photodyn Ther. 2018;23:362–4. https://doi.org/10.1016/j.pdpdt.2018.07.014.

34. Wang HW, Wang XL, Zhang LL, Guo MX, Huang Z. Aminolevulinic acid (ALA)-assisted photodynamic diagnosis of subclinical and latent HPV infection of external genital region. Photodiagn Photodyn Ther. 2008;5(4):251–5. https://doi.org/10.1016/j.pdpdt.2008.11.004.
35. Wang XL, Wang HW, Zhang LL, Guo MX, Su LN, Tao JN. 5-Aminolevulinic acid-mediated photodynamic diagnosis for condylomata acuminata. Chin J Dermatol. 2008;41(5):5.
36. Wang B, Shi L, Zhang YF, Zhou Q, Zheng J, Szeimies RM, et al. Gain with no pain? Pain management in dermatological photodynamic therapy. Br J Dermatol. 2017;177(3):656–65. https://doi.org/10.1111/bjd.15344.
37. Zhang HY, Shi L, Zhang YF, Wang PR, Zhang GL, Cao YJ, et al. Modified photodynamic therapy to minimize pain in the treatment of condylomata acuminata: a prospective, randomized, self-controlled study. Photodiagn Photodyn Ther. 2020;32:101915. https://doi.org/10.1016/j.pdpdt.2020.101915.
38. Wang XL, Xu SZ, Zhang CR. Treatment of recurrent condyloma acumninatumn by δ-aminolevulinic acid photodynamic therapy and micro- wave. Chin J Leprosy Skin Dis. 2002;1:20–1.
39. Huang JH, Zeng QH, Zuo CX, Yang SB, Xiang YP, Lu JY, et al. The combination of CO_2 laser vaporation and photodynamic therapy in treatment of condylomata acuminata. Photodiagn Photodyn Ther. 2014;11(2):130–3. https://doi.org/10.1016/j.pdpdt.2014.03.008.
40. Liao CH, Sun XF, Zhang GL, Zhang HY, Zhang LL, Wng XL. Advanced application of holmium: YAG laser combined ALA-PDT for the treatment of refractory condylomata acuminata in anal canal. Photodiagn Photodyn Ther. 2020;30:101696. https://doi.org/10.1016/j.pdpdt.2020.101696.
41. Lloyd KM. Multicentric pigmented Bowen's disease of the groin. Arch Dermatol. 1970;101(1):48–51.
42. Wade TR, Kopf AW, Ackerman AB. Bowenoid papulosis of the penis. Cancer. 1978;42(4):1890–903. https://doi.org/10.1002/1097-0142(197810)42:4<1890::aid-cncr2820420430>3.0.co;2-c.
43. Wang HW, Wang XL, Zhang CG, Le J. Analysis of 60 cases of Bowen's papulosis. Chin J Dermatol. 2004;37(6):368. https://doi.org/10.3760/j.issn:0412-4030.2004.06.025.
44. Munoz-Bello JO, Carrillo-Garcia A, Lizano M. Epidemiology and molecular biology of HPV variants in cervical cancer: the state of the art in Mexico. Int J Mol Sci. 2022;23(15):8566. https://doi.org/10.3390/ijms23158566.
45. Gross G, Hagedorn M, Ikenberg H, Rufli T, Dahlet C, Grosshans E, et al. Bowenoid papulosis. Presence of human papillomavirus (HPV) structural antigens and of HPV 16-related DNA sequences. Arch Dermatol. 1985;121(7):858–63. https://doi.org/10.1001/archderm.121.7.858.
46. Wang HW, Wang XL, Zhang CG. Detection of HPV16 and 18 in Bowen like papular lesions. Chin J Leprosy Skin Dis. 2008;24(3):181–2. https://doi.org/10.3969/j.issn.1009-1157.2008.03.006.
47. Rombaldi RL, Serafini EP, Villa LL, Vanni AC, Barea F, Frassini R, et al. Infection with human papillomaviruses of sexual partners of women having cervical intraepithelial neoplasia. Braz J Med Biol Res. 2006;39(2):177–87. https://doi.org/10.1590/s0100-879x2006000200003.
48. Porter WM, Francis N, Hawkins D, Dinneen M, Bunker CB. Penile intraepithelial neoplasia: clinical spectrum and treatment of 35 cases. Br J Dermatol. 2002;147(6):1159–65. https://doi.org/10.1046/j.1365-2133.2002.05019.x.
49. Wilkinson E, Kneale B, Lynch P. Report of the ISSVD Terminology Committee. J Reprod Med Obstetr Gynecol. 1986;31(10):973–4.
50. Darragh TM, Colgan TJ, Thomas Cox J, Heller DS, Henry MR, Luff RD, et al. The lower anogenital squamous terminology standardization project for HPV-associated lesions: background and consensus recommendations from the College of American Pathologists and the American Society for Colposcopy and Cervical Pathology. Int J Gynecol Pathol. 2013;32(1):76–115. https://doi.org/10.1097/PGP.0b013e31826916c7.
51. Bornstein J, Bogliatto F, Haefner HK, Stockdale CK, Preti M, Bohl TG, et al. The 2015 International Society for the Study of vulvovaginal disease (ISSVD) terminology of vulvar squamous intraepithelial lesions. J Low Genit Tract Dis. 2016;20(1):11–4. https://doi.org/10.1097/LGT.0000000000000169.
52. Lopez-Revilla R, Pineda MA, Ortiz-Valdez J, Sanchez-Garza M, Riego L. Human papillomavirus type 16 variants in cervical intraepithelial neoplasia and invasive carcinoma in san Luis Potosi City, Mexico. Infect Agent Cancer. 2009;4:3. https://doi.org/10.1186/1750-9378-4-3.
53. Darwich L, Canadas MP, Sirera G, Alameda F, Forcada P, Delas J, et al. Human papillomavirus genotype distribution and human papillomavirus 16 and human papillomavirus 18 genomic integration in invasive and in situ cervical carcinoma in human immunodeficiency virus-infected women. Int J Gynecol Cancer. 2011;21(8):1486–90. https://doi.org/10.1097/IGC.0b013e31822a0195.
54. Lv T, Wang HW, Wang XL,Yang LJ, Xiao Q, Guo MX. Retrospective analysis of four therapies for Bowen's papular disease. Chin J Dermatovenereol. 2010;24(2):126–8.
55. Rodolakis A, Diakomanolis E, Vlachos G, Iconomou T, Protopappas A, Stefanidis C, et al. Vulvar intraepithelial neoplasia (VIN)–diagnostic and therapeutic challenges. Eur J Gynecol Oncol. 2003;24(3–4):317–22.
56. Wang HW, Wang XL, Guo MX, Liu F, Le J. Observation of the therapeutic effect of imiquimod cream on Bowen like papular disease. Chin J Dermatol. 2007;40(2):80–2. https://doi.org/10.3760/j.issn:0412-4030.2007.02.005.

57. Wang XL, Xu SZ, Zhang CG, Wang HW. Mechanism exploration of photodynamic therapy with 5-aminolevulinic acid for the treatment of genital warts. Chin J Dermatovenereol. 2001;15(4):234–7. https://doi.org/10.3969/j.issn.1001-7089.2001.04.008.
58. Martin-Hirsch PL, Whitehurst C, Buckley CH, Moore JV, Kitchener HC. Photodynamic treatment for lower genital tract intraepithelial neoplasia. Lancet. 1998;351(9113):1403. https://doi.org/10.1016/s0140-6736(98)24019-0.
59. Fehr MK, Hornung R, Schwarz VA, Simeon R, Haller U, Wyss P. Photodynamic therapy of vulvar intraepithelial neoplasia III using topically applied 5-aminolevulinic acid. Gynecol Oncol. 2001;80(1):62–6. https://doi.org/10.1006/gyno.2000.6028.
60. Fehr MK, Hornung R, Degen A, Schwarz VA, Fink D, Haller U, et al. Photodynamic therapy of vulvar and vaginal condyloma and intraepithelial neoplasia using topically applied 5-aminolevulinic acid. Lasers Surg Med. 2002;30(4):273–9. https://doi.org/10.1002/lsm.10048.
61. Yang CH, Lee JC, Chen CH, Hui CY, Hong HS, Kuo HW. Photodynamic therapy for bowenoid papulosis using a novel incoherent light-emitting diode device. Br J Dermatol. 2003;149(6):1297–9. https://doi.org/10.1111/j.1365-2133.2003.05661.x.
62. Paoli J, Ternesten Bratel A, Lowhagen GB, Stenquist B, Forslund O, Wennberg AM. Penile intraepithelial neoplasia: results of photodynamic therapy. Acta Derm Venereol. 2006;86(5):418–21. https://doi.org/10.2340/00015555-0130.
63. Wang XL, Wang HW, Guo MX, Huang Z. Combination of immunotherapy and photodynamic therapy in the treatment of Bowenoid papulosis. Photodiagn Photodyn Ther. 2007;4(2):88–93. https://doi.org/10.1016/j.pdpdt.2007.01.002.
64. Welbourn H, Duthie G, Powell J, Moghissi K. Can photodynamic therapy be the preferred treatment option for anal intraepithelial neoplasia? Initial results of a pilot study. Photodiagn Photodyn Ther. 2014;11(1):20–1. https://doi.org/10.1016/j.pdpdt.2013.11.004.
65. Che QL, Li JP, Wang JY, Wang Q, Jiang LF, Li ZJ, et al. Therapeutic evaluation of 5-aminolevulinic acid-mediated photodynamic therapy in Bowenoid papulosis. Photodiagn Photodyn Ther. 2020;29:101635. https://doi.org/10.1016/j.pdpdt.2019.101635.
66. Akoel KM, Welfel J, Gottwald L, Suzin J. Photodynamic diagnosis of vulvar precancerous conditions and invasive cancers using 5-aminolevulinic acid. Ginekol Pol. 2003;74(9):662–5.
67. Wang XL, Wang HW, Zhang LL, Guo MX, Su J, Tao JN. Application of 5-aminolevulinic acid photodynamic therapy in the diagnosis of genital warts. Chin J Dermatol. 2008;41(5):296–300. https://doi.org/10.3321/j.issn:0412-4030.2008.05.006.
68. zur Hausen H. Papillomavirus infections–a major cause of human cancers. Biochim Biophys Acta. 1996;1288(2):55–78. https://doi.org/10.1016/0304-419x(96)00020-0.
69. Crawford LV. A study of human papilloma virus DNA. J Mol Biol. 1965;13(2):362–72. https://doi.org/10.1016/s0022-2836(65)80103-6.
70. Forman D, de Martel C, Lacey CJ, Soerjomataram I, Lortet-Tieulent J, Bruni L, et al. Global burden of human papillomavirus and related diseases. Vaccine. 2012;30(Suppl 5):12–23. https://doi.org/10.1016/j.vaccine.2012.07.055.
71. Dalstein V, Riethmuller D, Prétet J, Le Bail Carval K, Sautière J, Carbillet J, et al. Persistence and load of high-risk HPV are predictors for development of high-grade cervical lesions: a longitudinal French cohort study. Int J Cancer. 2003;106(3):396–403.
72. Arbyn M, Weiderpass E, Bruni L, de Sanjosé S, Saraiya M, Ferlay J, et al. Estimates of incidence and mortality of cervical cancer in 2018: a worldwide analysis. Lancet Glob Health. 2020;8(2):e191–203. https://doi.org/10.1016/s2214-109x(19)30482-6.
73. Wei L, Zhao Y, Shen D, Zhao F, Geng L, Bi H, et al. Expert consensus on cervical cancer screening and abnormal management in China (I). Chin Clin J Obstetr Gynecol. 2017;18(2):190–2. https://doi.org/10.13390/j.issn.1672-1861.2017.02.032.
74. Ref C. The discovery of HIV and cancerogenic human papilloma viruses. Unfallchirurg. 2008;111(12):1037–40. https://doi.org/10.1007/s00113-008-1536-3.
75. Egemen D, Cheung LC, Chen X, Demarco M, Perkins RB, Kinney W, et al. Risk estimates supporting the 2019 ASCCP risk-based management consensus guidelines. J Low Genit Tract Dis. 2020;24(2):132–43. https://doi.org/10.1097/lgt.0000000000000529.
76. Wei L, Shen D, Zhao F, Geng L, Bi H, Zhao Y, et al. Expert consensus on cervical cancer screening and abnormal management in China (II). Chin Clin J Obstetr Gynecol. 2017;18(3):286–8. https://doi.org/10.13390/j.issn.1672-1861.2017.03.041.
77. Øvestad I, Gudlaugsson E, Skaland I, Malpica A, Kruse A, Janssen E, et al. Local immune response in the microenvironment of CIN2-3 with and without spontaneous regression. Mod Pathol. 2010;23(9):1231–40.
78. Kriska T, Korytowski W, Girotti A. Role of mitochondrial cardiolipin peroxidation in apoptotic photokilling of 5-aminolevulinate-treated tumor cells. Arch Biochem Biophys. 2005;433(2):435–46.
79. Wang JY, Wang Q, Chen PJ, Li Q, Li ZJ, Xu MN, et al. Podophyllotoxin-combined 5-aminolevulinic acid photodynamic therapy significantly promotes HR-HPV-infected cell death. Photodermatol Photoimmunol Photomed. 2022;38(4):343–53. https://doi.org/10.1111/phpp.12754.
80. Li ZJ, Teng MZ, Wang YJ, Wang Q, Feng YJ, Xiao ZX, et al. The mechanism of 5-aminolevulinic acid photodynamic therapy in promoting endoplas-

mic reticulum stress in the treatment of HR-HPV-infected HeLa cells. Photodermatol Photoimmunol Photomed. 2021;37(4):348–59. https://doi.org/10.1111/phpp.12663.
81. Pahernik SA, Botzlar A, Hillemanns P, Dellian M, Kirschstein M, Abels C, et al. Pharmacokinetics and selectivity of aminolevulinic acid-induced porphyrin synthesis in patients with cervical intraepithelial neoplasia. Int J Cancer. 1998;78(3):310–4. https://doi.org/10.1002/(sici)1097-0215(19981029)78:3<310::Aid-ijc9>3.0.Co;2-y.
82. Hillemanns P, Korell M, Schmitt-Sody M, Baumgartner R, Beyer W, Kimmig R, et al. Photodynamic therapy in women with cervical intraepithelial neoplasia using topically applied 5-aminolevulinic acid. Int J Cancer. 1999;81(1):34–8.https://doi.org/10.1002/(sici)1097--0215(19990331)81:1<34::aid-ijc7>3.0.co;2-h.
83. Barnett AA, Haller JC, Cairnduff F, Lane G, Brown SB, Roberts DJ. A randomized, double-blind, placebo-controlled trial of photodynamic therapy using 5-aminolaevulinic acid for the treatment of cervical intraepithelial neoplasia. Int J Cancer. 2003;103(6):829–32. https://doi.org/10.1002/ijc.10888.
84. Bodner K, Bodner-Adler B, Wierrani F, Kubin A, Szölts-Szölts J, Spängler B, et al. Cold-knife conization versus photodynamic therapy with topical 5-aminolevulinic acid (5-ALA) in cervical intraepithelial neoplasia (CIN) II with associated human papillomavirus infection: a comparison of preliminary results. Anticancer Res. 2003;23(2c):1785–8.
85. Andikyan V, Kronschnabl M, Hillemanns M, Wang X, Stepp H, Hillemanns P. Fluorescence diagnosis with 5-ALA thermogel of cervical intraepithelial neoplasia. Gynakol Geburtshilfliche Rundsch. 2004;44(1):31–7. https://doi.org/10.1159/000074315.
86. Wang XL, Yao HX, Miao F, Wang L, Wang HW. 5-aminolevulinic acid photodynamic therapy for cervical intraepithelial neoplasia grade I. Chin J Clin. 2011;5(16):4751–5.
87. Miao F, Wang XL, Wang HW, Zhang LL, Guo MX, Zhang HQ. 5-aminolevulinic acid photodynamic treatment of high-risk cervical HPV infection. Chin J Dermatol Venereol. 2012;26(1):3.
88. Wu AY, Li Q, Ling JY, Gu LY, Hong ZB, Di W, et al. Effectiveness of photodynamic therapy in women of reproductive age with cervical high-grade squamous intraepithelial lesions (HSIL/CIN2). Photodiagn Photodyn Ther. 2021;36:102517. https://doi.org/10.1016/j.pdpdt.2021.102517.
89. Ma LY, Gao XR, Geng L, You K, Wu ZX, Li Y, et al. Efficacy and safety of photodynamic therapy mediated by 5-aminolevulinic acid for the treatment of cervical intraepithelial neoplasia 2: a single-center, prospective, cohort study. Photodiagn Photodyn Ther. 2021;36:102472. https://doi.org/10.1016/j.pdpdt.2021.102472.
90. Niu JX, Cheng MX, Hong ZB, Ling JY, Di W, Gu LY, et al. The effect of 5-aminolaevulinic acid photodynamic therapy versus CO(2) laser in the treatment of cervical low-grade squamous intraepithelial lesions with high-risk HPV infection: a nonrandomized, controlled pilot study. Photodiagn Photodyn Ther. 2021;36:102548. https://doi.org/10.1016/j.pdpdt.2021.102548.
91. Cai HH, Ma TT, Che YC, Wang YK, Wang CL, Yin GJ. Loop electrosurgical excision procedure followed by 5-aminolevulinic acid photodynamic therapy for cervical intraepithelial neoplasia, a report of six cases. Photodiagn Photodyn Ther. 2020;29:101650. https://doi.org/10.1016/j.pdpdt.2020.101650.
92. Maździarz A. Successful pregnancy and delivery following selective use of photodynamic therapy in treatment of cervix and vulvar diseases. Photodiagn Photodyn Ther. 2019;28:65–8. https://doi.org/10.1016/j.pdpdt.2019.07.004.
93. Yao HX, Zhang HY, Pu XW, Shi L, Zhang YF, Wang PR, et al. Photodynamic therapy combined with carbon dioxide laser for low-grade vaginal intraepithelial neoplasia: a retrospective analysis. Photodiagn Photodyn Ther. 2020;30:101731. https://doi.org/10.1016/j.pdpdt.2020.101731.
94. Chinese Society of Dermatology. Chinese guidelines on the clinical application of 5-aminolevulinic acid-based photodynamic therapy in dermatology (2021 edition). Chin J Dermatol. 2021;54(1):1–9.
95. Yamaguchi S, Tsuda H, Takemori M, Nakata S, Nishimura S, Kawamura N, et al. Photodynamic therapy for cervical intraepithelial neoplasia. Oncology. 2005;69(2):110–6. https://doi.org/10.1159/000087812.
96. Morison WL. Anti-viral treatment of warts. Br J Dermatol. 1975;92(1):97–9. https://doi.org/10.1111/j.1365-2133.1975.tb03040.x.
97. Stahl D, Veien NK, Wulf HC. Photodynamic inactivation of virus warts: a controlled clinical trial. Clin Exp Dermatol. 1979;4(1):81–5. https://doi.org/10.1111/j.1365-2230.1979.tb01594.x.
98. Ammann R, Hunziker T, Braathen LR. Topical photodynamic therapy in verrucae. A pilot study. Dermatology. 1995;191(4):346–7. https://doi.org/10.1159/000246597.
99. Stender IM, Na R, Fogh H, Gluud C, Wulf HC. Photodynamic therapy with 5-aminolaevulinic acid or placebo for recalcitrant foot and hand warts: randomized double-blind trial. Lancet. 2000;355(9208):963–6. https://doi.org/10.1016/s0140-6736(00)90013-8.
100. Wu MF, Lv T, Miao F, Wang XL, Liu YQ, Wang HW. Periungual and subungual warts successfully treated with combination of electric shaving, curettage, and photodynamic therapy. Photodermatol Photoimmunol Photomed. 2021;37(1):82–4. https://doi.org/10.1111/phpp.12599.
101. Fabbrocini G, Di Costanzo MP, Riccardo AM, Quarto M, Colasanti A, Roberti G, et al. Photodynamic therapy with topical delta-aminolaevulinic acid for the

treatment of plantar warts. J Photochem Photobiol B. 2001;61(1–2):30–4. https://doi.org/10.1016/s1011-1344(01)00141-5.

102. Mizuki D, Kaneko T, Hanada K. Successful treatment of topical photodynamic therapy using 5-aminolevulinic acid for plane warts. Br J Dermatol. 2003;149(5):1087–8. https://doi.org/10.1111/j.1365-2133.2003.05617.x.
103. Lu YG, Wu JJ, He Y, Yang HZ, Yang YD. Efficacy of topical aminolevulinic acid photodynamic therapy for the treatment of verruca planae. Photomed Laser Surg. 2010;28(4):561–3. https://doi.org/10.1089/pho.2009.2566.
104. Li Q, Jiao B, Zhou F, Tan Q, Ma Y, Luo L, et al. Comparative study of photodynamic therapy with 5%, 10% and 20% aminolevulinic acid in the treatment of generalized recalcitrant facial verruca plana: a randomized clinical trial. J Eur Acad Dermatol Venereol. 2014;28(12):1821–6. https://doi.org/10.1111/jdv.12319.
105. Morrow DI, Garland MJ, McCarron PA, Woolfson AD, Donnelly RF. Innovative drug delivery strategies for topical photodynamic therapy using porphyrin precursors. J Environ Pathol Toxicol Oncol. 2007;26(2):105–16. https://doi.org/10.1615/jenvironpatholtoxicoloncol.v26.i2.50.
106. Donnelly RF, McCarron PA, Morrow DI, Sibani SA, Woolfson AD. Photosensitizer delivery for photodynamic therapy. Part 1: topical carrier platforms. Expert Opin Drug Deliv. 2008;5(7):757–66. https://doi.org/10.1517/17425247.5.7.757.
107. Yoo KH, Kim BJ, Kim MN. Enhanced efficacy of photodynamic therapy with methyl 5-aminolevulinic acid in recalcitrant periungual warts after ablative carbon dioxide fractional laser: a pilot study. Dermatologic Surg. 2009;35(12):1927–32. https://doi.org/10.1111/j.1524-4725.2009.01307.x.
108. Stender IM, Lock-Andersen J, Wulf HC. Recalcitrant hand and foot warts successfully treated with photodynamic therapy with topical 5-aminolaevulinic acid: a pilot study. Clin Exp Dermatol. 1999;24(3):154–9. https://doi.org/10.1046/j.1365-2230.1999.00441.x.
109. Shi L, Luo M, Zhang FH, Zhang LL, Wang B, Liu P, et al. Photothermal therapy enhanced the effectiveness of imiquimod against refractory cutaneous warts through boosting immune responses. J Biophotonics. 2019;12(2):e201800149. https://doi.org/10.1002/jbio.201800149.
110. Xingfan Mo RL, Li J, Feng M, Chen X, Minzhi W, Zhao L. Clinical effect of surgical removal combined with 5-aminolevulinic acid photodynamic therapy for plantar warts. Chin J Med Aesth Cosmet. 2019;25(4):326–9. https://doi.org/10.3760/cma.j.issn.1671-0290.2019.04.020.
111. Wu LS, Chen WQ, Su J, Li FF, Chen ML, Zhu W, et al. Efficacy of the combination of superficial shaving with photodynamic therapy for recalcitrant periungual warts. Photodiagn Photodyn Ther. 2019;27:340–4. https://doi.org/10.1016/j.pdpdt.2019.06.021.
112. Hussein E, Zagho M, Nasrallah G, Elzatahry A. Recent advances in functional nanostructures as cancer photothermal therapy. Int J Nanomedicine. 2018;13:2897–906. https://doi.org/10.2147/ijn.S161031.
113. Richter K, H. M., Buchner J. The heat shock response: life on the verge of death. Mol Cell. 2010;40(2):253–66. https://doi.org/10.1016/j.molcel.2010.10.006.
114. Knavel EM, Brace CL. Tumor ablation: common modalities and general practices. Tech Vasc Interv Radiol. 2013;16(4):192–200. https://doi.org/10.1053/j.tvir.2013.08.002.
115. Zhang FH, Liu P, Zhang LL, Wu QQ, Wang B, Zhang GL, Wang PR, Zhou FF, Chen WR, Wang XL. A novel cosmetic and clinically practicable laser immunotherapy for facial verruca plana: intense pulsed light combined with BCG-PSN. Photodiagn Photodyn Ther. 2018;22:86–90. https://doi.org/10.1016/j.pdpdt.2018.02.003.

ALA-PDT in the Treatment of Diseases of Hair Follicles and Sebaceous Glands

9

Xiaojing Liu, Linglin Zhang, Yajing Cao, Zhi Cao, Jin Yang, Bo Wang, and Xiuli Wang

9.1 ALA-PDT for the Treatment of Acne Vulgaris

9.1.1 Introduction

Acne vulgaris is a chronic inflammatory skin condition affecting pilosebaceous glands and ranks eighth in global disease prevalence, predominantly impacting individuals aged 16–20 years. The recurring nature of acne, along with facial scarring and discoloration associated with moderate-to-severe cases, often leads to low self-esteem, anxiety, and depression, significantly affecting both physical and mental health. This condition imposes substantial physical, social, psychological, mental and economic burdens on affected individuals [1, 2].

The pathogenesis of acne is complex and multifactorial, involving sebaceous gland hyperplasia with excessive sebum production, follicular hyperkeratosis leading to sebaceous follicle obstruction, skin inflammation, and colonization of the sebaceous glands by microorganisms, particularly *Cutibacterium acnes* (*C. acnes*). These factors are interconnected, with abnormal sebaceous gland function and excessive lipid secretion serving as prerequisites for acne development. Genetic predispositions, environmental factors, and diet can increase androgen and insulin-like growth factor 1 (IGF-1) levels, leading to increased sebum production and altered lipid composition. These changes disrupt the follicular microenvironment, promote *C. acnes* growth, and inhibit gram-positive bacterial symbiosis, triggering innate immune responses and inflammation [3–6]. Early lipid and microecological shifts induce interleukin-1α (IL-1α)-mediated inflammation, causing abnormal keratinization of pilosebaceous ducts and microcomedone formation. The activation of Toll-like receptors (TLRs) further amplifies the inflammatory response and innate immunity, contributing to comedo development and aggravating *C. acnes* proliferation and sebum blockage [7]. Free fatty acids produced by *C. acnes* stimulate follicles, attracting neutrophils and worsening inflammation, eventually leading to T lymphocyte infiltration and the activation of acquired immunity. Prolonged inflammation can cause follicular wall rupture, allowing sebum, microorganisms, and keratin to penetrate the dermis, triggering a foreign body-like inflammatory reaction.

X. Liu · L. Zhang · Y. Cao · Z. Cao · J. Yang
X. Wang (✉)
Institute of Photomedicine, Shanghai Skin Disease Hospital, School of Medicine, Tongji University, Shanghai, China
e-mail: wangxiuli_1400023@tongji.edu.cn

B. Wang
Avera Medical Group Dermatology, Aberdeen, SD, USA

University of South Dakota, Vermillion, SD, USA
e-mail: makiwang@med.umich.edu

X. Wang, B. Wang (eds.), *Photodynamic Therapy in Dermatology*, https://doi.org/10.1007/978-981-96-8915-6_9

9.1.1.1 Clinical Manifestations

Acne commonly occurs on the forehead, cheeks, chest, shoulders, and back. The initial lesion is a conical papule on the hair follicle with a yellowish-white top and is composed of sebum and shed keratinocytes. Open comedones, caused by melanin deposition, represent early acne damage. As the condition progresses, inflammatory papules may develop, and pustules may form at the top. If inflammation continues, red nodules or cysts can appear. While acne lesions typically do not cause subjective symptoms, they may be painful when inflammation is pronounced.

The grade of acne vulgaris was divided into: mild (grade I): only comedones; moderate (grade II): inflammatory papules; moderate (grade III): pustules; and severe (grade IV): nodules and cysts.

9.1.1.2 Histopathology

The histopathological manifestations of early microcomedone include dilated follicular funnels containing keratinized epithelium and narrow follicular openings. Closed comedones are characterized by a dense cystic structure filled with keratinized debris, hair, and bacteria in the follicular lumen. Open comedones feature wide follicular openings with atrophied or absent sebaceous glands. As the follicular duct continues to expand, the follicular funnel ruptures, releasing its contents into the dermis, which triggers an inflammatory infiltration of neutrophils, lymphocytes, and mononuclear macrophages and may lead to a foreign body granuloma-like response or even scar formation.

9.1.2 Management

The principles for acne treatment focus on exfoliation, dissolving comedones, inhibiting sebum secretion, and addressing bacterial growth and inflammation. These include the use of systemic and topical medications, physical and chemical therapies, photodynamic therapy, and other methods.

9.1.2.1 Medical Therapy

Acne medications include both topical and systemic drugs. Topical treatments are the cornerstone of acne therapy and include retinoids, antimicrobial agents such as benzoyl peroxide, and antibiotics. Systemic treatments include oral tetracycline antibiotics such as doxycycline and minocycline, as well as oral isotretinoin. However, oral isotretinoin has a slow onset, requires prolonged use, and poses risks such as teratogenicity, craniosynostosis, and potential liver and lipid metabolism dysfunction, which limits its use, particularly in women of childbearing age and adolescents [8]. Systemic antibiotics, while effective, often cause gastrointestinal side effects, impact bone and tooth development, lead to photosensitivity, and contribute to antibiotic resistance, all of which restrict their clinical use [9].

9.1.2.2 Physical Treatment

As physiotherapy has advanced, phototherapies, particularly red and blue light, have become widely used in acne treatment. Since the 1990s, attempts have been made to use red and blue light in the treatment of acne. Meffert et al. reported that blue-light irradiation at a cumulative dose of 325 J/cm^2 could significantly improve the clinical symptoms of acne [10]. Papageorgiou et al. later demonstrated that low-dose multifrequency irradiation was more effective [11]. Early devices for red- and blue-light therapy were bulky and difficult to operate, limiting their use in acne treatment. Since 2006, the authors' group has been using red and blue light to treat mild and moderate acne and has achieved satisfactory clinical efficacy. Currently, LED light sources, which emit 415-nm blue light and 633-nm red light, are widely used in the clinic for their antibacterial, anti-inflammatory, and restorative effects, improving acne outcomes. In a 2021 randomized controlled trial, the authors' group reported that red- and blue-light therapies were similarly effective for mild-to-moderate acne, although red light caused fewer adverse effects, such as hyperpigmentation, making it the preferred choice [12]. Patients are recommended to undergo two to three treatments per week for 10–20 min each for 6–8 weeks to reduce inflammation effectively.

With home-use red- and blue-light devices and improved patient compliance, these therapies are expected to expand into home treatment [13, 14]. However, for patients with severe acne, the efficacy of red and blue light alone is limited.

9.1.3 ALA-PDT

ALA-PDT, a new type of phototherapy, has shown promising results in the treatment of moderate-to-severe acne following continuous exploration and optimization of therapeutic parameters.

An early study in 1990 revealed that porphyrins can accumulate in the sebaceous glands of mice after intraperitoneal ALA injection [15]. In 2000, Hongcharu et al. treated acne on the back via ALA-PDT and reported that the sebaceous glands were acutely damaged and reduced in size. After 20 weeks of multiple PDT treatments or 10 weeks after a single treatment, good clinical outcomes were obtained [16]. Itoh et al. successfully treated ten patients with facial acne after incubation with 20% ALA for 4 h and irradiation with halogen lamps (600–700 nm, 17 mW/cm^2, 13 J/cm^2), with effects lasting for 6 months [17]. However, research on the use of PDT for acne treatment has been limited since the following decade.

In 2009, the authors' group reported that the topical application of 10% ALA cream followed by 633-nm LED light source irradiation (100 mW/cm^2, 50–60 J/cm^2) was both safe and effective in treating severe facial acne, showing better short-term efficacy than oral isotretinoin. The team further detected PpIX fluorescence in acne lesions of varying severity, with stronger fluorescence observed in severe acne lesions. These findings suggest that ALA-PDT is particularly suitable for treating moderate-to-severe acne with inflammatory papules, pustules, and cysts. Previous studies have indicated that topical ALA mainly accumulates in the epidermis, with no significant PpIX accumulation in the dermis. While earlier researchers speculated that ALAs might enter the pilosebaceous unit via the sebaceous duct, convincing evidence was lacking. The authors' group, however, confirmed for the first time that intense PpIX fluorescence accumulates in the sebaceous glands of acne patient tissues via the sebaceous duct, thereby establishing sebaceous glands as the target tissue for ALA-PDT in treating moderate-to-severe acne [18].

The authors' team refined ALA-PDT treatment parameters for acne, recommending 3–5% ALA concentration, 3-h application time, and gradually increasing energy from 30 J/cm^2 to 70 J/cm^2. This protocol, validated through clinical applications, has become a foundation for treating moderate-to-severe acne in China. In 2013, a large multicenter study in China confirmed the efficacy of 5% ALA-PDT, leading to the establishment of national photodynamic therapy research centers [19]. In 2014, Professors Xiuli Wang, Heng Gu, and Heyi Zheng developed the first "Expert Consensus on the Clinical Application of ALA-PDT," reporting low ALA concentrations (5%) and short incubation times (1–3 h). International recognition followed, with the American Academy of Dermatology's 2016 guidelines highlighting PDT as the most evidence-supported light therapy for acne, referencing the team's research. In 2021, updated guidelines recommended 5% ALA, 1–1.5-h incubation, and LED red light at 40–100 mW/cm^2 and 60–126 J/cm^2 for optimal results.

In summary, while ALA-PDT shows promise in acne treatment, its underlying mechanisms require further investigation, and treatment parameters need refinement to maximize its efficacy (Figs. 9.1 and 9.2).

9.1.3.1 Potential Mechanisms of PDT for Treating Acne Vulgaris

The authors' group developed *in vitro* and animal models, including *C. acnes* and *Staphylococcus epidermidis* (*S. epidermis*), to investigate acne pathogenesis. To facilitate further research, they established immortalized human sebaceous gland cells (XL-i-20) derived from Chinese acne patients, providing a valuable model for clinical and basic studies. While the precise mechanism of ALA-PDT in acne treatment remains unclear, ALA-PDT is widely recognized to target the four primary pathogenic factors of acne vulgaris.

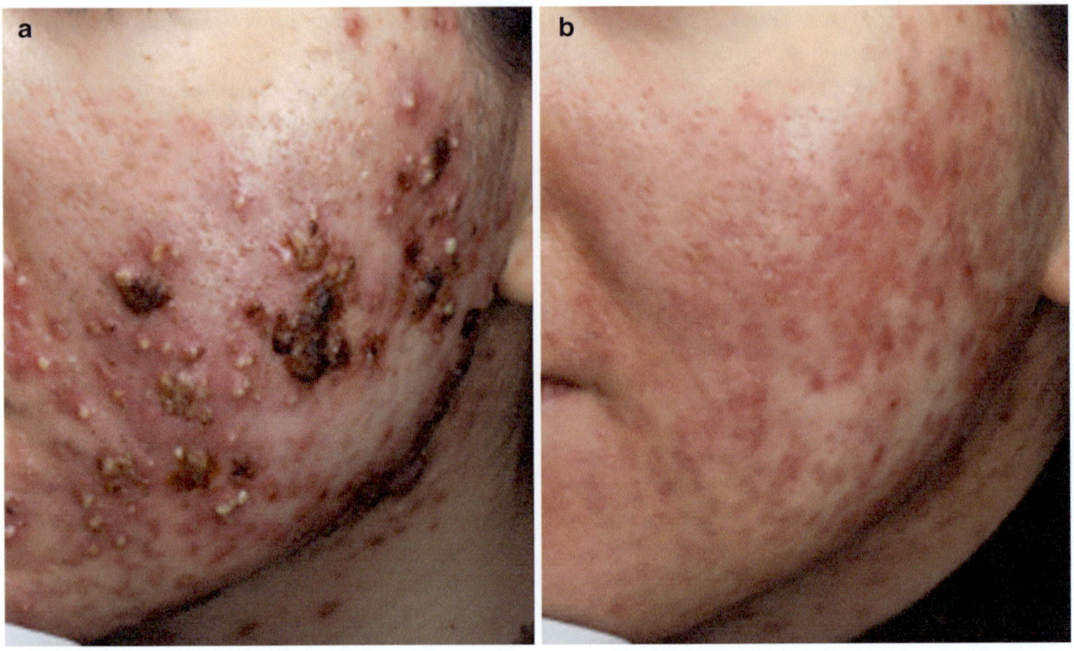

Fig. 9.1 ALA-PDT for severe acne (papulopustular acne): (**a**) before and (**b**) after

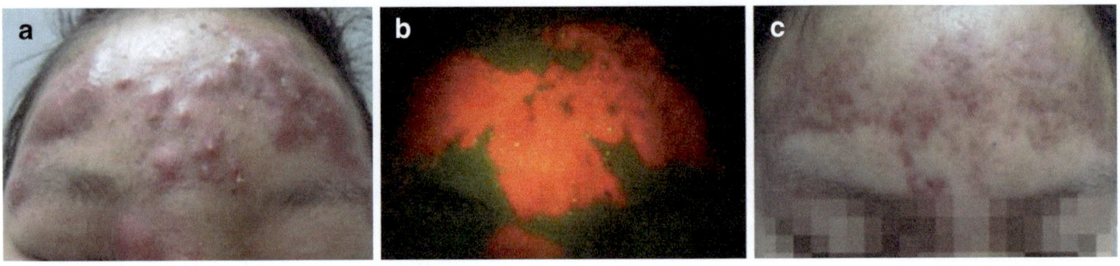

Fig. 9.2 ALA-PDT for severe acne (nodulocystic): (**a**) before ALA-PDT, (**b**) fluorescence detection after 1.5 h of incubation with ALA, and (**c**) cysts subsided at the 3-week follow-up after three sessions of ALA-PDT

ALA-PDT Reduces Sebum Secretion by Targeting Sebaceous Glands

The authors' group discovered that after ALA incubation, the compound enters the pilosebaceous unit via hair follicle opening and selectively accumulates in sebaceous glands (Fig. 9.3) [20]. This enrichment enables the photodynamic reaction to release substantial reactive oxygen species (ROS), which damage sebaceous glands, leading to reduced sebum secretion and gland atrophy. These findings provide direct evidence that the topical photosensitizer ALA can specifically target and be absorbed by sebaceous glands. Similarly, Hongcharu et al. demonstrated that ALA-PDT for back acne resulted in neutrophil infiltration around sebaceous glands, with 40% of the glands being destroyed or atrophied posttreatment. Three weeks later, the percentage of destroyed sebaceous glands increased to 55%, accompanied by a significant reduction in sebum production [18].

ALA-PDT inhibits sebum secretion by inducing sebaceous gland cell apoptosis. The authors' team demonstrated that ALA-PDT downregulates SREBP-1 expression in sebocytes by activating the AMPK pathway [21]. Jeong et al. reported that ALA-PDT induces apoptosis in sebaceous gland cells, although the number of apoptotic cells is not directly proportional to the ALA concentration [22]. Since ALA conversion

Fig. 9.3 PpIX fluorescence was enriched in sebaceous glands after 3 h of incubation with ALA

to PpIX primarily occurs in mitochondria, the apoptosis induced by ALA-PDT is linked mainly to mitochondria-dependent mechanisms, including mitochondrial membrane depolarization, cytochrome C release, and the activation of caspase-3 and caspase-9. Additionally, ALA-PDT induces sebaceous gland cell apoptosis by suppressing the Akt/Erk-mTOR-p70 S6K pathway and reduces sebum production by inhibiting the mTOR-SREBP-1/PPARγ signaling pathway [23].

ALA-PDT Increases the Microbial Diversity of the Pilosebaceous Gland Unit

The primary causative microorganisms of acne vulgaris are gram-positive bacteria, particularly *C. acnes* and *S. epidermidis*. *C. acnes* produces porphyrins, which appear as brick-red fluorescence under Wood's lamp, mainly on the nose and forehead [24]. While *C. acnes* is traditionally thought to be a key trigger for chronic inflammation in acne, this view is being reconsidered, as studies have shown no significant difference in *C. acnes* abundance between acne patients and non-acne patients [25]. Instead, the loss of skin microbial diversity and the activation of innate immunity are now considered primary factors in chronic acne inflammation [26, 27]. The authors' group reported that ALA-PDT inhibits *S. epidermidis* activity and biofilm formation. Recent studies have shown that ALA-PDT enhances microbial diversity in hair follicles and skin surfaces. Genome sequencing of severe acne patients by Tao et al. revealed a reduction in *C. acnes* and an increase in *Pseudomonas fluorescens* after 5% ALA-PDT, along with a decrease in functional genes related to energy metabolism and DNA replication [28]. Yang et al. also reported that ALA-PDT increased the diversity of the acne microbiome in the epidermis [29]. Therefore, ALA-PDT not only suppresses pathogenic microorganisms but also improves the microenvironment of the pilosebaceous unit by restoring microbial diversity.

ALA-PDT Improves Abnormal Keratinization of Hair Follicle Epithelial Cells

Recent studies have indicated that various pathogens can stimulate the epidermis and hair follicle epithelium, triggering the release of cytokines such as IL-1α, which promote keratinocyte proliferation and abnormal keratinization, leading to acne formation [7]. ALA is absorbed by keratinocytes and converted into PpIX [30]. In vitro studies suggest that ALA-PDT can improve abnormal keratinization in keratinocytes [31]. PDT-generated ROS may downregulate fibroblast growth factor receptor 2b (FGFR2b), a downstream target of protein kinase C (PKC), thereby reducing IL-1α expression and inhibiting keratinocyte proliferation and differentiation [32]. While Fabbrocini et al. reported 79% efficacy of ALA-PDT in treating comedones [33], Orringer et al. reported only a 7% improvement [34]. The authors' team also reported the limited efficacy of ALA-PDT for comedones, suggesting that its ability to correct pilosebaceous epithelial keratinization remains controversial and requires further investigation.

Immunomodulatory Effects of ALA-PDT

ALA-PDT has immunomodulatory effects on both normal skin and acne, with transient inflammation amplification commonly observed in severe acne patients posttreatment. This acute inflammatory response, characterized by erythema, edema, and pustules, is positively correlated with the efficacy of PDT [35]. The authors' group reported that ALA-PDT amplifies inflammation by up-regulating CXCL8 expression via the p38 pathway and inducing M1 macrophages polarization by TREM1/COX2 axis [36, 37]. In the first few days after treatment, keratinocytes and sebocytes produce cytokines that attract inflammatory cells, such as neutrophils, T lymphocytes, dendritic cells, and monocytes, contributing to the amplified inflammatory response. This immunomodulatory effect, marked by increased inflammation, is a key mechanism underlying the efficacy of ALA-PDT in treating severe acne. Acute inflammation typically begins to subside within 24 h posttreatment.

Two weeks after ALA-PDT treatment, the expression of TLR2 and TLR4 decreased by 50% and 30%, respectively [22]. Ma et al. reported that ALA-PDT reduced the upregulation of TLR2, TLR4, IL-1α, IL-8, and TNF-α in acne lesions and keratinocytes [38]. Wang et al. reported that ALA-PDT alleviated inflammation in *C. acnes*-infected sebaceous gland plaques in golden hamsters by downregulating NF-κB while upregulating STAT3, which has anti-inflammatory effects. It is speculated that ALA-PDT may induce IL-10 secretion, as confirmed by Byun's study [39]. Additionally, ALA-PDT alleviated inflammation by inhibiting *C. acnes*-induced iNOS, NO, and proinflammatory cytokines in HaCaT cells and mice while reducing the phosphorylation of p38, JNK, ERK, IKKα/β, and NF-κB p65. This leads to the inhibition of the NF-κB and p38 MAPK signaling pathways, thereby suppressing inflammation [38].

In summary, in the early stage of treatment, ALA-PDT targets keratinocytes and sebocytes, amplifying the inflammatory response and halting chronic inflammation by upregulating chemokines such as CXCL8 via p38 and other pathways, recruiting inflammatory cells such as T cells, B cells, neutrophils, and macrophages. In the later stages, ALA-PDT downregulates TLR expression by inhibiting the NF-κB and MAPK signaling pathways, ultimately controlling inflammation. Despite its efficacy, the immunomodulatory effects of ALA-PDT in acne treatment are complex, and the precise mechanisms remain unclear and require further investigation.

ALA-PDT Promotes Extracellular Matrix Remodeling

The authors' group reported that after ALA-PDT treatment, the patient's skin became more delicate and smoother, with an increased number of collagen and elastic fibers in the treated area, which were more densely arranged [40]. Previous studies have confirmed that *C. acnes* can induce the expression of MMP-9 and MMP-2 in keratinocytes and sebaceous gland cells, respectively, promoting the degradation of the extracellular matrix and exacerbating pilosebaceous gland disruption and *C. acnes* infection. Osiecka et al. reported that MMP-2 and MMP-9 were almost absent in acne lesions following PDT [41]. Our team discovered that low-dose ALA-PDT stimulates keratinocytes to release TGF-β1, which activates the TGF-β pathway in dermal fibroblasts, leading to collagen remodeling in the dermis [42], indicating that extracellular matrix remodeling may play a role in the effectiveness of ALA-PDT for treating acne (Fig. 9.4).

In summary, ALA-PDT effectively targets all four aspects of acne pathogenesis: it inhibits cell growth and proliferation by targeting hair follicles and sebaceous glands, suppresses follicular

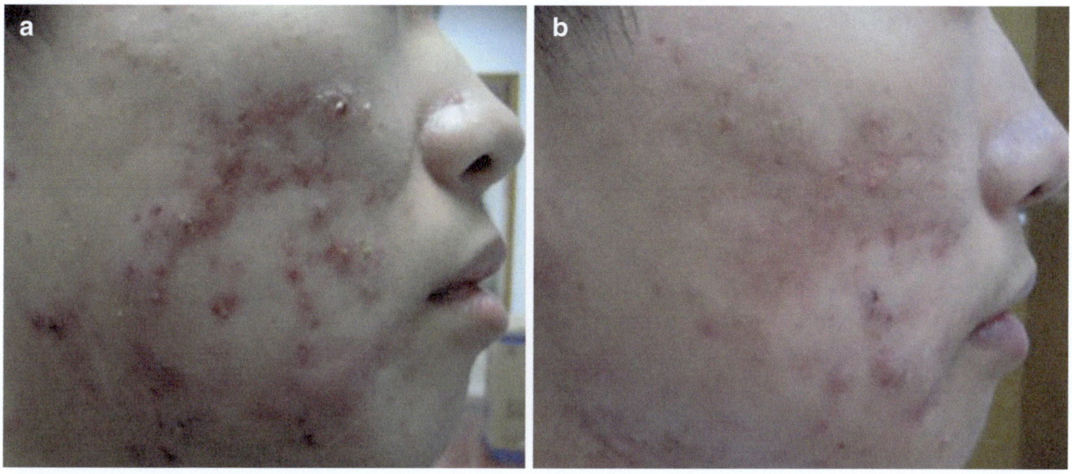

Fig. 9.4 ALA-PDT for severe acne patients with acne scars: (**a**) before ALA-PDT and (**b**) scar alleviation and finer skin after ALA-PDT

bacteria such as *C. acnes* while maintaining the microecology of pilosebaceous units, reverses follicular hyperkeratinization, reduces follicular obstruction, and modulates the inflammatory and immune responses associated with acne, with immune modulation being a key factor in treatment success. Additionally, ALA-PDT promotes extracellular matrix remodeling, enhances collagen synthesis, stimulates fibroblast proliferation, and provides cosmetic benefits, particularly for patients with scar-prone acne.

9.1.3.2 Clinical Application

Although the efficacy of ALA-PDT for moderate-to-severe acne is well established, its clinical practice varies across dermatology practices. Issues such as intolerable pain, "reactive acneiform eruption," and other adverse effects may hinder patients' acceptance and adherence to treatment. Recent studies, particularly clinical trials, have focused on determining the optimal treatment parameters and establishing standardized practices.

Photosensitizers

ALA is the only photosensitizer approved for clinical topical use in China, and it is commonly used in the form of creams, lotions, and thermosensitive gels. Cream is the most common form due to its ease of application; protective, hydrating, and lubricating effects; and good transdermal absorption. When ALA-PDT is used to treat skin lesions, cream is typically the preferred option. In Europe and the United States, ALA is used at concentrations ranging from 10% to 20% for acne treatment, but an early study by the authors' team revealed that 3%, 5%, and 10% ALA had similar efficacies for treating facial acne, with no significant difference between them [43]. Considering economic factors and potential side effects, low concentrations of ALA are recommended for clinical use.

Although oral ALA (10 mg/kg) has shown a 92% skin lesion clearance rate in some studies [44], it is rarely used for acne because of concerns over risks and local distribution.

In summary, 5% low-concentration ALA in cream or gel form is the preferred treatment for moderate-to-severe acne.

Light Sources

Light sources for the PDT treatment of acne are mainly divided into laser light sources and nonlaser light sources, including 500–1200-nm intense pulsed light (IPL), 630–635-nm red light, 405–420-nm blue light, and 585- or 595-nm pulsed dye lasers (PDLs). LED light, known for its good monochromaticity and narrow spectrum, is a cold light source that emits colored visible light directly without the need for filtering. Its stable energy output and large coverage area make LED light particularly effective for treating widespread acne lesions, which often affect the face, chest, and back. Thus, LED light is considered a suitable and efficient light source for acne PDT treatment.

In addition, the wavelength and light dose are crucial factors influencing the clinical efficacy of ALA-PDT. The light wavelength must align with the absorption spectrum of PpIX, typically approximately 410 nm, 505 nm, 540 nm, 580 nm, or 630 nm. While the 410-nm light in the Soret band is significantly stronger than the longer wavelength Q-band light, factors such as light penetration and dose must also be considered, as sebaceous glands are located 0.5–1 mm beneath the skin surface. For acne treatment, wavelengths of 550–700 nm at 15 J/cm^2 and 600–700 nm at 13 J/cm^2 have been used, with only the former proven to inhibit sebum secretion. Sakamoto et al. suggested that PDT works at two levels: low-energy irradiation improves bacterial growth, inflammation, and follicular hyperkeratosis, whereas higher energy targets sebaceous glands, reducing sebum secretion [45]. However, further clinical trials are needed to fully understand these effects. The main light sources used for acne are as follows:

Red Light

Compared with blue light, red light, typically in the 630–635-nm range, is within the Q band of the porphyrin absorption spectrum of *C. acnes* and offers deeper penetration, exceeding 6 mm, although it has a weaker photoactivation effect on PpIX. However, it effectively induces the PDT reaction, reduces inflammation in pilosebaceous glands, minimizes scar formation, and promotes tissue repair. Red light is the most widely used light source for clinical PDT in acne treatment and is often referred to as conventional PDT (C-PDT). Studies have shown that 5% ALA-PDT combined with red light results in an effectiveness rate of 85.71–95.23% after three sessions and during follow-up [46]. The "ALA-PDT Treatment Expert Consensus" in China recommends a red-light irradiation dose of 60–126 J/cm^2, with an energy density of 40–100 mW/cm^2, and treatment every 1–2 weeks, with no more than six sessions.

Blue Light

The narrow-spectrum blue light emits stable light at approximately 410 nm, which aligns with the Soret band absorption peak at 415 nm in the spectrum of the endogenous porphyrins of *C. acnes*. Porphyrins (fecal porphyrin III and protoporphyrin IX) are activated by blue light to release singlet oxygen and reactive oxygen radicals, producing a photodynamic effect. Terrell et al. initially used 20% ALA with blue light to successfully treat a patient with moderate acne [47]. Later, Taub et al. used blue-light PDT to treat multiple cases of acne, with an effective rate of more than 90%, and half of the patients had an improvement rate of more than 75% in terms of skin lesions [48]. Although blue-light PDT is more effective than blue light alone, its limited penetration depth still results in suboptimal outcomes [49]. Therefore, blue light is not recommended as the primary light source for ALA-PDT in the treatment of moderate-to-severe acne.

Intense Pulsed Light

The spectrum range of IPL is 400–1200 nm. Through its selective photothermal and photochemical effects, IPL can coagulate blood vessels, reduce postinflammatory erythema and hyperpigmentation, promote collagen tissue repair, and decrease neutrophil activity around acne lesions to help clear inflammation [50, 51]. Studies have shown that after 12 weeks of IPL-PDT treatment, the clearance rate of inflammatory lesions can reach 87.7–89.5%, which is significantly higher than the 66.8–74.0% clearance rate with IPL alone, with both methods effectively reducing sebum secretion. For noninflammatory lesions, the clearance rates are similar: 38% for IPL-PDT and 44% for IPL alone [52–55]. The authors' team compared C-PDT and IPL-PDT (12–15 J/cm^2), and both light sources were found to effectively treat moderate-to-severe acne. Considering the mild side effects of IPL, as well as its ability to reduce erythema and pigmentation, promote tissue repair, and offer better patient tolerance, IPL is recommended as a viable light source for ALA-PDT [56] (Fig. 9.5). For patients who experience pain with the C-PDT or have higher cosmetic expectations, IPL is an excellent alternative.

Pulsed Dye Laser

The 595-nm PDL is mostly used for the treatment of vascular diseases but has also been explored for acne treatment. A clinical study involving 19 patients with acne reported a skin lesion clearance rate of 77% with PDL-PDT [57]. Orringer et al. conducted a split-face study comparing PDL-PDT and a control group and reported that the PDL-PDT group had significantly fewer inflammatory lesions, such as pustules, and a significant reduction in postinflammatory erythema [34]. Another clinical trial comparing long-pulse width PDL-PDT with simple PDL revealed that the clearance rate of inflammatory lesions was greater than 70% for PDL-PDT, whereas it was 67% for simple PDL; however, both treatments had a 30% clearance rate for noninflammatory lesions, with patients expressing greater satisfaction on the PDL-PDT side [58]. The energy used during PDL treatment typically ranges from 7.0 J/cm^2 to 7.5 J/cm^2. However, research on PDL-PDT for moderate-to-severe acne remains limited, and the final efficacy of this treatment still requires further verification through more clinical trials.

Daylight

Daylight PDT (DL-PDT) is suitable for treating acne lesions located in exposed areas. Kwon et al. used a novel 1.5% 3-butenyl ALA applied to acne patients' faces every other day in the morning, followed by sunlight as the light source, for a total of 12 sessions. The results revealed that the clearance rates for inflammatory and noninflammatory skin lesions were 58.0% and 34.1%, respectively. Histopathological analysis revealed a reduction in IL-8, IL-1β, MMP-9, and NF-κB, suggesting that DL-PDT can reduce inflammation and clear acne lesions [59]. The authors' team also compared DL-PDT with red-light photodynamic therapy and reported that the clinical efficacy of DL-PDT was comparable, with an effective rate of 85% after 6 weeks, whereas C-PDT had a 92.3% efficacy rate, although DL-PDT caused only mild pain. However, severe hyperpigmentation cases have been reported [60] (Fig. 9.6); other recent research results have reached similar conclusions [61]. DL-PDT is simple, easy to perform, and offers good clinical efficacy with mild adverse reactions, making it useful for certain applications. However, its limitations include its dependence on weather and seasons, lack of scheduling control, and the requirement for continuous patient participation. Additionally, the long-term adverse effects are not fully understood, and large-scale clinical studies are needed for further evaluation.

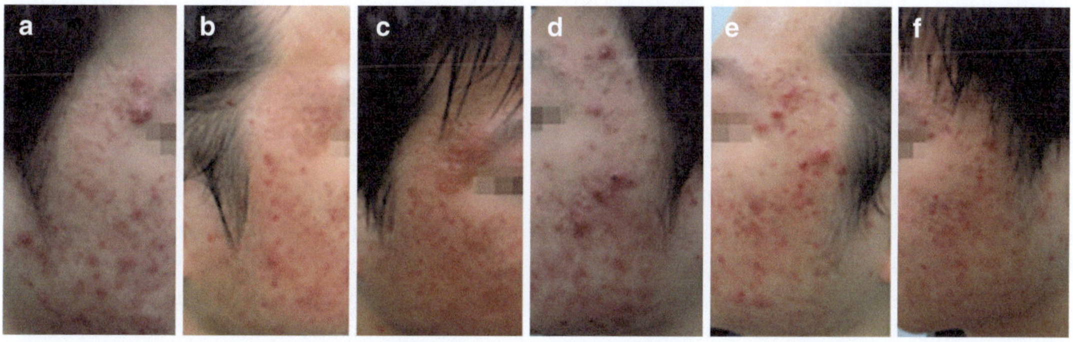

Fig. 9.5 Comparison of IPL-PDT and C-PDT for severe acne: (**a**–**c**) C-PDT, (**d**–**f**) IPL-PDT, (**a**, **d**) before treatment, (**b**, **e**) reduced nodules 2 weeks after treatment, and (**c**, **f**) 2 months after treatment, postinflammatory erythema with no obvious nodules or cysts

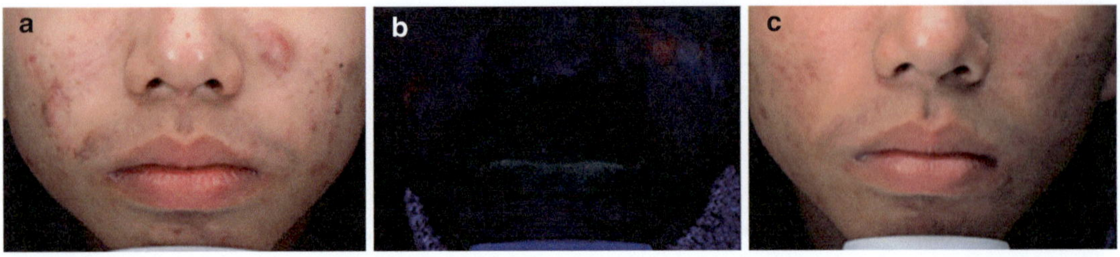

Fig. 9.6 DL-PDT for severe acne with cysts: (**a**) before DL-PDT, (**b**) brick-red fluorescence was observed after incubation with ALA for 30 min, and (**c**) transient hyperpigmentation on the left side of the face 2 weeks after two sessions of DL-PDT

Parameter Optimization

Modified Painless ALA-PDT (M-PDT)

The primary purposes of optimizing ALA-PDT for moderate-to-severe acne are modifying parameters and reducing adverse reactions. The authors' team designed a modified split-face M-PDT. In this study, on one side of the face, 5% ALA cream was incubated for 0.5 h without being wiped off, followed by red-light illumination at 150 J/cm^2 with a lower power density, referred to as M-PDT. On the other hand, 5% ALA cream was applied for 1.5 h and then wiped off, with red-light illumination at 50 J/cm^2 (C-PDT). The results revealed no significant difference in efficacy between the two groups, but the M-PDT group experienced almost no pain or adverse effects, with only mild erythema and edema and no severe hyperpigmentation. These findings suggest that a shorter duration of ALA application combined with an extended exposure time can maintain equivalent efficacy while effectively reducing pain and other side effects [62] (see Fig. 7.3 in Chap. 7). Therefore, the authors' group proposed M-PDT: 5% ALA cream was incubated for 0.5 h in the dark. When exposed to light (with a power density of 40 mW/cm^2 and an energy density of 150 J/cm^2), the photosensitizer remained on the skin surface. On the basis of these findings, the authors recommended the M-PDT as the first choice for acne treatment because of its good efficacy and mild side effects such as pain.

Optimization of the Illumination Strategy

Wu et al. compared a two-step illumination method (red-light irradiation at 40 mW/cm^2 for 5 min, followed by 80 mW/cm^2 for 15 min) with a three-step method (40 mW/cm^2 for 5 min, then 80 mW/cm^2 for 12.5 min, and back to 40 mW/cm^2 for 5 min) in the treatment of acne vulgaris. Both methods demonstrated equal efficacy, but patients treated with the three-step method reported lower visual analog pain scores (VASs) [63], suggesting that modifying the illumination strategy can increase patient comfort during PDT without compromising its therapeutic effect, providing new insights for optimizing PDT treatment.

In summary, red light at approximately 630 nm with stable energy is the recommended light source for clinical ALA-PDT in treating moderate-to-severe acne because of its deeper skin penetration and efficacy. IPL offers mild side effects and better patient tolerance but is costly, making it a suitable alternative. While DL-PDT is convenient and effective, the risk of severe hyperpigmentation limits its clinical use. M-PDT, which shortens the incubation time and extends the illumination duration, effectively reduces adverse reactions while maintaining therapeutic outcomes, making it a promising approach for optimizing ALA-PDT.

Combination Therapy Applications

Clinically, ALA-PDT alone is effective for treating moderate-to-severe acne, although some studies have explored its combination with oral minocycline or isotretinoin. Research indicates that combining oral minocycline with ALA-PDT yields better results compared to minocycline alone, although high-quality randomized controlled trials comparing combination therapy with ALA-PDT alone are still lacking [64, 65]. Minocycline may also reduce and shorten the acute inflammatory response after ALA-PDT, although its photosensitivity must be considered. A randomized controlled trial involving 70 patients revealed that ALA-PDT combined with isotretinoin achieved better efficacy and lower recurrence rates compared to ALA-PDT alone [66]. However, since isotretinoin influences keratinocyte proliferation and differentiation, it may exacerbate adverse reactions when combined with ALA-PDT, requiring clinicians to carefully manage potential side effects in combination therapies.

Indications

1. ALA-PDT is recommended for the treatment of moderate-to-severe acne and scar-prone acne.
2. ALA-PDT is recommended for patients who are resistant to other therapies or unable to tolerate systemic antibiotics and retinoids, with evidence-based support classified as Level I.
3. ALA-PDT is recommended for individuals unwilling to undergo oral or topical treatments or whose occupations make medical treatment impractical.

Protocol

Step 1. Cleansing: Thoroughly clean the lesions with detergent or clean water.

Step 2. Pretreatment: Ensure adequate pretreatment of acne lesions before ALA-PDT [67]. For larger cysts, techniques such as plum-blossom needling, microneedling, fractional lasers, or surgical incisions are recommended to increase drug absorption, light penetration, and cyst drainage after PDT. For patients undergoing multiple sessions, surface crusting should be removed before treatment to improve drug penetration.

Step 3. ALA application: ALA gel or a solution of a certain concentration was prepared, and ALA was evenly applied to the treatment area, avoiding the eyelids, cornea, and canthus. The mixture was incubated in darkness for 0.5–1.5 h as needed, after which the ALA was gently removed before illumination.

Step 4. Illumination: A suitable light source and parameters for PDT should be selected. Both the patient and operator should wear protective goggles during treatment.

Precautions

1. Provide thorough health education and confirm informed consent. Ensure that patients understand the mechanism, treatment steps, and potential adverse reactions of ALA-PDT, including pain, erythema, swelling, exudation, crust formation, dyspigmentation, scaling, dryness, etc.
2. ALA-PDT may trigger transient inflammatory reactions, such as reactive acne, which typically occur 1–2 days after the first session. This manifests as numerous pustules and worsened primary lesions. It usually resolves within 1–2 weeks without additional treatment, although temporary hyperpigmentation may persist longer. To prevent reactive acne in subsequent sessions, consider shortening the incubation time or reducing the light dosage.
3. Moisturizing and sun protection post-PDT can help alleviate adverse reactions and support skin barrier repair.
4. Regular follow-up: The therapeutic effects of ALA-PDT can last for several months. For patients with severe, recurrent acne, additional PDT sessions may be considered.
5. While ALA-PDT is effective for treating inflammatory grade II acne, owing to its cost and associated adverse reactions, it is not currently recommended for this severity level.

9.1.3.3 Recommended Protocols (Table 9.1)

As a treatment for moderate-to-severe acne, ALA-PDT offers several advantages, including rapid, safe, and effective lesion clearance; reduced recurrence and severity of inflammation; and the absence of systemic side effects. With ongoing efforts to optimize PDT, it is anticipated to become a first-line physical therapy for moderate-to-severe acne. Future advancements should focus on improving photosensitizers, developing novel photosensitizers, and refining treatment parameters to increase their efficacy and broaden the application of PDT in acne management.

Table 9.1 Recommendations for the PDT of acne vulgaris

Recommendation	The concentration and incubation time of ALA	Light sources	Illumination parameters	Treatment session
M-PDT	3–5% ALA cream; incubation for 0.5 h	LED red light (630–635 nm)	40–60 J/cm^2; 150 mW/cm^2	Every 1–2 weeks
C-PDT	3–5% ALA cream; incubation for1–1.5 h	LED red light (630–635 nm)	40–100 J/cm^2; 60–126 mW/cm^2	Every 1–2 weeks
IPL-PDT	3–5% ALA cream; incubation for 0.5–1 h	IPL (400–1200 nm)	15–17 J/cm^2	Every 2–3 weeks
DL-PDT	3–5% ALA cream; incubation for 0.5–1 h	Daylight (295–2500 nm)	Expose to daylight for 1 h	Every 1–2 weeks

9.2 ALA-PDT for the Treatment of Hidradenitis Suppurativa

9.2.1 Introduction

Hidradenitis suppurativa (HS), also known as acne inversa (AI), is a chronic, painful, and debilitating inflammatory skin disease that affects hair follicles and is characterized by a relapsing and remitting course. It typically manifests after puberty with deep-seated, painful, and inflamed lesions in apocrine gland-bearing areas such as the axillae, groin, and perineum [68]. HS significantly impacts patients' quality of life, with approximately 50% experiencing moderate-to-severe depression and anxiety [69, 70].

9.2.1.1 Clinical Features

HS is characterized by chronic, painful nodules, abscesses, suppurating sinus tracts and tunnels, and double- and multiended comedones with significant scarring in intertriginous areas [71]. The disease initiates with follicular hyperkeratosis and blockage of the follicular opening, leading to retention of follicular contents and subsequent deep follicular and perifollicular inflammation. This process results in recurrent abscesses, sinus tracts, fistulas, and scarring. HS lesions are typically associated with severe pain, significantly impacting patients' quality of life.

The Hurley staging system is the most commonly used method for classifying HS severity and guiding treatment selection. It consists of three stages: Stage I, characterized by single or multiple isolated abscesses without sinus tracts or scarring; Stage II, defined by recurrent abscesses with one or more sinus tracts and scarring separated by areas of normal skin; and Stage III, involving diffuse boils with multiple interconnected sinus tracts and no intervening normal skin [72]. In addition to Hurley staging, the modified Sartorius score provides a more detailed, open-ended assessment of disease intensity, whereas the International Hidradenitis Suppurativa Severity Score System (IHS4) offers a dynamic evaluation of HS severity, incorporating lesion count and extent of inflammation [73, 74].

9.2.1.2 Etiology and Pathogenesis

The etiology and pathogenesis of hidradenitis suppurativa (HS) remain incompletely understood, but it is currently considered a result of the interplay between genetic predisposition and environmental factors [73, 75]. A positive family history has been reported in 30–40% of HS patients [76, 77], and various mutations in γ-secretase components, such as *NCSTN*, *PSENEN*, *PSEN1*, and *POGLUT1*, indicate genetic heterogeneity of HS [78]. Risk factors include nicotine use, hormonal influences, obesity, mechanical friction, and skin microbiota dysbiosis [79–81]. Histologically, HS is driven by follicular hyperkeratosis, leading to hair follicle rupture and subsequent apocrine gland inflammation characterized by elevated levels of IL-1β, IL-17, and TNF-α. Upon follicular rupture, stem cells from the follicular bulge proliferate, forming epithelial strips that contribute to sinus tract development. HS has been proposed as a subtype of autoinflammatory keratinization disease [82]. Heterozygous loss-of-function mutations in genes encoding γ-secretase, including NCSTN,

PSENEN, PSEN1, and POGLUT1, which lead to hyperkeratosis, dysfunctional follicular differentiation, and cyst formation through the impaired Notch signaling pathway, have been identified in HS patients [83–86]. In addition, Psen1−/Psen2−, Psen1−, Ncstn+/− and Notch1−/Notch2− mice mimic the phenotype of human HS, indicating a role of abnormal keratinization in the pathogenesis of HS. Additionally, the HS samples presented increased levels of IL-1β, IL-36, caspase-1, and NLRP3, along with Th17/Treg axis dysregulation, highlighting the role of autoinflammation. The association of HS with immune-mediated conditions such as inflammatory bowel disease (IBD) and pyoderma gangrenosum (PG) and the efficacy of biologics targeting TNF-α, IL-1, IL-23, and IL-17A in treating moderate-to-severe HS further underscore its link to aberrant keratinization and autoinflammation.

9.2.2 Management

Treatment options for HS include antibiotics, biologics, lasers, surgery, and photodynamic therapy (PDT). These treatments (Table 9.2) should be tailored or used in combination on the basis of disease severity and the patient's condition.

9.2.3 Photodynamic Therapy (PDT)

On the basis of the pathogenesis of HS and the therapeutic mechanisms of PDT, this treatment may exert multiple beneficial effects, including selective destruction of cells within HS lesions, modulation of the inflammatory response, bacterial eradication, and disruption of biofilms [88].

9.2.3.1 ALA/MAL-PDT

Over the years, numerous case reports and small-scale clinical studies have been conducted on PDT activated by different light sources for treating HS, yielding mixed results. In 2004, Gold M et al. treated four cases of recalcitrant HS with blue-light ALA-PDT, applying 20% ALA for 15–30 min followed by blue-light irradiation for an average of 18 min. The treatment intervals were 1–2 weeks, with three to four treatments in total. At the 3-month follow-up, 75–100% lesion clearance was achieved, and three patients experienced no recurrence within 3 years [89]. Schweiger's study also showed promising results, with 12 HS patients treated with blue light or IPL light sources weekly for 4 weeks and 3 patients achieving complete lesion clearance [90]. However, contrasting outcomes were observed in other studies. In 2005, Strauss et al. treated four patients with recalcitrant HS with 20% ALA and light sources of 633 nm or 570–670 nm, but none of these patients achieved significant improvement, and two patients experienced worsening. All four reported discomfort, such as burning and stinging, causing one patient to discontinue treatment. This raised questions about the efficacy of ALA-PDT for HS [91]. In 2006, Rivard and Ozong treated two HS patients with blue-light ALA-PDT, but despite some improvement, they concluded that ALA-PDT did not "cure" the patients [92]. The authors' group also observed limited outcomes when treating three Hurley stage III HS patients with red-light ALA-PDT in 2016, suggesting that while ALA-PDT may be effective for Hurley stages I and II, its limited efficacy in stage III could be due to scar formation and tissue fibrosis that hinder the absorption of ALA/MAL and light penetration, warranting further investigation into its use for HS.

9.2.3.2 Surgery Combined with PDT

Surgery and PDT are complementary treatments for HS, with surgery assisting in the absorption of ALA and light penetration, while PDT helps reduce postsurgical complications and clears hidden lesions. Wenbo Bu et al. treated seven HS patients via surgery combined with PDT (S-PDT). For Hurley stage I patients, simple surgical incisions and drainage were performed, whereas stage II and III patients underwent surgical incisions, drainage, and removal of necrotic tissues. After surgery, the lesion was covered with 20% ALA solution for 3 h, followed by irradiation with 635-nm LED light (80 mW/cm^2) for 20 min. Stage I patients received two sessions of ALA-PDT, whereas stage II and III patients received four sessions, with treatment intervals of 7–10 days. At the 6- to 12-month follow-up, the lesions had com-

Table 9.2 Management of HS

Treatment	Hurley stage	Mechanism	Recommended dosing
Antibiotics			
Topical antibiotics			
Clindamycin	I, II	Antibacterial	1% solution or cream, BID for 3 months
Systemic antibiotics			
Tetracycline	I, II	Antibacterial	500 mg BID for 4 months
Clindamycin Rifampicin	I–III	Antibacterial	Clindamycin: 300 mg BID Rifampicin: 600 mg daily or 300 mg BID For 10 weeks
Rifampin Moxifloxacin Metronidazole	I–III	Anti-inflammatory, antimicrobial	Rifampin: 300 mg BID Moxifloxacin: 400 mg daily Metronidazole: 500 mg TID
Ertapenem	II, III	Antibacterial	1 g IV daily
Non-biologic systemic agents			
Glucocorticoids	II, III	Immunosuppressant Antiproliferative	Short term for flares or therapeutic bridge: 0.5–1.0 mg/kg daily Adjunct therapy: 10 mg daily
Dapsone (DDS)	I, II	Anti-inflammatory	50–200 mg daily for 1–48 months
Anti-androgen contraceptives	I, II	Antiandrogenic	Variable, daily
Cyclosporine	II, III	Immunomodulator	5–6 mg/kg daily
Biologic systemic agents			
Adalimumab	II, III	TNF-α inhibitor	40 mg SQ weekly
Infliximab	II, III	TNF-α inhibitor	5–10 mg/kg IV q4–8 weeks
Secukinumab	II, III	IL-17 inhibitor	300 mg SQ q2 weeks
Bimekizumab	II, III	IL-17 inhibitor	320 mg SQ q2 weeks
Brodalumab	II, III	IL-17R antagonist	210 mg/1.5 mL SQ q2 weeks [87]
Anakinra	II, III	IL-1-inhibitor	100 mg SQ daily
Ustekinumab	II, III	IL-12/IL-23 inhibitor	45/90 mg SQ q12 weeks
Procedural therapy			
Intralesional triamcinolone	I–III	Anti-inflammatory	10–40 mg/mL
Laser			
Nd:YAG laser	II, III	Follicular destruction	40–50 J/cm^2, 10-mm spot size, 20 ms for skin types I–III 25–35 J/cm^2, 10-mm spot size, 35 ms for skin types IV–VI
Carbon dioxide laser	II, III	Lesion ablation	A fluence of 55 W with a 0.2- to 1-mm spot size
Surgery			
Wide excision	II, III	Lesion excision	NA
Unroofing/deroofing	I–III	Tissue-saving, partial Lesion excision	NA
Incision and drainage	I–III	Lesion drainage	NA

pletely disappeared without recurrence [93]. The authors' group also achieved satisfactory outcomes with S-PDT every 2 weeks, where refractory lesions such as cysts, sinus tracts, and scarring were initially removed by surgical incisions, followed by red-light ALA-PDT (Fig. 9.7).

9.2.3.3 Intralesional PDT (I-PDT)

Intralesional PDT (I-PDT) has also yielded more promising results than PDT alone, possibly because of the deeper penetration of the photosensitizer and light into tissue. In Valladares-Narganes's study, 27 patients with HS and

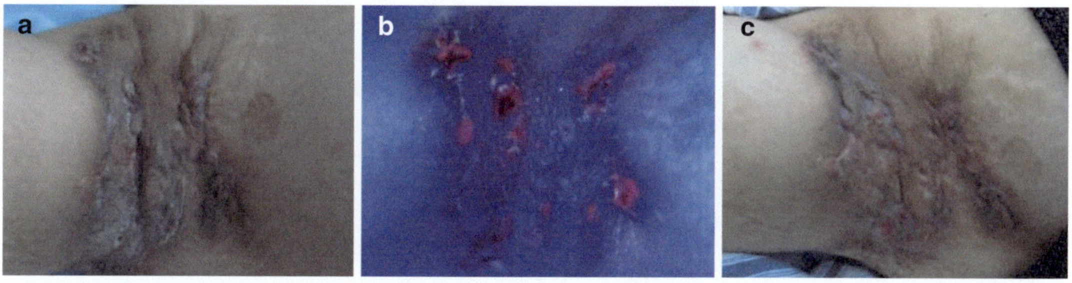

Fig. 9.7 ALA-PDT treatment of a Hurley stage II patient with HS: (**a**) before surgical treatment, (**b**) fluorescence detection after 4 h of ALA, and (**c**) after surgery combined with ALA-PDT treatment

long-standing sinus tracts underwent I-PDT for one to three sessions. A 1% ALA solution was administered at 0.2 mL/cm^3 into the fistulas, which were subsequently incubated for 3 h, followed by intralesional irradiation with a 630-nm laser diode at 1 W/cm^3 for 3 min. I-PDT was especially effective for single or isolated fistulas, with improvement after a single session, whereas more sessions were required for multiple, interconnected fistulas. Mild-to-moderate pain was reported (VAS score < 6), and at the 6-month follow-up, 37% of patients achieved complete responses, 41% had good responses, and 19% had partial responses. Compared with surgery, I-PDT is well tolerated, effective, and less invasive, particularly for isolated fistulas [94]. Subsequent studies confirmed the efficacy and safety of I-PDT with larger sample sizes, highlighting that ALA enhances light absorption by tissues, resulting in promising efficacy with lower light energy and shorter incubation times [95, 96]. A retrospective study by Garcias-Ladaria J et al. investigated 117 nodal and fistula lesions in 42 HS patients. Two hours later, 2% ALA gel or 1% ALA solution was administered to the lesions, followed by intralesional irradiation (0.4-mm diffusion fiber of a 630-nm semiconductor laser, 1.4 W, energy density 168 J/cm^2). Three months after treatment, 22.2% of the lesions subsided, 62.4% improved, and 15.4% remained unchanged. Adverse effects included burning (45.3%) and abscess formation (6.8%). I-PDT is considered more effective for multiple nodular skin lesions because it improves photosensitizer absorption and light penetration, although its ideal efficacy for Hurley stage III HS patients with combined fistulas/sinus tracts remains unclear [97].

9.2.3.4 Methylene Blue Photodynamic Therapy (MB-PDT)

Fadel et al. applied methylene blue photodynamic therapy (MB-PDT) to treat 11 HS patients with photosensitizers of MB (free MB, FMB) and liposomes of MB (methylene blue niosomal, NMB) in a single-blind, randomized, comparative study. After a 30-min incubation of MB, patients were treated with IPL (630–1200 nm, 20-ms pulse duration, and 25 J/cm^2 fluence) twice a month for up to 6 months. The results showed that NMB-PDT had better clinical efficacy than FMB-PDT did, reducing skin lesions by 77.3% compared with 44.1% for FMB. Both treatments had mild adverse effects, with no pain or hyperpigmentation observed. The NMB group experienced a longer remission period, with no recurrence within 6 months, whereas three patients in the FMB group relapsed after 6 months [98]. Considering the penetration depth of the IPL and the photosensitive feature of MB, the efficacy of this method needs to be further confirmed. Agut-Busquet et al. retrospectively analyzed seven cases of HS treated with MB intradermal injection photodynamic therapy (MB-I-PDT), where 1% MB solution was injected into the lesions under ultrasound guidance, followed by 635-nm LED light irradiation 15 min later. The results revealed that at 1 month posttreatment, six patients improved, and at the 6-month follow-up, five patients experienced sustained remission of lesions in the treated area [99]. Gamissans et al. conducted a retrospective cross-sectional study of 41 HS cases via the same approach and reported that 58.5% of lesions had a maximum diameter reduction of ≥75%, 22% had a reduction of 50–75%, and 19.5% had a reduction of <50%, with a 12.5% recurrence rate [99].

9.2.4 Recommended Regimes

As HS lesions are deep-seated and prone to forming sinus tracts and scarring, the penetration depth of topical photosensitizers and light is often limited, which can hinder the full effectiveness of ALA-PDT (MAL-PDT) in treating HS. On the basis of clinical experience and a review of previous literature, ALA-PDT is considered a potential alternative for treating Hurley stage I and II HS patients, particularly those who have failed standard therapies or refuse surgery. However, for Hurley stage III patients, mono-ALA-PDT is not recommended because scarring and tissue fibrosis impede photosensitizer absorption and light penetration. To enhance efficacy, ALA intralesional PDT (ALA-I-PDT) or ALA-PDT combined with surgery are recommended, as they can overcome these limitations. Although methylene blue (MB) PDT has shown good results, MB is not approved in China, so ALA remains the preferred option. On the basis of clinical experience and studies on ALA-PpIX fluorescence kinetics in conditions such as condyloma acuminatum and acne, the authors believe that the 1% ALA concentration used in other studies may be too low, and further research is needed to identify the optimal concentration for ALA-I-PDT. Additionally, owing to the hyperinflammatory nature of HS, combining PDT with systemic therapies or novel biologics may be necessary for better outcomes, and this is an area that the authors' team is currently exploring.

9.3 ALA-PDT for the Treatment of Rosacea

9.3.1 Introduction

Rosacea is a chronic, recurrent inflammatory dermatosis that primarily affects the midfacial skin and eyes [100]. During the 1800s, advancements in clinical illustrations significantly contributed to the formalization of dermatology as a distinct medical field. These high-quality images play a pivotal role in distinguishing rosacea from acne at an early stage [101]. The term "rosacea" was first introduced in 1828.

9.3.1.1 Epidemiology

The prevalence of rosacea varies widely across populations, ranging from less than 1% to 22% [102]. In 2019, a census conducted across 15 communities in Changsha, South Central China, revealed rosacea in 3.48% of the study population on the basis of skin examinations performed by board-certified dermatologists [103]. The condition is more commonly diagnosed in women than in men and is particularly prevalent among fair-skinned individuals of Celtic origin [102]. Although rosacea may occur at any age, it typically begins after the age of 30 [104].

9.3.1.2 Triggers and Pathogenesis

Rosacea can be triggered or aggravated by a variety of factors, including emotional stress, spicy foods, hot drinks, high temperatures, alcohol consumption, light exposure, and menopause. Although its exact pathogenesis remains unclear, multiple factors are believed to contribute to its development, including genetic predisposition, dysregulation of the innate immune system, overgrowth of commensal skin organisms, aberrant neurovascular signaling, and impaired skin barrier function, all of which may collectively drive the clinical manifestations of rosacea [105].

Genetic Factors

The genetics of rosacea are poorly understood, but gene variants, susceptibility, and associations with autoimmune diseases suggest a genetic predisposition to the condition [106]. Strong evidence for this predisposition includes a high incidence of familial history, links to autoimmune disorders, and the identification of specific genetic variants [106]. One of the most compelling indicators is the high prevalence of rosacea among individuals of northern European descent, particularly those of Celtic ancestry. However, despite these associations, knowledge of the genetic factors involved in rosacea remains limited, and further research is needed to clarify the genetic components contributing to its development.

Neurovascular Dysregulation

Two subfamilies of transient receptor potential (TRP) cation channels have been implicated in the pathogenesis of rosacea because of their roles in sensory and inflammatory signaling. The first group includes vanilloid (TRPV) receptors, specifically TRPV1 to TRPV4, whereas the second group consists of ankyrin (TRPA) channels, with TRPA1 thought to play a significant role in the disorder. Although the exact signaling pathways of these receptors remain unclear, they are known to be activated by stimuli such as heat and inflammation, which may contribute to hallmark rosacea symptoms such as flushing and burning [105].

Microorganisms [105]

Microorganisms are hypothesized to contribute to rosacea pathogenesis, although their exact role remains unclear. Compared with individuals without rosacea, those with rosacea have a greater density of Demodex mites on their facial skin, suggesting a potential role in its development. Compared with nonhemolytic isolates from healthy skin, *Staphylococcus epidermidis* isolates from pustules in papulopustular rosacea (PPR) patients have shown beta-hemolytic properties and produce different proteins at 37 °C. Both *Demodex folliculorum* and *S. epidermidis* may contribute to rosacea by stimulating toll-like receptor 2 (TLR2). The involvement of *Helicobacter pylori* in rosacea remains uncertain, although the high prevalence of *H. pylori* seropositivity in rosacea populations suggests a possible link. Additionally, *Bacillus oleronius,* a nonmotile, gram-negative, endospore-forming bacterium, has been isolated from *D. folliculorum* mites in rosacea patients. Neutrophils exposed to *B. oleronius* from healthy individuals exhibit increased production of inflammatory mediators such as matrix metalloproteinase-9 (MMP-9), tumor necrosis factor (TNF), and interleukin-8, similar to the inflammatory profile observed in the PPR.

Dysregulation of the Innate Immune System

Patients with rosacea exhibit increased baseline expression of cathelicidin and kallikrein 5 (KLK5), the serine protease responsible for cleaving cathelicidin into its active peptide form, LL-37. KLK5 and LL-37 are more abundant in rosacea skin than in healthy skin, and their forms differ. In rosacea, LL-37 is processed into shorter fragments that regulate key processes such as leukocyte chemotaxis, angiogenesis, and extracellular matrix component expression. Additionally, elevated levels of toll-like receptor 2 (TLR2), which activates KLK5, are observed in rosacea patients, along with increased matrix metalloproteinases that further activate KLK5, contributing to the inflammatory and vascular abnormalities characteristic of the disease.

Abnormal Barrier Function

The skin of patients with rosacea has increased transepidermal water loss and decreased epidermal hydration. These changes may be related to increased serine protease levels in rosacea and can be reversed with treatment.

9.3.1.3 Histopathology [105]

The histopathological findings in different rosacea subtypes are often nonspecific, making biopsy necessary only when the diagnosis is uncertain or when other conditions must be ruled out. In erythematotelangiectatic rosacea (ETR), histology typically shows superficial vasodilation and a mild lymphohistiocytic infiltrate, occasionally with plasma cells. Papulopustular rosacea (PPR) presents with a perivascular and perifollicular inflammatory infiltrate in the superficial and mid-dermis and is composed of lymphocytes, neutrophils, and plasma cells. Pustular lesions exhibit superficial neutrophil accumulation that extends beyond the follicle, unlike acne vulgaris. In phymatous rosacea, the histopathological features include sebaceous gland hyperplasia, follicular plugging, telangiectasia, dermal thickening, fibrosis, and large deposits of dermal mucin.

9.3.1.4 Diagnosis and Classification

Rosacea is a chronic inflammatory skin disease that primarily affects the centrofacial region, including the zygoma, cheeks, glabella, chin, and nose; some cases involve the eyes or periocular area and rarely occur outside the face. Its main clinical manifestations include persistent erythema, flushing, papules, pustules, telangiectasia, and skin hypertrophy. Patients may also experience skin sensitivity symptoms such as burning, stinging, edema, dryness, and ocular symptoms such as foreign body sensation, photosensitivity, itching, and general discomfort.

In 2002, the National Rosacea Society (NRS) established the National Rosacea Society Expert Committee (NRSEC) to create a standardized classification system for diagnosing and investigating the manifestations and relationships of various rosacea subtypes and potential variants [107] (Table 9.3). To improve the system's effectiveness for clinicians and researchers, the committee updated the method for assessing the severity of rosacea in 2004 [108].

As clinical practice has intensified, researchers have recognized the limitations of subtype-based classification, highlighting the need for a more patient-centered approach. Subtype classifications may not encompass the full range of clinical presentations and can complicate severity assessment. In contrast, a phenotype-based approach could enhance patient outcomes by addressing individual clinical presentations and concerns. Therefore, there is a clear need to move beyond traditional subtype classification. In 2017, according to the Global ROSacea Consensus, ROSCO [109] recommended shifting from a subtype-based approach to a phenotype-based method for diagnosing, classifying, and managing rosacea, aligning with the NRS update [104]. This new phenotypic approach focuses on diagnosis and treatment based on the characteristics presented by the patient rather than categorizing them into specific subtypes. This shift aims to facilitate more targeted treatments for rosacea. The diagnostic criteria for ROSCO require at least one diagnostic phenotype or two major phenotypes to diagnose rosacea (Table 9.4).

9.3.2 Treatment [100]

The symptoms of rosacea can be reduced or controlled through a combination of topical and systemic therapies; light, laser, and energy-based devices; and proper skin care and lifestyle management. The current therapeutic strategy for rosacea focuses on alleviating clinical symptoms, reducing disease recurrence, and improving patients' quality of life.

9.3.2.1 Education [110]

Patient education on trigger avoidance and proper skin care techniques, such as moisturizing and sun protection, is a crucial nonpharmacologic first step in managing rosacea. When specific triggers or exacerbating factors are identified, avoidance can help control symptoms. Additionally, proper skin care is essential for maintaining remission and alleviating rosacea symptoms. Regular skin care practices, including mild cleansing, moistening, and sun protection, have been shown to significantly improve skin hydration, reduce both objective and subjective skin sensitivity, and enhance overall skin health.

Table 9.3 Subtypes and variants of rosacea and their characteristics [107]

Subtype	Characteristics
ETR	Flushing and persistent central facial erythema with or without telangiectasia
PPR	Persistent central facial erythema with transient, central-facial papules or/and pustules
Phymatous	Thickening skin, surface irregularities and enlargement. May occur on the nose, chin, forehead, cheeks, or ears
Ocular	Foreign body sensation in the eye, burning or stinging, dryness, itching, ocular photosensitivity, blurred vision, telangiectasia of the sclera or other parts of the eye, or periorbital edema
Granulomatous	Noninflammatory; hard; brown, yellow, or red cutaneous papules; or nodules of uniform size

Table 9.4 ROSCO diagnostic, major and minor features of rosacea [109]

Diagnostic[a]	Major[b]	Minor
Persistent centrofacial erythema associated with periodic intensification by potential trigger factors	Flushing/transient centrofacial erythema Inflammatory papules and pustules Telangiectasia	Burning sensation of the skin Stinging sensation of the skin Edema Dry sensation of the skin
Phymatous changes	Ocular manifestations • Lid margin telangiectasia • Blepharitis • Keratitis/conjunctivitis/ sclerokeratitis	

[a] Phymatous changes are individually diagnostic of rosacea, and persistent centrofacial erythema associated with periodic intensification by potential trigger factors is a minimum diagnostic feature of rosacea
[b] If either flushing/transient erythema, inflammatory papules/pustules, telangiectasia, or ocular manifestations were present, the addition of any other major phenotype could be diagnostic of rosacea

9.3.2.2 Pharmacologic Treatments

Topical Medications [110]

Topical treatments approved by the US Food and Drug Administration for rosacea include topical sodium sulfacetamide, azelaic acid, metronidazole, and the alpha-adrenergic agonist brimonidine. Off-label treatments that have shown some benefit in treating rosacea in smaller case series include topical retinoids, topical calcineurin inhibitors, topical macrolides, benzoyl peroxide, topical permethrin cream, and ivermectin cream. Sodium sulfacetamide, in particular, is especially useful for patients with rosacea who also have concomitant seborrheic dermatitis.

Systemic Medications [110]

Tetracyclines, specifically doxycycline, improve rosacea symptoms through anti-inflammatory dosing by decreasing matrix metalloproteinase expression, downregulating inflammatory cytokines, reducing reactive oxygen species levels, and inhibiting nitric oxide-mediated vasodilation. Isotretinoin may be effective in treating severe, recalcitrant papulopustular rosacea by downregulating TLR2 expression. Beta-blockers, which act by vasoconstricting dermal blood vessels, have been shown to decrease erythema and flushing in some patients with rosacea.

9.3.2.3 Surgery [111]

Surgical treatment for rosacea aims to remove hypertrophied sebaceous glands and normalize the nasal contour. Surgical methods can be divided into two main groups: complete excision and incomplete excision, followed by reepithelialization of the remaining glandular epithelium. Incomplete excision methods include cryosurgery, dermabrasion, laser ablation, and electrosurgery.

9.3.2.4 Botulinum Toxin Type A

Botulinum toxin type A (BoNT-A) is a potent neurotoxin produced by *Clostridium botulinum* that inhibits the release of acetylcholine (ACh) from presynaptic vesicles. In addition to blocking ACh, BoNT-A also modulates several other neuropeptides, including substance P (SP), calcitonin gene-related peptide (CGRP), and vasoactive intestinal peptide (VIP). As ACh and VIP are key mediators of vasodilation and flushing, the inhibition of their release provides a plausible mechanism for the effectiveness of BoNT-A in treating rosacea [112].

9.3.2.5 Light, Laser, and Other Energy-Based Device Therapies [113]

These include intense pulsed light, pulsed dye lasers, CO_2 lasers or erbium lasers, 1064-nm ND:YAG lasers, visible light, radiofrequency, and photodynamic therapy.

9.3.3 ALA/MAL-PDT

9.3.3.1 Therapeutic Mechanism

Although the exact mechanism of ALA-PDT (aminolevulinic acid photodynamic therapy) in treating rosacea remains unclear, some research suggests that it may impact factors such as Demodex mites, bacteria, and immune regulation [114, 115]. Additionally, porphyrins tend to accumulate more in the follicular sebaceous gland unit, which makes it an important target structure for ALA-PDT in the treatment of rosacea.

Inhibition of Demodex and other microorganisms: Previous studies have confirmed that PDT has a positive effect on Demodex infection, potentially by directly killing Demodex mites through local immunomodulation or by inhibiting them via activation of endogenous porphyrins [115]. PDT may also help reduce the inflammatory response of rosacea by targeting and destroying other microorganisms, such as *Staphylococcus epidermidis* [116].

The immunomodulatory effects of PDT include a broad range of immunomodulatory effects, with sublethal levels of PDT capable of regulating immune cell functions, including cell signaling, cytokine types and secretion levels, and the expression of immune cell surface molecules [114]. In addition, PDT has the ability to selectively kill activated T cells [117] and increase the production of the matrix metalloproteinases MMP-1 and MMP-3 in fibroblasts [118]. These factors may partially explain the immunomodulatory effects of PDT in rosacea. However, the exact treatment mechanism of PDT for rosacea remains unclear, and further research is needed to clarify its role.

9.3.3.2 Clinical Application

PDT has not only antitumor effects but also anti-inflammatory and immunomodulatory effects, making it a potential treatment for inflammatory skin diseases [114]. Researchers worldwide have explored the use of MAL-PDT for the treatment of rosacea, with the first clinical study dating back to 2005, when Nybaek and Jemec used MAL-PDT to treat four rosacea patients and reported that three experienced remission [119]. These findings suggest that PDT is an effective option for select cases of rosacea. In 2006, Katz et al. [120] reported a case of a 45-year-old woman with rosacea who had failed standard treatments and received six sessions of ALA-PDT. Improvement was observed after the second treatment and was "excellent" by the sixth session, with no flares 1 month posttreatment. In 2007, Bryld et al. [121] treated 17 patients with rosacea with the MAL-PDT, and 10 had good results, 4 had fair results, and 3 had poor results. In 2011, Baglieri et al. [122] treated a 50-year-old patient with refractory granulomatous rosacea via six sessions of ALA-PDT (20% ALA, incubated for 3 h, 630 nm, light dose of 40 J/cm^2, 2-week intervals). The patients improved after three treatments and achieved a "good" outcome by the sixth, without adverse effects. In 2016, Friedmann et al. [123] explored the treatment of rosacea with ALA-PDT using different light sources. The study involved 30 rosacea patients whose lesions were incubated with 20% ALA for 1 h. Four different combinations of blue light, red light, intense pulsed light, and dye lasers were used as treatment light sources. The patients received one to six sessions of PDT, with an average of 1.3 ± 0.9 treatments. All patients showed mild-to-moderate improvement, and there was no significant difference in the curative effect among the different light source groups.

Recent studies in China have evaluated the clinical efficacy and safety of PDT for the treatment of rosacea, suggesting its potential as a therapeutic option. Preliminary trials have shown that ALA-PDT can alleviate inflammatory lesions in the Chinese population [124, 125]. Fan et al. treated 20 patients with ETR and PPR using a 5% 5-ALA emulsion applied under occlusion for 2 h, followed by LED red-light irradiation (100 mW/cm^2, 80–90 J/cm^2, 635 ± 15 nm) for 15 min over four sessions at 10-day intervals. All patients showed gradual clinical improvement, with subjective symptoms such as flushing, itching, tingling, and burning significantly relieved, and no recurrence was observed 24 weeks posttreatment. Similarly, Sun et al. [125] treated seven cases of ETR and ten cases of PPR with ALA-PDT, reporting a total effective rate (≥50% improvement) of 64.71% after three sessions. These findings highlight ALA-PDT as a safe and effective option for the management of rosacea (Table 9.5).

Table 9.5 Studies of PDT in rosacea

Photosensitizer	Number of cases	Types	Result	References
MAL	4	ETR/PPR	Three cases were in complete remission, of which one case had no recurrence at 9-month follow-up, and the other two cases had a 3-month remission	[119]
	17	/	Most patients receiving PDT can stop or significantly reduce other treatments, and the duration of remission ranges from approximately 3 months to 2 years	[121]
ALA	20	ETR/PPR	The objective symptoms of all patients were significantly alleviated compared to baseline. No recurrence at 24 weeks	[124]
	17	ETR/PPR	Effective rate of three treatments (≥50% improvement) was 64.71%. The total effective rate of seven cases of ET was 57.14%, of ten cases of PP was 70%	[125]
	1	ETR/PPR	Total of six sessions, the improvement was significant after the second treatment, and was considered to be "significant" after final treatment. There was no recurrence	[120]
	1	Gr	Total of six sessions, the lesions were significantly improved after the third treatment, and were evaluated as "good" after the sixth treatment	[122]
	30	ETR/PPR/Rh	The average course of treatment was 1.3 ± 0.9 times. The average improvement was 1.7 points (mild-to-moderate improvement), and there was no significant difference among all the groups	[123]
	20	ETR/PPR	16 (80%) patients in the ALA-PDT group achieved treatment success, with the clearance rates of papulopustular lesions of 85%	[126]

Tetracyclines, particularly minocycline, are currently considered the most effective and well-researched therapy for rosacea, with minocycline recommended for severe papulopustular rosacea (PPR). While ALA-PDT has shown potential in alleviating rosacea symptoms, there is a lack of comparative studies with first-line treatments and limited data on adverse reactions, making its clinical application uncertain. To address this, the authors compared the efficacy and safety of modified ALA-PDT and oral minocycline in the treatment of moderate-to-severe rosacea [126]. A total of 44 patients with rosacea were recruited for this single-center, randomized, evaluator-blind, controlled study. Forty-one patients completed the treatment, with 21 receiving oral minocycline (100 mg daily for 8 weeks) and 20 receiving modified ALA-PDT (5% ALA incubated for 30 min, followed by irradiation with 630-nm LED red light at 30 mW/cm^2 for 1 h, with a total energy density of 108 J/cm^2) at intervals of 1–2 weeks for three to five sessions. At the end of treatment, 80% of ALA-PDT patients and 81% of minocycline patients achieved treatment success, with papulopustular lesion clearance rates of 85% and 89%, respectively. The lesion count reduction and median change in the rosacea-specific quality of life score in the ALA-PDT group were not inferior to those in the minocycline group. By week 12 posttreatment, recurrence occurred in 5% of ALA-PDT patients compared with 25% in the minocycline group (p = 0.18), and by week 24, the recurrence rates were 15% and 40%, respectively. The adverse reactions in the ALA-PDT group were primarily acute inflammatory responses, all of which were manageable and resolved spontaneously (Fig. 9.8).

9.3.3.3 Recommended Treatment Regimens

To date, owing to the lack of convincing clinical research, the above clinical research parameters can only be used as a reference.

9.3.3.4 Adverse Reactions

Rosacea is easily triggered or worsened by various physical and environmental factors. In treating patients with actinic keratosis (AK) and

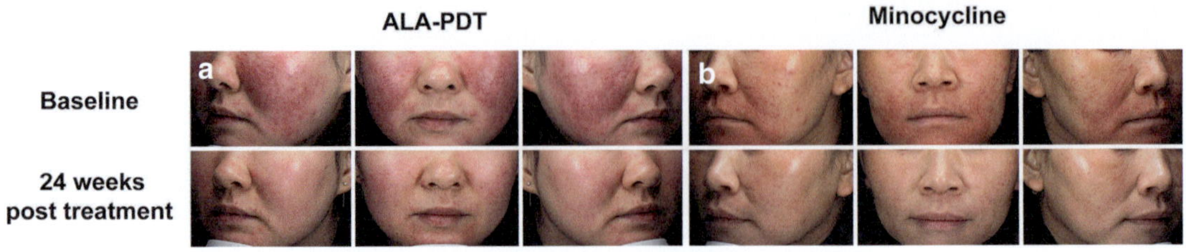

Fig. 9.8 Representative images of patients treated with ALA-PDT and minocycline

rosacea using ALA-PDT, the authors' team reported that parameters used for AK often led to excessive skin inflammation in these patients, likely due to skin barrier disruption, vascular dysfunction, and Demodex death [127]. Conventional ALA-PDT doses can provoke significant inflammatory responses, exacerbating symptoms such as flushing. Therefore, selecting appropriate treatment parameters is crucial to avoid aggravating inflammation.

While ALA-PDT offers a noninvasive alternative for rosacea management, its clinical parameters require further optimization and validation. Overall, determining the best ALA-PDT settings for the treatment of rosacea remains a priority for future research.

9.4 ALA-PDT for the Treatment of Alopecia

9.4.1 Introduction

Alopecia is a prevalent and debilitating dermatological condition that, while not life-threatening, significantly impacts patients' quality of life, self-esteem, and social functioning. Its recurrent nature and time-consuming treatments further increase the disease burden, often causing substantial psychological distress [4]. With the growing public emphasis on physical health and aesthetics, alopecia has garnered increased attention, making its treatment a research focus in recent years.

Alopecia can be classified into noncicatricial and cicatricial types on the basis of whether permanent hair follicle damage occurs. Common noncicatricial types include androgenetic alopecia (AGA), alopecia areata, telogen effluvium, and trichotillomania, whereas cicatricial alopecia encompasses lymphocytic, neutrophilic, mixed, and nonspecific subtypes [1, 2]. Recently, PDT has been explored as a treatment for noncicatricial alopecia, with preliminary observations also suggesting potential efficacy in treating cicatricial alopecia.

9.4.1.1 Nonicatricial Alopecia

Androgenetic alopecia (AGA) is an androgen-dependent hair loss disorder characterized by the progressive miniaturization of hair follicles and affects both men and women. The condition has a strong genetic predisposition, and factors such as dietary imbalances and sleep deprivation can trigger or worsen it. Studies have demonstrated that increased androgen receptor density and/or heightened activity of type II 5-α reductase in the scalps of AGA patients lead to an abnormal amplification of local androgen effects. This suppresses the activation, division, and differentiation of hair follicle stem cells, resulting in a shortened anagen phase, a prolonged telogen phase, and a decreased anagen-to-telogen ratio. Over time, the hair follicles progressively shrink and may eventually atrophy and disappear. Clinically, AGA presents as a receding frontal and temporal hairline, with thinning and reduced hair density at the vertex, often accompanied by excessive scalp oil secretion.

Alopecia areata is an organ-specific autoimmune disorder mediated by T lymphocytes, affecting individuals of all ages but primarily young adults, with equal incidence in men and women. While its exact etiology remains unclear, genetic predisposition and immune dysregulation are strongly implicated [3]. Research suggests that during the anagen phase of normal hair growth, the follicle bulb possesses immune privilege. However, in alopecia areata, this privilege is compromised, as hair follicles express human leukocyte antigens (HLA-A, HLA-B, HLA-C, and HLA-DR), leading to an attack by cytotoxic T lymphocytes on hair matrix cells. This immune response causes hair loss without destroying the normal follicular structure, thereby preventing scarring or permanent tissue damage. Clinically, alopecia areata presents as well-defined, round or oval patches of hair loss, which can affect any hair-bearing area of the body. In severe cases, the disease may progress to alopecia totalis or alopecia universalis.

9.4.1.2 Cicatricial Alopecia

Folliculitis decalvans is a form of cicatricial folliculitis characterized by the destruction of hair follicles, resulting in permanent hair loss. It affects both men and women and can occur in any hair-bearing area, although the vertex and occipital scalp are most commonly involved. While the exact etiology is unknown, it is thought to be associated with *Staphylococcus aureus* infection and localized immune dysregulation of the scalp. Clinically, it presents with follicular papules, pustules, perifollicular erythema, and hyperkeratosis. A hallmark feature is "tufted hair," where multiple hair shafts emerge from a single follicular opening. In advanced stages, small, irregular patches of cicatricial alopecia develop, which may coalesce into larger, more extensive areas of permanent hair loss.

9.4.2 Treatment of Alopecia

9.4.2.1 Treatment for Non-Cicatricial Alopecia

Treatment for AGA The treatment of AGA should begin early for optimal outcomes and typically involves a combination of oral and topical medications, physical therapies, and hair transplantation. The FDA has approved oral finasteride and topical minoxidil (2% or 5%) as first-line treatments. Finasteride, a 5-α reductase inhibitor, decreases dihydrotestosterone (DHT) levels in the scalp, thereby reducing androgenic suppression of hair follicles and promoting regrowth. Minoxidil, a potassium channel blocker, stimulates hair follicle epithelial cell proliferation, improves scalp blood flow, and supports follicle growth, although its exact mechanism is unclear. For female AGA, oral spironolactone, cyproterone, and dutasteride, which have antiandrogenic properties, are effective options [5]. Chinese herbal formulations have also shown potential benefits and are often used alongside conventional therapies. Hair transplantation techniques, such as follicular unit transplantation, have become standardized, but pre- and postoperative use of oral or topical medications is crucial for maintaining native hair growth.

Emerging therapies, such as photobiomodulation, which involves prolonged low-dose red-light exposure, and platelet-rich plasma (PRP) injection, which delivers growth factors to the scalp, have shown promise in activating hair follicle stem cells and promoting regeneration. However, further high-quality research is needed to confirm their efficacy and safety.

The treatments for alopecia areata are quite diverse, including oral and topical medical local therapy, contact sensitization, physical therapy, and biologics, although none can fully prevent or cure the condition. Treatment efficacy varies among individuals, and recurrence is common, often necessitating a tailored or combined approach [6, 7].

Oral treatments include glucocorticoids, cyclosporine, methimazole, and traditional Chinese medicine formulations. Oral glucocorticoids are typically reserved for severe or rapidly progressing cases. Cyclosporine is an option for adults over 20 years of age with total alopecia and no family history of atopy, whereas methimazole may be considered for adolescents aged 13–18 years with severe forms. Topical treatments involve glucocorticoids applied directly or via intralesional injections to reduce inflammation, minoxidil for hair regrowth, anthralin for its anti-inflammatory and immunosuppressive effects, and contact sensitizers to induce local contact dermatitis, stimulating hair regeneration.

Physical therapies include 308-nm excimer light, narrow-band UVB, and photobiomodulation. Emerging treatments such as platelet-rich plasma (PRP) injections and novel biological agents have also shown promise in recent studies.

9.4.2.2 Treatment for Cicatricial Alopecia

The treatment of folliculitis decalvans is challenging, with the primary goal being to prevent the progression from early follicular papules and pustules to irreversible alopecia. For localized lesions, topical antibiotics and glucocorticoids are commonly used, whereas extensive lesions often require systemic antibiotics and glucocorticoids, which are sometimes combined with retinoids, sulfone, zinc, and/or topical tacrolimus. Recently, some evidence has suggested that ALA-PDT may be effective in managing folliculitis decalvans, but owing to the rarity of this condition, clinical studies and case reports remain limited, and robust evidence-based data are still lacking.

9.4.3 Mechanisms of ALA-PDT in Alopecia

9.4.3.1 The Follicular Sebaceous Gland Unit Is One of the Main Targets of ALA-PDT

ALA-PDT has been clinically applied to treat diseases involving hair follicle sebaceous gland units. The authors' group successfully captured brick-red fluorescence images of these units via fluorescence diagnostic techniques in a previous study, confirming that the fluorescence originated from PpIX, a metabolite of ALA absorbed into the tissue. These findings further demonstrated that ALA is selectively absorbed by the hair follicle sebaceous gland unit, suggesting that this structure is a primary target for ALA-PDT treatment [8].

9.4.3.2 ALA-PDT Activates Follicular Stem Cells

Animal experiments by Carrasco et al. revealed that low levels of ROS can promote cell proliferation, with a significant increase in the number of proliferating cells within mouse skin hair follicles after PDT treatment, thereby stimulating hair growth [9]. Jin et al. further revealed that low-dose ROS reduce β-catenin degradation by activating the PI3K/AKT/GSK-3β signaling pathway in hair follicle stem cells, while also increasing Wnt protein expression and secretion. This transient expansion of progenitor cells enhances the Wnt/β-catenin signaling pathway, promoting the activation of hair follicle stem cells and progenitor cells and ultimately facilitating the transition of hair follicles into the growth phase [10].

9.4.3.3 ALA-PDT Inhibits Sebaceous Gland Hyperplasia and Sebum Secretion

The authors' group reported a significant reduction in sebum secretion in patients treated with ALA-PDT. These findings confirm that ALA-PDT can inhibit sebaceous gland hyperplasia and decrease sebaceous secretion, providing a theoretical basis for its potential to alleviate the clinical symptoms of excessive scalp sebum secretion in AGA patients.

9.4.3.4 ALA-PDT Has Antimicrobial and Immunomodulatory Effects

Certain types of alopecia, such as folliculitis decalvans, are associated with local infections, particularly *S. aureus*, and scalp immune abnormalities. ALA-PDT has demonstrated potent anti-infection properties and the ability to enhance the local immune response, providing a theoretical basis for its efficacy in treating infection-related alopecia. However, the exact mechanisms underlying these effects remain unclear and require further investigation [11, 12].

9.4.3.5 ALA-PDT Regulates the Skin Microenvironment

Numerous studies have demonstrated that ALA-PDT exerts regulatory effects on various cell types, including keratinocytes, fibroblasts, immune cells, sebaceous cells, hair follicle stem cells, and lymphatic and vascular endothelial cells. By promoting the resolution of chronic inflammation and delaying skin aging, ALA-PDT helps regulate the skin microenvironment and maintain homeostasis, potentially creating favorable conditions for hair growth.

9.4.4 Clinical Application of ALA-PDT in Alopecia

9.4.4.1 ALA-PDT for the Treatment of Noncicatricial Alopecia

The application of ALA-PDT in the treatment of AGA The effectiveness of ALA-PDT in treating AGA remains unclear. To investigate its potential, the authors' group conducted an exploratory study using C57BL/6 mice as an animal model. Following back depilation, the mice were treated with ALA-PDT at three different light doses: high (15 J/cm^2), medium (10 J/cm^2), and low (5 J/cm^2). The results revealed that hair density and length were significantly greater in the ALA-PDT groups than in the control group, with no significant differences observed among the different light doses. However, adverse reactions such as local erosion, ulceration, and scabbing occurred in the high- and medium-dose groups, whereas the low-dose group presented no noticeable side effects. This preliminary study suggested that low-dose ALA-PDT may promote hair growth with a favorable safety profile.

In 2017, the authors conducted the first randomized, placebo-controlled split-scale clinical study on the efficacy and safety of low-dose ALA-PDT for treating AGA in six patients with stage III–V AGA. A 5% ALA solution was applied and incubated for 3 h in the dark, followed by LED red light (630 ± 5 nm) exposure at 90 mW/cm^2 with an energy density of 60 J/cm^2, which was administered every 2 weeks for six cycles. During follow-up, hair density initially decreased on the ALA-PDT-treated side, similar to the early shedding phase seen with minoxidil, before returning to baseline, suggesting an effect on the hair growth cycle. However, 12 weeks after the final treatment, hair density did not significantly differ from that of the red-light control group, possibly due to the small sample size and short follow-up. This pioneering study demonstrated the feasibility of ALA-PDT for AGA and highlighted the need for further research with optimized parameters, larger sample sizes, and longer observation periods to validate its potential.

ALA-PDT has been applied in the treatment of alopecia areata, although its efficacy remains controversial (Table 9.6). Most studies have focused on patients resistant to conventional therapies, making treatment more challenging, and many have not optimized ALA-PDT parameters or included long follow-up periods, contributing to the uncertainty surrounding its effectiveness. Future research aimed at optimizing treatment parameters, shortening treatment intervals, increasing treatment frequency, and extending follow-up periods may provide stronger evidence for the efficacy of ALA-PDT in managing alopecia areata.

Current reports suggest that PDT treatment can improve symptoms of folliculitis decalvans, including pain, erythema, cysts, and pustules, with hair loss being controlled and long-term relief being achieved (Table 9.7). Adverse reactions, such as reversible erythema, pigmentation, a burning sensation, and mild pain, are generally mild. However, a small number of patients showed no significant improvement or experienced worsening of symptoms. Overall, the available reports are limited and primarily consist of case studies. Larger, randomized controlled clinical trials are needed in the future to confirm the efficacy and safety of PDT for treating folliculitis decalvans.

On the basis of the above evidence, the authors' group designed a photodynamic device to promote hair growth and applied for a patent (patent No. ZL201710046464.X). This patent established a complete technical system for the clinical exploration and application of PDT in the area of hair regrowth.

9.4.4.2 Recommended Protocol

Owing to a lack of convincing clinical studies, the above clinical research parameters can serve only as a reference. Further well-designed clini-

Table 9.6 Current reports on the treatment of alopecia areata with PDT

Authors, year	Cases	Parameters					Efficacy
		Photosensitizers, incubation period	Light sources	Light doses	Treatment frequency	Pretreatment	
Bissonnette et al., 2000 [128]	6	5%,10%, 20%ALA, 3 h	600–700 nm	Starting with 10 J/cm^2, and add 5 J/cm^2 every 2 weeks	Once every 2 weeks for 20 times	/	No significant hair growth
Fernández-Guarino et al., 2008 [129]	6	MLA, 3 h	630 nm	37 J/cm^2 7.5 min	Once every 4 weeks for 4–12 times	/	One case with alopecia areata of the beard got complete regrowth, two cases showed growth of some thin hair over <10
Yoo et al., 2010 [130]	8	MAL, 3 h	630 nm	37 J/cm^2 7.5 min	Once every 4 weeks 3 times	Microneedle	No significant hair growth
Giorgio CM et al., 2020 [131]	41	10%ALA, 2 h	630 nm	37 J/cm^2 8 min	Once every 3 weeks 6 times	Microneedle	PDT alone: 2 (2/15) patients achieved complete hair regrowth, 5 (5/15) patients had improvement of ≥50% of the treated areas. 1 (1/15) patient had improvement of <50% PDT combined with microneedling:Three (3/17) patients had complete hair regrowth, seven (7/17) patients had improvement of ≥50% of the treated areas, and six (6/17) had improvement of <50%
Linares-González et al., 2020 [132]	1	ALA, 3 h	630 nm	37 J/cm^2 7.5 min	Once every 4 weeks 6 times	/	Complete hair regrowth

Table 9.7 Current reports on the treatment of folliculitis decalvans with PDT

Authors, year	Cases	Parameters Photosensitizers, incubation period	Light sources	Light doses	Treatment frequency	Efficacy
Castaño-Suárez et al., 2012 [133]	1	MAL, 3 h	630 nm	37 J/cm² 7.5 min	Three cycles of PDT at 8-week intervals, each cycle involved two treatment sessions 2 weeks apart	Significant improvement; remained disease-free 12 months after last cycle
Miguel-Gomez et al., 2015 [134]	10	MAL, 3 h	630 nm	37 J/cm²	Four sessions of PDT at 4-week intervals	Nine (9/10) patients achieved clinical improvement, among which one patient remained disease free at 35 months after the last treatment
Burillo-Martinez et al., 2016 [135]	3	MAL, 3 h	630 nm	37 J/cm²	PDT once every 2 weeks, 2 PDT sessions per cycle. Repeat cycle every 4–6 weeks for 3–8 total cycles	Two patients showed mild improvement immediately after PDT sessions, but relapse early; remaining patients displayed worsening of the condition.
Collier et al., 2018 [136]	1	Porfimer sodium, 1 mg/kg	630 nm	100–140 J/cm²	Once every 4 months for 4 cycles	Significant improvement; the condition was stable at 20 months after PDT
Lin et al., 2020 [137]	1	5% ALA, 3 h	633 nm ± 3 nm	80 J/cm² 20 min	Once every 2 weeks for 4 cycles	Significant improvement; the condition was stable at 1 year follow-up
Yang et al., 2021 [138]	13	10% ALA, 3 h	633 nm	100 mW/cm² 30 min	Once every 10–14 days 3 times	Seven cases improved significantly and six cases improved moderately followed the first PDT. At 1 year after the last PDT, nine (9/13) cases werestable and the other four4 cases relapsed
Le Calvé et al., 2021 [139]	4	MAL, 30 min	635 nm	12–37 J/cm² 2.5 h	Once every 1–4 weeks 3 times	All cases got improved, but one case experienced slight progression in the center of alopecia area. The condition of all the four cases were stable at 4 months to 2 years follow-up

cal studies are needed to optimize these parameters.

9.4.4.3 Adverse Reactions and Complications

The adverse reactions of ALA-PDT in the treatment of alopecia are generally mild due to the relatively low light dose and photosensitizer concentration. The most common side effect is a mild burning sensation, while erythema and pigmentation may occur posttreatment. Erythema typically appears immediately after the procedure and subsides within 5 days, whereas pigmentation resolves completely within 3 months after treatment cessation.

Overall, ALA-PDT is safe and well tolerated in alopecia treatment. In conclusion, ALA-PDT offers a safe, noninvasive treatment option for alopecia, but its clinical parameters need further optimization, and its long-term efficacy requires confirmation through additional studies.

References

1. Zaenglein AL. Acne vulgaris. N Engl J Med. 2018;379(14):1343–52. https://doi.org/10.1056/NEJMcp1702493.
2. Layton AM, Thiboutot D, Tan J. Reviewing the global burden of acne: how could we improve care to reduce the burden? Br J Dermatol. 2021;184(2):219–25. https://doi.org/10.1111/bjd.19477.
3. Common JEA, Barker JN, van Steensel MAM. What does acne genetics teach us about disease pathogenesis? Br J Dermatol. 2019;181(4):665–76. https://doi.org/10.1111/bjd.17721.
4. Mirdamadi Y, Thielitz A, Wiede A, Goihl A, Papakonstantinou E, Hartig R, et al. Insulin and insulin-like growth factor-1 can modulate the phosphoinositide-3-kinase/Akt/FoxO1 pathway in SZ95 sebocytes in vitro. Mol Cell Endocrinol. 2015;415:32–44. https://doi.org/10.1016/j.mce.2015.08.001.
5. Clayton RW, Gobel K, Niessen CM, Paus R, van Steensel MAM, Lim X. Homeostasis of the sebaceous gland and mechanisms of acne pathogenesis. Br J Dermatol. 2019;181(4):677–90. https://doi.org/10.1111/bjd.17981.
6. Zouboulis CC. Endocrinology and immunology of acne: two sides of the same coin. Exp Dermatol. 2020;29(9):840–59. https://doi.org/10.1111/exd.14172.
7. Selway JL, Kurczab T, Kealey T, Langlands K. Toll-like receptor 2 activation and comedogenesis: implications for the pathogenesis of acne. BMC Dermatol. 2013;13:10. https://doi.org/10.1186/1471-5945-13-10.
8. DiGiovanna JJ, Langman CB, Tschen EH, Jones T, Menter A, Lowe NJ, et al. Effect of a single course of isotretinoin therapy on bone mineral density in adolescent patients with severe, recalcitrant, nodular acne. J Am Acad Dermatol. 2004;51(5):709–17. https://doi.org/10.1016/j.jaad.2004.04.032.
9. Garner SE, Eady A, Bennett C, Newton JN, Thomas K, Popescu CM. Minocycline for acne vulgaris: efficacy and safety. Cochrane Database Syst Rev. 2012;8:CD002086. https://doi.org/10.1002/14651858.CD002086.pub2.
10. Meffert H, Gaunitz K, Gutewort T, Amlong UJ. Therapy of acne with visible light. Decreased irradiation time by using a blue-light high-energy lamp. Dermatol Monatsschr. 1990;176(10):597–603.
11. Papageorgiou P, Katsambas A, Chu A. Phototherapy with blue (415 nm) and red (660 nm) light in the treatment of acne vulgaris. Br J Dermatol. 2000;142(5):973–8. https://doi.org/10.1046/j.1365-2133.2000.03481.x.
12. Li J, Li J, Zhang L, Liu X, Cao Y, Wang P, et al. Comparison of red light and blue light therapies for mild-to-moderate acne vulgaris: a randomized controlled clinical study. Photodermatol Photoimmunol Photomed. 2022;38(5):459–64. https://doi.org/10.1111/phpp.12769.
13. Lee SY, You CE, Park MY. Blue and red light combination LED phototherapy for acne vulgaris in patients with skin phototype IV. Lasers Surg Med. 2007;39(2):180–8. https://doi.org/10.1002/lsm.20412.
14. Kwon HH, Lee JB, Yoon JY, Park SY, Ryu HH, Park BM, et al. The clinical and histological effect of home-use, combination blue–red LED phototherapy for mild-to-moderate acne vulgaris in Korean patients: a double-blind, randomized controlled trial. Br J Dermatol. 2013;168(5):1088–94. https://doi.org/10.1111/bjd.12186.
15. Divaris DX, Kennedy JC, Pottier RH. Phototoxic damage to sebaceous glands and hair follicles of mice after systemic administration of 5-aminolevulinic acid correlates with localized protoporphyrin IX fluorescence. Am J Pathol. 1990;136(4):891–7.
16. Hongcharu W, Taylor CR, Chang Y, Aghassi D, Suthamjariya K, Anderson RR. Topical ALA-photodynamic therapy for the treatment of acne vulgaris. J Invest Dermatol. 2000;115(2):183–92. https://doi.org/10.1046/j.1523-1747.2000.00046.x.
17. Itoh Y, Ninomiya Y, Tajima S, Ishibashi A. Photodynamic therapy of acne vulgaris with topical delta-aminolaevulinic acid and incoherent light in Japanese patients. Br J Dermatol. 2001;144(3):575–9. https://doi.org/10.1046/j.1365-2133.2001.04086.x.
18. Ding HL, Wang XL, Wang HW, Huang Z. Successful treatment of refractory facial acne using repeat short-

cycle ALA-PDT: case study. Photodiagn Photodyn Ther. 2011;8(4):343–6. https://doi.org/10.1016/j.pdpdt.2011.07.003.
19. Ma L, Xiang LH, Yu B, Yin R, Chen L, Wu Y, et al. Low-dose topical 5-aminolevulinic acid photodynamic therapy in the treatment of different severity of acne vulgaris. Photodiagn Photodyn Ther. 2013;10(4):583–90. https://doi.org/10.1016/j.pdpdt.2013.06.007.
20. Ding HL, Wang XL, Wang HW, et al. Successful treatment of refractory facial acne using repeat short-cycle ALA-PDT: case study. Photodiagn Photodyn Ther. 2011;8(4):343–6.
21. Yang J, Shi L, Xu D, Liu J, Zhang L, Liu X, et al. 5-Aminolaevulinic acid photodynamic therapy suppresses lipid secretion of primary sebocytes through AMPK/SREBP-1 pathway. Photodiagn Photodyn Ther. 2021;36:102537. https://doi.org/10.1016/j.pdpdt.2021.102537.
22. Jeong E, Hong JW, Min JA, Lee DW, Sohn MY, Lee WJ, et al. Topical ALA-photodynamic therapy for acne can induce apoptosis of Sebocytes and downregulate their TLR-2 and TLR-4 expression. Ann Dermatol. 2011;23(1):23–32. https://doi.org/10.5021/ad.2011.23.1.23.
23. Tuo J, Wang Q, Zouboulis CC, Liu Y, Ma Y, Ma L, et al. ALA-PDT suppressing the cell growth and reducing the lipogenesis in human SZ95 sebocytes by mTOR signaling pathway in vitro. Photodiagn Photodyn Ther. 2017;18:295–301. https://doi.org/10.1016/j.pdpdt.2017.03.006.
24. Shu M, Kuo S, Wang Y, Jiang Y, Liu YT, Gallo RL, et al. Porphyrin metabolisms in human skin commensal Propionibacterium acnes bacteria: potential application to monitor human radiation risk. Curr Med Chem. 2013;20(4):562–8. https://doi.org/10.2174/0929867311320040007.
25. Fitz-Gibbon S, Tomida S, Chiu BH, Nguyen L, Du C, Liu M, et al. Propionibacterium acnes strain populations in the human skin microbiome associated with acne. J Invest Dermatol. 2013;133(9):2152–60. https://doi.org/10.1038/jid.2013.21.
26. Dagnelie MA, Montassier E, Khammari A, Mounier C, Corvec S, Dreno B. Inflammatory skin is associated with changes in the skin microbiota composition on the back of severe acne patients. Exp Dermatol. 2019;28(8):961–7. https://doi.org/10.1111/exd.13988.
27. Ramasamy S, Barnard E, Dawson TL Jr, Li H. The role of the skin microbiota in acne pathophysiology. Br J Dermatol. 2019;181(4):691–9. https://doi.org/10.1111/bjd.18230.
28. Tao S, Wang Z, Quan C, Ge Y, Qian Q. The effects of ALA-PDT on microbiota in pilosebaceous units of patients with severe acne: a metagenomic study. Photodiagn Photodyn Ther. 2021;33:102050. https://doi.org/10.1016/j.pdpdt.2020.102050.
29. Yang Y, Tao S, Zeng R, Zheng H, Ge Y. Modulation of skin microbiome in acne patients by aminolevulinic acid-photodynamic therapy. Photodiagn Photodyn Ther. 2021;36:102556. https://doi.org/10.1016/j.pdpdt.2021.102556.
30. Yang J, Chen AC, Wu Q, Jiang S, Liu X, Xiong L, et al. The influence of temperature on 5-aminolevulinic acid-based photodynamic reaction in keratinocytes in vitro. Photodermatol Photoimmunol Photomed. 2010;26(2):83–8. https://doi.org/10.1111/j.1600-0781.2010.00495.x.
31. Orringer JS, Hammerberg C, Hamilton T, Johnson TM, Kang S, Sachs DL, et al. Molecular effects of photodynamic therapy for photoaging. Arch Dermatol. 2008;144(10):1296–302. https://doi.org/10.1001/archderm.144.10.1296.
32. Gozali MV, Yi F, Zhang JA, Liu J, Wu HJ, Xu Y, et al. Photodynamic therapy inhibit fibroblast growth factor-10 induced keratinocyte differentiation and proliferation through ROS in fibroblast growth factor receptor-2b pathway. Sci Rep. 2016;6:27402. https://doi.org/10.1038/srep27402.
33. Fabbrocini G, Cacciapuoti S, De Vita V, Fardella N, Pastore F, Monfrecola G. The effect of aminolevulinic acid photodynamic therapy on microcomedones and macrocomedones. Dermatology. 2009;219(4):322–8. https://doi.org/10.1159/000252854.
34. Orringer JS, Sachs DL, Bailey E, Kang S, Hamilton T, Voorhees JJ. Photodynamic therapy for acne vulgaris: a randomized, controlled, split-face clinical trial of topical aminolevulinic acid and pulsed dye laser therapy. J Cosmet Dermatol. 2010;9(1):28–34. https://doi.org/10.1111/j.1473-2165.2010.00483.x.
35. Shi L, Yang J, Zhang L, Zhang Y, Yan G, Zhang H, et al. A prospective study of adverse reactions of ALA-PDT for acne vulgaris. Photodiagn Photodyn Ther. 2022;38:102752. https://doi.org/10.1016/j.pdpdt.2022.102752.
36. Zhang L, Yang J, Liu X, Xu D, Shi L, Liu J, et al. 5-Aminolaevulinic acid photodynamic therapy amplifies intense inflammatory response in the treatment of acne vulgaris via CXCL8. Exp Dermatol. 2021;30(7):923–31. https://doi.org/10.1111/exd.14357.
37. Liu P, Liu XJ, Zhang LL, Wang PR, Zeng QY, Wang XL, et al. ALA-PDT augments intense inflammation in the treatment of acne vulgaris by COX2/TREM1 mediated MI macrophage polarization. Biochem Pharmacol. 2023;208:115403. https://doi.org/1016/j.bop.2022.115403.
38. Ma Y, Chen Q, Liu Y, Wang Q, Huang Z, Xiang L. Effects of 5-aminolevulinic acid photodynamic therapy on TLRs in acne lesions and keratinocytes cocultured with P. Acnes. Photodiagn Photodyn Ther. 2016;15:172–81. https://doi.org/10.1016/j.pdpdt.2016.07.002.
39. Byun JY, Lee GY, Choi HY, Myung KB, Choi YW. The expressions of TGF-beta(1) and IL-10 in cultured fibroblasts after ALA-IPL photodynamic

treatment. Ann Dermatol. 2011;23(1):19–22. https://doi.org/10.5021/ad.2011.23.1.19.
40. Ji J, Zhang LL, Ding HL, Wang HW, Huang Z, Wang XX, et al. Comparison of 5-aminolevulinic acid photodynamic therapy and red light for treatment of photoaging. Photodiagn Photodyn Ther. 2014;11(2):118–21. https://doi.org/10.1016/j.pdpdt.2014.02.007.
41. Osiecka B, Jurczyszyn K, Symonowicz K, Bronowicz A, Ostasiewicz P, Czapinska E, et al. In vitro and in vivo matrix metalloproteinase expression after photodynamic therapy with a liposomal formulation of aminolevulinic acid and its methyl ester. Cell Mol Biol Lett. 2010;15(4):630–50. https://doi.org/10.2478/s11658-010-0033-1.
42. Wang P, Han J, Wei M, Xu Y, Zhang G, Zhang H, et al. Remodeling of dermal collagen in photoaged skin using low-dose 5-aminolevulinic acid photodynamic therapy occurs via the transforming growth factor-beta pathway. J Biophotonics. 2018;11(6):e201700357. https://doi.org/10.1002/jbio.201700357.
43. Wang XL, Wang HW, Zhang LL, Guo MX, Huang Z. Topical ALA PDT for the treatment of severe acne vulgaris. Photodiagn Photodyn Ther. 2010;7(1):33–8. https://doi.org/10.1016/j.pdpdt.2010.01.003.
44. Kimura M, Itoh Y, Tokuoka Y, Kawashima N. Delta-aminolevulinic acid-based photodynamic therapy for acne on the body. J Dermatol. 2004;31(12):956–60. https://doi.org/10.1111/j.1346-8138.2004.tb00637.x.
45. Sakamoto FH, Torezan L, Anderson RR. Photodynamic therapy for acne vulgaris: a critical review from basics to clinical practice: part II. Understanding parameters for acne treatment with photodynamic therapy. J Am Acad Dermatol. 2010;63(2):195–211. https://doi.org/10.1016/j.jaad.2009.09.057.
46. Ma Y, Liu Y, Wang Q, Ren J, Xiang L. Prospective study of topical 5-aminolevulinic acid photodynamic therapy for the treatment of severe adolescent acne in Chinese patients. J Dermatol. 2015;42(5):504–7. https://doi.org/10.1111/1346-8138.12836.
47. Terrell S, Aires D, Schweiger ES. Treatment of acne vulgaris using blue light photodynamic therapy in an African-American patient. J Drugs Dermatol. 2009;8(7):669–71.
48. Taub AF. Photodynamic therapy for the treatment of acne: a pilot study. J Drugs Dermatol. 2004;3(6):10–4.
49. Akaraphanth R, Kanjanawanitchkul W, Gritiyarangsan P. Efficacy of ALA-PDT vs blue light in the treatment of acne. Photodermatol Photoimmunol Photomed. 2007;23(5):186–90. https://doi.org/10.1111/j.1600-0781.2007.00303.x.
50. Barakat MT, Moftah NH, El Khayyat MA, Abdelhakim ZA. Significant reduction of inflammation and sebaceous glands size in acne vulgaris lesions after intense pulsed light treatment. Dermatol Ther. 2017;30(1):12418. https://doi.org/10.1111/dth.12418.
51. Prieto VG, Diwan AH, Shea CR, Zhang P, Sadick NS. Effects of intense pulsed light and the 1,064 nm Nd:YAG laser on sun-damaged human skin: histologic and immunohistochemical analysis. Dermatologic Surg. 2005;31(5):522–5. https://doi.org/10.1111/j.1524-4725.2005.31154.
52. Mei X, Shi W, Piao Y. Effectiveness of photodynamic therapy with topical 5-aminolevulinic acid and intense pulsed light in Chinese acne vulgaris patients. Photodermatol Photoimmunol Photomed. 2013;29(2):90–6. https://doi.org/10.1111/phpp.12031.
53. Oh SH, Ryu DJ, Han EC, Lee KH, Lee JH. A comparative study of topical 5-aminolevulinic acid incubation times in photodynamic therapy with intense pulsed light for the treatment of inflammatory acne. Dermatologic Surg. 2009;35(12):1918–26. https://doi.org/10.1111/j.1524-4725.2009.01315.x.
54. Yeung CK, Shek SY, Bjerring P, Yu CS, Kono T, Chan HH. A comparative study of intense pulsed light alone and its combination with photodynamic therapy for the treatment of facial acne in Asian skin. Lasers Surg Med. 2007;39(1):1–6. https://doi.org/10.1002/lsm.20469.
55. Rojanamatin J, Choawawanich P. Treatment of inflammatory facial acne vulgaris with intense pulsed light and short contact of topical 5-aminolevulinic acid: a pilot study. Dermatologic Surg. 2006;32(8):991–6. https://doi.org/10.1111/j.1524-4725.2006.32221.x.
56. Zhang L, Wu Y, Zhang Y, Liu X, Wang B, Wang P, et al. Topical 5-aminolevulinic photodynamic therapy with red light vs intense pulsed light for the treatment of acne vulgaris: a spilit face, randomized, prospective study. Dermatoendocrinol. 2017;9(1):e1375634. https://doi.org/10.1080/19381980.2017.1375634.
57. Alexiades-Armenakas M. Long-pulsed dye laser-mediated photodynamic therapy combined with topical therapy for mild to severe comedonal, inflammatory, or cystic acne. J Drugs Dermatol. 2006;5(1):45–55.
58. Haedersdal M, Togsverd-Bo K, Wiegell SR, Wulf HC. Long-pulsed dye laser versus long-pulsed dye laser-assisted photodynamic therapy for acne vulgaris: a randomized controlled trial. J Am Acad Dermatol. 2008;58(3):387–94. https://doi.org/10.1016/j.jaad.2007.11.027.
59. Kwon HH, Moon KR, Park SY, Yoon JY, Suh DH, Lee JB. Daylight photodynamic therapy with 1.5% 3-butenyl 5-aminolevulinate gel as a convenient, effective and safe therapy in acne treatment: a double-blind randomized controlled trial. J Dermatol. 2016;43(5):515–21. https://doi.org/10.1111/1346-8138.13191.
60. Zhang L, Zhang Y, Liu X, Shi L, Wang P, Zhang H, et al. Conventional versus daylight photodynamic therapy for acne vulgaris: a randomized and prospective clinical study in China. Photodiagn Photodyn

Ther. 2020;31:101796. https://doi.org/10.1016/j.pdpdt.2020.101796.
61. Artzi O, Sprecher E, Koren A. A split-face clinical trial of conventional red-light photodynamic therapy versus daylight photodynamic therapy for acne vulgaris. J Cosmet Dermatol. 2021;20(12):3924–30. https://doi.org/10.1111/jocd.14359.
62. Zhang Y, Zhang H, Zhang L, Wang P, Shi L, Zhang G, et al. Modified 5-aminolevulinic acid photodynamic therapy to reduce pain in the treatment of moderate to severe acne vulgaris: a prospective, randomized, split-face study. J Am Acad Dermatol. 2021;84(1):218–20. https://doi.org/10.1016/j.jaad.2020.04.146.
63. Wu HE, Liu YB, Cui L, Xu GJ, Sun XD. Three-step irradiance schedule versus two-step irradiance schedule for pain control during topical 5-aminolevulinic acid-photodynamic therapy of facial acne in Chinese patients: a prospective randomized comparative study. Lasers Surg Med. 2022;54(2):224–9. https://doi.org/10.1002/lsm.23464.
64. Guo K, Zhu D, Lu Z, Pan Y, Deng H. Effect of minocycline hydrochloride combined with photodynamic therapy on skin barrier function of patients with acne. Am J Transl Res. 2021;13(7):8427–32.
65. Xu X, Zheng Y, Zhao Z, Zhang X, Liu P, Li C. Efficacy of photodynamic therapy combined with minocycline for treatment of moderate to severe facial acne vulgaris and influence on quality of life. Medicine. 2017;96(51):e9366. https://doi.org/10.1097/MD.0000000000009366.
66. Liu L, Liu P, Wei G, Meng L, Zhang C, Zhang C. Combination of 5-Aminolevulinic acid photodynamic therapy and isotretinoin to treat moderate-to-severe acne. Photodiagn Photodyn Ther. 2021;34:102215. https://doi.org/10.1016/j.pdpdt.2021.102215.
67. Shi L, Yang Y, Zhang L, Yan J, Zhang H, Li C, et al. Efficacy and therapeutic reactions of tri-needle-pretreatment combined with painless ALA-PDT for the treatment of moderate-to-severe acne vulgaris: a randomized controlled trial. Photodiagn Photodyn Ther. 2022;37:102680. https://doi.org/10.1016/j.pdpdt.2021.102680.
68. Goldburg SR, Strober BE, Payette MJ. Hidradenitis suppurativa: epidemiology, clinical presentation, and pathogenesis. J Am Acad Dermatol. 2020;82(5):1045–58. https://doi.org/10.1016/j.jaad.2019.08.090.
69. Butt M, Rigby A, Leslie DL, Foulke GT, Flamm A, Kirby JS, et al. Associations of internalized skin bias with age, adverse psychopathology, and health-related quality of life among patients with hidradenitis suppurativa: a cross-sectional analysis. JAMA Dermatol. 2022;158(4):432–8. https://doi.org/10.1001/jamadermatol.2022.0248.
70. Machado MO, Stergiopoulos V, Maes M, Kurdyak PA, Lin PY, Wang LJ, et al. Depression and anxiety in adults with hidradenitis suppurativa: a systematic review and meta-analysis. JAMA Dermatol. 2019;155(8):939–45. https://doi.org/10.1001/jamadermatol.2019.0759.
71. Nguyen TV, Damiani G, Orenstein LAV, Hamzavi I, Jemec GB. Hidradenitis suppurativa: an update on epidemiology, phenotypes, diagnosis, pathogenesis, comorbidities and quality of life. J Eur Acad Dermatol Venereol. 2021;35(1):50–61. https://doi.org/10.1111/jdv.16677.
72. Sartorius K, Lapins J, Emtestam L, Jemec GB. Suggestions for uniform outcome variables when reporting treatment effects in hidradenitis suppurativa. Br J Dermatol. 2003;149(1):211–3. https://doi.org/10.1046/j.1365-2133.2003.05390.x.
73. Sabat R, Jemec GBE, Matusiak L, Kimball AB, Prens E, Wolk K. Hidradenitis suppurativa. Nat Rev Dis Primers. 2020;6(1):18. https://doi.org/10.1038/s41572-020-0149-1.
74. Zouboulis CC, Tzellos T, Kyrgidis A, Jemec GBE, Bechara FG, Giamarellos-Bourboulis EJ, et al. Development and validation of the international hidradenitis Suppurativa severity score system (IHS4), a novel dynamic scoring system to assess HS severity. Br J Dermatol. 2017;177(5):1401–9. https://doi.org/10.1111/bjd.15748.
75. Vazquez BG, Alikhan A, Weaver AL, Wetter DA, Davis MD. Incidence of hidradenitis suppurativa and associated factors: a population-based study of Olmsted County, Minnesota. J Invest Dermatol. 2013;133(1):97–103. https://doi.org/10.1038/jid.2012.255.
76. Ingram JR. The genetics of hidradenitis suppurativa. Dermatol Clin. 2016;34(1):23–8. https://doi.org/10.1016/j.det.2015.07.002.
77. von der Werth JM, Williams HC. The natural history of hidradenitis suppurativa. J Eur Acad Dermatol Venereol. 2000;14(5):389–92. https://doi.org/10.1046/j.1468-3083.2000.00087.x.
78. Frew JW, Vekic DA, Woods J, Cains GD. A systematic review and critical evaluation of reported pathogenic sequence variants in hidradenitis suppurativa. Br J Dermatol. 2017;177(4):987–98. https://doi.org/10.1111/bjd.15441.
79. Yu W, Barrett J, Liu P, Parameswaran A, Chiu ES, Lu CP. Novel evidence of androgen receptor immunoreactivity in skin tunnels of hidradenitis suppurativa: assessment of sex and individual variability. Br J Dermatol. 2021;185(4):855–8. https://doi.org/10.1111/bjd.20520.
80. Boer J, Nazary M, Riis PT. The role of mechanical stress in hidradenitis suppurativa. Dermatol Clin. 2016;34(1):37–43. https://doi.org/10.1016/j.det.2015.08.011.
81. Bukvic Mokos Z, Mise J, Balic A, Marinovic B. Understanding the relationship between smoking and hidradenitis Suppurativa. Acta Dermatovenerol Croat. 2020;28(1):9–13.
82. Nomura T. Hidradenitis Suppurativa as a potential subtype of autoinflammatory keratinization disease. Front Immunol. 2020;11:847. https://doi.org/10.3389/fimmu.2020.00847.

83. Li A, Peng Y, Taiclet LM, Tanzi RE. Analysis of hidradenitis suppurativa-linked mutations in four genes and the effects of PSEN1-P242LfsX11 on cytokine and chemokine expression in macrophages. Hum Mol Genet. 2019;28(7):1173–82. https://doi.org/10.1093/hmg/ddy414.
84. Zhang X, Sisodia SS. Acne inversa caused by missense mutations in NCSTN is not fully compatible with impairments in notch signaling. J Invest Dermatol. 2015;135(2):618–20. https://doi.org/10.1038/jid.2014.399.
85. Ingram JR, Wood M, John B, Butler R, Anstey AV. Absence of pathogenic gamma-secretase mutations in a South Wales cohort of familial and sporadic hidradenitis suppurativa (acne inversa). Br J Dermatol. 2013;168(4):874–6. https://doi.org/10.1111/bjd.12048.
86. Nomura Y, Nomura T, Suzuki S, Takeda M, Mizuno O, Ohguchi Y, et al. A novel NCSTN mutation alone may be insufficient for the development of familial hidradenitis suppurativa. J Dermatol Sci. 2014;74(2):180–2. https://doi.org/10.1016/j.jdermsci.2014.01.013.
87. Navrazhina K, Frew JW, Grand D, Williams SC, Hur H, Gonzalez J, et al. Interleukin-17RA blockade by brodalumab decreases inflammatory pathways in hidradenitis suppurativa skin and serum. Br J Dermatol. 2022;187(2):223–33. https://doi.org/10.1111/bjd.21060.
88. Tricarico PM, Zupin L, Ottaviani G, Rupel K, Celsi F, Genovese G, et al. Photobiomodulation as potential novel third line tool for noninvasive treatment of hidradenitis suppurativa. G Ital Dermatol Venereol. 2020;155(1):88–98. https://doi.org/10.23736/S0392-0488.19.06247-3.
89. Gold M, Bridges TM, Bradshaw VL, Boring M. ALA-PDT and blue light therapy for hidradenitis suppurativa. J Drugs Dermatol. 2004;3(1 Suppl):S32–5.
90. Schweiger ES, Riddle CC, Aires DJ. Treatment of hidradenitis suppurativa by photodynamic therapy with aminolevulinic acid: preliminary results. J Drugs Dermatol. 2011;10(4):381–6.
91. Strauss RM, Pollock B, Stables GI, Goulden V, Cunliffe WJ. Photodynamic therapy using aminolaevulinic acid does not lead to clinical improvement in hidradenitis suppurativa. Br J Dermatol. 2005;152(4):803–4. https://doi.org/10.1111/j.1365-2133.2005.06475.x.
92. Rivard J, Ozog D. Henry ford hospital dermatology experience with Levulan Kerastick and blue light photodynamic therapy. J Drugs Dermatol. 2006;5(6):556–61.
93. Bu W, Xu X, Wang Y, Huang L, Zeng R, Chen X, et al. Surgery combined with photodynamic therapy for the treatment of hidradenitis Suppurativa: a report of 7 cases. Photodiagn Photodyn Ther. 2017;18:46–9. https://doi.org/10.1016/j.pdpdt.2017.01.176.
94. Valladares-Narganes LM, Rodriguez-Prieto MA, Blanco-Suarez MD, Rodriguez-Lage C, Garcia-Doval I. Treatment of hidradenitis suppurativa with intralesional photodynamic therapy using a laser diode attached to an optical cable: a promising new approach. Br J Dermatol. 2015;172(4):1136–9. https://doi.org/10.1111/bjd.13385.
95. Suarez-Valladares MJ, Rodriguez-Prieto MA, Serra-Llusa R. Penetration of 630 nm laser and 5-aminolevulinic acid in tissue with intralesional photodynamic therapy. Photodiagn Photodyn Ther. 2016;16:166–8. https://doi.org/10.1016/j.pdpdt.2016.09.006.
96. Suarez Valladares MJ, Eiris Salvado N, Rodriguez Prieto MA. Treatment of hidradenitis suppurativa with intralesional photodynamic therapy with 5-aminolevulinic acid and 630 nm laser beam. J Dermatol Sci. 2017;85(3):241–6. https://doi.org/10.1016/j.jdermsci.2016.12.014.
97. Garcias-Ladaria J, Corral-Magana O, Del Pozo LJ, Martin-Santiago A. Intralesional photodynamic therapy in hidradenitis suppurativa: getting closer to the target. Photodiagn Photodyn Ther. 2021;34:102339. https://doi.org/10.1016/j.pdpdt.2021.102339.
98. Fadel MA, Tawfik AA. New topical photodynamic therapy for treatment of hidradenitis suppurativa using methylene blue niosomal gel: a single-blind, randomized, comparative study. Clin Exp Dermatol. 2015;40(2):116–22. https://doi.org/10.1111/ced.12459.
99. Agut-Busquet E, Romani J, Gilaberte Y, Garcia-Malinis A, Ribera-Pibernat M, Luelmo J. Photodynamic therapy with intralesional methylene blue and a 635 nm light-emitting diode lamp in hidradenitis suppurativa: a retrospective follow-up study in 7 patients and a review of the literature. Photochem Photobiol Sci. 2016;15(8):1020–8. https://doi.org/10.1039/c6pp00082g.
100. Schaller M, Almeida LMC, Bewley A, Cribier B, Del Rosso J, Dlova NC, et al. Recommendations for rosacea diagnosis, classification and management: update from the global ROSacea COnsensus 2019 panel. Br J Dermatol. 2020;182(5):1269–76. https://doi.org/10.1111/bjd.18420.
101. Cribier B. Medical history of the representation of rosacea in the 19th century. J Am Acad Dermatol. 2013;69(6 Suppl 1):S2–S14. https://doi.org/10.1016/j.jaad.2013.04.046.
102. van Zuuren EJ. Rosacea. N Engl J Med. 2017;377(18):1754–64. https://doi.org/10.1056/NEJMcp1506630.
103. Li J, Wang B, Deng Y, Shi W, Jian D, Liu F, et al. Epidemiological features of rosacea in Changsha, China: a population-based, cross-sectional study. J Dermatol. 2020;47(5):497–502. https://doi.org/10.1111/1346-8138.15301.
104. Gallo RL, Granstein RD, Kang S, Mannis M, Steinhoff M, Tan J, et al. Standard classification and pathophysiology of rosacea: the 2017 update by the National Rosacea Society expert committee. J Am

Acad Dermatol. 2018;78(1):148–55. https://doi.org/10.1016/j.jaad.2017.08.037.
105. Two AM, Wu W, Gallo RL, Hata TR. Rosacea: part I. Introduction, categorization, histology, pathogenesis, and risk factors. J Am Acad Dermatol. 2015;72(5):749–58. https://doi.org/10.1016/j.jaad.2014.08.028.
106. Awosika O, Oussedik E. Genetic predisposition to rosacea. Dermatol Clin. 2018;36(2):87–92. https://doi.org/10.1016/j.det.2017.11.002.
107. Wilkin J, Dahl M, Detmar M, Drake L, Feinstein A, Odom R, et al. Standard classification of rosacea: report of the National Rosacea Society Expert Committee on the classification and staging of rosacea. J Am Acad Dermatol. 2002;46(4):584–7. https://doi.org/10.1067/mjd.2002.120625.
108. Wilkin J, Dahl M, Detmar M, Drake L, Liang MH, Odom R, et al. Standard grading system for rosacea: report of the National Rosacea Society Expert Committee on the classification and staging of rosacea. J Am Acad Dermatol. 2004;50(6):907–12. https://doi.org/10.1016/j.jaad.2004.01.048.
109. Tan J, Almeida LM, Bewley A, Cribier B, Dlova NC, Gallo R, et al. Updating the diagnosis, classification and assessment of rosacea: recommendations from the global ROSacea COnsensus (ROSCO) panel. Br J Dermatol. 2017;176(2):431–8. https://doi.org/10.1111/bjd.15122.
110. Two AM, Wu W, Gallo RL, Hata TR. Rosacea: part II. Topical and systemic therapies in the treatment of rosacea. J Am Acad Dermatol. 2015;72(5):761–70. https://doi.org/10.1016/j.jaad.2014.08.027.
111. Tuzun Y, Wolf R, Kutlubay Z, Karakus O, Engin B. Rosacea and rhinophyma. Clin Dermatol. 2014;32(1):35–46. https://doi.org/10.1016/j.clindermatol.2013.05.024.
112. Zhang H, Tang K, Wang Y, Fang R, Sun Q. Use of botulinum toxin in treating rosacea: a systematic review. Clin Cosmet Investig Dermatol. 2021;14:407–17. https://doi.org/10.2147/CCID.S307013.
113. Loyal J, Carr E, Almukhtar R, Goldman MP. Updates and best practices in the management of facial erythema. Clin Cosmet Investig Dermatol. 2021;14:601–14. https://doi.org/10.2147/CCID.S267203.
114. Reinhard A, Sandborn WJ, Melhem H, Bolotine L, Chamaillard M, Peyrin-Biroulet L. Photodynamic therapy as a new treatment modality for inflammatory and infectious conditions. Expert Rev Clin Immunol. 2015;11(5):637–57. https://doi.org/10.1586/1744666X.2015.1032256.
115. Gilaberte Y, Frias MP, Rezusta A, Vera-Alvarez J. Photodynamic therapy with methyl aminolevulinate for resistant scalp folliculitis secondary to demodex infestation. J Eur Acad Dermatol Venereol. 2009;23(6):718–9. https://doi.org/10.1111/j.1468-3083.2009.03171.x.
116. Li X, Guo H, Tian Q, Zheng G, Hu Y, Fu Y, et al. Effects of 5-aminolevulinic acid-mediated photodynamic therapy on antibiotic-resistant staphylococcal biofilm: an in vitro study. J Surg Res. 2013;184(2):1013–21. https://doi.org/10.1016/j.jss.2013.03.094.
117. Darvekar S, Juzenas P, Oksvold M, Kleinauskas A, Holien T, Christensen E, et al. Selective killing of activated T cells by 5-aminolevulinic acid mediated photodynamic effect: potential improvement of extracorporeal photopheresis. Cancer. 2020;12(2):377. https://doi.org/10.3390/cancers12020377.
118. Karrer S, Bosserhoff AK, Weiderer P, Landthaler M, Szeimies RM. Keratinocyte-derived cytokines after photodynamic therapy and their paracrine induction of matrix metalloproteinases in fibroblasts. Br J Dermatol. 2004;151(4):776–83. https://doi.org/10.1111/j.1365-2133.2004.06209.x.
119. Li A, Fang R, Mao X, Sun Q. Photodynamic therapy in the treatment of rosacea: a systematic review. Photodiagn Photodyn Ther. 2022;38:102875. https://doi.org/10.1016/j.pdpdt.2022.102875.
120. Katz B, Patel V. Photodynamic therapy for the treatment of erythema, papules, pustules, and severe flushing consistent with rosacea. J Drugs Dermatol. 2006;5(2 Suppl):6–8.
121. Bryld LE, Jemec GB. Photodynamic therapy in a series of rosacea patients. J Eur Acad Dermatol Venereol. 2007;21(9):1199–202. https://doi.org/10.1111/j.1468-3083.2007.02219.x.
122. Baglieri F, Scuderi G. Treatment of recalcitrant granulomatous rosacea with ALA-PDT: report of a case. Indian J Dermatol Venereol Leprol. 2011;77(4):536. https://doi.org/10.4103/0378-6323.82420.
123. Friedmann DP, Goldman MP, Fabi SG, Guiha I. Multiple sequential light and laser sources to activate aminolevulinic acid for rosacea. J Cosmet Dermatol. 2016;15(4):407–12. https://doi.org/10.1111/jocd.12231.
124. Fan L, Yin R, Lan T, Hamblin MR. Photodynamic therapy for rosacea in Chinese patients. Photodiagn Photodyn Ther. 2018;24:82–7. https://doi.org/10.1016/j.pdpdt.2018.08.005.
125. Sun Y, Chen L, Zhang Y, Gao X, Wu Y, Chen H. Topical photodynamic therapy with 5-aminolevulinic acid in Chinese patients with rosacea. J Cosmet Laser Ther. 2019;21(4):196–200. https://doi.org/10.1080/14764172.2018.1502455.
126. Yang J, Liu X, Cao Y, Wang P, Zhang H, Chen Q, et al. 5-Aminolevulinic acid photodynamic therapy versus minocycline for moderate-to-severe rosacea: a single-center, randomized, evaluator-blind controlled study. J Am Acad Dermatol. 2023;89(4):711–8. https://doi.org/10.1016/j.jaad.2023.06.027.
127. Liu P, Liu X, Wang P, Zhang L, Hu C, Yang X, et al. Inflammation burst after 5-aminolevulinic acid-photodynamic therapy for the treatment of actinic keratosis complicating rosacea: a case report. Photodiagn Photodyn Ther. 2022;39:102897. https://doi.org/10.1016/j.pdpdt.2022.102897.

128. Bissonnette R, Shapiro J, Zeng H, McLean DI, Lui H. Topical photodynamic therapy with 5-aminolaevulinic acid does not induce hair regrowth in patients with extensive alopecia areata. Br J Dermatol. 2000;143(5):1032–5. https://doi.org/10.1046/j.1365-2133.2000.03783.x.
129. Fernández-Guarino M, Harto A, García-Morales I, Pérez-García B, Arrazola JM, Jaén P. Failure to treat alopecia areata with photodynamic therapy. Clin Exp Dermatol. 2008;33(5):585–7. https://doi.org/10.1111/j.1365-2230.2008.02712.x.
130. Yoo KH, Lee JW, Li K, Kim BJ, Kim MN. Photodynamic therapy with methyl 5-aminolevulinate acid might be ineffective in recalcitrant alopecia totalis regardless of using a microneedle roller to increase skin penetration. Dermatologic Surg. 2010;36(5):618–22. https://doi.org/10.1111/j.1524-4725.2010.01515.x.
131. Giorgio CM, Babino G, Caccavale S, Russo T, De Rosa AB, Alfano R, et al. Combination of photodynamic therapy with 5-aminolaevulinic acid and microneedling in the treatment of alopecia areata resistant to conventional therapies: our experience with 41 patients. Clin Exp Dermatol. 2020;45(3):323–6. https://doi.org/10.1111/ced.14084.
132. Linares-González L, Ródenas-Herranz T, Sáenz-Guirado S, Ruiz-Villaverde R. Successful response to photodynamic therapy with 5-aminolevulinic acid nanoemulsified gel in a patient with universal alopecia areata refractory to conventional treatment. Dermatol Ther. 2020;33(3):e13416. https://doi.org/10.1111/dth.13416.
133. Castaño-Suárez E, Romero-Maté A, Arias-Palomo D, Borbujo J. Photodynamic therapy for the treatment of folliculitis decalvans. Photodermatol Photoimmunol Photomed. 2012;28(2):102–4. https://doi.org/10.1111/j.1600-0781.2011.00639.x.
134. Miguel-Gomez L, Vano-Galvan S, Perez-Garcia B, Carrillo-Gijon R, Jaen-Olasolo P. Treatment of folliculitis decalvans with photodynamic therapy: results in 10 patients. J Am Acad Dermatol. 2015;72(6):1085–7. https://doi.org/10.1016/j.jaad.2015.02.1120.
135. Burillo-Martinez S, Maroñas-Jimenez L, Palencia-Pérez SI, Vanaclocha-Sebastián F, López-Gómez S. Failure of photodynamic therapy (PDT) in 3 patients with folliculitis decalvans. J Am Acad Dermatol. 2016;74(4):e69–70. https://doi.org/10.1016/j.jaad.2015.09.075.
136. Collier NJ, Allan D, Diaz Pesantes F, Sheridan L, Allan E. Systemic photodynamic therapy in folliculitis decalvans. Clin Exp Dermatol. 2018;43(1):46–9. https://doi.org/10.1111/ced.13238.
137. Lin X, Zhou S, Wang X, Zhu X. Aminolevulinic acid photodynamic therapy for folliculitis decalvans: a case report. Dermatol Ther. 2020;33(3):e13358. https://doi.org/10.1111/dth.13358.
138. Yang L, Chen J, Tong X, Gao L, Ding S, Guo A. Photodynamic therapy should be considered for the treatment of folliculitis decalvans. Photodiagn Photodyn Ther. 2021;35:102356. https://doi.org/10.1016/j.pdpdt.2021.102356.
139. Le Calvé C, Abi-Rached H, Vicentini C, Maire C, Delaporte E, Mordon S, et al. Treatment of folliculitis decalvans by photodynamic therapy using a new light-emitting device: a case series of 4 patients. JAAD Case Rep. 2021;17:69–72. https://doi.org/10.1016/j.jdcr.2021.09.026.

ALA-PDT in the Treatment of Skin Aging

10

Peiru Wang, Yu Yan, Yuling Yang, Bo Wang, and Xiuli Wang

10.1 Introduction

The skin is the largest organ in the human body and serves as a crucial physical and immune barrier that maintains homeostasis between the internal and external environments. Skin aging is a key aspect of the overall aging process, and the incidence of age-related skin conditions has been steadily increasing [1]. The signs of skin aging include wrinkles, sallowness, rough texture, mottled pigmentation, increased fragility, and impaired wound healing. Along with these cosmetic changes, skin aging is also characterized by a decline in essential functions, such as the skin's barrier and immune functions. In addition to causing aesthetic concerns, skin aging is closely linked to the onset and progression of various geriatric skin diseases and skin cancers [2]. Therefore, intervening in and delaying skin aging play a significant role in preventing precancerous lesions and skin tumors in elderly individuals, thereby enhancing their overall health, quality of life, and dignity.

P. Wang (✉) · Y. Yan · Y. Yang · X. Wang
Institute of Photomedicine, Shanghai Skin Disease Hospital, School of Medicine, Tongji University, Shanghai, China
e-mail: wangpeiru@tongji.edu.cn; 2231159@tongji.edu.cn; wangxiuli_1400023@tongji.edu.cn

B. Wang
Avera Medical Group Dermatology, Aberdeen, SD, USA

University of South Dakota, Vermillion, SD, USA
e-mail: makiwang@med.umich.edu

10.1.1 Classification and Presentation of Skin Aging

Skin aging can be categorized into two types: endogenous aging and exogenous aging. Endogenous aging, also referred to as intrinsic aging or natural senescence, is the result of the natural aging process and is typically associated with increasing age [3]. In contrast, exogenous aging is caused by external environmental factors such as ultraviolet (UV) radiation, smoking, pollution, malnutrition, and exposure to chemical substances. Among these, UV radiation is the most significant contributor to exogenous skin aging, and as such, the term photoaging is often used interchangeably with exogenous aging [4, 5]. Visible changes in skin appearance and tissue structure due to photoaging tend to occur earlier and are more pronounced than those caused by endogenous aging. The mechanisms underlying skin aging include DNA damage, protein folding dysfunction, depletion of stem cells, a decline in mitochondrial function, accumulation of inflammatory factors, and a reduced nutrient supply [5, 6].

Clinical manifestations of endogenous skin aging include dryness, increased scaling, skin

X. Wang, B. Wang (eds.), *Photodynamic Therapy in Dermatology*,
https://doi.org/10.1007/978-981-96-8915-6_10

laxity and brittleness, reduced elasticity, and the appearance of fine lines, with a skin pattern typically maintained and a grayish–white skin tone [3]. In contrast, photoaged skin shows more pronounced changes, such as increased laxity, deep wrinkles, a leathery appearance, heightened pigmentation, dilated blood vessels, altered or absent skin patterns, and a yellowish-gray tone. Prolonged UV exposure leads to the accumulation of reactive oxygen species (ROS) and an increase in matrix metalloproteinases (MMPs) that promote dermal matrix degradation [7]. This exposure significantly increases the risk of actinic keratosis (AK), which is considered the critical step in the progression from photodamaged skin to squamous cell carcinoma (SCC) [8]. Additionally, many AKs and nonmelanoma skin cancers (NMSCs), collectively referred to as actinic field damage, are commonly found in photodamaged skin [9].

Endogenous skin aging is characterized by a slowed turnover of keratinocytes, reduced fibroblast functionality, and histopathological changes such as thinning of the epidermis and dermis, as well as a reduction in collagen, elastic fibers, lymphatic vessels, and blood vessels. In contrast, the histopathological changes in photoaged skin are more complex, including abnormal thickening of the stratum corneum, hypertrophy of the spinous layer, flattening of the epidermis–dermis junction, uneven distribution of melanocytes, and a reduction in dermal fibroblasts. Fractionated collagen fibers may be disordered, with elastic fibers becoming fragmented and clumped. Additionally, there is increased deposition of glycosaminoglycans; infiltration of hypertrophic mast cells, neutrophils, and monocytes in the dermis; a decrease in the number but dilation of blood vessels; and a reduction in the number of lymphatic vessels [10–13].

10.1.2 Common Strategies for Skin Rejuvenation

The goal of skin rejuvenation is to slow the aging process and restore a youthful appearance and functionality to the skin. Currently, various antiaging methods, including preventive measures, strategies to slow the aging process, and even attempts to reverse aging, have emerged in the medical field. These approaches have led to the development of diverse antiaging treatments, which can be categorized into protective products, topical medications, oral medications, chemical and physical exfoliation treatments, photothermal therapies, and injectable treatments. Among these methods, PDT stands out as a form of photothermal therapy.

UV protection: Minimizing excessive exposure to UV radiation is crucial for preventing skin photoaging. Key strategies include physical sun protection, such as wearing protective clothing and the regular use of topical sunscreen products. In recent years, oral photoprotective agents have also gained attention. These include vitamin derivatives such as β-carotene, anthocyanins, lycopene, and lutein, as well as antioxidants such as flavonoids, polyphenols, resveratrol, and omega-3 polyunsaturated fatty acids, all of which contribute to enhancing the skin's defense against UV damage [14].

Medication therapy: Medication therapy for skin aging primarily involves oral antioxidants, including coenzyme Q10, superoxide dismutase, catalase, lutein, vitamins C and E, and omega-3 polyunsaturated fatty acids. These agents work by neutralizing reactive oxygen species, reducing the activation of the MAPK pathway, and decreasing collagen degradation mediated by matrix metalloproteinases (MMPs). Systemic hormone replacement therapy in menopausal women also has antiaging effects by maintaining the activity of epidermal keratinocytes and dermal fibroblasts. Topical medications with antiaging effects include (1) antioxidants such as vitamin C, vitamin B, vitamin E, and polyphenols and (2) agents promoting collagen and elastin synthesis, such as retinoic acid and its derivatives, salicylic acid, etc. Both systemic and topical medications exhibit slow onset, limited efficacy, and challenges in long-term adherence.

Chemical and physical exfoliation treatments include various chemical peels that use acids such as trichloroacetic acid, fruit acids, salicylic acid, and microdermabrasion. These treatments promote the shedding of aged keratinocytes, accelerating epidermal cell turnover and stimulating fibroblast proliferation and activity in the dermis, which increases the synthesis of dermal collagen and elastic fibers. These methods primarily target the exfoliation of the epidermis and are effective for addressing pigmentation and superficial wrinkles caused by photoaging. However, their efficacy is limited for severe skin photoaging or natural aging, and there is a risk of residual pigmentation.

Photothermal therapy targets skin aging markers such as pigments, blood vessels, and collagen via the use of light-induced heat to improve pigmentation, dilated capillaries, skin laxity, and wrinkling. These methods can be categorized into nonablative and ablative photothermal therapies on the basis of the extent of damage. Nonablative photothermal therapy, such as intense pulsed light (IPL) and PDT, causes minimal damage and is milder. It targets vessels with pulsed dye lasers (585 nm), pigments with KTP532 lasers, alexandrite lasers (755 nm), and picosecond lasers (755 nm), and collagen with nonablative fractional lasers such as 1540 nm, 1550 nm, 1565 nm lasers, and honeycomb picosecond lasers. Ablative fractional lasers, including the 10,600-nm CO_2 laser and 2940-nm erbium laser, promote collagen synthesis through controlled damage, rejuvenating the skin but increasing the risk of scarring and pigmentation due to deeper damage. Additionally, radiofrequency treatments such as Thermage®, Thermolift®, and focused ultrasound can stimulate collagen remodeling for skin tightening, although their effects are more prominent in the deep dermis, with a limited impact on the epidermis and a risk of burns during treatment.

PDT is a promising drug–device combination treatment that offers several advantages over traditional methods, such as being nonablative, having low toxicity, good local selectivity, and reproducibility, and having few side effects and drug resistance. Both clinical and basic studies have confirmed the effectiveness of PDT as an antiaging agent. In 2002, Ruiz-Rodriguez et al. introduced the concept of photodynamic skin rejuvenation [15], and since then, PDT has gained significant attention for treating skin photoaging and rejuvenation, with reports of its remarkable cosmetic benefits for photodamaged skin. In previous studies, our research group applied PDT to treat photoaging skin in various areas, such as the forearms, face, and neck, and found that it improved skin photoaging [16–19]. The rejuvenating effects of PDT are long-lasting, with continuous improvement in wrinkles observed even 2 years after treatment [16]. The European Dermatology Forum (EDF) Guidelines recommend topical PDT for skin rejuvenation with a Grade A recommendation and level I evidence [20].

Injectable therapies include (1) neurotoxin agents such as botulinum toxin for improving dynamic wrinkles; (2) injectable filling agents such as hyaluronic acid for reducing wrinkles; and (3) injection of active nutritional factors, commonly referred to as or mesoplasty, to increase fibroblast activity and improve the state of aging skin, including growth factors, amino acids, and autologous platelet-rich plasma [21]. However, injectable treatments are invasive and carry a risk of infection.

10.2 ALA-PDT Mechanisms in Skin Rejuvenation

PDT is a noninvasive approach based on the application of photosensitizers to skin lesions followed by irradiation with light sources [15, 22]. ALA, a second-generation photosensitizer developed in recent years, serves as a precursor in hemoglobin synthesis within the body. Although ALA is naturally present in cells in very small amounts and is not photosensitive by itself, exogenous ALA can penetrate the stratum corneum and sebaceous units, where it is converted into photosensitive porphyrin compounds such as PpIX. When irradiated with specific wavelengths of light, these compounds undergo a photodynamic reaction, producing singlet oxygen and other biological effects [23]. The main mechanism of skin rejuvenation involves the removal of senescent cells while also indirectly remodeling the dermal extracellular matrix by the secretion of cytokines into dermal cells [24]. PDT not only enhances the function of keratinocytes (KCs) and fibroblasts (FBs) but also modulates the skin microenvironment, ultimately reversing skin aging (Fig. 10.1).

10.2.1 Epidermal Reconstruction by ALA-PDT

Intrinsic skin aging is characterized by skin thinning and reduced proliferation of KCs and FBs. Low-dose photodynamic therapy (PDT) using 0.1 mM methyl 5-aminolevulinate hydrochloride (MAL) and 3.72 J/cm^2 red light was found to mildly increase endogenous reactive oxygen species (ROS) levels, thereby promoting the proliferation of human immortalized keratinocytes (HaCaT) cells. However, higher concentrations of MAL (0.5 mM or 1 mM) inhibited HaCaT cell growth. Further studies revealed that transient cyclin D1 expression, driven by SRC kinase activity, stimulated KC growth [25], suggesting that ALA-PDT may similarly enhance KC proliferation through low-dose ROS. Consistent with these findings, the authors administered three low-dose ALA-PDT treatments to 15-month-old naturally aging SKH-1 mice, resulting in increased epidermal thickness and enhanced cell proliferation [13].

Orringer et al. treated 25 adult volunteers with forearm photoaging via ALA combined with a pulsed dye laser and reported a reduction in pho-

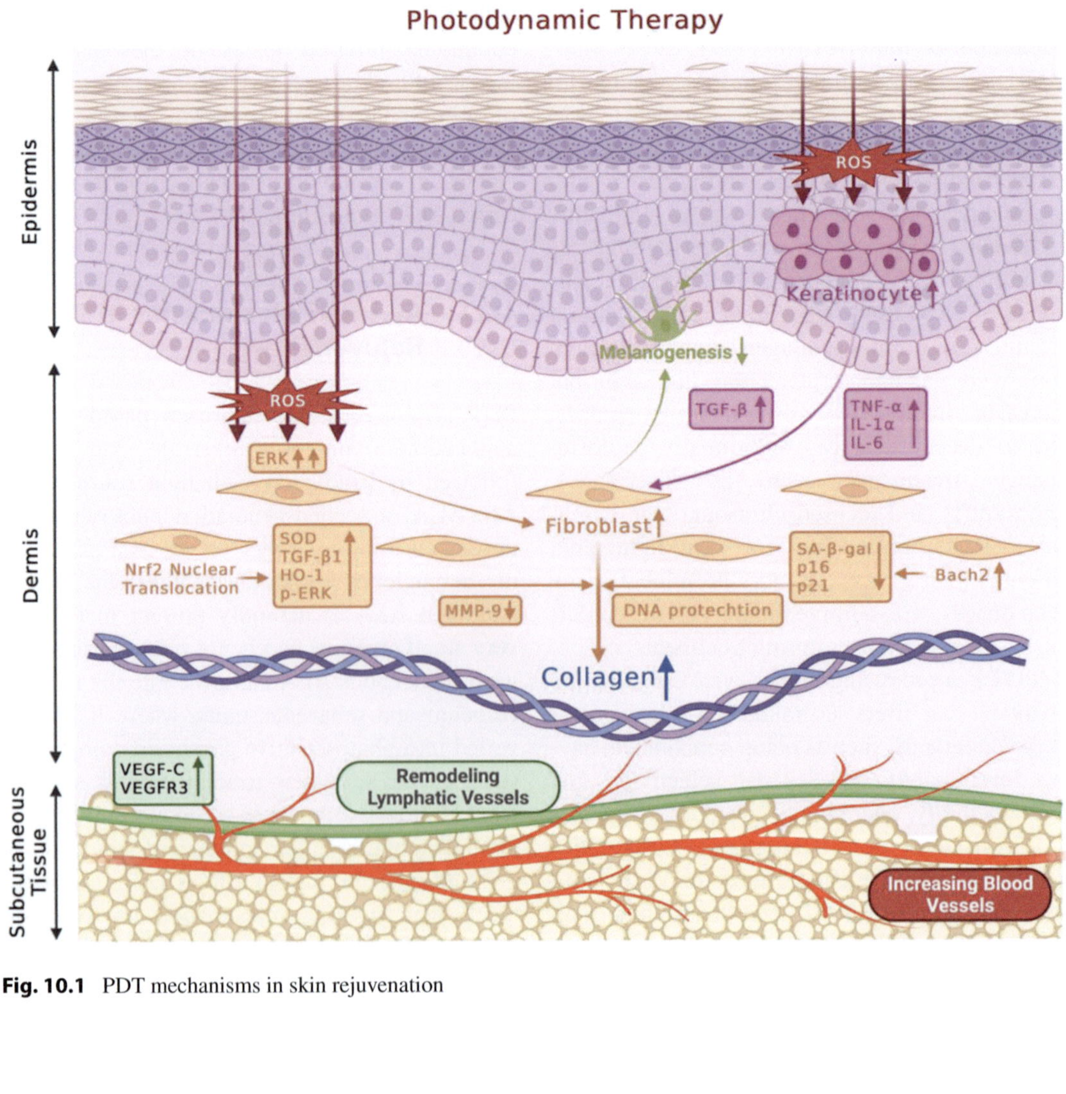

Fig. 10.1 PDT mechanisms in skin rejuvenation

todamaged cells, a significant decrease in p53 expression (an early marker of epidermal carcinogenesis), and a greater than fivefold increase in the proliferation marker Ki-67 ($P < 0.05$). Additionally, epidermal reconstruction occurred, with a greater than 1.4-fold increase in epidermal thickness ($P < 0.05$) [26]. However, the effects of ALA-PDT on Ki-67 in photodamaged skin remain inconsistent. Bagazgoitia et al. reported that PDT reduced both Ki-67 and p53 expression, suggesting a reversal of the carcinogenic process and a link to the tumor microenvironment (TME) in photodamaged skin [27].

10.2.2 Dermal Reconstruction by ALA-PDT

Many studies have confirmed that PDT can increase collagen production. Fink-Puches et al. reported significant fibrosis and histopathological alterations in the dermis in 1998, suggesting that ALA-PDT increases collagen production [28]. A subsequent split-face study by Marmur et al. confirmed the findings of Fink-Puches, who reported a notable increase in type I collagen fibers in the ALA-IPL group [29]. Similarly, Szeimies et al. demonstrated increased collagen production and reduced solar elastosis after three consecutive MAL-PDT sessions with red light across the entire photodamaged area [30]. These histological findings support the notion that PDT improves photoaged skin by remodeling the dermal matrix.

Jang et al. investigated the molecular mechanisms underlying photorejuvenation following PDT in dermal fibroblasts and reported that PDT-generated ROS activate the extracellular signal-regulated kinase (ERK) pathway, leading to increased fibroblast proliferation and motility [31]. Prolonged ERK activation upregulated MMP-3 and collagen type Iα expression, whereas NAC (an antioxidant) inhibited both fibroblast proliferation and ERK activation, indicating that low ROS levels resulting from low-dose PDT have growth-promoting effects. These findings suggest that the intracellular ROS generated by low-level PDT can activate the MAPK and ERK pathways, stimulating fibroblast activity, enhancing collagen synthesis, and contributing to skin rejuvenation.

10.2.3 Crosstalk Between Keratinocytes and Fibroblasts

Research has established that crosstalk between KCs and FBs regulates collagen synthesis [32]. Kim et al. explored keratinocyte–fibroblast interactions during PDT for photoaging and revealed that cytokines secreted by KCs post-PDT, such as IL-1α, IL-6, and TNF-α, reduce MMP-1 expression and increase collagen type Iα expression, indicating that PDT indirectly promotes collagen synthesis in FBs via KC-derived cytokines [33]. The same team reported that PDT reduced melanogenesis in melanocytes (MCs) through paracrine effects from KCs and FBs, improving mottled hyperpigmentation in photodamaged skin [34]. Wang et al. demonstrated that low-dose ALA-PDT (<2 J/cm^2) enhances FB collagen synthesis and proliferation via TGF-β activation from KCs, promoting dermal collagen synthesis in a photoaged mouse model [35]. Interestingly, red PpIX fluorescence was primarily observed in the epidermis and hair follicles, with a minimal presence in the dermis, indicating that low-dose ALA-PDT remodeled dermal collagen indirectly.

10.2.4 Reduction in Oxidative Stress

Chen et al. demonstrated that the antioxidant effects of low-dose PDT on UV-induced photoaging in human dermal fibroblasts (HDFs) are significantly mediated by nuclear factor erythroid 2-related factor 2 (Nrf2) [36]. Following ALA-PDT treatment (0.1 mmol/L ALA and 21 J/cm^2 red light), superoxide dismutase (SOD) activity increased, and Nrf2 translocated into the nucleus, leading to the upregulation of TGF-β1 and collagen types I and III, whereas MMP-9 expression decreased. These molecular changes promoted collagen remodeling and mitigated oxidative stress in HDFs. Notably, when Nrf2 was knocked down, both the antioxidative effects and collagen synthesis were significantly reduced, underscoring the pivotal role of Nrf2 in the photorejuvenation process.

10.2.5 Prevention of DNA Damage

Bach2, a key regulator of cell senescence and DNA damage, has been implicated in ALA-PDT treatment of skin photoaging both in vivo and in vitro. Low-dose PDT was shown to increase Bach2 accumulation, which coincided with a reduction in senescence-associated β-galactosidase (SA-β-gal) activity and decreased expression of the senescence markers p16 and p21 in photodamaged fibroblasts [24]. Furthermore, silencing Bach2 induced cellular senescence, whereas Bach2 knockdown combined with PDT led to a further decrease in SA-β-gal activity, highlighting Bach2's crucial role in mitigating cellular senescence and enhancing the antiaging effects of PDT.

10.2.6 Improving the Skin Microenvironment by ALA-PDT

Remodeling lymphatic vessels: Recent studies have highlighted the multifaceted effects of low-dose ALA-PDT on skin rejuvenation. One study demonstrated that low-dose ALA-PDT (3% ALA, 6.0 J/cm^2 red light) significantly increased lymphatic vessel density and function in intrinsically aged SKH-1 mice [13]. This treatment not only improved skin thickness and smoothness but also enhanced lymphatic drainage, as evidenced by the Evans blue assay. Mechanistically, this LV remodeling was mediated via the VEGF-C/VEGFR3 pathway, accompanied by increased VE-cadherin expression, which contributed to improved lymphatic function.

Remodeling the cutaneous immune microenvironment: A recent human single-cell sequencing study revealed that ALA-PDT could rejuvenate the cutaneous immune microenvironment by partially reversing immunosenescence and alleviating the immunosuppressive state in photoaged skin. The therapy improved immune cell function, reduced cellular senescence, and mitigated hypoxia and reactive oxygen species (ROS) levels in immune cells. Notably, it increases the activity of immune receptors and increases the proportion of naïve T cells while also enhancing the functionality of various immune cells, including T cells, macrophages, Langerhans cells, dendritic cells, and mast cells, thereby promoting a more robust and youthful immune response in the skin [37].

10.3 Clinical Application

The absorption spectrum of PpIX spans the entire visible range, making various light sources suitable for PDT, including light-emitting diodes (LEDs), intense pulsed light (IPL), pulsed dye lasers (PDLs), and light-emitting lamps. In recent years, daylight-PDT and sequential combination therapies have also been explored for skin rejuvenation. Clinical studies have demonstrated the effectiveness of PDT in improving signs of photoaging, with outcomes varying with the light source used, as summarized in Tables 10.1 and 10.2.

10.3.1 Indications and Contraindications

PDT is suitable for individuals with various signs of skin aging, including wrinkles, epidermal thinning, pigmentation, and telangiectasia. However, it is contraindicated in individuals with known allergies to photosensitizers or photosensitive conditions, particularly porphyria, active connective tissue diseases, solar urticaria, or polymorphic light eruption.

Table 10.1 Summary of studies on PDT with a single light source in photorejuvenation

Light source and parameters	PS (incubation time)	Study design	Patient characteristics	Sessions (follow-up)	Assessment	Side effects	Results	References
IPL (515–1200 nm, 23–28 J/cm^2, double pulse of 2.4 and 4 ms)	Topical 5-ALA solution (30–60 min)	Prospective, randomized, controlled, split-face study	20 patients with at least a modest degree of photoaging	Three split-face treatments with IPL and IPL-ALA, two sessions with IPL only (1 month)	Global photodamage, fine lines, mottled pigmentation, tactile roughness, and sallowness (on a scale of 0–4)	Erythema, edema, scaling and dryness is more frequent in ALA-IPL side	ALA-IPL vs IPL: 80% vs 45% for the improvement of photoaging ($p = 0.008$), 85% vs 20% for mottled pigmentation ($p < 0.001$), 60% vs 25% for fine lines ($p = 0.008$)	Dover et al. [22]
IPL (550 nm and 570 nm, 34 J/cm^2, double pulsing with a 20-m/s delay)	ALA (30–60 min)	Prospective, randomized, controlled, split-face study	16 patients with mild-to-moderate photodamage and at least three facial AKs	Three sessions (1 and 3 months)	Score of tactile skin roughness, crow's feet appearance, mottled hyperpigmentation, facial telangiectasias, and facial AKs	Erythema and edema	Short-contact ALA-IPL vs IPL: 55% vs 29.5% for the improvement of crow's feet appearance, 55% vs 29.5% for mottled pigmentation, 60.3% vs 37.2% for mottled hyperpigmentation	Gold et al. [38]

(continued)

Table 10.1 (continued)

Light source and parameters	PS (incubation time)	Study design	Patient characteristics	Sessions (follow-up)	Assessment	Side effects	Results	References
IPL (530–750 nm, 7 J/cm², double pulses of 2.5 ms, delay 10 ms); (400–720 nm, 3.5 J/cm², long pulse duration of 30 ms)	0.5% liposome encapsulated 5-ALA (1 h)	Randomized, prospective, split face study	37 healthy female patients	Three sessions (3-month)	Fitzpatrick wrinkle scale	No side effects were observed	C-PDT vs PDT-alone: 1.2 vs 1.1 for reduction of periorbital wrinkles, 0.8 vs 0.7 for reduction of perioral wrinkles ($p = 0.224$)	Bjerring et al. [39]
IPL (500–670 and 870–1400 nm, 23–30 J/cm²)	5% ALA (2 h)	Comparative split-face study	16 Japanese women with slight-to-mild facial photodamage	Three sessions (1 and 3 months)	Mottled pigmentation, crow's feet appearance, fine lines, tactile roughness and sallowness (on a five-point scale)	IPL-ALA-PDT-treated side showed mild-to-severe symptoms of pain, burning sensation or erythema	No significant difference of the reduction in the photoaging score between the two sides, but 75% of subjects felt better on the PDT-treated side than IPL-treated side	Kosaka et al. [40]
IPL (20, 25, 40, and 50 J/cm²)	ALA (2 h)	Randomized, controlled study	24 patients with five or more AK lesions and moderate-to-severe photodamage	One session (5–7 days and 8 weeks)	Nine-point photonumeric Griffiths scale for photodamage	Erythema, crusts erosion, edema	40 and 50 J/cm² have better efficacy for AK ($p = 0.018$ and 0.016), but no significant improvement of photodamaged skin	Haddad et al. [41]
IPL (400–720 nm, 3.5 J/cm² energy and 30 ms duration) long pulsed Nd:YAG laser (61.8–83.9 J/cm²)	0.5% liposome-encapsulated 5-ALA (applied every 5 min in 1 h)	Randomized controlled split face study	12 patients with two or more scores of periorbital wrinkles	Three sessions (12 weeks after last session)	Fitzpatrick wrinkle classification system (FWCS)	Five patients reported transient erythema	IPL-PDT vs LPNY: 0.9 vs 0.3 for lateral periorbital wrinkles ($p = 0.02$) (IPL-PDT showed better results than LPNY)	Shin et al. [42]

IPL (≥600 nm, 16.2 J/cm², three passes, ellipse flex PPT)	1% MAL (3 h)	Prospective, randomized, placebo-controlled, monocentric, within-patient, observer blinded	37 patients with 1–4 AK and severe photodamaged skin on the dorsal hands	Three treatments of MAL-IPL and placebo-IPL (10 weeks)	Complete AK clearance per hand, neocollagenesis of subepidermal collagen, mottled pigmentation, overall appearance and wrinkles	The incidence of mild erythema, scaling, and crusting is significantly higher in MAL-IPL group	MAL-IPL vs placebo-IPL: 2.4 ± 2.0 vs 2.1 ± 2.1 for improvement in mottled pigmentation ($p = 0.032$), 2.2 ± 1.7 vs 1.8 ± 1.7 for improvement in overall appearance ($p = 0.042$)	Kohl et al. [43]
IPL (615 nm, 40 J/cm², double pulse, 4 ms)	20% ALA (4 h)	Uncontrolled	17 patients with varying degrees of photodamage and AKs	Two sessions (1 and 3 months)	Pigmentary alterations, scarring	Erythema and edema with crusting in 10 days	Distinct improvement of skin texture, no pigmentary alterations or scarring and reduction of 91% of AK lesions	Ruiz-Rodriguez et al. [15]
IPL (420–720 nm, 3.5 J/cm² energy and 30-ms duration single spots for a total of 10.5 J/cm² energy)	0.5% ALA in spray formulation (applied every 5 min in 1 h)	Uncontrolled	30 healthy volunteers	Three sessions (1 week and 3 months)	Wrinkle depth by modified Fitzpatrick wrinkle scale (MFWS)	No side effects were observed during and after treatment	The average overall improvement was greater for periorbital (73%) than for nasolabial wrinkles (50%)	Piccioni et al. [44]

(continued)

Table 10.1 (continued)

Light source and parameters	PS (incubation time)	Study design	Patient characteristics	Sessions (follow-up)	Assessment	Side effects	Results	References
VPL (610–950 nm, 80 J/cm^2, double pulsed at 40 J/cm^2) LED (50 mW/cm^2, 37 J/cm^2)	16% MAL (3 h)	Prospective, randomized, controlled split-face study	25 patients with mild-to-moderate AK (forehead and scalp)	One session (2 weeks, 3 months)	Sense of pain (primary outcome measure), lesion response, cosmesis and patient satisfaction (secondary outcome measures)	Pain, redness, hypopigmentation, crusting, and burning sensation	VPL and LED are equivalent in AK clearance and cosmetic effects, but VPL cause significantly less pain than LED ($p < 0.001$)	Babilas et al. [45]
Red light (Aktilite®; Galderma, 8 min at 37 J/cm^2)	0.5 g MAL (3 h)	Prospective, double-blind, double-arm, randomized, placebo-controlled trial	65 patients with a symmetrical photodamage grade of 2 or 3	Two sessions (1 month)	Dover modified global Photodamage severity score and histological changes	Erythema, edema, scaling, and dryness is more frequent in ALA-IPL side	There was an increase in dermal thickness ($P < 0.01$) and improvement in collagen, elastic tissue and perifollicular fibrosis after the treatment of MAL plus red light	Sanclemente et al. [46]
Red light (630 nm, 37 J/cm^2)	MAL (3 h)	Prospective, controlled study	26 patients with photodamaged skin and multiple facial AK	Three sessions (3 months)	Five-point scale for photodamage, number of AKs, histopathological and immunohistochemical changes	Erythema and edema is common, and crusts and erosions resolved within 1 week	Photodamaged skin achieved significant improvement in the global score ($P < 0.001$)	Szeimies et al. [30]
Red light or blue light	MAL (3 h)	Prospective, single center trial	18 patients with moderate-to-severe photodamage of the head or upper trunk	One session (0, 2, 7, and 30 days)	Signs of photodamage	Mild erythema	No significant difference between blue and red light in efficacy	Palm et al. [47]

Red light (630 nm, 50 mW/cm^2)	10% ALA (2 h)	Comparative, controlled study	14 patients with photoaging skin	Two sessions with PDT and 12 sessions with red light alone (2 weeks and 4 weeks)	Signs of photodamage, SC hydration, TEWL, L*a*b* values	Mild erythema	Noticeable and more prominent improvement in tactile roughness and hyperpigmentation, significant improvement in SC hydration ($P = 0.002$) and TEWL ($P < 0.001$) after two-session PDT	Ji et al. [17]
Red light (630 nm, 60 J/cm^2) IPL (520–1200 nm, 60 J/cm^2)	5% ALA (2 h)	Randomized, double-blinded and controlled prospective study	14 patients with photoaging skin	Two sessions (4 and 8 weeks)	Signs of photodamage, SC hydration, TEWL, color coordinates (L*a*b* values), MI, EI, skin elasticity	Pain, erythema, edema, and hyperpigmentation	The SC hydration, L* value, elasticity and thickness increased, whereas the TEWL and MI value decreased. Red-light-PDT and IPL-PDT group were more obvious than IPL group ($P < 0.05$)	Zhang et al. [18]

Table 10.1 (continued)

Light source and parameters	PS (incubation time)	Study design	Patient characteristics	Sessions (follow-up)	Assessment	Side effects	Results	References
Red light (633 nm ± 6 nm, 36 J/cm^2, Omnilux, British)	10% ALA (3 h)	Retrospective study	10 patients with AK	Several sessions until lesions achieved complete response (1, 6, and 24 months)	Global scores of photoaging (GSP)	Pain	GSP scores in 1 month ($p < 0.05$) and 6 months ($p < 0.01$) were significant lower than at baseline. The significant improvement of fine lines ($p < 0.05$), mottled pigmentation ($p < 0.05$) lasted for 24 months	Zhang et al. [16]
Blue light (417 ± 5 nm, 16 min and 40 s, 10 J/cm^2)	20% δ-ALA solution (1, 2, or 3 h)	Spilt-face, placebo-controlled RCT	18 patients with at least four facial AKs and mild-to-moderate diffuse facial photodamage	One sessions (1 day, 1 week, 1 month, and 5 months)	Eight-point Griffiths score index in specific features and 6-grade of global cosmetic improvements	Mild to moderate pain during treatment and moderate phototoxic effects for 1 week	At 1 and 5 months there was a significant effect of fine wrinkling ($P < 0.002$), sallowness ($P < 0.001$), mottled pigmentation ($P = 0.05$)	Touma et al. [48]
PDL (595 nm, 4–7.5 J/cm^2 fluences, 10 ms pulse duration, 10-mm spot size)	20% ALA (3 h or overnight)	Prospective, controlled study	41 patients between 35 and 91 years old with AKs	One session (10 days,2 months, 4 months, 6 months and 8 months)	The cleared percentage of AKs	Slight pain; slight-to-moderate erythema	PDL-PDT achieved 90% reduction of AK lesion at 4-months follow-up and excellent posttreatment cosmesis	Alexiades-Armenakas et al. [49]

Indoor daylight (400–700 nm, 120 min, 52.3 J/cm^2) Red light (630 ± 5 nm, 8 min, 37 J/cm^2)	MAL (30 min)	Comparative, intrapatient, split-face, randomized clinical trial	43 patients with more than 5 AKs lesions on the face or scalp	Two sessions (3 months)	The number and area of AKs and four categories of cosmetic outcome	cPDT was more painful than idlPDT	Roughness ($P <$ 0.001) and erythema ($P <$ 0.001) of the cosmetic outcome had a significant improvement, the scores of global photodamage, fine lines, mottled pigmentation, tactile roughness, and sallowness were not significantly different in two groups	Arisi et al. [50]
Daylight (10,000 lux) AFL (single pass, 22% density, 7.5–37.5 J/cm^2, 10–50 J/cm^2, 12.5–25 J/cm^2, and 7–30 J/cm^2)	MAL (30 min)	Randomized, side-by-side, single-blind trial	18 patients with symmetrical AKs and photodamage	One session (3 months)	AK clearance, global photodamage and telangiectasia, dyspigmentation and skin texture on a four-point severity scale	AFL-PDT vs MD-PDT: pain (mean 3 vs 5, $P = 0.002$), crusting (1 vs 0, $P = 0.004$), erythema (3 vs 2, $P = 0.002$) on day 1	AFL-PDT vs MD-PDT:AK clearance (81% vs 60%, $P < 0.001$), improvement in skin texture ($P = 0.001$) and dyspigmentation ($P = 0.003$), higher preference of patients (12 vs 4, $P = 0.077$)	Wenande et al. [51]

(continued)

Table 10.2 Summary of studies on the use of PDT with multiple light sources for photorejuvenation

Light sources	PS (incubation time)	Study design	Patient characteristics	Sessions (follow-up)	Assessment	Side effects	Results	References
IPL + red light	20% ALA (1 h)	Prospective, controlled study	21 patients with a maximum of four nonhyperkeratotic AKs	One session (3 months and 6 months)	Five-point standardized photoaging scale	Fine, discreet, hyperpigmented crusting	The global photoaging scores, including fine lines, mottled pigmentation, sallowness, tactile roughness, and telangiectasias improved significantly ($p < 0.05$ vs baseline) ($p < 0.05$ vs 3 months)	Clementoni et al. [52]
Blue light + PDL, blue light + IPL, blue light + PDL + IPL, or blue light + red light + PDL + IPL	20% ALA (1 h)	Retrospective, single-center study	96 patients with Fitzpatrick skin types I–III	Several (one to three) sessions per patient preference	0 = none, 1 = mild, 2 = moderate/good, 3 = excellent for improvement in photodamage or overall skin quality	Erythema, acne flares, peeling, and pain	Mean degree of photodamage improvement was 1.7 ± 0.5, mean improvement of overall skin quality was 1.8 ± 0.2. There were no significant difference among groups	Friedmann et al. [53]
Red light + IPL, red light alone	10% ALA gel (30 min)	Single-site prospective, randomized, intraindividual split chest pilot study	18 patients with moderate-to-severe photodamage	Two sessions (1, 4, 12, and 24 weeks)	Global aesthetic improvement scale (GAIS)	No local or systemic adverse effects were reported	ALA-PDT + IPL vs ALA-PDT: 3.57 ± 0.09 vs 2.89 ± 0.09 of mean GAIS scores	Abrouk et al. [54]
PDL, PDL + blue light, IPL, and IPL + blue light	20% ALA (2 h)	Prospective study	220 patients with either photodamage or AK (126 received treatment for photodamage)	One session (1 month)	Improvement of photodamage on a scale of 0–4	No side effects were reported	PDL vs PDL + blue light vs IPL vs IPL + blue light: 1.5 vs 1.8 vs 2.9 vs 3.0 of improvement score at 1-month follow-up	Abrouk et al. [55]

10.3.2 Selection and Application of Photosensitizers

5-Aminolevulinic acid (5-ALA, Levulan® Kerastick or other ALA formulation) and methyl aminolevulinate (MAL, Metvix® 160 mg/g cream) are the most commonly used photosensitizers in dermatology [56]. ALA is a precursor of PpIX in the heme biosynthesis pathway, whereas MAL, an ester of ALA, converts to PpIX within target cells [57, 58]. ALA concentrations typically range from 0.5% to 20%. In a controlled study of red-light PDT for forearm photoaging, the authors reported that after 2 h of incubation, the PpIX fluorescence was greater in the 10% and 20% ALA groups than in the 5% ALA group, with no significant difference between the 10% and 20% groups [59]. However, PDT treatment with 10% and 20% ALA cream resulted in increased local pain, erythema, edema, and post-treatment pigmentation. To reduce these adverse effects, novel ALA-based photosensitizers, such as 0.5% ALA liposomal spray and 2% ALA gel containing hyaluronic acid, have been reported for PDT rejuvenation [60, 61].

On the basis of early-stage basic and clinical research, as well as patient experiences, the authors' group recommended that low-dose PDT treatment be used in clinical practice, with an ALA concentration of 5%–10% and an incubation time of 2 h in the dark. For daylight PDT (DL-PDT) and modified painless photodynamic therapy (M-PDT), the incubation time can be reduced to just 30 min.

10.3.3 Light Sources for PDT

ALA can be activated to promote the photodynamic reaction when exposed to an appropriate wavelength of light. Various light sources, including LEDs, IPL, PDL, and daylight, have been utilized to trigger this photodynamic action. Recently, studies have explored the synergistic efficacy of multiple light sources in sequential combination modalities of PDT [54, 55].

The Red-Light PDT FDA has approved the therapeutic protocol of LED-generated red light combined with MAL to treat minimally to moderately thick actinic keratosis (AK) on the scalp and face. The longer the wavelength of a light source is, the deeper it penetrates skin tissues. Red light (630–700 nm) can reach the dermis and stimulate fibroblast proliferation [62]. As a result, red light is frequently used in PDT for treating AK and photoaging. The commonly used regimens for photoaging treatment with red-light PDT are listed in Table 10.3.

A randomized controlled trial (RCT) demonstrated significant improvements on the MAL plus red-light treatment side compared with the placebo plus red light side, with notable improvements in fine lines, mottled hyperpigmentation, tactile roughness, sallowness, and erythema, although telangiectasia was unaffected [63]. Facial global photodamage improved in 68.8% of the patients, and 29.2% succeeded in the MAL-red light group, whereas the placebo group

Table 10.3 ALA-PDT-recommended antiaging regimens

		ALA				Illumination dose	
Treatment regimen	Pretreatment method	Dosage form	Concentration (%)	Light source	Application time (h)	Power density (mW/cm^2)	Energy density (J/cm^2)
C-PDT	Clean the skin	Creams, gels, or solutions	5–10	Red light	3–6	40–100	80–120
M-PDT	Clean the skin	Creams, gels, or solutions	5–10	Red light	0.5	40	100–150

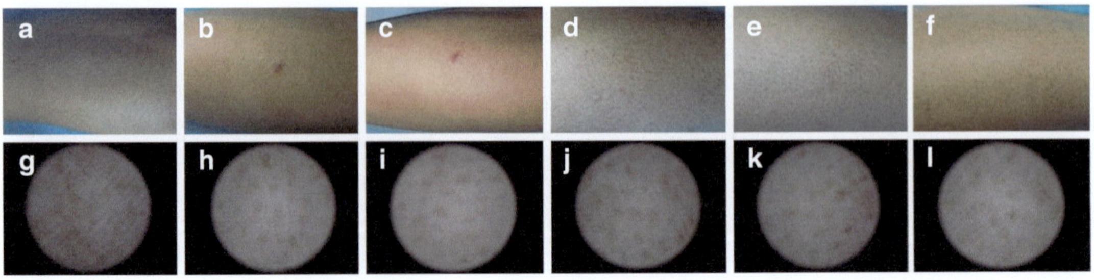

Fig. 10.2 Clinical (upper row) and dermoscopic (lower row) appearance of photoaged skin on the forearm after red-light-PDT and red light alone. Compared with red-light treatment, red-light-PDT improved the firmness and pigmentation of photoaged forearm skin more strongly. (**a**, **g**) Before red-light PDT treatment, (**b**, **h**) after 4 weeks of red-light-PDT treatment, (**c**, **i**) after 6 weeks of red-light PDT treatment, (**d**, **j**) before red-light treatment, (**e**, **k**) after 4 weeks of red-light treatment, and (**f**, **l**) after 6 weeks of red-light treatment

showed no improvement. However, adverse effects were more common on the MAL-red light side. A comparative study also revealed that the combination of ALA and red light was more effective than red light alone, with both groups showing increases in collagen and elastic fiber density [17] (Fig. 10.2). Another RCT revealed a significant increase in dermal thickness in photodamaged skin after MAL plus red-light treatment in a split-face, placebo-controlled model [46]. Histopathological improvements were observed in collagen, elastic tissue, and perifollicular fibrosis, but the results were not statistically significant.

Numerous studies have demonstrated the cosmetic benefits of PDT for facial photoaging, and skin rejuvenation of the neck has also been reported. Zhang et al. investigated the use of red-light PDT, and their findings revealed that IPL-PDT had better skin rejuvenation effects than IPL treatment alone on neck skin [18] (Fig. 10.3). Since the skin on the neck is thinner than that on the face or upper arms, adverse reactions such as erythema and hyperpigmentation occur more frequently. However, exposure to light alone and PDT did not affect the function or size of the thyroid.

Pretreatment to maximize photosensitizer penetration has been explored to improve the effectiveness of PDT. In a randomized study involving 15 patients, ablative fractional laser resurfacing (AFXL) prior to 3-h MAL application combined with red-light irradiation led to improvements in AK and photoaging, such as skin texture and pigmentation. However, this approach also increases the incidence of acute reactions and long-term adverse effects [64]. Another RCT using a fractional 1927-nm thulium laser (TL) consistently concluded that combining TL with PDT enhanced the antiphotoaging effects, particularly with respect to skin texture [65].

A retrospective clinical study investigated the long-term (over 12 months) rejuvenating effect of low-dose ALA-PDT with red light (36 J/cm^2) as the light source on photoaging in Chinese patients [16] (Fig. 10.4). The study revealed that improvements in mottled pigmentation and fine lines lasted for up to 24 months, demonstrating that PDT with a red LED produced a prolonged antiphotoaging effect.

Another FDA-approved PDT regimen for AK is the combination of ALA and blue light (400–480 nm). While blue light is less commonly used for treating skin cancers because of its shorter wavelength, several studies have demonstrated its efficacy for photoaging [47, 48, 66]. One case report revealed that PDT with blue light effectively treated multiple nonhyperkeratotic AKs and improved the appearance of photodamaged skin, including increased skin elasticity and decreased skin thickness [66]. Touma et al. reported a nearly 90% clearance rate of AK and significant improvements in mottled hyperpigmentation, skin quality, sallowness, and fine wrinkles after one session of ALA-PDT with blue light. However, coarse wrinkling does not improve with a single treatment [48]. PDT with

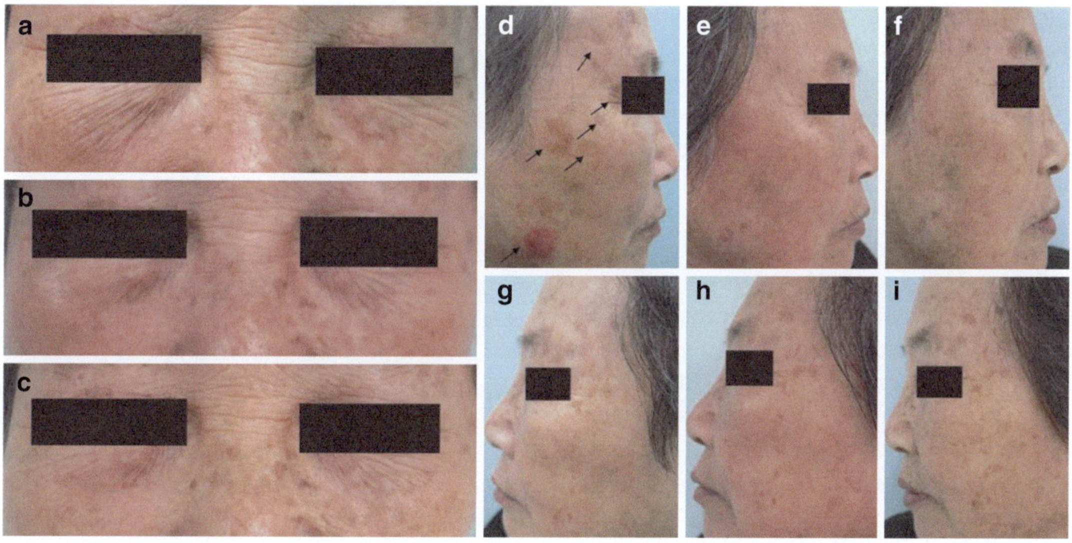

Fig. 10.3 Red-light-PDT has a long-lasting effect on skin wrinkles. The right side was subjected to PDT regional surface treatment, and the wrinkled area was treated at the same time. The left side was only treated with AK lesions, the wrinkled area was not treated, and the wrinkles and pigmentation on the right side were significantly reduced. (**a**, **d**, **g**) Before treatment and (**b**, **e**, **h**) 6 months after treatment, fine lines, facial pigmentation, and AK lesions (indicated by black arrows) improved on the right side of the face, and fine lines and pigmentation could still be observed on the left side. (**c**, **f**, **i**) Wrinkles and pigmentation continued to improve after 2 years of treatment

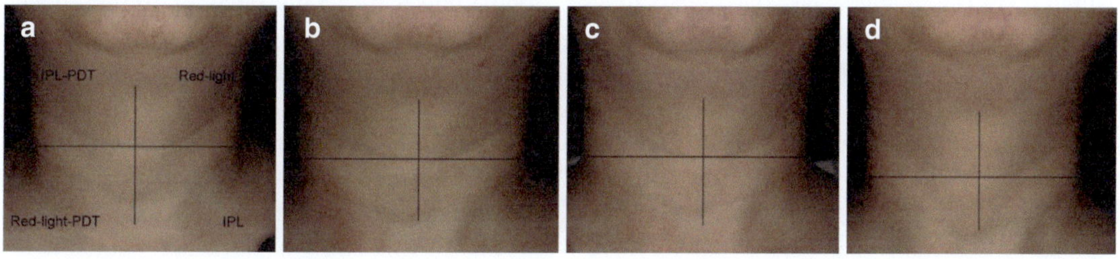

Fig. 10.4 Improving the photoaging of neck skin after treatment with red light, red-light-PDT, IPL-PDT, and IPL alone. (**a**) 0 weeks: the skin on the neck before treatment shows the characteristic appearance of photoaging; (**b**) 4 weeks after the first treatment. Significant pigmentation in the red-light PDT-treated area; (**c**) 8 weeks: 4 weeks after the second treatment. Fine and deep wrinkles and pigmentation in the IPL-PDT-treated area were visibly improved. There was little to no pigmentation in the red-light PDT area; (**d**) 12 weeks: 8 weeks after the second treatment. Red-light PDT and IPL-PDT are more effective than IPL alone in improving pigmentation and coarse wrinkles of photoaging skin on the neck. Red-light PDT is not as effective as IPL-PDT in improving photoaging skin on the neck

an LED as the light source is suitable for patients with AK and photoaging. A study comparing blue and red light for the treatment of photodamaged skin revealed that both protocols had equivalent effectiveness and moderate adverse effects [47], suggesting that more studies are needed to compare their skin rejuvenation effects.

PDT with Intense Pulsed Light The first report of PDT and IPL was by Ruiz-Rodriguez et al. in 2002, coining the term "photodynamic photorejuvenation" [15] and demonstrating a 90% clearance rate of AK lesions with excellent cosmetic outcomes, including no pigmentation or scarring. IPL alone stimulates the recovery process by promoting new collagen formation and enhancing dermal remodeling, leading to improved skin elasticity and reduced fine wrinkles. When combined with PDT, IPL enhances these effects, resulting in synergistic benefits. Compared with IPL treatment alone, split-face studies have shown that IPL-PDT offers superior cosmetic improvements in terms of global photoaging scores [22, 40], mottled pigmentation [22, 38], fine lines [22], crow's feet, skin roughness, and telangectasias [38]. However, it does not significantly change tactile roughness or sallowness [22, 40]. Compared with placebo-IPL, IPL-PDT also significantly improves mottled pigmentation and overall appearance, particularly on the atrophic skin of the dorsal hand, but does not result in major differences in skin roughness or wrinkle size and depth [43]. Kosaka et al. demonstrated that the IPL-ALA-PDT protocol is effective for Asian patients with darker skin [40]. Even a short application of ALA (30–60 min) followed by exposure to IPL results in more significant improvements in photoaging than IPL alone [38]. Despite its practicality and safety for skin rejuvenation, IPL-PDT should be used cautiously in the beard area of male patients because of the potential destruction of hair follicles.

A study evaluated wrinkle reduction after treatment with a new 0.5% ALA spray encapsulated in liposomes combined with IPL-PDT. At the end-of-treatment visit, significant improvements were observed, with a 73% reduction in periorbital wrinkles and a 50% reduction in nasolabial wrinkles. The less pronounced improvement in nasolabial wrinkles may be attributed to thicker skin or richer facial expression in that area [44]. Additionally, Shin et al. confirmed that IPL-PDT resulted in a more significant reduction in lateral periorbital wrinkles than did the long-pulsed Nd:YAG laser (0.9 vs 0.3) [42].

To enhance photosensitizer penetration into the epidermis and optimize ALA activation for treating photodamaged skin, microneedling devices are combined with PDT. A microneedle roller is used to penetrate the epidermal-dermal barrier, followed by ALA incubation and irradiation with IPL and red light. Significant improvements in global photoaging scores, including fine lines, mottled pigmentation, sallowness, tactile roughness, and telangiectasias, were observed at 3 and 6 months after therapy [52].

IPL devices use flash lamps and cutoff filters to emit polychromatic light of a determined wavelength spectrum (500–1200 nm), pulse duration, pulse interval, and fluency. A wavelength above approximately 600 nm is suitable for the combination of PDT and IPL [67]. Babilas et al. conducted a prospective RCT examining the effectiveness and pain of a new IPL system, variable pulsed light (VPL), and reported that VPL caused less pain than the red LED system because of shorter illumination times [45]. Short pulse durations help reduce pain. Haddad et al. compared IPL systems with different fluences (20, 25, 40, and 50 J/cm^2) for AK and photodamage and reported that higher fluences (40 and 50 J/cm^2) were more effective for detecting AK but not for improving photodamaged skin [41]. A randomized split-face study investigated two IPL systems and revealed that after three continuous treatments, the C-PDT (530–750 nm, 7 J/cm^2, double pulses of 2.5 ms, delay of 10 ms)-treated side presented a more significant improvement in wrinkles and telangiectasias than did the PDT alone-treated side (400–720 nm, 3.5 J/cm^2, long pulse duration of 30 ms). The authors suggested that widening the wavelength range and reducing the light dose did not improve wrinkle reduction but that this modality is particularly suitable for darker skin types [39]. Despite numerous studies, the optimal IPL-PDT regimen remains uncertain owing to variations in IPL parameters across different studies.

PDT with pulsed dye lasers (PDLs) combined with photosensitizers is effective for skin rejuvenation, particularly for treating vascular lesions such as telangiectasias and rosacea. A prospective, controlled study demonstrated the safety and efficacy of PDL-PDT for treating AK and photodamaged skin [49]. Forty-one patients with AKs underwent either a 3-h or overnight ALA incubation followed by PDL (595 nm, 4–7.5 J/cm^2 fluences, 10 ms pulse duration, 10 mm spot size). At all follow-ups, approximately 90% of the AKs on the head were cleared after a single treatment. No significant differences in safety or efficacy were observed between the 3-h and overnight incubation times, indicating that the PDL offers reduced pain and shorter incubation durations. Additionally, PDL-mediated PDT improved posttreatment cosmesis, with a lower risk of hypopigmentation and scarring.

A comparative study involving 25 patients with photodamaged forearms treated with ALA-PDL-PDT demonstrated significant epidermal and dermal remodeling. Biopsy samples from the laser-irradiated areas showed increased epidermal proliferation, as evidenced by increased Ki67 expression and increased collagen production in both the epidermis and dermis. Immunohistochemical analysis revealed that the expression of type I and III procollagen genes in the ALA-PDT-PDL group was approximately double that in the PDL-alone group, indicating a synergistic effect between PDL and ALA in promoting skin rejuvenation and remodeling [26].

Daylight-PDT (DL-PDT) offers a convenient and effective treatment for AK and actinic field damage by utilizing sunlight as a light source. An initial RCT comparing MAL incubation followed by either red LED light or daylight showed that DL-PDT was not inferior to conventional PDT (cPDT) in efficacy but caused significantly less pain [68]. A split-face trial of 43 patients with more than five AK lesions and photodamage on the face or scalp revealed comparable reductions in AK number and area between cPDT and indoor-daylight PDT (idlPDT). Both treatments significantly improved roughness and erythema, with 70.7% of patients preferring idlPDT because of its reduced pain [50]. Additionally, pretreatment with ablative fractional laser (AFL) or microdermabrasion (MD) enhances DL-PDT efficacy, with AFL providing superior improvements in depigmentation ($P = 0.003$) and skin texture ($P = 0.001$) compared with MD-PDT [51]. However, to prevent UV-induced damage, patients should apply physical sunscreen to all sun-exposed areas before photosensitizer application. Overall, DL-PDT is a painless, effective option for treating extensively photodamaged skin.

PDT with combination therapy: Recent studies have explored the efficacy of combining multiple light sources with PDT for photoaging. A retrospective study of 96 patients revealed no significant differences in outcomes for actinically damaged skin treated with ALA-PDT using various light sources, including blue light sequentially with red light, PDL, and/or IPL, although the results were limited by uneven patient numbers and follow-up times [53]. In a split-chest study, 18 subjects receiving 10% ALA gel with IPL plus red light (ALA-IPL-PDT) on one side achieved significantly better global aesthetic improvement (GAIS: 3.57 ± 0.09) than did those receiving ALA-PDT alone (2.89 ± 0.09), with a single ALA-IPL-PDT session yielding results comparable to those of multiple sessions of PDT or IPL alone [54]. Another prospective study comparing light source combinations (PDL, PDL + blue light, IPL, IPL + blue light) revealed that IPL with blue light achieved the greatest improvement, with a GAIS score of 3.0 [55]. The wavelength of blue light targets the PpIX absorption peak (417 nm), while IPL may provide additional benefits, such as increased penetration depth and selective photothermolysis of melanin. Although PDT with sequential combination therapy results in a greater financial burden, it should be noted that a single treatment combining PDT with multiple light sources achieved equivalent cosmetic outcomes to several sessions of IPL or PDT alone, implying that PDT with multiple light sources may produce an intensive effect and lead to more favorable cosmetic results. Moreover, the sequential use of different light sources may take advantage of the synergy of their unique mechanisms of action and cover the simultaneous targets of multiple PpIX absorption peaks, leading to improved efficacy.

10.4 Adverse Effects

Pain during PDT was once a significant concern, but with optimized protocols, it has become a less severe side effect. Compared with conventional red LED light, daylight-PDT has been shown to be more tolerable, with fewer reports of discomfort [50]. Common inflammatory reactions, including erythema, edema, and desquamation, are well documented and primarily result from phototoxic effects [69]. Shortening the incubation time has been suggested as a potential strategy to mitigate these adverse effects. Future research should focus on developing modified PDT protocols with minimal side effects to enhance their use for aesthetic purposes.

10.5 Precautions

After applying photosensitizers, patients should follow medical advice and remain indoors as much as possible for 24–48 h post-PDT to prevent phototoxic reactions. During this period, they should avoid sun exposure and, for at least 2 weeks, use sunscreen with an SPF of 30 or higher when outdoors, along with physical protection such as hats and sunglasses. If makeup is necessary, the use of nonirritating cosmetics in combination with sunscreen is recommended; however, if redness, swelling, or stinging occurs, makeup should be avoided.

In summary, ALA-PDT is an effective treatment for skin aging, significantly reducing the risk of photoaging-related precancers and skin cancer. It offers a safe and reproducible skin rejuvenation option with long-lasting results. By selecting the appropriate light source and adjusting the ALA concentration, incubation time, and light parameters, PDT can achieve optimal skin rejuvenation with minimal side effects. Future advancements in user-friendly photosensitizers, simplified home-use photodynamic devices, and innovative technologies are expected to expand the application and accessibility of PDT for skin rejuvenation.

References

1. Deo MS, Kerse N, Vandal AC, Jarrett P. Dermatological disease in the older age group: a cross-sectional study in aged care facilities. BMJ Open. 2015;5(12):e009941. https://doi.org/10.1136/bmjopen-2015-009941.
2. Passeron T, Lim HW, Goh CL, Kang HY, Ly F, Morita A, et al. Photoprotection according to skin phototype and dermatoses: practical recommendations from an expert panel. J Eur Acad Dermatol Venereol. 2021;35(7):1460–9. https://doi.org/10.1111/jdv.17242.
3. Rittié L, Fisher G. Natural and sun-induced aging of human skin. Cold Spring Harb Perspect Med. 2015;5(1):a015370. https://doi.org/10.1101/cshperspect.a015370.
4. Tobin D. Introduction to skin aging. J Tissue Viability. 2017;26(1):37–46. https://doi.org/10.1016/j.jtv.2016.03.002.
5. Fitsiou E, Pulido T, Campisi J, Alimirah F, Demaria M. Cellular senescence and the senescence-associated secretory phenotype as drivers of skin Photoaging. J Invest Dermatol. 2021;141(4 s):1119–26. https://doi.org/10.1016/j.jid.2020.09.031.
6. Pilkington SM, Bulfone-Paus S, Griffiths CEM, Watson REB. Inflammaging and the skin. J Invest Dermatol. 2021;141(4 s):1087–95. https://doi.org/10.1016/j.jid.2020.11.006.
7. Yaar M, Gilchrest BA. Photoageing: mechanism, prevention and therapy. Br J Dermatol. 2007;157(5):874–87. https://doi.org/10.1111/j.1365-2133.2007.08108.x.
8. Oppel T, Korting HC. Actinic keratosis: the key event in the evolution from photoaged skin to squamous cell carcinoma. Therapy based on pathogenetic and clinical aspects. Skin Pharmacol Physiol. 2004;17(2):67–76. https://doi.org/10.1159/000076016.
9. Philipp-Dormston WG, Sanclemente G, Torezan L, Tretti Clementoni M, Le Pillouer-Prost A, Cartier H, et al. Daylight photodynamic therapy with MAL cream for large-scale photodamaged skin based on the concept of 'actinic field damage': recommendations of an international expert group. J Eur Acad Dermatol Venereol. 2016;30(1):8–15. https://doi.org/10.1111/jdv.13327.
10. Sawane M, Kajiya K. Ultraviolet light-induced changes of lymphatic and blood vasculature in skin and their molecular mechanisms. Exp Dermatol. 2012;21(Suppl 1):22–5. https://doi.org/10.1111/j.1600-0625.2012.01498.x.
11. Wlaschek M, Tantcheva-Poór I, Naderi L, Ma W, Schneider LA, Razi-Wolf Z, et al. Solar UV irradiation and dermal photoaging. J Photochem Photobiol B. 2001;63(1–3):41–51. https://doi.org/10.1016/s1011-1344(01)00201-9.
12. Jakic B, Kerjaschki D, Wick G. Lymphatic capillaries in aging. Gerontology. 2020;66(5):419–26. https://doi.org/10.1159/000508459.
13. Yang Y, Shen S, Cao Y, Wang D, Kang Z, Wang P, et al. Remodeling lymphatic vessels in intrinsically aged skin on SKH-1 mouse using low dose 5-aminolevulinic acid photodynamic therapy via VEGF-C/VEGFR3 pathway. Photodiagn Photodyn Ther. 2022;2022:102851. https://doi.org/10.1016/j.pdpdt.2022.102851.
14. Dermatology Development Committee of the Dermatologist Branch of the Chinese Medical Doctor Association. Expert consensus on skin sun protection. Chin J Dermatol. 2017;50(5):316–20. https://doi.org/10.3760/cma.j.issn.0412-4030.2017.05.002.
15. Ruiz-Rodriguez R, Sanz-Sanchez T, Cordoba S. Photodynamic photorejuvenation.

Dermatologic Surg. 2002;28(8):742–4. https://doi.org/10.1046/j.1524-4725.2002.02018.x.
16. Zhang L, Zhao Z, Wang P, Zhang G, Wang B, Shi L, et al. Long-term improvement on photoaging after ALA photodynamic therapy for actinic keratosis: a retrospective study. Photodiagn Photodyn Ther. 2021;33:102181. https://doi.org/10.1016/j.pdpdt.2021.102181.
17. Ji J, Zhang LL, Ding HL, Wang HW, Huang Z, Wang XX, et al. Comparison of 5-aminolevulinic acid photodynamic therapy and red light for treatment of photoaging. Photodiagn Photodyn Ther. 2014;11(2):118–21. https://doi.org/10.1016/j.pdpdt.2014.02.007.
18. Zhang HY, Ji J, Tan YM, Zhang LL, Wang XJ, Wang PR, et al. Evaluation of 5-aminolevulinic acid-mediated photorejuvenation of neck skin. Photodiagn Photodyn Ther. 2014;11(4):498–509. https://doi.org/10.1016/j.pdpdt.2014.10.003.
19. Li J, Zhang Y, Zhang G, Zhang L, Zhou Z, Wang P, et al. Modified painless photodynamic therapy for facial multiple actinic keratosis in China: a prospective split-face control study. Lasers Surg Med. 2023;55(10):871–9. https://doi.org/10.1002/lsm.23728.
20. Morton CA, Szeimies RM, Basset-Seguin N, Calzavara-Pinton P, Gilaberte Y, Haedersdal M, et al. European dermatology forum guidelines on topical photodynamic therapy 2019 part 1: treatment delivery and established indications - actinic keratoses, Bowen's disease and basal cell carcinomas. J Eur Acad Dermatol Venereol. 2019;33(12):2225–38. https://doi.org/10.1111/jdv.16017.
21. Chaudhary M, Khan A, Gupta M. Skin aging: pathophysiology and current market treatment approaches. J Curr Aging Sci. 2020;13(1):22–30. https://doi.org/10.2174/1567205016666190809161115.
22. Dover JS, Bhatia AC, Stewart B, Arndt KA. Topical 5-aminolevulinic acid combined with intense pulsed light in the treatment of photoaging. Arch Dermatol. 2005;141(10):1247–52. https://doi.org/10.1001/archderm.141.10.1247.
23. Shi L, Wang H, Chen K, Yan J, Yu B, Wang S, et al. Chinese guidelines on the clinical application of 5-aminolevulinic acid-based photodynamic therapy in dermatology (2021 edition). Photodiagn Photodyn Ther. 2021;35:102340. https://doi.org/10.1016/j.pdpdt.2021.102340.
24. Wang M, Yang X, Chang L, Chen J, Luo J, Wu Y, et al. Low-level PDT treatment modulated photoaging mediated by UVA irradiation through regulating Bach2. Photodiagn Photodyn Ther. 2020;29:101606. https://doi.org/10.1016/j.pdpdt.2019.101606.
25. Blazquez-Castro A, Carrasco E, Calvo MI, Jaen P, Stockert JC, Juarranz A, et al. Protoporphyrin IX-dependent photodynamic production of endogenous ROS stimulates cell proliferation. Eur J Cell Biol. 2012;91(3):216–23. https://doi.org/10.1016/j.ejcb.2011.12.001.
26. Orringer JS, Hammerberg C, Hamilton T, Johnson TM, Kang S, Sachs DL, et al. Molecular effects of photodynamic therapy for photoaging. Arch Dermatol. 2008;144(10):1296–302. https://doi.org/10.1001/archderm.144.10.1296.
27. Bagazgoitia L, Cuevas Santos J, Juarranz A, Jaen P. Photodynamic therapy reduces the histological features of actinic damage and the expression of early oncogenic markers. Br J Dermatol. 2011;165(1):144–51. https://doi.org/10.1111/j.1365-2133.2011.10270.x.
28. Fink-Puches R, Soyer HP, Hofer A, Kerl H, Wolf P. Long-term follow-up and histological changes of superficial nonmelanoma skin cancers treated with topical delta-aminolevulinic acid photodynamic therapy. Arch Dermatol. 1998;134(7):821–6. https://doi.org/10.1001/archderm.134.7.821.
29. Marmur ES, Phelps R, Goldberg DJ. Ultrastructural changes seen after ALA-IPL photorejuvenation: a pilot study. J Cosmet Laser Ther. 2005;7(1):21–4. https://doi.org/10.1080/14764170051003725.
30. Szeimies RM, Torezan L, Niwa A, Valente N, Unger P, Kohl E, et al. Clinical, histopathological and immunohistochemical assessment of human skin field cancerization before and after photodynamic therapy. Br J Dermatol. 2012;167(1):150–9. https://doi.org/10.1111/j.1365-2133.2012.10887.x.
31. Jang YH, Koo GB, Kim JY, Kim YS, Kim YC. Prolonged activation of ERK contributes to the photorejuvenation effect in photodynamic therapy in human dermal fibroblasts. J Invest Dermatol. 2013;133(9):2265–75. https://doi.org/10.1038/jid.2013.25.
32. Nowinski D, Lysheden AS, Gardner H, Rubin K, Gerdin B, Ivarsson M. Analysis of gene expression in fibroblasts in response to keratinocyte-derived factors in vitro: potential implications for the wound healing process. J Invest Dermatol. 2004;122(1):216–21. https://doi.org/10.1046/j.0022-202X.2003.22112.x.
33. Kim SK, Koo GB, Kim YS, Kim YC. Epithelial–mesenchymal interaction during photodynamic therapy-induced photorejuvenation. Arch Dermatol Res. 2016;308(7):493–501. https://doi.org/10.1007/s00403-016-1666-3.
34. Kim SK, Oh SJ, Park SY, Kim WJ, Kim YS, Kim YC. Photodynamic therapy inhibits melanogenesis through paracrine effects by keratinocytes and fibroblasts. Pigment Cell Melanoma Res. 2018;31(2):277–86. https://doi.org/10.1111/pcmr.12658.
35. Wang P, Han J, Wei M, Xu Y, Zhang G, Zhang H, et al. Remodeling of dermal collagen in photoaged skin using low-dose 5-aminolevulinic acid photodynamic therapy occurs via the transforming growth factor-β pathway. J Biophotonics. 2018;11(6):e201700357. https://doi.org/10.1002/jbio.201700357.
36. Chen J, Luo J, Tan Y, Wang M, Liu Z, Yang T, et al. Effects of low-dose ALA-PDT on fibroblast photoaging induced by UVA irradiation and the

underlying mechanisms. Photodiagn Photodyn Ther. 2019;27:79–84. https://doi.org/10.1016/j.pdpdt.2019.05.006.
37. Yan Y, Yan G, Cao Z, Wang B, Zeng Q, Shi L, et al. Single cell transcriptome profiling reveals cutaneous immune microenvironment remodeling by photodynamic therapy in photoaged skin. Front Immunol. 2023;14:1183709. https://doi.org/10.3389/fimmu.2023.1183709.
38. Gold MH, Bradshaw VL, Boring MM, Bridges TM, Biron JA. Split-face comparison of photodynamic therapy with 5-aminolevulinic acid and intense pulsed light versus intense pulsed light alone for photodamage. Dermatologic Surg. 2006;32(6):795–801.; discussion 801-793. https://doi.org/10.1111/j.1524-4725.2006.32163.x.
39. Bjerring P, Christiansen K, Troilius A, Bekhor P, de Leeuw J. Skin fluorescence controlled photodynamic photorejuvenation (wrinkle reduction). Lasers Surg Med. 2009;41(5):327–36. https://doi.org/10.1002/lsm.20781.
40. Kosaka S, Yasumoto M, Akilov OE, Hasan T, Kawana S. Comparative split-face study of 5-aminolevulinic acid photodynamic therapy with intense pulsed light for photorejuvenation of Asian skin. J Dermatol. 2010;37(12):1005–10. https://doi.org/10.1111/j.1346-8138.2010.00946.x.
41. Haddad A, Santos ID, Gragnani A, Ferreira LM. The effect of increasing fluence on the treatment of actinic keratosis and photodamage by photodynamic therapy with 5-aminolevulinic acid and intense pulsed light. Photomed Laser Surg. 2011;29(6):427–32. https://doi.org/10.1089/pho.2009.2733.
42. Shin HT, Kim JH, Shim J, Lee JH, Lee DY, Lee JH, et al. Photodynamic therapy using a new formulation of 5-aminolevulinic acid for wrinkles in Asian skin: a randomized controlled split face study. J Dermatolog Treat. 2015;26(3):246–51. https://doi.org/10.3109/09546634.2014.933163.
43. Kohl E, Popp C, Zeman F, Unger P, Koller M, Landthaler M, et al. Photodynamic therapy using intense pulsed light for treating actinic keratoses and photoaged skin of the dorsal hands: a randomized placebo-controlled study. Br J Dermatol. 2017;176(2):352–62. https://doi.org/10.1111/bjd.14970.
44. Piccioni A, Fargnoli MC, Schoinas S, Suppa M, Frascione P, Ginebri A, et al. Efficacy and tolerability of 5-aminolevulinic acid 0.5% liposomal spray and intense pulsed light in wrinkle reduction of photodamaged skin. J Dermatolog Treat. 2011;22(5):247–53. https://doi.org/10.3109/09546634.2011.590791.
45. Babilas P, Knobler R, Hummel S, Gottschaller C, Maisch T, Koller M, et al. Variable pulsed light is less painful than light-emitting diodes for topical photodynamic therapy of actinic keratosis: a prospective randomized controlled trial. Br J Dermatol. 2007;157(1):111–7. https://doi.org/10.1111/j.1365-2133.2007.07959.x.
46. Sanclemente G, Correa LA, Garcia JJ, Barrera M, Villa JF, Garcia HI. Methyl aminolevulinate plus red light vs. placebo plus red light in the treatment of photodamaged facial skin: histopathological findings. Clin Exp Dermatol. 2012;37(4):379–86. https://doi.org/10.1111/j.1365-2230.2011.04249.x.
47. Palm MD, Goldman MP. Safety and efficacy comparison of blue versus red light sources for photodynamic therapy using methyl aminolevulinate in photodamaged skin. J Drugs Dermatol. 2011;10(1):53–60.
48. Touma D, Yaar M, Whitehead S, Konnikov N, Gilchrest BA. A trial of short incubation, broad-area photodynamic therapy for facial actinic keratoses and diffuse photodamage. Arch Dermatol. 2004;140(1):33–40. https://doi.org/10.1001/archderm.140.1.33.
49. Alexiades-Armenakas MR, Geronemus RG. Laser-mediated photodynamic therapy of actinic keratoses. Arch Dermatol. 2003;139(10):1313–20. https://doi.org/10.1001/archderm.139.10.1313.
50. Arisi M, Rossi MT, Spiazzi L, Guasco Pisani E, Venturuzzo A, Rovati C, et al. A randomized split-face clinical trial of conventional vs indoor-daylight photodynamic therapy for the treatment of multiple actinic keratosis of the face and scalp and photoaging. J Dermatolog Treat. 2021;33(4):2250–6. https://doi.org/10.1080/09546634.2021.1944594.
51. Wenande E, Phothong W, Bay C, Karmisholt KE, Haedersdal M, Togsverd-Bo K. Efficacy and safety of daylight photodynamic therapy after tailored pretreatment with ablative fractional laser or microdermabrasion: a randomized, side-by-side, single-blind trial in patients with actinic keratosis and large-area field cancerization. Br J Dermatol. 2019;180(4):756–64. https://doi.org/10.1111/bjd.17096.
52. Clementoni MT, Roscher MB, Munavalli GS. Photodynamic photorejuvenation of the face with a combination of microneedling, red light, and broadband pulsed light. Lasers Surg Med. 2010;42(2):150–9. https://doi.org/10.1002/lsm.20905.
53. Friedmann DP, Goldman MP, Fabi SG, Guiha I. Multiple sequential light and laser sources to activate aminolevulinic acid in the treatment of photodamage: a retrospective study. J Cosmet Laser Ther. 2015;17(5):252–8. https://doi.org/10.3109/14764172.2015.1022187.
54. Abrouk M, Dong J, Waibel JS. Medical and aesthetic improvement of photodamaged skin by the combination of intense pulsed light and photodynamic therapy with 10% aminolevulinic acid hydrochloride gel. Lasers Surg Med. 2022;54(1):62–5. https://doi.org/10.1002/lsm.23460.
55. Abrouk M, Gianatasio C, Li Y, Waibel JS. Prospective study of intense pulsed light versus pulsed dye laser with or without blue light in the activation of PDT for the treatment of actinic keratosis and photodamage. Lasers Surg Med. 2022;54(1):66–73. https://doi.org/10.1002/lsm.23492.
56. Morton CA, Szeimies RM, Basset-Seguin N, Calzavara-Pinton PG, Gilaberte Y, Haedersdal M,

et al. European dermatology forum guidelines on topical photodynamic therapy 2019 part 2: emerging indications - field cancerization, photorejuvenation and inflammatory/infective dermatoses. J Eur Acad Dermatol Venereol. 2020;34(1):17–29. https://doi.org/10.1111/jdv.16044.
57. Rick K, Sroka R, Stepp H, Kriegmair M, Huber RM, Jacob K, et al. Pharmacokinetics of 5-aminolevulinic acid-induced protoporphyrin IX in skin and blood. J Photochem Photobiol B. 1997;40(3):313–9. https://doi.org/10.1016/s1011-1344(97)00076-6.
58. Siddiqui MA, Perry CM, Scott LJ. Topical methyl aminolevulinate. Am J Clin Dermatol. 2004;5(2):127–37. https://doi.org/10.2165/00128071-200405020-00006.
59. Zhang G, Cao Z, Wang P, Zhu L, Zhang L, Zho Z, et al. Comparison of efficacy, adverse effects and costs between 20% ALA-PDT and 10% ALA-PDT for the treatment of actinic keratosis in Chinese patients. Photodiagn Photodyn Ther. 2020;31:101605. https://doi.org/10.1016/j.pdpdt.2019.101605.
60. Huang A, Nguyen JK, Austin E, Mamalis A, Cohen M, Semkhayev B, et al. Facial rejuvenation using photodynamic therapy with a novel preparation of ALA and hyaluronic acid in young adults. Arch Dermatol Res. 2020;312(8):567–73. https://doi.org/10.1007/s00403-020-02038-5.
61. de Leeuw J, van der Beek N, Bjerring P, Neumann HAM. Photodynamic therapy of acne vulgaris using 5-aminolevulinic acid 0.5% liposomal spray and intense pulsed light in combination with topical keratolytic agents. J Eur Acad Dermatol Venereol. 2010;24(4):460–9. https://doi.org/10.1111/j.1468-3083.2009.03447.x.
62. Roberts DW, Olson JD, Evans LT, Kolste KK, Kanick SC, Fan X, et al. Red-light excitation of protoporphyrin IX fluorescence for subsurface tumor detection. J Neurosurg. 2018;128(6):1690–7. https://doi.org/10.3171/2017.1.JNS162061.
63. Sanclemente G, Medina L, Villa JF, Barrera LM, Garcia HI. A prospective split-face double-blind randomized placebo-controlled trial to assess the efficacy of methyl aminolevulinate + red-light in patients with facial photodamage. J Eur Acad Dermatol Venereol. 2011;25(1):49–58. https://doi.org/10.1111/j.1468-3083.2010.03687.x.
64. Togsverd-Bo K, Haak CS, Thaysen-Petersen D, Wulf HC, Anderson RR, Haedersdal M. Intensified photodynamic therapy of actinic keratoses with fractional CO2 laser: a randomized clinical trial. Br J Dermatol. 2012;166(6):1262–9. https://doi.org/10.1111/j.1365-2133.2012.10893.x.
65. Hendel K, Mogensen M, Wenande E, Dierickx C, Haedersdal M, Togsverd-Bo K. Fractional 1,927 nm thulium laser plus photodynamic therapy compared and combined for photodamaged decollete skin: a side-by-side randomized controlled trial. Lasers Surg Med. 2020;52(1):44–52. https://doi.org/10.1002/lsm.23194.
66. Gold MH. The evolving role of aminolevulinic acid hydrochloride with photodynamic therapy in photoaging. Cutis. 2002;69(6 Suppl):8–13.
67. Karrer S, Kohl E, Feise K, Hiepe-Wegener D, Lischner S, Philipp-Dormston W, et al. Photodynamic therapy for skin rejuvenation: review and summary of the literature–results of a consensus conference of an expert group for aesthetic photodynamic therapy. J Dtsch Dermatol Ges. 2013;11(2):137–48. https://doi.org/10.1111/j.1610-0387.2012.08046.x.
68. Wiegell SR, Haedersdal M, Philipsen PA, Eriksen P, Enk CD, Wulf HC. Continuous activation of PpIX by daylight is as effective as and less painful than conventional photodynamic therapy for actinic keratoses; a randomized, controlled, single-blinded study. Br J Dermatol. 2008;158(4):740–6. https://doi.org/10.1111/j.1365-2133.2008.08450.x.
69. Ibbotson SH, Wong TH, Morton CA, Collier NJ, Haylett A, McKenna KE, et al. Adverse effects of topical photodynamic therapy: a consensus review and approach to management. Br J Dermatol. 2019;180(4):715–29. https://doi.org/10.1111/bjd.17131.

ALA-PDT for the Treatment of Other Cutaneous Diseases

11

Yunfeng Zhang, Jianhua Huang, Hongwei Wang, Qihang Chang, Guolong Zhang, Zijun Zhao, Bo Wang, and Xiuli Wang

11.1 ALA-PDT for the Treatment of Leukoplakia

11.1.1 Introduction

Leukoplakia is a disorder characterized by the appearance of white patches on mucosal surfaces, most commonly in the oral cavity and external genitalia. These patches result from excessive keratinization and epithelial hyperplasia and carry a significant risk of malignant transformation into squamous cell carcinoma. In China, the cancer transformation rate for oral leukoplakia (OLK) ranges between 4% and 18% [1, 2]. OLK is predominantly observed in middle-aged and older adults, with a slightly higher prevalence in males. The risk of malignancy is influenced by factors such as size, location, clinical presentation, and degree of epithelial dysplasia. Vulvar leukoplakia typically affects postmenopausal women and commonly involves areas such as the clitoris, inner labia minora, and vaginal mucosa. In cases of bladder leukoplakia, patients may experience urinary tract symptoms, although these symptoms are nonspecific and can mimic conditions such as chronic cystitis, glandular cystitis, urethritis, or overactive bladder [3]. Moreover, colon leukoplakia is often asymptomatic in its early stages and is usually detected incidentally during colonoscopy [4].

The histopathological features of leukoplakia include epithelial hyperplasia with hyperkeratosis and/or parakeratosis [5]. Epithelial proliferation occurs in two distinct forms: simple proliferation and atypical proliferation. Simple proliferation is characterized by basal cell hyperplasia and acanthosis, occasionally accompanied by multinucleated cells, increased mitotic activity, nuclear hyperchromasia, prominent nucleoli within the spinous layer, and disruption of basal cell polarity. In contrast, atypical proliferation presents more pronounced basal cell stratification, polarity disorders, nuclear hyperchromasia, dysplastic nuclei, and increased mitotic activity. Additionally, atypical proliferation may exhibit pathological features such as an increased nuclear-to-cytoplasmic ratio, reduced cell adhesion, prominent nucleoli, and dyskeratosis, all of which are associated with a greater risk of malignant transformation.

Y. Zhang · Q. Chang · G. Zhang · Z. Zhao · X. Wang
Institute of Photomedicine, Shanghai Skin Disease Hospital, School of Medicine, Tongji University, Shanghai, China
e-mail: wangxiuli_1400023@tongji.edu.cn

J. Huang · H. Wang (✉)
Department of Dermatology, Huadong Hospital, Fudan University, Shanghai, People's Republic of China

B. Wang
Avera Medical Group Dermatology, Aberdeen, SD, USA

University of South Dakota, Vermillion, SD, USA
e-mail: makiwang@med.umich.edu

X. Wang, B. Wang (eds.), *Photodynamic Therapy in Dermatology*,
https://doi.org/10.1007/978-981-96-8915-6_11

Leukoplakia is linked to factors such as mechanical stimulation, poor hygiene, and chronic inflammation. Recent studies have suggested that leukoplakia is associated with coinfection with human papillomavirus (HPV), EB virus, and *Candida albicans* [6]. Diagnosis typically involves a combination of clinical examination and histopathological evaluation. However, distinguishing leukoplakia from other conditions that can affect mucous membranes, such as vitiligo, lichen sclerosus, neurodermatitis, lichen planus, and secondary syphilis mucosal plaques, is essential.

11.1.2 Treatment Methods

The treatment options for leukoplakia include laser therapy, cryotherapy, and surgical resection. However, previous studies have been limited by the absence of rigorous randomized controlled clinical trials, resulting in uncertain efficacy. Long-term follow-up studies have not identified a definitive method to prevent leukoplakia recurrence or reduce malignancy.

11.1.2.1 Surgery

Currently, there is no universally accepted standardized diagnosis and treatment protocol for leukoplakia aimed at reducing oral recurrence and malignancy. Surgical resection and biopsy are widely acknowledged as diagnostic and therapeutic approaches for suspected cases of leukoplakia malignancy [7]. In cases of OLK, the skin lesions and surrounding areas often demonstrate a "field cancerization" phenomenon, where one or several cloned or tumor cells with genetic mutations identical to lesions are present in the seemingly normal surrounding tissues, contributing to postoperative recurrence or malignancy. This recurrence, often due to residual lesions after surgery, carries a greater risk of cancer transformation [8, 9]. Holmstrup et al. reported that 33% of recurrent leukoplakia cases following surgery ultimately progressed to cancer [10]. Therefore, comprehensive postoperative histopathological examination of all excised tissues and margins is essential to ensure maximal removal of diseased tissue, and close postoperative monitoring of patients is imperative.

11.1.2.2 Laser Therapy

Laser therapy offers several advantages over surgical treatment, including reduced bleeding, minimal scar formation, decreased pain and swelling, and shorter operation times. Various types of lasers can be clinically employed to treat OLK, such as CO_2 lasers, Nd:YAG lasers, KTP lasers, semiconductor lasers and Er:YAG lasers (erbium lasers) [11]. However, existing studies on the evidence that laser intervention prevents cancer occurrence are insufficient, highlighting the need for multicenter, prospective, randomized controlled clinical trials to further ascertain the long-term efficacy and recurrence rate of laser treatment.

11.1.2.3 Medication Therapy

There have been reports of the use of topical retinoids in the treatment of leukoplakia, but their efficacy remains unclear. In clinical practice, a small number of doctors use topical treatments such as imiquimod to reduce the recurrence rate of mucosal vitiligo. However, there is currently a lack of prospective, randomized controlled clinical studies confirming the effectiveness of these treatments.

11.1.2.4 Photodynamic Therapy

As a novel treatment approach, photodynamic therapy (PDT) offers unique advantages, including preservation of tissue integrity, reduced recurrence rates, and the potential for repeated treatments. PDT has found applications in a variety of skin conditions, including skin cancers, and its treatment mechanism is further elaborated upon in Chap. 2.

Systemic PDT Systemic PDT was first utilized for treating leukoplakia in 1993 when Grant et al. applied it to 11 patients with "field cancerization" of OLK, all of whom were confirmed to have early-stage infiltrating squamous cell carcinoma alongside leukoplakia. Owing to the extensive nature of the lesions, surgery was not feasible. Patients received 2 mg/kg Photofrin systemically, followed by red-light irradiation (50–100 J/cm^2) after 48 h. During treatment, patients experienced itching and pain and were managed with oral analgesics, and necrosis developed in the treated area within 3–4 days, which took 3–5 weeks to heal completely. At 6–8 weeks posttreatment, complete remission occurred in ten patients, with one showing residual white patches. After 12 months, two patients experienced white patch recurrence, but no progression to cancer was noted. This study highlights PDT as a promising treatment for early invasive malignant tumors and concurrent precancerous conditions [12].

In 1996, Fan KF et al. employed systemic 5-aminolevulinic acid photodynamic therapy (ALA-PDT) to treat OLK. Eighteen patients with histologically confirmed precancerous and malignant oral lesions received 60 mg/kg ALA orally (dissolved in orange juice and administered at 0, 1, and 2 h), followed by irradiation with a 628-nm laser at 100 J/cm^2 or 200 J/cm^2. Significant systemic discomfort occurred during treatment, including nausea and vomiting in six patients, which resolved within 24 h, and one case of photosensitivity lasted more than 48 h. Posttreatment biopsies revealed epidermal necrosis ranging from 0.1 mm to 1.3 mm in depth in all patients. At 12 weeks, biopsies of 12 consenting patients presented normal tissue pathology, whereas other patients presented seemingly normal epidermis but declined biopsy [13]. These findings highlight the efficacy of systemic PDT but underscore the need for methods to mitigate its side effects.

Local PDT To mitigate systemic side effects such as skin phototoxicity associated with systemic PDT, researchers have explored localized ALA-PDT for treating OLK. In 2004, Tsai JC and colleagues treated 33 cases of oral lesions, including 24 cases of OLK, 5 cases of oral proliferative verrucous leukoplakia (OPVL), 2 cases of erythroplakia, and 1 case of verrucous carcinoma. A 20% ALA solution was applied to the lesions for 2 h, followed by 635-nm LED light irradiation at 100 J/cm^2 once a week for three sessions, covering normal tissue at the periphery. Among the OLK patients, 3 achieved complete resolution, 9 achieved partial improvement, and 12 achieved no improvement. Among the OPVL patients, 4 achieved complete resolution and 1 achieved partial improvement. The erythroplakia patients and the verrucous carcinoma patients achieved partial remission. Patients reported a mild burning sensation during light exposure but tolerated the treatment well without anesthesia or analgesics. These findings highlight the potential of localized ALA-PDT for treating OLK, emphasizing the need for further clinical research to refine treatment parameters [14].

Treatment Parameters of Local ALA-PDT In 2007, Chen et al. compared the effects of different ALA-PDT treatment frequencies on OLK. Sixty-five patients received once-weekly treatments, while another 32 received treatments twice weekly. Both groups were treated with a 20% ALA solution applied for 1.5–2 h, followed by 635 ± 5-nm LED red-light irradiation at 100 mW/cm^2. Patients underwent one to six treatments, with an average of 3.5 sessions. In the once-weekly group, 5 patients achieved complete regression, 33 achieved partial remission, and 27 experienced no improvement. In the 2-weekly group, 11 patients achieved complete regression and 21 achieved partial remission. Clinical outcomes were significantly better in the 2-weekly group, highlighting the potential benefit of increased treatment frequency for OLK [15].

In 2011, Kawczyk Krupka et al. compared the efficacy and adverse reactions of ALA-PDT and cryotherapy for OLK. The ALA-PDT group included 48 patients treated biweekly with 635 nm red-light irradiation at 100 J/cm^2. After six to eight treatments, 35 patients (72.9%)

achieved complete remission, whereas 13 (27.1%) experienced relapse within 6 months. The cryotherapy group consisted of 37 patients treated every 3 weeks; 33 (89.2%) achieved complete remission, of whom 9 (24.3%) experienced recurrence after six to eight treatments. While the efficacy and recurrence rates were similar between the groups, the cryotherapy group reported more severe pain, whereas tolerability was better in the ALA-PDT group. These results suggest that ALA-PDT is a viable alternative treatment for OLK [16].

In 2015, Selvam et al. treated five patients with OLK via ALA-PDT with 10% ALA, a 635-nm red-light source with a light dose of 100 J/cm^2. Patients underwent six to eight treatments, all of which resulted in recovery without significant adverse effects. Additionally, no recurrences were observed during the 1-year follow-up period [17].

In 2019, the National Clinical Research Center for Oral Diseases from the Chinese Academy of Medical Sciences proposed guidelines for managing OLK on the basis of clinical experience and a systematic literature review. These guidelines recommended photodynamic therapy (PDT) as a first-line treatment option for specific types of OLK. The protocol suggested applying a 20% ALA solution externally for 2–3 h, followed by LED red-light irradiation at 100 J/cm^2, with treatments conducted every 2–3 weeks. This framework provides clinical practitioners with a standardized approach for treating OLK effectively [18].

Local ALA-PDT Combined with Other Methods For patients with refractory leukoplakia in specific areas or with extensive lesions, the efficacy of PDT alone may be limited, necessitating combined treatment approaches. In 2017, the authors' group managed a challenging case involving extensive lesions across multiple areas, including the right corner of the mouth, buccal mucosa, gums, and labial mucosa, with pronounced keratinization. Pathological diagnosis confirmed OLK, and surgical or laser interventions were deemed impractical because of the complexity of the oral cavity. Initial treatment with two rounds of ALA-PDT (10% ALA applied for 3 h, followed by 635-nm LED red-light irradiation at 100 J/cm^2 every 2 weeks) showed limited efficacy. To enhance treatment, a CO_2 laser was used to excise the visible keratinized areas, improving ALA absorption, as confirmed by fluorescence analysis, which revealed increased PpIX intensity after laser treatment. After two combined treatments, significant lesion reduction was noted, although certain areas remained resistant. Ultimately, six rounds of CO_2 laser therapy combined with PDT achieved complete lesion clearance (Fig. 11.1), with no recurrence observed during a 14-month follow-up [19].

These findings highlight the potential of combination therapy, such as CO_2 lasers with PDT, for managing extensive skin lesions with pronounced keratinization. Additionally, further exploration of alternative combined approaches is crucial for improving clinical outcomes.

11.1.3 Conclusions

In summary, although numerous treatment methods are available for leukoplakia, high-quality evidence-based studies remain scarce. ALA-PDT is a promising option for OLK treatment because of its noninvasive approach, minimal invasiveness, and lack of scar formation. For patients with extensive lesions and marked keratinization, combination therapies, including CO_2 or holmium lasers, may further enhance treatment outcomes.

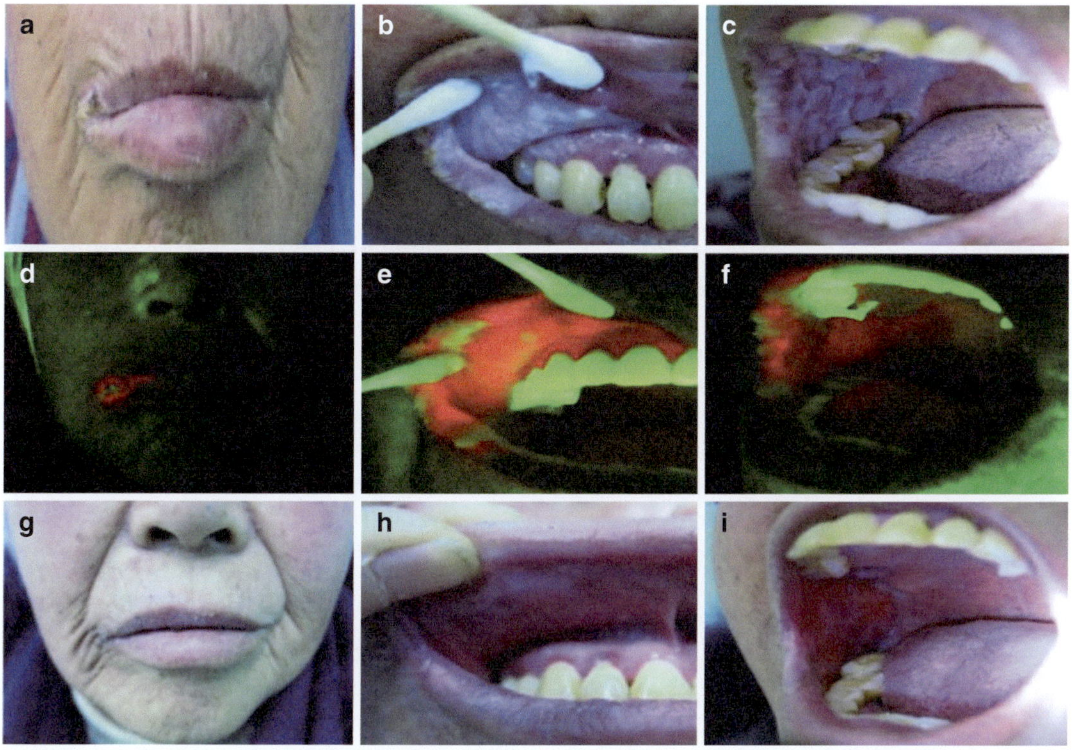

Fig. 11.1 ALA-PDT for extensive refractory OLK. (**a–c**) Large white hyperkeratotic plaques can be seen in the oral cavity before treatment. (**d–f**) After ALA was applied 3 h externally, the visible skin lesions presented brick-red fluorescence. (**g–i**) After six treatments with a CO_2 laser combined with ALA-PDT, the oral endothelial damage completely disappeared

11.2 ALA-PDT for the Treatment of Lichen Sclerosus

11.2.1 Overview of Lichen Sclerosus

Lichen sclerosus is a chronic inflammatory skin disease with an unclear etiology, although studies suggest that higher levels of tissue-specific antibodies, such as circulating extracellular matrix protein antibodies, are present in affected patients. Many individuals with lichen sclerosus also have autoimmune diseases such as thyroid disorders, vitiligo, and lichen planus, supporting the theory that it is an autoimmune condition. Hallopeau and Darier first reported and named the disease 'lichen sclerosus' in the nineteenth century [20]. This condition is not rare, and its varied clinical manifestations often lead to missed or incorrect diagnoses. Lichen sclerosus can be classified into anogenital and extragenital forms [21]. Approximately 3.5–5% of women with anogenital lichen sclerosus and 4–5% of men with genital lichen sclerosus may develop squamous cell carcinoma, rarely other skin tumors, such as verrucous carcinoma, melanoma, or basal cell carcinoma, may also occur. Thus, both female anogenital and male genital lichen sclerosus require active treatment and lifelong follow-up [21, 22].

11.2.1.1 Clinical Features

Adult Female Anogenital Lichen sclerosus lesions in female adults commonly affect the interlabial sulci, labia minora, clitoris, and perineum, with involvement of the mucocutaneous junction and rare involvement of other genital mucosal areas. The lesions typically appear as ivory-white, flat papules and plaques with epidermal atrophy, and in extramucosal areas, follicular plugging may be present, often accompanied by ecchymosis, hyperkeratosis, fissures, and erosions. Itching is the primary symptom, and in severe cases, it can significantly impact sleep quality. Some patients may be asymptomatic, with lesions discovered during a physical exam. Pain can arise from erosions or fissures, and scarring may lead to clitoral burying and fusion of the labia minora to the labia majora. In advanced cases, the labia minora may be lost, and significant narrowing of the vaginal introitus can occur.

Child Female Anogenital Lichen sclerosus lesions in juvenile females present similarly to those in adult females but with more prominent ecchymosis and increased perianal involvement. Constipation may occur as a secondary symptom due to pain caused by fissures. It is crucial to distinguish lichen sclerosus in juvenile females from sexual abuse, as ecchymosis can be misleading. While sexual abuse may trigger or exacerbate lichen sclerosus through the Koebner phenomenon, not all cases of lichen sclerosus in young females are linked to abuse, necessitating careful evaluation and diagnosis.

Adult Male Anogenital Lichen sclerosus in adult males commonly affects the prepuce, coronary sulcus, and glans penis, with perianal involvement being rare. The clinical manifestations are similar to those observed in adult females. When the urethral opening and urethra are involved, scarring can lead to urethral stricture, causing changes in the urinary stream. Common symptoms include foreskin tightness, phimosis, erectile dysfunction, and pain during erections, although itching is not a prominent symptom in this population.

Child Male Anogenital In male children, genital lichen sclerosus is more likely to occur in the foreskin, and phimosis is common.

Extragenital Lesions of Lichen Sclerosus This typically occurs on the upper trunk, axillae, buttocks, and lateral thighs, although rarer sites include the mouth, face, scalp, hands, feet, and nails. The lesions usually appear as porcelain-white patches or plaques, often accompanied by ecchymosis. The Koebner phenomenon is common and occurs at sites of compression, surgical scars, radiation scars, or trauma. Extragenital lichen sclerosus must be differentiated from morphea to ensure accurate diagnosis.

11.2.1.2 Histopathology

Histopathological examination is recommended when the clinical presentation is atypical, and a multisite biopsy should be conducted if there is suspicion of neoplastic changes. Early-stage pathological changes typically include interfacial dermatitis, with pronounced hyperkeratosis, particularly at follicular openings, which may lead to follicular plugging. Epidermal atrophy, flattening of the epidermal processes, basal cell edema, and liquefaction are commonly observed. Additionally, there is noticeable edema and hyalinization of superficial dermal collagen, along with a band-like lymphocytic infiltrate.

11.2.2 Treatment

Spontaneous regression of lichen sclerosus is rare, making early diagnosis, timely treatment, lifelong follow-up, and cancer prevention crucial, particularly for genital lichen sclerosus. Severe cases can lead to disruptive atrophy, sexual dysfunction, and even squamous cell carcinoma. Conventional treatment strategies include: (1) reducing local skin irritation and using topical moisturizers; (2) applying topical treatments such as potent or superpotent corticosteroids, calcineurin inhibitors, 5-fluorouracil, tretinoin, testosterone, or progesterone; (3) using cryotherapy or CO_2 lasers for hyperkeratinized lesions; and (4) surgery for severe phimosis, precancerous lesions, or squamous cell carcinoma. Lifelong follow-up is essential to monitor for complications.

11.2.3 ALA-PDT

11.2.3.1 Mechanisms

A number of studies have shown that ALA-PDT is effective for treating lichen sclerosus [23–27]. Local immune dysfunction caused by vasodilation and lymphocyte extravasation in lichen sclerosus lesions is a potential causative factor, and ALA-PDT can be therapeutic by promoting collagen formation and reducing lymphocyte extravasation [28].

11.2.3.2 Clinical Efficacy

In 1999, Hillemanns et al. first reported the effectiveness of ALA-PDT in treating vulvar lichen sclerosus in 12 female patients. After one to three sessions of PDT, 10 patients experienced significant improvement in itching at 6–8 weeks posttreatment, with relief lasting up to 6 months [24]. In 2014, the authors conducted a prospective, randomized clinical trial to compare ALA-PDT with topical potent corticosteroids for treating vulvar lichen sclerosus [29]. Forty-three patients, averaging 51.4 years of age, were randomly assigned to either the ALA-PDT group or the topical corticosteroid group. In the ALA-PDT group, a 10% ALA cream was applied to the lesion and surrounding area for 3 h, followed by irradiation with a 633-nm semiconductor laser. Patients underwent four treatments at 2-week intervals. The corticosteroid group received 0.05% clobetasol propionate cream daily for 8 weeks. The results revealed that the complete response rate in the ALA-PDT group (14/20) was double that in the corticosteroid group (7/20) (Fig. 11.2). After 6 months, 13 of the 14 cured patients in the ALA-PDT group did not relapse, whereas all 7 cured patients in the corticosteroid group relapsed. The recurrence rate in the ALA-PDT group was significantly lower than that in the corticosteroid group.

Topical potent corticosteroids are the conventional first-line treatment for lichen sclerosus, but recurrence is common after drug withdrawal, and long-term use can lead to skin atrophy and secondary infections. ALA-PDT has a long-lasting effect, a high cure rate, and a low recurrence rate in treating lichen sclerosus, with additional antitumor and anti-infection properties, making it a safe and effective alternative [30]. However, conventional ALA-PDT (C-PDT) can cause significant pain in patients with genital lichen sclerosus, who often require local anesthesia. In 2017, the authors' group introduced modified painless photodynamic therapy (M-PDT) for treating genital lichen sclerosus, which resulted in no noticeable pain during treatment while maintaining efficacy comparable to that of C-PDT.

11.2.3.3 Recommended Protocols

Both the C-PDT and M-PDT can be used for the treatment of lichen sclerosus. For pain-sensitive patients, the M-PDT is preferred. The specific protocol is shown in Table 11.1.

ALA-PDT is an effective treatment for lichen sclerosus, offering faster results than topical corticosteroids and providing protection against secondary fungal and viral infections. Modified painless photodynamic therapy (M-PDT) is a promising approach that reduces pain and is likely to be increasingly used to treat lichen sclerosus. Regular lifelong follow-up is essential for all patients, and surgery should be considered if there is a risk of cancer development.

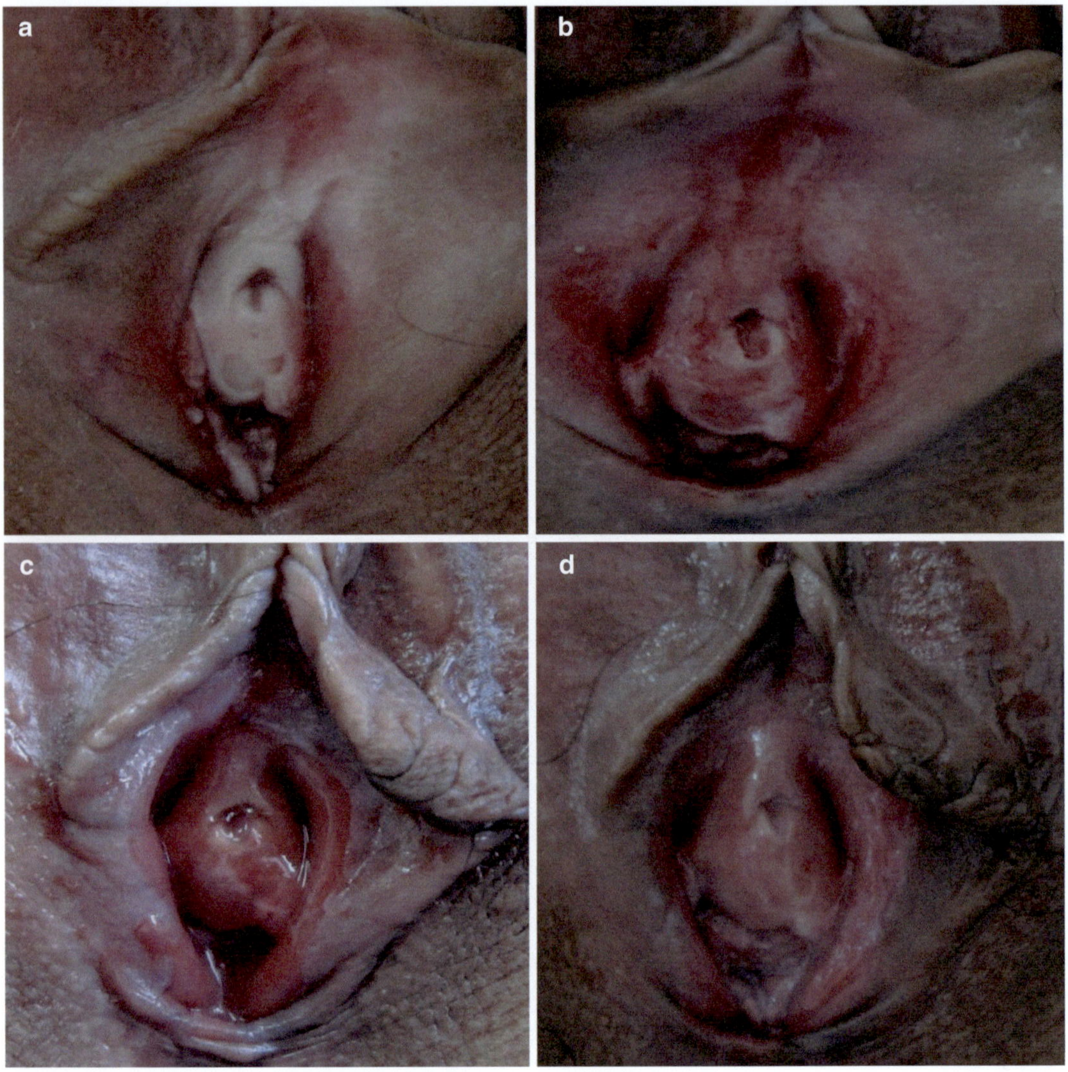

Fig. 11.2 Photographs of vulvar lichen sclerosus before and after ALA-PDT. (**a**) Hyperkeratosis, atrophy, sclerosis, and hypopigmentation were observed before treatment. (**b**) After 2 weeks of the first ALA-PDT treatment, hyperkeratosis, atrophy, sclerosis, and hypopigmentation improved, and telangiectasia was visible. (**c**) The lesion disappeared at 2 weeks after four sessions of ALA-PDT. (**d**) There was no recurrence at the 6-month follow-up after treatment

Table 11.1 Recommended protocols for the treatment of lichen sclerosus with ALA-PDT[a]

Recommendation	Pretreatment	Formulated ALA		Incubation time (h)	Dose of light	
		ALA formulation	ALA concentration (%)		Energy density (J/cm²)	Power density (mW/cm²)
C-PDT	Clean, plum needle	Creams or solutions	10–20	3–6	100–200	60–150
M-PDT	Same	Same	Same	0.5–1	Same	28–40

[a] Interval: 1–2 weeks

11.3 ALA-PDT for the Treatment of Chronic Wounds

11.3.1 Introduction

Chronic refractory wounds are wounds with multifactorial causes that show no signs of healing despite treatment for more than a month, affecting an estimated eight million people globally [31]. In the United States and Europe, chronic wounds impact approximately 2% of the population, with the prevalence increasing with age and higher risks among individuals with diabetes and obesity. These wounds have complex mechanisms, are challenging to treat, and often lead to prolonged disability, increased risk of medical complications, and diminished quality of life. They also impose significant social and economic burdens on patients, families, and society.

11.3.1.1 Etiology Classification

Multiple factors contribute to poor wound healing, including systemic and local factors.

Systemic factors include age, obesity, malnutrition, medications (corticosteroids, hydroxyurea, methotrexate, chemotherapies, immunosuppressives, BCG vaccination), chronic medical conditions (diabetes mellitus, hypertension, blood disorders, autoimmune conditions, neuropathic conditions, cardiac failure, hypoxia, endocrine disorders, vascular disease, diabetes, cancer, and immunosuppression), and habits (smoking and alcohol consumption).

Local factors include (1) trauma (such as sharp injuries, radiation, electric shock, compression, and burns), vascular diseases (such as varicose veins, thromboembolic vasculitis, and variant vasculitis), neuropathy (including diabetic peripheral neuropathy, Lyme disease, and uremia), infections (bacterial, fungal, viral, tuberculosis, and atypical mycobacteria), and inappropriate local treatments (such as excessive debridement, unsuitable dressings, or wounds that are excessively dry or wet).

11.3.1.2 Clinical Manifestations

Venous leg ulcers (VLUs) commonly arise from factors such as trauma, lower extremity surgery, and deep vein thrombosis, with a prevalence of 1–1.5%. These ulcers are typically located between the middle of the calf and approximately 1 in below the medial ankle. They may present as single or multiple irregular, shallow lesions with red granulation or yellow fibrous tissue. Associated features include varicosities, pitting edema, stasis dermatitis, hemosiderin pigmentation, and lipodermatosclerosis. Patients often report symptoms such as leg heaviness, swelling, and pain after prolonged standing, which improve with elevation.

Diabetic foot ulcer (DFU) commonly occurs at pressure-prone sites such as soles and is often associated with limb deformities, limited joint mobility, peripheral neuropathy, or angiopathic changes. Peripheral neuropathy causes distal numbness or paresthesia, whereas autonomic nerve defects result in reduced sweating, altered blood flow regulation, impaired distal oxygenation, and warm, pink, dry, cracked skin on the distal extremities. These factors predispose patients to frequent infections, with 50–60% of DFU patients showing signs of infection upon hospital admission.

Malignant wounds: A significant percentage of cancer patients develop malignant wounds, including squamous cell carcinoma, basal cell carcinoma, malignant fibrosarcoma, leiomyosarcoma, Kaposi's sarcoma, melanoma, Merkel cell carcinoma, and cutaneous large lymphoma [32]. Pain is the most prevalent symptom and may manifest as persistent, breakthrough, incident, or spontaneous pain. Exudation, primarily serous fluid, occurs in 14.6% of malignant wounds, with some patients presenting with purulent discharge. Additionally, 10.4% of malignant wounds are associated with unpleasant odors, described as "fishy," or resembling "spoiled meat," whereas 5.2% involve pruritus or itchiness, and 4.2% result in bleeding [33].

Pressure ulcers (PUs) are localized areas of tissue necrosis caused by unrelieved pressure, shear, or friction, are often exacerbated by factors such as excessive moisture, and typically occur over bony prominences. They are classified into four stages on the basis of depth: Stage I involves localized skin thickening or nonblanchable erythema; Stage II presents as partial-thickness loss with red or pink wound surfaces, potentially accompanied by blisters or ruptures; Stage III features full-thickness skin loss with visible subcutaneous fat but no exposure of bone, tendon, or muscle; and Stage IV involves full-thickness tissue loss with exposure of bone, tendon, or muscle [32].

11.3.2 Conventional Treatment

11.3.2.1 Local Treatment

Debridement: It is essential in treating chronic wounds, as necrotic tissue hinders healing [34]. Common methods include surgical, autolytic, biologic, and mechanical debridement. Surgical debridement rapidly removes necrotic tissue via scissors, scalpels, or curettes under anesthesia. Autolytic debridement relies on endogenous enzymes such as proteolytic, fibrinolytic, and collagenolytic enzymes to degrade necrotic tissue. Mechanical debridement employs hydrotherapy, whirlpool, pulsed irrigation, waterjet irrigation, ultrasound, or high-pressure irrigation to remove adhesions and necrotic tissue from the wound surface.

Topical antimicrobial agents play a vital role in treating chronic wounds because of their broad-spectrum antimicrobial and anti-infective properties. Examples include sodium hypochlorite (0.5–5.25%), which inactivates ulcer microorganisms [35]; chlorhexidine, a cationic surfactant effective against most gram-positive and gram-negative bacteria [36]; and povidone iodine, which enhances the bactericidal effect of iodine by forming a thin bactericidal film on the skin, facilitating iodine penetration and release.

Topical antibiotics should be selected on the basis of bacterial culture results and drug sensitivity. Mupirocin provides broad-spectrum antibacterial coverage against common skin pathogens and is effective for primary and secondary skin infections. Fusidic acid is antibacterial against *Streptococcus dermatophilus*, *Staphylococcus*, *Corynebacterium microti*, and *Propionibacterium acnes* infections and especially has strong antibacterial effects against enzyme-producing *Staphylococcus aureus* and methicillin-resistant *Staphylococcus aureus* [37].

Dressings are essential for managing chronic ulcers by controlling infection, maintaining a moist environment, promoting gas exchange, removing exudates, and protecting new tissue. Various types of dressings include silver dressings, moisture-retentive films, foam dressings, and hydrogels. Silver dressings offer antimicrobial activity by binding to bacterial envelopes and DNA, disrupting cellular functions, and preventing DNA transcription. The 2012 International Consensus Guidelines on the Use of Silver-Containing Products recommend silver dressings for infected wounds [38]. Various types of silver-containing dressings have strong antimicrobial capacity, a broad antimicrobial spectrum, long-lasting antimicrobial activity, high safety, good antimicrobial properties, and are not easy to induce drug resistance. These dressings provide strong antimicrobial capacity, broad-spectrum activity, long-lasting effects, high safety, and minimal risk of inducing drug resistance. Moisture-retentive films made from semipermeable polyurethane or synthetic materials allow oxygen flow, prevent water vapor buildup, act as microbial barriers, and promote healing. Foam dressings, with an absorbent inner layer and a semipermeable outer layer, are ideal for high-exudate wounds and absorb fluids while maintaining a moist environment and preventing bacterial invasion. Hydrogel, a high-water-content polymer, is moisturizing, cooling, pain reliant, and anti-inflammatory, making it suitable for dry wounds, thermal burns, and graft donor sites, although it has poor adsorption and weak bacterial barrier properties.

Hyperbaric oxygen therapy: There is strong evidence that hyperbaric oxygen therapy (HBOT) reduces the risk of amputation in individuals with DFU by promoting partial and complete healing of problematic wounds. HBOT involves compressing pure oxygen at a minimum of 1.4 atmospheres over the entire body. This therapy helps the body combat infections in hypoxic soft tissue, reduces inflammation, enhances perfusion, and accelerates wound healing by improving the ability of white blood cells to phagocytose pathogens, promoting collagen aggregation and crosslinking, stimulating neovascularization in the wound bed, and recruiting and releasing stem cells into the circulation [39].

Vacuum-assisted closure (VAC) therapy is an innovative approach to promote wound healing. The vacuum system aids in the debridement of necrotic tissue, enhances tissue perfusion, creates a closed, moist environment, and reduces wound edema through the application of negative pressure. This improved local wound environment fosters the formation of healthy granulation tissue. The microdeformational forces generated by the VAC system stimulate healthy granulation tissue growth, whereas the macrodeformational forces produce strain contraction at the wound edges, tightening them and reducing the wound size. Consequently, VAC therapy creates optimal conditions for wound healing [40].

For patients with large or difficult-to-heal ulcers, especially those with exposed bones, joints, tendons, or those requiring long-term dressing changes, surgery may be considered once the patient's systemic condition is stable and infection is controlled. Surgical options include free skin grafting after ulcer excision, local skin flap transfer, and muscle flap transfer. Skin grafting involves covering the wound with normal or artificial skin to accelerate healing. Common surgical techniques include mesh skin grafting, punctate skin grafting, epidermal implantation within the granulation tissue, and free flap transplantation.

Traditional Chinese medicine (TCM) offers a unique approach to treating chronic wounds on the basis of the theory that their pathogenesis stems from the accumulation of dampness, heat, and toxicity due to stagnation in the veins and channels, with an inability to expel these harmful factors. Common TCM treatment methods include compression therapy, hoop therapy, leakage stain therapy, and techniques to prevent decay and promote muscle growth. Frequently used medicinal formulations include Ruyi Jinhuang powder, sugar Astragalus combination, muscle growth cream, comfrey oil gauze, and skin growth cream, among others.

Physiotherapy can enhance the skin repair process by generating thermal effects that relax blood vessels, increase the blood supply to the ulcerated tissue, increase the collagen content, and promote the regeneration of basal granulation tissue. Techniques used in physiotherapy for wound healing include microwave thermotherapy, semiconductor lasers, helium-neon lasers, pulsed ND:YAG lasers, infrared therapeutic devices, and ultrasound therapies.

11.3.2.2 Systemic Treatment

Chronic wounds are common in elderly individuals and are often associated with systemic underlying conditions such as hypoproteinemia, cardiac insufficiency, connective tissue diseases, diabetes, malnutrition, and infections. Therefore, actively treating primary diseases and comorbidities is crucial for promoting chronic wound healing and improving microcirculation. Herbal treatments such as *Salvia miltiorrhiza* and Rhizoma ligustici wallichii can also support this process.

11.3.3 ALA-PDT

11.3.3.1 Mechanism

The difficulty in chronic wound healing is due primarily to various factors, with infection being the most significant, as it keeps wounds stuck in a prolonged inflammatory state. The rise of multidrug-resistant (MDR) bacteria exacerbates this issue, leading to antibiotic failure and the emergence of superbacteria, which pose major challenges in managing chronic ulcers. PDT has shown promising potential in treating chronic wounds because of its effects, including antibacterial activity and the upregulation of growth factor and matrix metalloproteinase expression, making it an increasingly recognized option for wound healing.

Antimicrobial activity: The antimicrobial mechanism of PDT involves the generation of reactive oxygen species (ROS) when photosensitizers that are incubated in the dark are activated by specific wavelengths of light. This process results in the apoptosis or necrosis of pathogens.

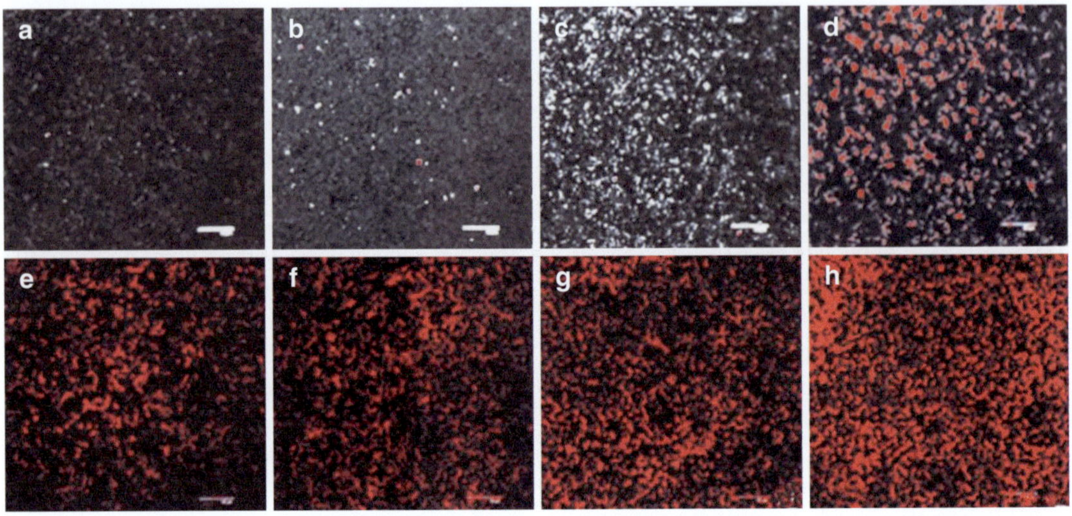

Fig. 11.3 Incubation of ALA and *Staphylococcus epidermidis*. Brick-red fluorescence occurred after incubation of *S. epidermidis* with 50 mmol/L ALA, and the fluorescence gradually increased with increasing incubation time. (**a–h**) Brick-red fluorescence images of PpX after 3, 5, 8, 12, 16, 18, 20, and 24 h of coincubation, respectively (×400)

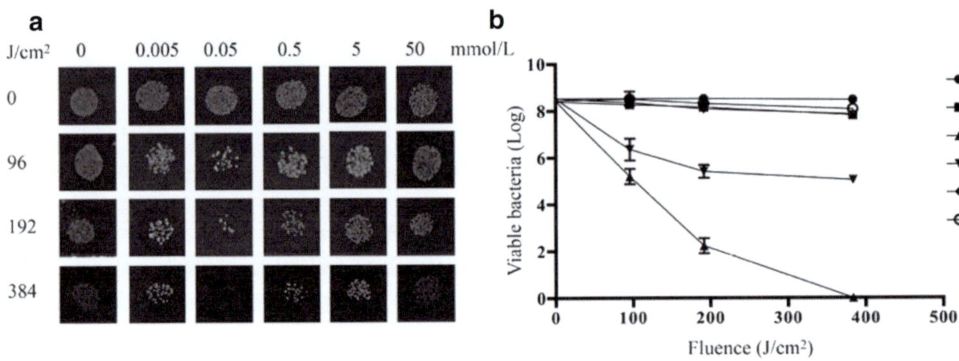

Fig. 11.4 Effects of ALA-PDT on MRSA. (**a**) Different concentrations of ALA were incubated in the dark for 4 h, and colonies were counted after exposure to light at 0, 96, 192, and 384 J/cm^2. (**b**) The survival colony count at 0.05 mmol/L ALA and 384 J/cm^2; the MRSA bacteria were completely inactivated. * indicates $P < 0.05$ compared with 0 mmol/L

In 2012, the authors' group studied the antibacterial mechanism of ALA-PDT against skin pathogenic bacteria and reported that ALA could be taken up by *Staphylococcus epidermidis* (*S. epidermidis*), with ALA-PDT significantly inhibiting bacteria [41] (Fig. 11.3). Furthermore, ALA-PDT was shown to be effective against drug-resistant bacteria, including methicillin-resistant *Staphylococcus aureus* (MRSA) [42] (Fig. 11.4). Dai et al. used polyethylenimine (PEI)-ce6 as a photosensitizer for the photodynamic treatment of bruising ulcer infections in mice, leading to an effective reduction in MRSA on the ulcer surface [43]. Additionally, PDT using toluidine blue O (TBO) as a photosensitizer and He-Ne as a light source successfully inactivated 34 strains of *Staphylococcus aureus* and 8 strains of MRSA isolated from patients' wounds [44].

Induction of acute inflammation is a complex process involving cytokines critical to wound repair and is a key stage in regulating cell differentiation. Either excessive or insufficient inflammation hinders healing [45]. Acute inflammation, which is the initial response to injury, involves the accumulation of neutrophils in tissues and ends once tissue repair is complete, promoting infection control and injury repair [46]. In contrast, chronic inflammation, often caused by persistent microbial infections [47], is characterized by the infiltration of monocytes, macrophages, and lymphocytes, leading to prolonged and difficult-to-heal wounds [48] activates the immune system by inducing a local acute inflammatory response. Following PDT, the levels of inflammatory factors such as IL-1β and TNF-α increase significantly, with TNF-α promoting the activation of neutrophils at the lesion site and the aggregation of monocytes, macrophages, and mast cells to activate CD8+ T cells to clear dead cells. These proinflammatory factors decrease after 1 week [49]. The authors' group reported that ALA-PDT activates the NLRP3 inflammasome, significantly increasing IL-1r1 and IL-1β levels, indicating the role of PDT in amplifying the local inflammatory response [50].

Triggering: proliferation PDT effectively promotes cell migration and epithelialization in newly formed fibrocytes, fibrin, and granulation tissue. It upregulates the expression of various growth factors, such as transforming growth factor (TGF)-β1 and β3, epidermal growth factor (EGF), basic fibroblast growth factor (bFGF), and vascular endothelial growth factor (VEGF). The authors' group reported that ALA-PDT increased the release of TGF-β1 from keratinocytes by activating the TGF-β pathway and stimulating collagen expression in human dermal fibroblasts. Animal studies further confirmed that ALA-PDT remodeled collagen in the mouse dermis and improved skin photoaging (Fig. 11.5) [51]. In a mouse skin ulcer model treated with ALA-PDT, the authors' group reported significantly increased expression of TGF-β1, bFGF, and VEGF via immunohistochemistry, qPCR,

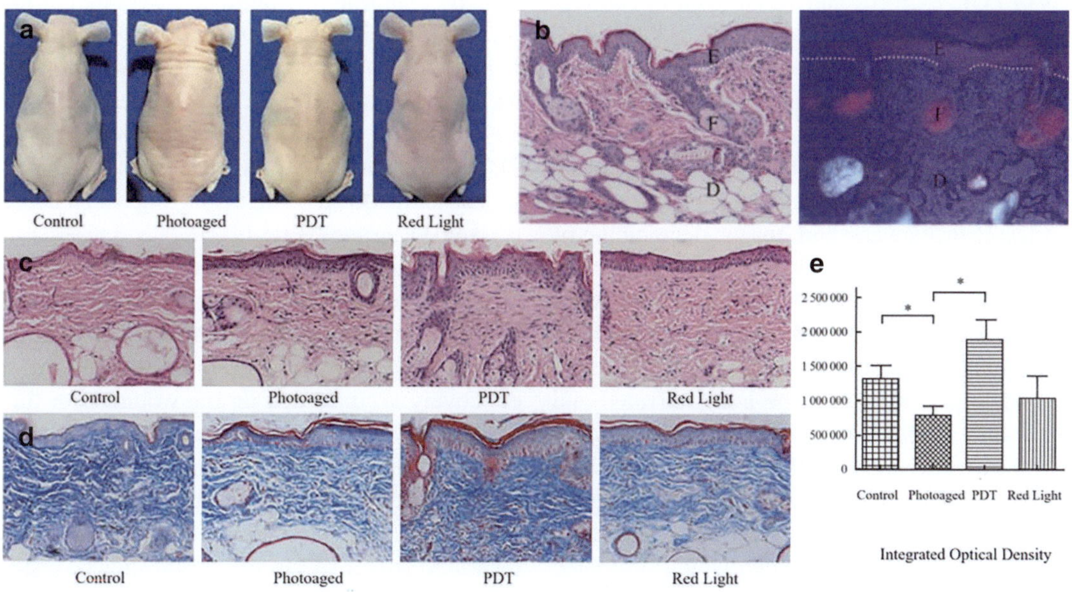

Fig. 11.5 Remodeling of dermal collagen in photoaged mice by ALA-PDT. (**a**) Skin morphology of SKH-1 mice in the control group, photoaging group, PDT group, and red-light group. (**b**) After 3% ALA was applied for 3 h, PpIX fluorescence in SKH-1 mice was detected via fluorescence microscopy (*E* = epidermis, *D* = dermis, *F* = hair follicle). (**c**) H&E staining revealed increased collagen regeneration in the PDT group compared with the other groups. (**d**) Masson staining revealed increased collagen content in the PDT group (×400). (**e**) Masson staining revealed increased integrated optical density of dermal collagen in the PDT group. * indicates $P < 0.05$

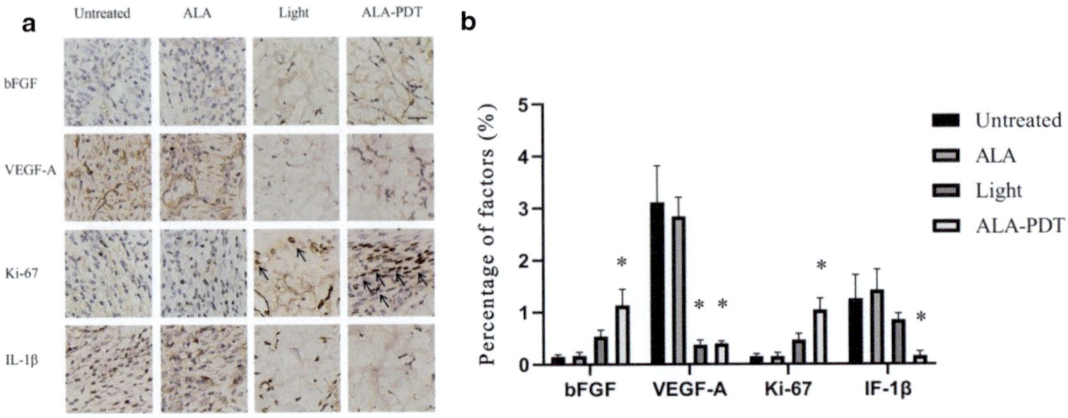

Fig. 11.6 Effects of ALA-PDT on bFGF, VEGF-A, Ki-67, and IL-1β. (**a**) Immunohistochemical images of bFGF, VEGF-A, Ki-67, and IL-13 expression on the 14th day after treatment of the wounds. (**b**) bFGF and Ki-67 expression was increased, and IL-1β expression was inhibited in the ALA-PDT and red-light groups; bar = 50 μm. *$P < 0.05$

and ELISA [52, 53] (Fig. 11.6). Additionally, PDT mediated by sinoporphyrin sodium (DVDMS) has been shown to be effective in treating burn wounds infected with multidrug-resistant *Staphylococcus aureus*, with higher levels of FGF, TGF-β1, and VEGF than in controls [54]. Semiconductor laser PDT, which uses Huangbai-solution compounds to treat infected bedsores, also significantly promoted EGF expression [55].

The matrix metalloproteinase (MMP) family consists of calcium-dependent, zinc-containing proteases that are essential for the degradation of the extracellular matrix (ECM). They play a critical role in all stages of wound healing by regulating the wound matrix, facilitating cell migration, and promoting tissue remodeling. During tissue remodeling, MMPs must be both activated and expressed. ALA-PDT has been shown to upregulate the expression of MMP1 and MMP3 in fibroblasts. After 48 h of ALA-PDT irradiation, the mRNA levels of MMP1 and MMP3 increased by 2.4- and 4.3-fold, respectively, which promoted collagen degradation and ECM remodeling [56].

11.3.3.2 Treatment Parameters

The efficacy of ALA-PDT strongly depends on the therapeutic parameters, and the appropriate parameters are adopted for different diseases.

Previous studies on ALA-PDT for wound treatment have used varying concentrations of ALA, typically ranging from 10% to 20%, on the basis of the concentrations used for other diseases. However, there is a lack of research specifically exploring the optimal concentration for chronic wounds [57]. In a study by the authors' group, four wounds of the same size were created on the backs of the mice, and 0%, 3%, 10%, or 30% ALA gel was applied for 3 h prior to ALA-PDT. The results revealed that the healing rate was faster in the 10% and 30% groups than in the 0% and 3% groups (Fig. 11.7).

For example, Morimoto et al. reported significant brick-red fluorescence on the wound surface 24 h after the intraperitoneal injection of an ALA solution in a mouse model, indicating that ALA effectively accumulated on the wound after this period [58]. Similarly, the authors' group studied fluorescence under a Wood lamp at 0 h, 3 h, 6 h, and 9 h after applying ALA gel to the back wounds of mice. The fluorescence intensity was measured with a spectrometer and showed a significant increase at 3 h postapplication, reaching a peak at 6 h before gradually decreasing. These findings support the clinical practice of applying ALA for 3 h [52] (Fig. 11.8).

Power, irradiance and fluence light power, irradiance (power density), energy density, light

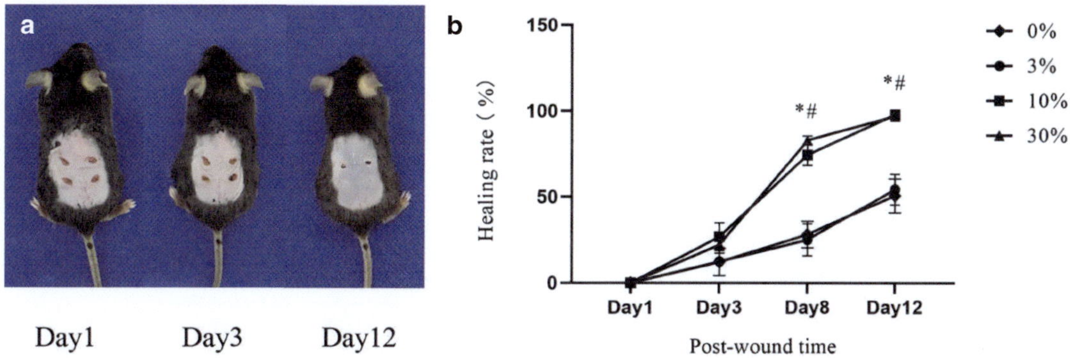

Fig. 11.7 Exploration of ALA concentration in ALA-PDT treatment of skin ulcers. (**a**) The 30% and 10% ALA treatments were more effective than the 3% ALA treatment. (**b**) Quantitative analysis revealed that after the same 25 J/cm^2, the wound healing rates of the 10% and 30%ALA groups were significantly faster than those of the 0% and 3% ALA groups. * indicates 30% compared with 0% $P < 0.05$; # indicates $P < 0.05$ compared with 10% and 0%

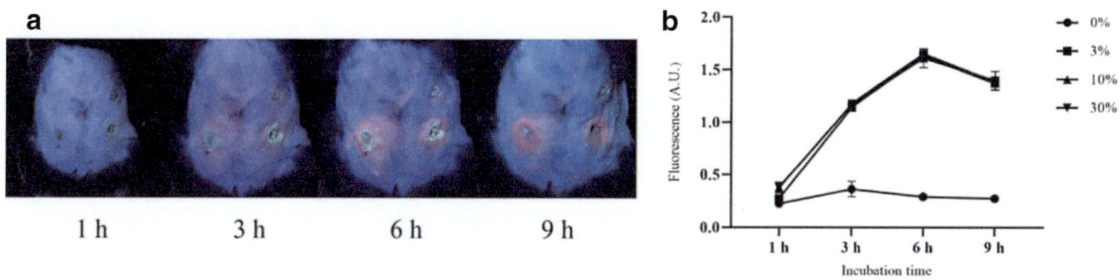

Fig. 11.8 Exploration of the effects of ALA incubation on the ALA-PDT of wounds. (**a**) Fluorescence images of PpIX coated with ALA at different concentrations and at different time points. (**b**) Fluorescence spectrometer data showing the fluorescence intensity values of 3%, 10% and 30% ALA at different times

exposure time and light mode all influence the efficacy of PDT. In the authors' study, different doses of 0 J/cm^2, 25 J/cm^2, 50 J/cm^2, and 100 J/cm^2 were administered to wounds on the backs of the mice, with the 25 J/cm^2 group showing the best therapeutic effect [52] (Fig. 11.9). This is attributed to the dual effects of reactive oxygen species (ROS): excessive ROS cause oxidative stress, damaging cell DNA, proteins, and lipids and leading to cell necrosis [59], whereas lower ROS levels act as second messengers, regulating pathways such as the AMPK/Akt, NF-κB, and p38 MAPK pathways and promoting better bio-activation [60]. In a study by Sahu et al., 60 J/cm^2 PDT reduced NF-κB and p38 MAPK levels, decreased neutrophil infiltration, and enhanced angiogenesis, whereas 120 J/cm^2 PDT had the opposite effects [61]. Similarly, Chiu applied indocyanine to mouse wounds and irradiated them with 0 J/cm^2, 5 J/cm^2, and 15 J/cm^2, finding that 5 J/cm^2, which produces lower ROS levels, activated downstream signaling pathways and promoted cell migration [62]. These findings suggest that increased light energy may not be favorable for activating healing pathways.

The wavelength is another critical factor in PDT, as it should align with the absorption spectrum of the chosen photosensitizer, with each photosensitizer corresponding to a specific wavelength. Longer wavelengths, such as red and infrared, offer stronger tissue penetration, with red light at 630 nm being commonly used in ALA-PDT for solid tumors because of its ability to penetrate deeper into tissues. Conversely, blue

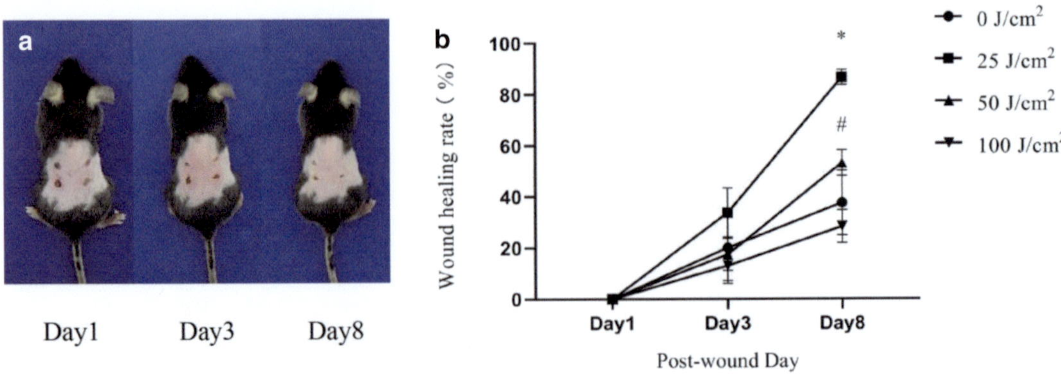

Fig. 11.9 Exploration of the effects of light dose in ALA-PDT treatment of wounds. (**a**) Healing of wounds in mice treated with different energy densities. (**b**) Faster wound healing at 25 J/cm^2 and 50 J/cm^2 than at 0 J/cm^2 and 100 J/cm^2, * indicates that when 25 J/cm^2 was compared with the untreated group, $P < 0.05$; # indicates that $P < 0.05$ when 50 J/cm^2 was compared with the untreated group

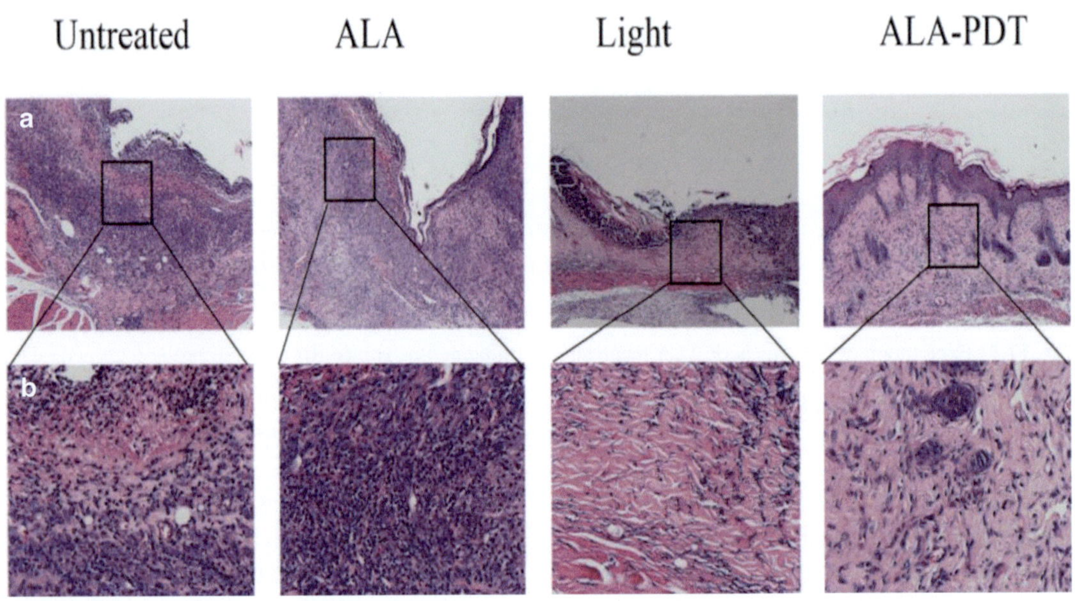

Fig. 11.10 Histopathology of mouse wounds after different treatments. Compared with those in the untreated and ALA groups, there were fewer inflammatory and increased collagen bundles in the red light and ALA-PDT groups. (**a**) 100× and (**b**) 400×

light has weaker penetration but can generate antibacterial activity by activating endogenous microbial porphyrins, reducing the number of MRSA bacteria by nearly 1 log under 50 J/cm^2 of blue-light irradiation [63]. Red light, especially in the 620–720 nm range, is widely used for wound treatment because it can reach deeper tissues, reduce microorganisms, promote DNA synthesis, enhance cell migration, and facilitate wound healing [64]. In the authors' study on mouse wounds, 630-nm red light promoted collagen and capillary hyperplasia, further supporting its effectiveness in wound healing [53] (Fig. 11.10).

11.3.3.3 Antibacterial Effects of PDT

The broad spectrum of ALA-PDT does not induce drug resistance, making it a promising nonantibiotic treatment strategy for a variety of drug-resistant bacteria. In 2012, the authors' group conducted an in vitro antibacterial study of ALA-PDT [41]. Under light doses of 30 J/cm^2, 50 J/cm^2, 70 J/cm^2, 90 J/cm^2, and 100 J/cm^2, the viable colony numbers of *S. epidermidis* were 172.8 ± 3.9 × 10^3 CFU/m^2, 96.0 ± 2.9 × 10^3 CFU/mL, 59.2 ± 3.3 × 10^3 CFU/mL, 10.8 ± 1.7 × 10^3 CFU/mL, and 0.5 ± 0.6 × 10^3 CFU/mL, respectively. At 100 J/cm^2, *S. epidermidis* was completely suppressed. At 10 mmol/L, 20 mmol/L, 30 mmol/L, 40 mmol/L, and 50 mmol/L, the numbers of viable bacteria were 162.5 ± 4.8 × 10^3 CFU/mL, 97.0 ± 5.7 × 10^3 CFU/mL, 57.0 ± 3.2 × 10^3 CFU/mL, 19.0 ± 1.9 × 10^3 CFU/mL, and 0.5 ± 0.6 × 10^3 CFU/mL, respectively. Statistical differences were found between the different concentration groups. The authors' group further explored the role of ALA-PDT on *S. epidermidis* biofilms [65]. After incubation at 50 mmol/L for 16 h, the number of surviving *S. epidermidis* gradually decreased with increasing light dose. Under illuminations of 100 J/cm^2, 200 J/cm^2, and 300 J/cm^2, the number of surviving colonies was 210 ± 7.55 × 10^5, 91 ± 1.53 × 10^5, and 16 ± 1.52 × 10^5, respectively, with significant differences observed between the negative control group and the single red-light irradiation group.

Scanning electron microscopy revealed that after ALA-PDT, the biofilm structure became loose, blurred, or disappeared, revealing a single colony distribution (Fig. 11.11). In 2019, the authors' group studied the bactericidal and antibacterial effects of ALA-PDT on MRSA in an in vitro experiment [42]. Under 384 J/cm^2 illumination, the microbial viability of ALA at 0.005 mM, 0.05 mM, 0.5 mM, 5 mM, and 50 mM decreased by 0.65 log, 8.47 log, 3.44 log, 0.62

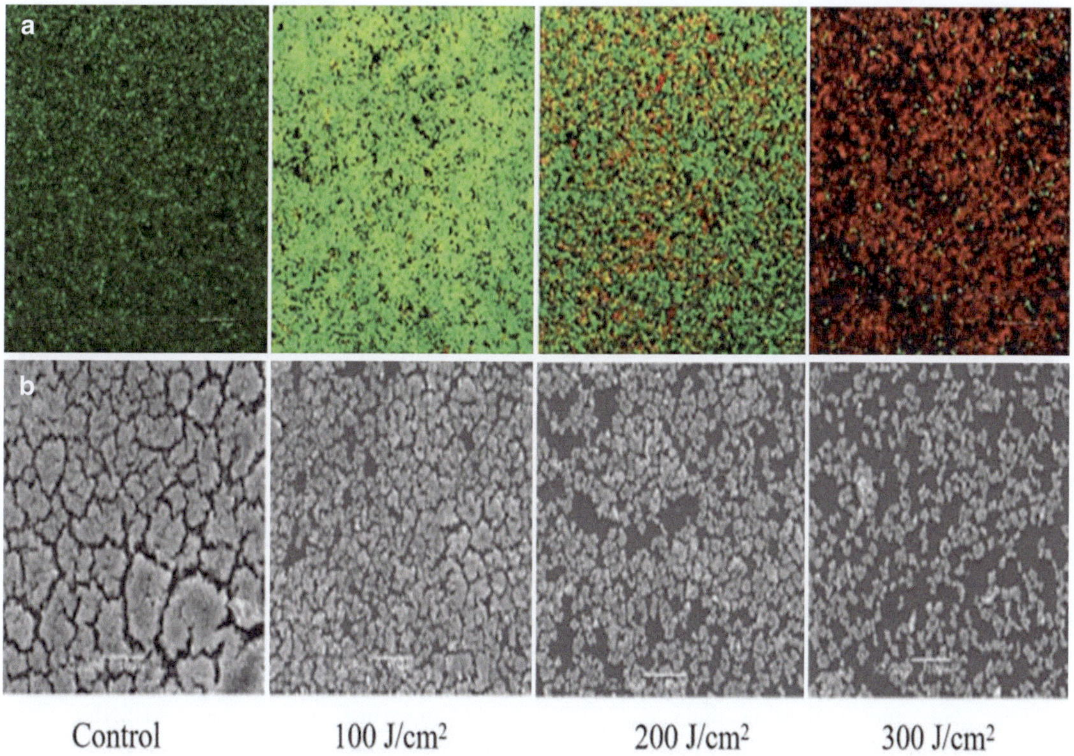

Fig. 11.11 Effects of ALA-PDT on biofilms. (**a**) Under a fluorescence microscope, the number of dead red bacteria in the biofilm increased after ALA-PDT. (**b**) Under an electron microscope, the structure of the biofilm gradually became loose, and the bacteria exhibited a single colony distribution

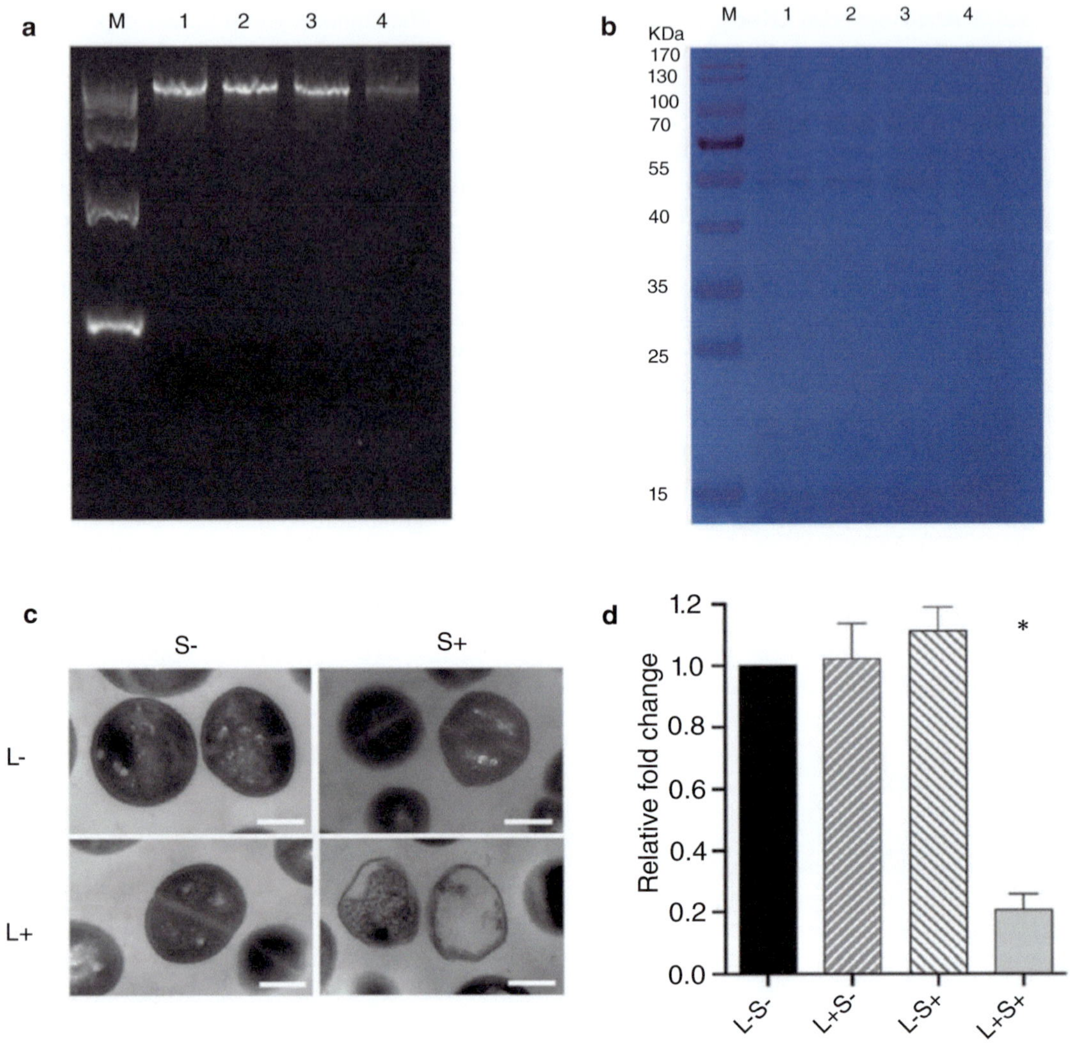

Fig. 11.12 Effects of ALA-PDT on the MRSA genome, cell protein, cell membrane, cytoplasm, and *nuc* genes. (**a**) Agarose gel electrophoresis revealed that ALA-PDT damaged the whole genome of bacteria. (**b**) Polyacrylamide gel electrophoresis revealed that ALA-PDT damaged the MRSA protein. (**c**) Transmission electron microscopy revealed a thin, irregular envelope, sparse cytoplasm, and leakage; bar: 500 μm. (**d**) qRT–PCR results revealed that ALA-PDT significantly inhibited *nuc* gene expression; $^*P < 0.05$

log, and 0.40 log, respectively, with MRSA almost completely eliminated at 0.05 mM. Electron microscopy revealed ruptured cell membranes and loose cytoplasm. qPCR revealed a 0.74-fold reduction in the transcription level of the MRSA-specific gene *nuc*, indicating that ALA-PDT effectively killed MRSA by destroying its cell membrane, cytoplasm, and nucleic acids (Fig. 11.12). Liu et al. reported that ALA-PDT had antibacterial effects on *Streptococcus pneumoniae* plankton and biofilms [66]. Under conditions of 400–780 nm and 100 mW/cm^2, the bacterial survival rate decreased with increasing ALA concentration. The survival of *Streptococcus pneumoniae* isolates ATCC700603, nonextended-spectrum β-lactamase (ESBL), and ESBL-producing isolates decreased by 3.68 log, 3.17 log, and 3.20 log, respectively. The amount of viable bacteria in the biofilm decreased by 3.09 log, 1.92 log, and 2.28 log, respectively.

After treatment with ALA-PDT (10 mM ALA, 633 ± 10 nm, 80 mW/cm^2, illumination for 60 min) on clinically isolated vancomycin-resistant Enterococcus (VRE), the survival rate of clinically isolated vancomycin-resistant Enterococcus (VRE) decreased by 5.37 log [67]. Hsieh compared different concentrations of ALA (1.0 mM, 2.5 mM, 5.0 mM, and 10.0 mM) with *S. aureus* and *Pseudomonas aeruginosa* (*P. aeruginosa*) in a dark room for 60 min and then irradiated the mixture with 630 nm red light at 216 J/cm^2, observing complete inactivation of *S. aureus* and a significant reduction in *P. aeruginosa* activity at 1.0 mM and 162 J/cm^2 [68].

In vivo research demonstrated the efficacy of ALA-PDT in promoting wound healing in MRSA-infected models [53] (Figs. 11.13 and 11.14). The authors' group established an infected wound mouse model and divided the wounds into untreated, ALA, red light, and ALA-PDT groups. In the ALA-PDT group, 10% ALA solution was applied, followed by 25 J/cm^2 (635 nm) illumination, resulting in a 2.05 log bacterial reduction on the wound surface by day

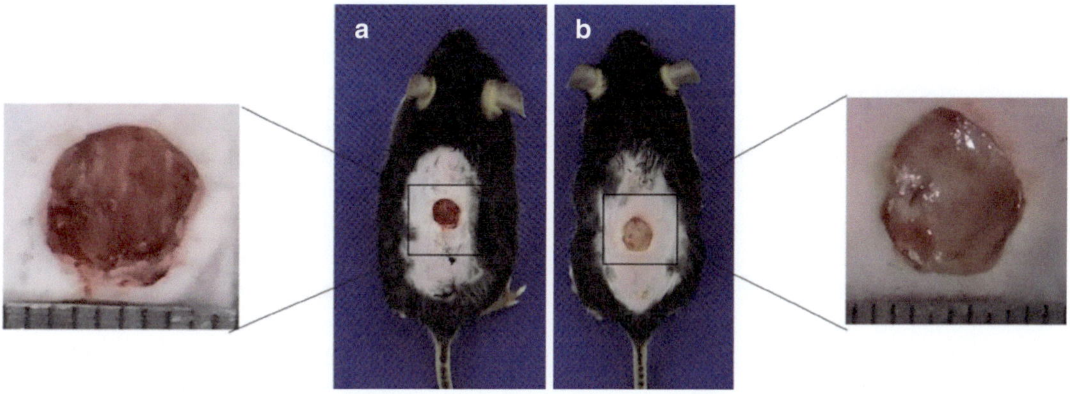

Fig. 11.13 Establishment of an infected wound model. (**a**) Wounds from uninfected mice were cleaner. (**b**) Wounds from infected mice were obviously red, swollen and exuded, with purulent secretions

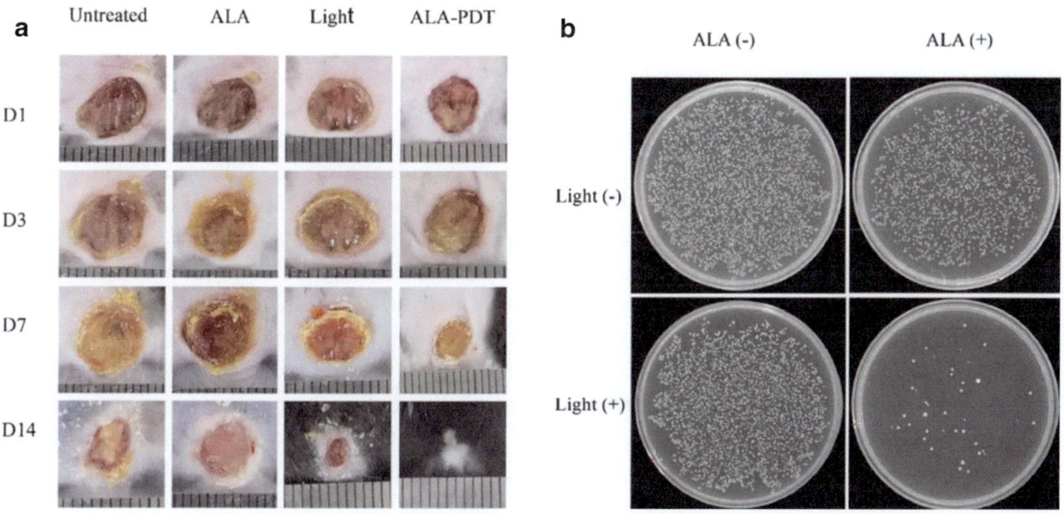

Fig. 11.14 Healing rates of wounds treated with ALA-PDT and the effects of ALA-PDT on the amount of bacteria present in the wounds. (**a**) Wound areas at days 1, 3, 7, and 14. (**b**) The number of bacterial colonies in the ALA-PDT group was significantly lower than that in the other three groups

2, along with histological evidence of re-epithelialization, increased microvessels and collagen, and reduced inflammatory cell infiltration. Morimoto et al. evaluated ALA-PDT via intraperitoneal ALA (0 mg/kg, 50 mg/kg, or 200 mg/kg) and 410 nm irradiation at 164.5 mW/cm^2 and reported that the 200 mg/kg and 50 J/cm^2 treatments reduced the wound size by an average of 5.4% by day 13 [58]. Epidermal stem cells (EpSCs), located in the hair follicle and interfollicular epidermis, are activated and migrate toward wound centers to accelerate epithelialization and regeneration. The ROS produced by PDT regulate intracellular signaling, enhancing EpSC differentiation, proliferation, and migration. Yang et al. applied 3% ALA to skin incisions wrapped in polyurethane for 3 h and irradiated them with LED red light (635 nm, 6 J/cm^2), finding that ALA-PDT significantly increased epithelial migration [69]. By day 5, the average epithelial lengths in the control, red light, ALA, and ALA-PDT groups were 296.63 μm, 326.91 μm, 486.04 μm, and 563.34 μm, respectively, highlighting the superior epithelialization effect of ALA-PDT.

11.3.3.4 Clinical Research on the Effects of PDT on Chronic Wounds

A 2015 randomized controlled clinical study evaluated ALA-PDT for chronic lower limb wounds infected with *P. aeruginosa* and involved 26 patients divided into ALA-PDT and red-light groups [70]. The ALA-PDT group received 20% ALA solution for 1.5 h followed by 630 nm red light at 80 J/cm^2 per session, once weekly for two sessions. At 24 h posttreatment, the bacterial count in the ALA-PDT group significantly decreased to $6.3 \times 10^5 \pm 1.7 \times 10^6$ CFU/cm^2 compared with that in the pretreatment group, whereas the red-light group presented no significant bacterial reduction ($3.4 \times 10^7 \pm 7.1 \times 10^7$ CFU/cm^2). By day 7, wound healing in the ALA-PDT group was markedly better, with average wound sizes decreasing from 12.72 ± 8.58 cm^2 to 3.4 ± 3.4 cm^2, whereas it was reduced from 11.85 ± 6.83 cm^2 to 7.8 ± 4.9 cm^2 in the red-light group. Transient redness, swelling, and pain lasting 1–3 days were noted in the ALA-PDT group. Li et al. treated five diabetic foot patients with ALA-PDT (20% ALA for 4 h, 635 nm, 100 mW/cm^2, 120 J/cm^2) combined with antibiotics weekly for three sessions, achieving complete ulcer healing, negative bacterial cultures, and good tolerability, although some patients experienced transient skin burning and local wound reactions [71]. Similar clinical studies abroad have demonstrated the effectiveness of ALA-PDT in treating chronic skin ulcers.

Krupkau et al. compared ALA-PDT with octenidine gel in patients with chronic lower limb ulcers and divided 20 patients into two groups. The ALA-PDT group received 20% ALA for 4 h followed by 630 nm red-light irradiation at 80 J/cm^2 for ten sessions. ALA-PDT demonstrated superior antibacterial effects, with four patients achieving a complete response, four with a partial response, and two with no response over an 8-month follow-up. Grandi et al. treated 19 patients with chronic lower limb wounds with 20% ALA liposome gel and 630-nm red light at 80 J/cm^2 weekly, reducing the wound area from 4479.9 ± 345.5 mm^3 to 3459 ± 190.3 mm^3 after three sessions [72]. ALA-PDT (20% ALA incubation for 2 h, blue-light irradiation) also successfully treated a scalp ulcer from erosive pustular skin disease in a 61-year-old woman after one session, with healing observed at 4 months [73]. In terms of tumor ulcers, the authors' group treated an 85-year-old cSCC patient with left forehead ulceration with surgical excision combined with ALA-PDT once a week, achieving wound healing after three sessions over 2 months (Fig. 11.15). In a rare case of *Mycobacterium parascrofulaceum* skin infection, the authors' group used ALA-PDT (20% ALA for 3 h, 630 nm, 180 J/cm^2) weekly, successfully healing the patient after five treatments with no recurrence after 1 year, marking a significant first application of ALA-PDT in such infections [74] (Fig. 11.16).

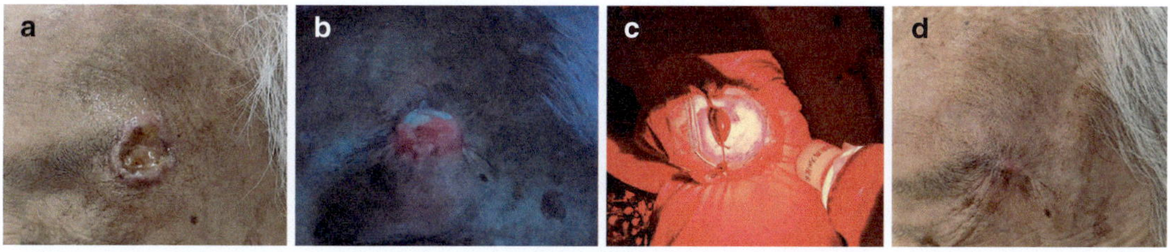

Fig. 11.15 ALA-PDT for cSCC. (**a**) Left forehead cSCC before treatment. (**b**) After surgical resection of the tumor lesion, brick-red fluorescence could be observed under a wood lamp 3 h after external application of ALA cream. (**c**) During ALA-PDT treatment. (**d**) The tumor was cured after three treatments with ALA-PDT

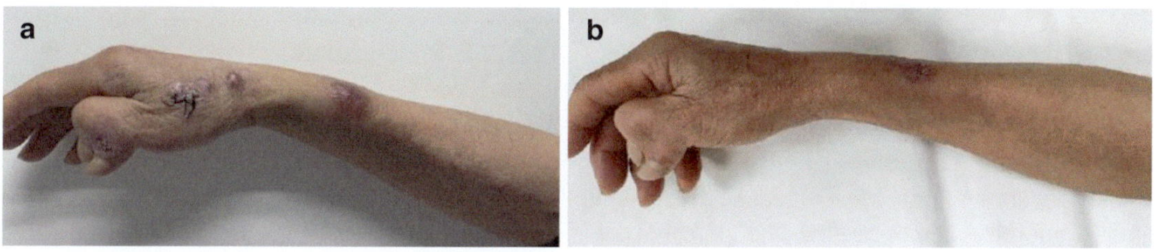

Fig. 11.16 ALA-PDT for the treatment of *Mycobacterium parascrofulaceum* infection of the skin. (**a**) *Mycobacterium parascrofulaceum* of skin prior to ALA-PDT and (**b**) no recurrence at the 1-year follow-up after ALA-PDT

11.3.4 PDT with Other Photosensitizers

Indocyanine green (ICG) is a near-infrared spectroscopic photosensitizer with strong absorptivity near 800 nm, enabling deep tissue penetration (up to 6 mm) to treat infections in deeper tissues effectively. Topaloglu et al. investigated the effect of ICG-PDT (808 nm, 450 J/cm^2) on bruising wounds in rats infected with multidrug-resistant *S. aureus*. They divided the wounds into groups treated with ICG-PDT, laser irradiation, ICG alone, or a combination of neither. The ICG concentrations tested were 500 μg/mL, 1000 μg/mL, and 2000 μg/mL, and the samples were illuminated for 15 min following a 3-min incubation. The results showed that ICG-PDT reduced bacterial loads by approximately 90%, whereas no significant bacterial reduction occurred in the groups treated with ICG or laser alone [75]. Dai et al. explored the efficacy of PEI-ce6-PDT on skin ulcers in mice infected with MRSA. Wounds were subjected to various energy densities (0–360 J/cm^2) via a 660 ± 15 nm laser, with 400 mM PEI-ce6 as the photosensitizer. A fluence-dependent reduction in bacterial load was observed, with the highest dose resulting in an average 2.7 log reduction in MRSA, demonstrating the potential of PEI-ce6-PDT in addressing resistant bacterial infections [43]. Garcia et al. evaluated the effects of toluidine blue (TBO)-mediated PDT on mouse wounds. Using a low-intensity aluminum arsenide laser (685 nm, 4.5 J/cm^2), they reported significant collagen fiber deposition, alignment, and neovascularization after 7 days of treatment. This outcome highlights the capacity of PDT to promote wound healing by enhancing structural and vascular regeneration [76]. PDT has also shown promise in treating chronic wounds in human patients. In a study involving 42 patients with pressure ulcers, phellodendron liquid-mediated PDT significantly improved epithelialization rates compared with those of controls [55]. The PDT group underwent two daily treatments with Huangbai liquid compound and 635 nm semiconductor laser irradiation (100 J/cm^2) over two 7-day courses. The epithelialization rates in the PDT group were 12.4% and 34.7% at days 7 and 14, respectively, whereas they were 5.1% and 10.5%, respectively, in the control group, indicating substantial therapeutic benefits. ShengTaiBuFen (STBF), a chlorophyll-derived photosensitizer with a wide absorption spectrum,

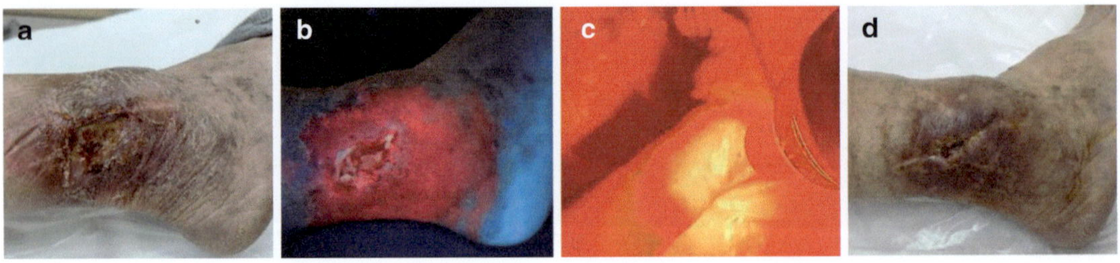

Fig. 11.17 STBF-PDT for the treatment of leg wounds. (**a**) Chronic wound of the right calf. (**b**) Brick-red fluorescence could be observed under a wood lamp after the STBF solution was applied for 1 h. (**c**) During STBF-PDT. (**d**) The wound significantly improved after 2 months of STBF-PDT treatment

has also shown efficacy in treating leg wounds. For the STBF-PDT, 0.5 mg/mL STBF solution was applied to the wound surface for 1 h before red-light irradiation (630 nm, 80 J/cm^2) was applied weekly for six sessions. Most ulcers nearly healed after 2 months, demonstrating the potential of STBF-PDT in chronic wound management [77] (Fig. 11.17). Other photosensitizer-mediated PDTs, such as polyl-L-lysine coupled chlorine P6 (pl-cp6) and zinc(II) phthalocyanine derivatives (RLP068/Cl), also have significant effects on chronic wounds. Pl-cp6-PDT (200 μM pl-cp6 after 30 min, 660 ± 25 nm; 100 mW/cm^2, 120 J/cm^2) can inhibit collagen degradation caused by bacterial infection; enhance epithelialization, hydroxyproline content and collagen remodeling; and accelerate the repair of bacterium-infected mouse ulcers [78]. RLP068/Cl-PDT (75 μM RLP068/Cl, 15 min of incubation, 690 ± 15 nm, 100 mW/cm^2, 84 J/cm^2) can be used for the antibacterial treatment of wounds [79]. PDT mediated by hypericin-laden nanocores (HY-NPs) could also provide antibacterial and therapeutic effects on wounds [80].

11.3.5 Recommended Scheme for ALA-PDT

11.3.5.1 Indications

Patients with chronic skin ulcers unresponsive to conventional treatments or coinfected with drug-resistant organisms who are not photosensitive.

11.3.5.2 Procedures

1. Perform debridement to remove necrotic tissue and scabs from the wound surface.
2. The wound area was measured prior to ALA-PDT, the required amount of 20% ALA solution was estimated on the basis of the ulcer size, and the samples were prepared accordingly. A gauze piece sufficient to cover the wound was soaked with ALA solution and applied to the wound surface, and for deeper wounds or sinuses, ALA-soaked strips were gently inserted into the ulcer before being wrapped for 3 h.
3. After the application, the gauze was removed, and the excess ALA solution was gently wiped off with sterile gauze.
4. The illumination parameters were set to 50–100 mW/cm^2, 630 nm, delivering 60–100 J/cm^2 per session on the basis of infection severity and ulcer depth, maintaining an irradiation distance of 10–20 cm.
5. Ensure that both the operator and the patient wear protective goggles during the procedure to safeguard their eyes.
6. Treatment was repeated every 4–7 days depending on the severity and depth of the ulcer, and any adverse reactions were recorded in detail.
7. After treatment, a routine wound dressing was applied via sterile gauze or an external wound dressing while adhering strictly to aseptic procedures.

11.3.5.3 Precautions

1. Ensure patient education and obtain signed informed consent prior to treatment.
2. The acute inflammatory reaction following PDT typically resolves independently within 1 week.
3. Inquire about the patient's pain levels during treatment and adjust treatment parameters as needed on the basis of the therapeutic response and any adverse reactions.
4. Regular follow-up is essential to monitor progress and any potential complications.

11.3.6 Conclusion

Both basic research and clinical applications have demonstrated the potential of ALA-PDT in wound treatment; however, clinicians must continue to gather and refine their experience with its clinical use, optimizing parameters to consistently improve its effectiveness.

11.4 PDT for Cutaneous Fungal Infections

11.4.1 Introduction

Cutaneous fungal infections are classified into superficial mycosis and subcutaneous mycosis. Superficial mycosis refers to a disease of superficial tissues caused by pathogenic or opportunistic fungi that infect the stratum corneum, mucous membranes, and appendages of the skin, such as nails, toenails, or hair. It includes conditions such as dermatophytosis, superficial candidiasis, and pityriasis versicolor. Subcutaneous mycoses, on the other hand, are chronic granulomatous infections affecting the skin and subcutaneous tissues; these infections are typically caused by fungi and include conditions such as sporotrichosis, chromoblastomycosis, and *Candida* granulomas [81].

Cutaneous fungal infections are widespread globally, affecting an estimated 20–25% of the population, particularly in tropical and subtropical regions [82]. While these infections are rarely fatal, they significantly impact an individual's quality of life and lead to a variety of comorbid symptoms, making them a public health concern. The prevalence of these infections varies by region and is influenced by factors such as age, sex, education, lifestyle, hygiene practices, immune response, fungal virulence, and socioeconomic status [83]. The increasing incidence of conditions such as AIDS, cancer, diabetes, and hematological disorders, along with the widespread use of broad-spectrum antibiotics, immunosuppressants, and glucocorticoids, has contributed to an increase in the incidence of cutaneous fungal infections [84].

11.4.2 Approaches

Pharmacological treatment is the primary approach for managing cutaneous fungal infections, with antifungal drugs such as imidazoles, arylamines, morpholinoids, echinocandins, and polyenes being commonly used [85].

For patients with early and mild superficial fungal infections, such as tinea pedis, tinea corporis, tinea cruris, and pityriasis versicolor, topical treatments are preferred. Commonly used topical antifungal drugs include imidazoles such as miconazole and bifonazole; arylamines such as terbinafine and buspirone; and morpholines such as amorolfine. These medications are recommended to be used for the full course of treatment and at the full dosage. For patients with extensive involvement, poor response to topical treatments, recurrent infections, or systemic diseases such as diabetes mellitus or AIDS, or those unwilling to use topical treatments, oral antifungal therapy or combination therapy is advised. Common oral antifungal agents include itraconazole (100–200 mg daily, twice a day for 1–2 weeks) and terbinafine (250 mg daily for 1–2 weeks, not recommended for pityriasis versicolor). Treatment failure and recurrence rates are high due to substandard treatment or poor patient compliance [86–88].

Oral antifungal medications are preferred for treating fungal infections of skin appendages, such as onychomycosis and tinea capitis. Terbinafine and itraconazole are first-line drugs, whereas fluconazole is considered a second-line option. The duration of treatment is adjusted on the basis of clinical manifestations and mycological findings, typically requiring 2–4 months of oral therapy for nail fungal diseases. If there is no significant improvement in clinical or mycological conditions after 1 month of oral treatment for tinea capitis, extending the treatment duration or switching oral medications may be necessary. In addition to oral medications, combination therapy, which may include combining oral treatments with topical therapies or adjunctive measures such as nail avulsion, medication under occlusion, nail grinding, and PDT, is recommended [89, 90].

Subcutaneous mycosis can be classified into various types on the basis of the pathogens involved, including cutaneous blastomycosis, sporotrichosis, fusarium, *Candida* granuloma, mycetoma, rhinosporidiosis, hyalotrichosis, aspergillosis, and Majocchi's granuloma [91]. Systemic antifungal therapy is the primary treatment for these diseases, with common drugs including azoles (itraconazole, voriconazole, and posaconazole), arylamines (terbinafine), and polyenes (amphotericin B). The duration of treatment is guided by clinical improvement and mycological findings, and therapy can be discontinued only once the lesions have resolved and mycological tests are negative. Owing to the long and challenging treatment course for these diseases, a combination of oral antifungal medications and adjunctive therapies, such as surgical resection and PDT, is recommended [92–94].

The prolonged duration of oral antifungal therapy, along with potential side effects and drug interactions, leads some patients to refuse or be unable to undergo oral treatment. This makes the management of onychomycosis, tinea capitis, and subcutaneous fungal infections more challenging in clinical practice. Additionally, the slow development of new antifungal drugs and the ongoing emergence of drug-resistant strains further complicate the clinical treatment of these infections [95, 96].

11.4.3 ALA-PDT

Although the therapeutic potential of PDT in antimicrobial treatments dates back to the early 1900s [97], research in this area has been slow, with an increased focus on antifungal applications only in recent decades [98]. Current studies primarily investigate the effects of PDT on dermatophytes, candidiasis, and certain deep-seated fungi using photosensitizers such as methylene blue (MB), ALA, and ALA methyl ester (MAL). In clinical practice, PDT is used mainly as an adjunctive treatment for refractory fungal infections, including nail fungal diseases, tinea capitis, and subcutaneous fungal infections, and offers advantages such as minimal toxic side effects, safety, reliability, and high reproducibility. In 2007, the authors' group explored the use of ALA-PDT for treating superficial fungal diseases, confirming its efficacy. However, ALA-PDT is considered an alternative treatment for severe, complicated, or drug-intolerant cases, given its clinical convenience and cost-effectiveness.

11.4.3.1 Mechanism

In vitro and in vivo studies have demonstrated that the antifungal action of PDT occurs through four main mechanisms: a Type I reaction, where the photosensitizer interacts with a substrate to generate free radicals and oxygen molecules, which react to produce reactive oxygen species (ROS), leading to fungal apoptosis and necrosis [99]; a Type II reaction, where energy is transferred from the photosensitizer to oxygen molecules, resulting in the formation of singlet oxygen ($^1O_2$), which damages the fungus [100]; a Type III reaction, where photosensitizers act as sensitizers of antioxidant carriers, reducing the natural free radical content in target cells and promoting the production of more $^1O_2$; and a Type IV reaction, which involves the combination of the photosensitizer with the target after photoexcitation. Type I and II reactions cause indirect damage, whereas types III and IV reactions lead to secondary effects from photosensitizer activation [101, 102]. PDT inhibits the growth of fungi such as *Candida*, dermatophytes, *Sporothrix*, *Botrytis cinerea*, and *Malassezia* by disrupting their cell wall structure and can also inhibit the formation of *Candida* biofilms [103–105]. In addition to direct antifungal action, PDT can recruit immune cells, promote local neutrophil and lymphocyte infiltration and enhance antifungal immunity [106, 107].

11.4.3.2 Clinical Efficacy

Superficial fungal infection: Tinea pedis, a superficial fungal infection affecting the interdigital, plantar, and lateral margins of the foot, is caused primarily by dermatophytes. The mainstay of treatment is topical antifungal medications, with oral antifungal therapy recommended for patients with severe or recurrent infections. Sotiriou applied ALA-PDT to treat 10 patients with interdigital tinea pedis, using 20% ALA cream as the photosensitizer, followed by irradiation with 570–670 nm red light at an energy dose of 50 J/cm^2 (irradiance: 50 mW/cm^2) after 3 hs of application. After three treatments, six patients had negative mycological tests, and after 2 months of follow-up, only three remained mycologically negative [108]. Calzavara Pinton et al. treated nine patients with interdigital tinea pedis using 20% ALA cream as a photosensitizer and red-light irradiation (575–700 nm) with an energy dose of 75 J/cm^2 and a power density of 100 mW/cm^2 after 4 h of topical application. After four treatments, six patients experienced clinical improvement and negative mycological tests, with a 67% remission rate. However, four patients relapsed within 2 months, and only two patients remained in clinical remission with negative mycological tests, resulting in a 22% clinical remission rate [109]. Both studies noted local erythema and pain during light exposure. These studies confirm the efficacy of PDT in treating tinea pedis, although the recurrence rate remains similar to that of conventional drug treatments.

Tinea cruris is a dermatophyte infection affecting the groin, perineum, perianal area, and buttocks. Topical antifungal medications are the first-line treatment, with oral antifungals recommended for severe or recurrent cases. In 2007, the authors' group used ALA-PDT to treat 5 patients with tinea cruris; 10% ALA cream was applied externally for 3 h, followed by 635 nm red-light irradiation at a power density of 50 mW/cm^2 and a fluence of 100 J/cm^2. Treatment was performed once every 2 weeks for a total of two sessions. After 1 month of follow-up, three patients had positive fungal examinations (Fig. 11.18). In 2009, Sotiriou treated 10 male patients with tinea cruris using 20% ALA cream applied externally for 4 h, followed by 570–670 nm red-light irradiation at 50 J/cm^2 and 50 mW/cm^2. After the first treatment, two patients had negative mycological tests, and after the second treatment, six more patients tested negative. After 2 months of follow-up, four patients had positive fungal tests, and only four remained negative. Patients experi-

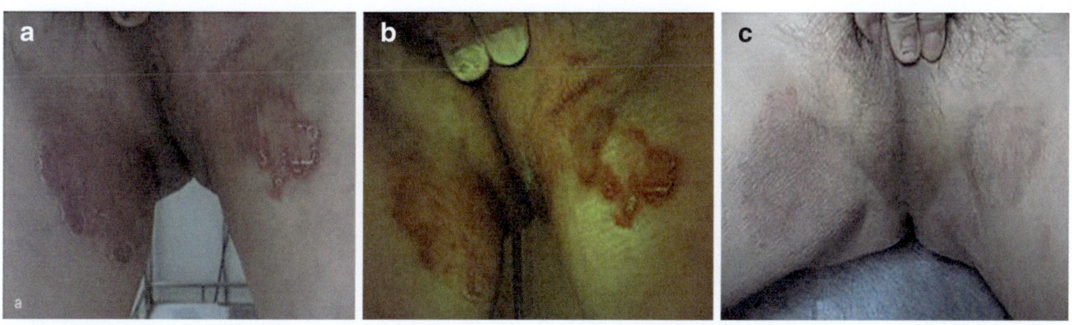

Fig. 11.18 Improvement after two sessions of ALA-PDT. (**a**) Before treatment. (**b**) Brick-red fluorescence could be observed after the external application of 10% ALA cream for 3 h. (**c**) The symptoms improved after two ALA-PDT treatments

enced burning pain and tingling during treatment, with local erythema appearing 3–4 days post-treatment [110].

Pityriasis versicolor is a chronic, recurrent superficial fungal infection caused by *Malassezia* affecting the stratum corneum. Kim used ALA-PDT to treat a patient under these conditions; 20% ALA cream was applied externally for 4 h, followed by 670 nm red-light irradiation. The treatment consisted of two sessions at 2-week intervals, with a fluence of 70–80 J/cm^2 during the first session and 80–90 J/cm^2 during the second session. After two treatments, the lesions healed, and no recurrence was observed after 3 months, with no reported discomfort [111].

Fungal infections of the skin, such as tinea capitis, a dermatophyte infection of the hair and scalp, are commonly observed in children, and its incidence has increased with increasing household pets. While systemic antifungal drugs are the first choice for treatment, the long duration of therapy and potential drug side effects pose challenges. Kerion, a severe form of tinea capitis, results from an intense inflammatory response to the infecting fungus or irregular treatment, often leading to more severe symptoms and prolonged treatment [90]. The authors' group treated a 2-year-old child with scalp kerion who had experienced hepatic injury from oral terbinafine. The child was treated with 20% ALA solution applied externally for 3 h, followed by irradiation with 635-nm red light at 100 J/cm^2 for 20 min, with a follow-up treatment 2 weeks later. After 1 month, the skin lesions had healed, fungal tests were negative, and there was no recurrence at 6 months (Fig. 11.19) [112]. Another study of a 3-year-old child treated with ALA-PDT alone reported a cure after two treatments (Fig. 11.20). A 10-year-

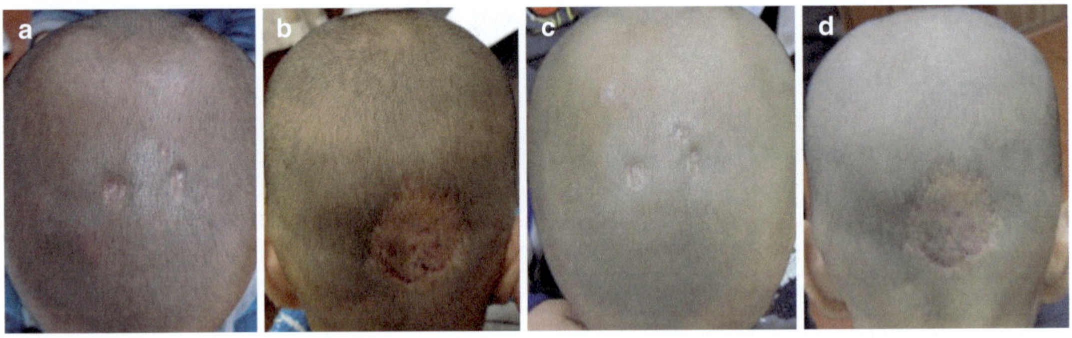

Fig. 11.19 A 2-year-old child with tinea capitis cured after two treatments with ALA-PDT. (**a**) Red nodules on the vertex scalp before ALA-PDT. (**b**) Alopecia and scarring over the occipital scalp before ALA-PDT. (**c**) Scalp lesions after two sessions of ALA-PDT. (**d**) Lesions of the occipital scalp after two sessions of ALA-PDT

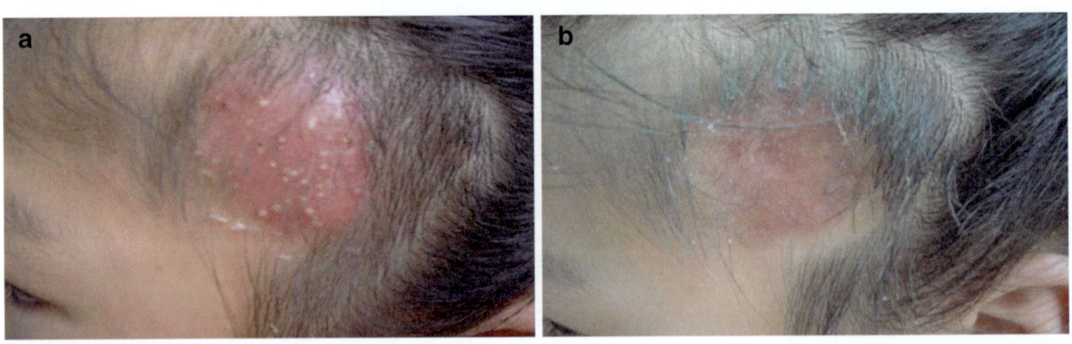

Fig. 11.20 A 3-year-old child with kerion cured after two treatments with ALA-PDT alone. (**a**) Before ALA-PDT and (**b**) after ALA-PDT

old child with kerion was cured by using ALA-PDT in combination with itraconazole (Fig. 11.21). A 4-year-old child with kerion was treated with oral terbinafine (at 125 mg/day) in combination with ALA-PDT (20% ALA cream, 2 h of incubation, 635 nm red light, 10 min of irradiation, 60 J/cm^2, 200 mW/cm^2).

There was no significant discomfort during the treatment. At the 4-week follow-up, more than 90% of the rash had subsided, new hair growth was observed in the area of the original damage, and fungal microscopy was negative. As a result, oral terbinafine tablets were discontinued (Fig. 11.22). No recurrence was noted during

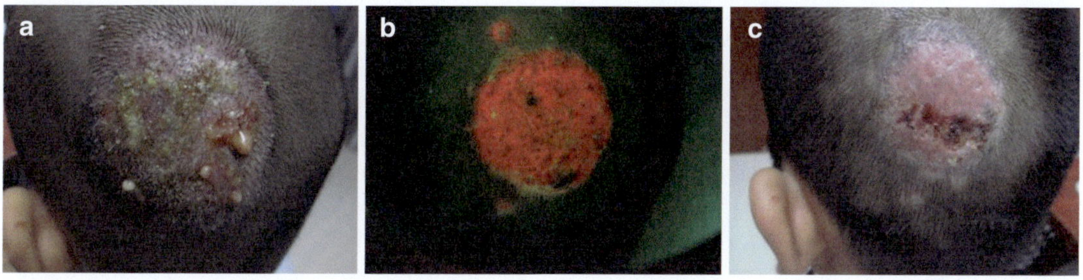

Fig. 11.21 ALA-PDT treatment in a 10-year-old child with kerion. (**a**) Before treatment. (**b**) After application of ALA cream, the lesion showed brick-red fluorescence. (**c**) Symptomatic improvement after 2 weeks of ALA-PDT combined with itraconazole

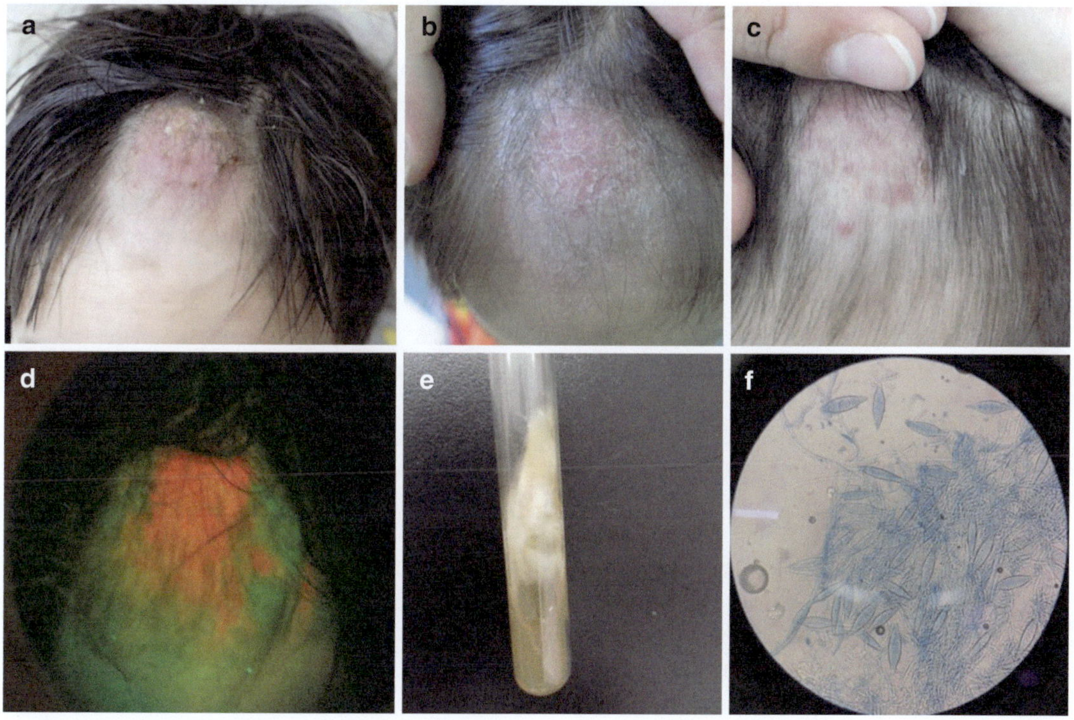

Fig. 11.22 A 4-year-old child with tinea capitis was cured after one ALA-PDT. (**a**) Before treatment. (**b**) After 2 weeks of ALA-PDT treatment. (**c**) After 4 weeks of ALA-PDT treatment. (**d**) After incubation with ALA, distinct brick-red fluorescence was observed. (**e**) White woolly colonies from fungal culture. (**f**) Microscopic analysis revealed spores and hyphae with a thick septum (×400)

the 8-week follow-up period after treatment [113].

Onychomycosis is one of the most common nail diseases and is caused by infections of the nail plate by organisms such as *dermatophytes*, *Candida*, and non-dermatophyte moulds. Although oral antifungal drugs are the preferred treatment, onychomycosis remains challenging because of prolonged treatment duration and potential side effects [89]. As an adjuvant therapy, PDT has been increasingly studied, with photosensitizers such as MAL, methylene blue (MB), ALA, Rose Bengal, and curcumin [111, 114, 115]. One of the largest studies on ALA-PDT for onychomycosis compared it to 5% amorolfine. In this open-label study, 56 patients with bilateral hallux onychomycosis were treated with either ALA-PDT (group A) or 5% amorolfine (group B), with both groups pretreated with a CO_2 fractional laser on one side of the nails. The ALA-PDT group was treated with 20% ALA cream and red-light irradiation (630 nm, 75 J/cm^2) every 3 weeks for a total of six treatments. After 3 months, 53% of the PDT group and 50% of the amorolfine group had negative fungal tests, indicating no significant difference. At 9 months posttreatment, 27% of the patients in the PDT group and 16% of those in the amorolfine group remained fungal free. This study demonstrated no significant advantage of ALA-PDT over 5% amorolfine [116]. Sotiriou treated 30 patients with subungual onychomycosis via a combination of 20% urea application followed by ALA-PDT with 20% ALA cream and red-light irradiation (570–670 nm, 40 J/cm^2). After 12 months, 43.3% of patients achieved complete remission or significant improvement, although the efficacy decreased to 36.6% at 18 months because of relapses [117]. Watanabe also reported successful ALA-PDT treatments in two patients with subungual onychomycosis, where 630-nm red light with an energy density of 100 J/cm^2 was applied after 5 h of 20% ALA incubation for six to seven sessions. Both patients remained fungal free after 3–6 months of follow-up, although they experienced pain during the treatments [118].

Subcutaneous mycosis is a chronic granulomatous inflammation caused by fungal infections of the skin and subcutaneous tissues, with a variety of causative organisms and localized infections, making clinical treatment challenging. Oral administration of antifungal drugs on the basis of drug sensitivity tests is the preferred treatment, but adjuvant therapies such as surgical excision and PDT have also been recommended. PDT is particularly effective for treating subcutaneous tissue granulomas because of its low toxicity and selective destruction of tissue. Case reports have highlighted the successful use of PDT for treating sporotrichosis, chromoblastomycosis, phaeohyphomycosis, *Candida* granulomas, and Majocchi granulomas [94]. The most commonly used photosensitizer is 10–20% ALA, and the light source is typically 630–635-nm red light with an energy range of 70–100 J/cm^2.

The authors' group successfully used ALA-PDT to treat a case of *Candida* granuloma on the right hand, applying 10% ALA cream externally for 4 h, followed by 630 nm red-light irradiation with a power density of 100 mW/cm^2 and an energy density of 360 J/cm^2. Treatment was repeated after 20 days, and 2 months later, the lesions had completely healed with no discomfort during treatment [119]. Additionally, ALA-PDT was successfully used to treat Majocchi's granuloma in a 73-year-old patient caused by *Trichophyton tonsurans* infection, for which oral or topical antifungal therapy failed. After 3 h of 10% ALA cream application, the patient underwent 635-nm red-light irradiation (100 mW/cm^2, 120 J/cm^2), and the scalp lesions were cured after three sessions, with no recurrence observed during a 3-month follow-up (Fig. 11.23) [107].

11.4.4 PDT with Other Photosensitizers

In addition to ALA, phenothiazines and other porphyrin-based photosensitizers, such as methylene blue (MB) and toluidine blue O (TBO), have been used to treat cutaneous fungal infections

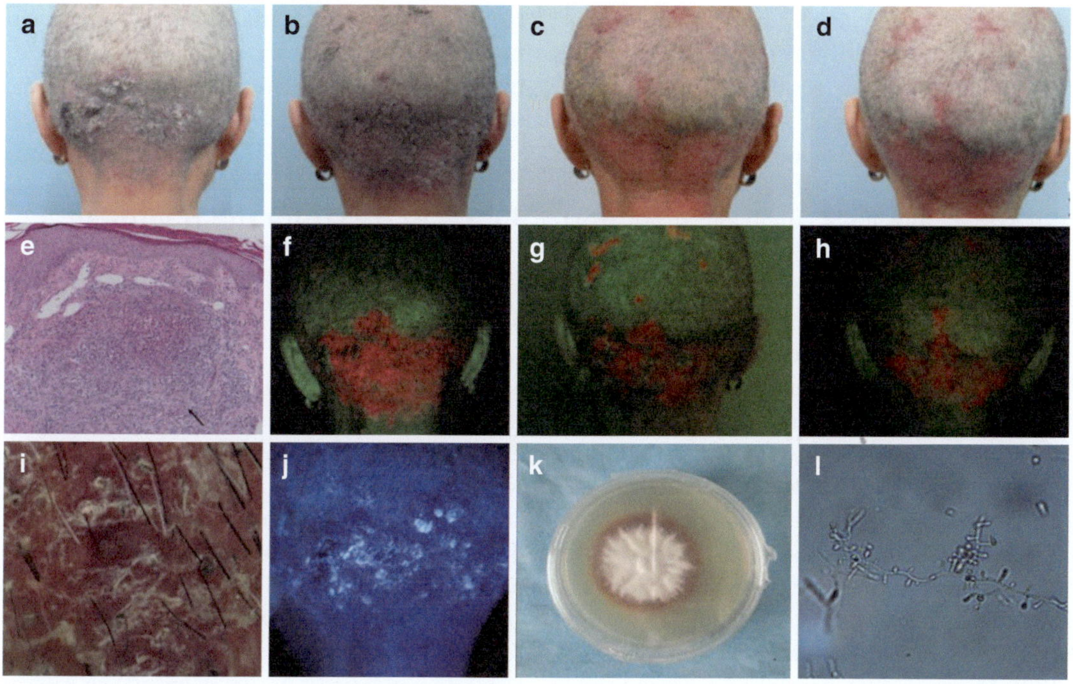

Fig. 11.23 ALA-PDT in a patient with Majocchi's granuloma. (**a**) Before treatment. (**b**) After the first treatment. (**c**) After the second treatment. (**d**) After the third treatment. (**e**) Pathology before ALA-PDT treatment revealed dense mixed infiltration in the dermis (H&E staining, ×100). (**f**) After initial incubation with ALA, distinctive brick-red fluorescence was observed, suggesting selective lesional ALA absorption. (**g**) After the second incubation with ALA, fluorescence decreased, indicating improvement of the lesion. (**h**) After the third incubation with ALA, fluorescence further decreased. (**i**) Dermoscopy revealed unstructured erythema of the occipital scalp accompanied by pustules and nodules with surface scales. (**j**) Bright white fluorescence of the lesion surface under Wood's lamp. (**k**) White, fluffy, radiating colonies on fungal culture. (**l**) Budding spores and hyphae under a microscope (×400)

because their permeability in the skin and nail plate is greater than that of ALA. Alberdi treated five female patients with dorsal disseminated pityriasis versicolor via MB-PDT, applying 2% MB solution for 3 min followed by (630 ± 5)-nm red-light irradiation at an energy density of 37 J/cm^2 for six treatments at 2-week intervals, achieving a 100% clinical remission rate with no recurrence in 6 months of follow-up and minimal side effects [120]. Natthamon used MB-PDT to treat nondermatophyte onychomycosis, first removing toenails with 40% urea wrap, incubating them with 1% MB solution for 3–5 min, and irradiating them with 630–640 nm red light (150 mW/cm^2, 120 J/cm^2) once every 2 weeks for six sessions, resulting in better results than those obtained with 5% amorolfine [114]. Garcia-Malinis successfully treated a patient with *Sporothrix schenckii* by incubating the lesion with 1% MB solution for 30 min followed by 2 h of sunlight exposure, which was repeated every 2 weeks for six sessions [121].

Porphyrin photosensitizers increase fungal cell membrane permeability under light exposure, disrupting physiological metabolism and causing fungal death. MAL, a lipophilic ester derivative of ALA, has demonstrated comparable therapeutic efficacy to ALA [122]. Navarro-Bielsa treated 20 onychomycosis patients with a combination of oral or topical antifungal drugs, 40% urea for nail removal, and MAL-PDT. After the application of 16% MAL cream for 3 h, 630-

nm red-light irradiation (37 J/cm^2) was administered every 1–2 weeks for 3–15 sessions on the basis of the response, resulting in clinical and mycological efficiencies of 80% and 60%, respectively, after 6 months [115]. Lee used MAL-PDT for six patients with recurrent *Malassezia* folliculitis, applying 16% MAL cream for 3 h and puncturing cystic or nodular lesions with a 1–2 mm needle to enhance MAL penetration, followed by 630 nm red-light irradiation (37 J/cm^2) every 2 weeks for three sessions. After 1 month, five patients experienced clinical improvement, with inflammation and lesions subsiding, and only one relapse occurred after 3 months; no significant adverse reactions were observed during treatment [123].

Phthalocyanine photosensitizers, known for their strong hydrophobicity, require liposome encapsulation or sulfonation to improve water solubility, limiting their use as antifungal agents [124]. Morgado et al. developed a water-soluble nanoemulsion (NE) encapsulating aluminum-phthalocyanine chloride (AICIPc-NE), which offers improved penetration and reduced staining compared with traditional photosensitizers. In a study involving 20 patients with nail fungal disease, 40% urea solution was applied for 1 week to enhance nail plate permeability, followed by the external application of 65 μm AICIPc-NE for 15 min and illumination with 660-nm light (30.9 J/cm^2, 51.5 mW/cm^2) every 15 days. Among the 16 patients who completed treatment (averaging 4.45 ± 1.76 sessions), 40% achieved negative mycological results and 60% achieved clinical remission 1 month posttreatment [125].

11.4.5 Conclusion

In summary, PDT is a less toxic, safe, reliable, and reproducible treatment option that can serve as an adjunctive or alternative therapy for patients intolerant of prolonged oral antifungal medications or those with drug-resistant fungal infections. However, the absence of large-scale randomized controlled trials limits the confirmation of its long-term efficacy and safety in treating cutaneous fungal infections, highlighting the need for further research.

11.5 ALA-PDT for the Treatment of Lichen Planus

11.5.1 Overview of Lichen Planus

Lichen planus (LP) is an idiopathic inflammatory disease of the skin and mucosa with an unclear etiology and a pathogenesis linked to various factors, such as infections, autoimmune conditions, stress, medications, localized skin diseases, metabolic or endocrine disorders, and dental materials. LP affects 1–2% of the population, with the prevalence of oral LP (OLP) ranging from 0.89% to 1.27% [126–129]. Mucosal involvement, particularly oral lesions, occurs in more than 75% of cutaneous LP cases, although only 10–20% of patients with initial oral lesions develop cutaneous involvement. Notably, 0.04–1.74% of OLP cases may progress to oral cancer [126].

11.5.1.1 Clinical Features

LP typically affects middle-aged individuals and can involve the skin, hair follicles, nails, and mucous membranes. The primary lesions are small, polygonal or rounded, purplish-red, flat-topped papules with well-defined borders. Some lesions are umbilicated, with a smooth, shiny, waxy surface featuring small white puncta or a network of fine white lines, known as "Wickham striae." Lesions may appear in a linear array along areas of trauma or scratches, referred to as the Koebner phenomenon. Pruritus is the main symptom, and the disease duration varies depending on the variant, with some lesions resolving within a year while others persist. Clinical variants include acute or subacute generalized LP, linear LP, annular LP, hypertrophic LP, atrophic LP, lichen planopilaris, bullous LP, actinic LP, LP pemphigoides, and LP pigmentosus.

11.5.1.2 Pathology

The histopathological features of LP include orthokeratosis, focal thickening of the granular cell layer, irregular acanthosis, and "sawtooth" rete ridges. There is liquefactive degeneration of the basal cell layer and a band-like lymphocytic infiltrate at the dermal–epidermal junction. Colloidal (Civatte) bodies may be present in the lower epidermis and superficial lamina propria and are often accompanied by pigmentary incontinence.

11.5.2 Treatment

The primary goals of LP treatment are to shorten the disease course and alleviate symptoms. Current therapies include the following: (1) topical therapies, such as corticosteroids to relieve itching and tretinoin to reduce hyperkeratosis, (2) systemic therapies, including systemic immunosuppressants and corticosteroid pulse therapy for refractory cases, and (3) physical therapy, such as laser therapy, cryotherapy, radiation therapy, and narrowband ultraviolet therapy, which are employed for hypertrophic, venous proliferative, and oral erosive lesions. However, these treatments often have limited efficacy and may cause side effects, such as immunosuppression. As a result, alternative treatments such as ALA-PDT are gaining recognition for managing LP.

11.5.3 ALA-PDT

11.5.3.1 Clinical Application

In 1999, Kirby et al. first reported the application of ALA-PDT in the treatment of hypertrophic lichen planus of the penis [130]. A 20% ALA emulsifying ointment was applied to the affected area, incubated in the dark for 4 h, and then irradiated with a patented nonlaser light source (Paterson-Whitehurst lamp) at 630 nm. The dose was 50 J/cm^2 at a fluence rate of 55 mW/cm^2. The patient received two treatments spaced 2 weeks apart, resulting in complete lesion resolution with no recurrence at the 6-month follow-up. Despite this initial success, similar reports remained scarce for an extended period.

In 2015, the authors' group conducted clinical research on ALA-PDT for treating lichen planus (LP) in 7 patients with 17 lesions. A 10% ALA cream was applied to the lesions and surrounding skin (0.5 cm margin, 1 mm thickness), followed by 3 h of light-protected incubation and red-light PDT at 635 nm with a dose of 100 J/cm^2. Lidocaine was used for local anesthesia to manage pain. After four treatments, complete clearance was achieved for 13 lesions across 5 patients, whereas partial responses were observed for 4 lesions in 2 patients. Notably, three previously corticosteroid-treated and relapsed lesions achieved complete clearance after one ALA-PDT session. No recurrences occurred in lesions with complete clearance during the 6-month follow-up, and the treatment demonstrated cosmetic benefits. In 2018, the authors reported a case of penile LP combined with condyloma acuminata, which was initially misdiagnosed as bowenoid papulosis. After confirming the diagnosis, ALA-PDT was applied with 635 nm red light at 100 J/cm^2, resulting in complete lesion clearance after two treatments at 2-week intervals, with no recurrence at the 2-year follow-up, confirming the safety and efficacy of ALA-PDT for LP and condyloma acuminata [131].

OLP requires effective treatment due to the risk of malignant transformation in longstanding, nonhealing cases. ALA-PDT has been proven effective for treating skin precancers, and its efficacy in OLP was investigated by Maloth et al. in a clinical study involving 8 patients with 20 OLP lesions [132]. The patients were divided into two groups: one received ALA-PDT (420 nm, >300 J/cm^2), and the other received topical corticosteroids. After 4 weeks, 80% of the lesions in the ALA-PDT group improved, a result comparable to that of the corticosteroid group. In a separate study, Magdalena et al. evaluated ALA-PDT in 50 patients with 124 reticular OLP lesions (aged 26–84 years) [133]. After ten sessions of ALA-PDT (630 nm, 150 J/cm^2), 109 lesions improved, with 46 completely cleared. After 12 months, the average reduction in the lesion area was 78.7%. A systematic review and meta-analysis by He et al. revealed that ALA-PDT was more effective than methylene blue PDT (MB-PDT) and that

Table 11.2 Recommended protocol for the treatment of LP with ALA-PDT

ALA formulation			Dose of light	
ALA formulation	ALA concentration (%)	Incubation time (h)	Energy density (J/cm^2)	Power density (mW/cm^2)
Cream	10	3–6	100–200	60–150

topical ALA produced better results than oral MB rinses [134].

11.5.3.2 Recommended Protocols

The recommended protocol for the treatment of LP with ALA-PDT is shown in Table 11.2.

- Interval: 2 weeks.
- Frequency: three times or achieving complete clearance.
- Pretreatment: Plum-needle pretreatment can be applied for thicker lesions.
- Efficacy evaluation: Clinical manifestation and pathological examination.
- Endpoint: Curing confirmed by histopathology.

11.5.4 PDT with Other Photosensitizers

Other photosensitizers used in PDT for treating OLP include MB, hexyl 5-aminolevulinate hydrochloride (HAL), MAL, chlorin-e-6-photolon, and toluidine blue [135–140].

HAL, a derivative of ALA, shares similar drug metabolism properties and has recently shown promise in treating genital erosion lichen planus (GELP). Helgesen et al. conducted a study involving 12 patients with GELP [141], which were divided into two groups, with either 6.25 mg/mL or 50 mg/mL HAL applied for 3 h. The biodistribution of HAL, measured by photoactive protoporphyrin IX (PpIX), was assessed via noninvasive fluorescence measurements, which revealed that 6.25 mg/mL HAL for 3 h was sufficient for effective absorption and conversion of HAL to PpIX in submucosal inflammatory and epithelial cells. This led to a randomized clinical trial with 40 female patients with GELP, who were divided into a HAL-PDT group (6.25 mg/mL HAL, 633 nm, 75 J/cm^2) and a corticosteroid group. After 6 weeks, both groups showed similar reductions in clinical scores (25% vs 22%, $P = 0.787$), with a slight difference at 24 weeks (35% vs 38%, $P = 0.801$). The HAL-PDT group, however, reported significantly less corticosteroid use and experienced fewer side effects, suggesting that HAL-PDT is as effective as corticosteroids for GELP while avoiding the long-term side effects of corticosteroid use [142].

In 2006, Aghahosseini et al. treated 13 patients with 26 OLP lesions via MB-PDT [135], where patients gargled with a 5% methylene blue solution for 5 min, followed by laser irradiation (632 nm, 120 J/cm^2). Significant improvements were observed in 16 lesions, with 4 lesions completely resolved. Significant reductions in sign and symptom scores were observed after 1 week and at follow-up sessions up to 12 weeks, with an average lesion size reduction of 44.3%. Later, the same protocol was used to treat 5 OLP lesions in 2 patients, yielding 80% improvement. In 2012, Sadaksharam et al. further confirmed the safety and efficacy of MB-PDT in 20 patients with OLP [137], showing effective lesion improvement without major side effects. A 12-week single-blind randomized trial by Kamil et al. in 2014 compared MB-PDT (640 nm, 120 J/cm^2) with topical corticosteroids in 30 patients with bilateral erythematous or erosive OLP. Both treatments were effective, with no significant difference between the two [143]. In 2017, Mostafa et al. conducted a randomized study on 20 patients with erosive OLP and reported that MB-PDT (660 nm, 100–130 mW/cm^2) was more effective than topical corticosteroids in pain relief and lesion clearance [144].

Finally, in 2020, Wafaa Saleh et al. recruited 20 patients with erosive OLP and compared MB-PDT with topical betamethasone valerate ointment [145]. The MB-PDT showed better results, with greater improvement than corticosteroids between time zero and the fourth week of treatment.

In 2013, Sobaniec et al. treated 23 patients with 48 OLP lesions via chlorin-e-6-phototherapy with red light (660 nm, 90 J/cm^2) for ten sessions at 2-week intervals [138]. The lesions were categorized by size, with 40 located on the lining mucosa and 8 on the gums and tongue. Significant reductions in lesion size (averaging 55%) were observed, with the best results for the lining mucosa (57.6%). However, lesions on the masticatory mucosa were significantly less common (30%). In the same year, Kvaal et al. treated 14 patients with OLP via MAL-PDT (600–660 nm, 75 J/cm^2), which resulted in significant improvement in OLPs after a single treatment session [139]. This improvement lasted up to 4 years, revealing the lasting effect of the MAL-PDT. Additionally, Jajarm et al. [140] and Mirza et al. [146] treated 25 and 45 patients with atrophic OLP, respectively, via toluidine blue PDT. Patients in the PDT group received topical application of 50 μL toluidine blue (1 mg/mL), followed by laser irradiation (630 nm, 10 mW/cm^2). Compared with the other two groups, the PDT group presented significantly better results, although the corticosteroid group experienced greater pain relief.

In summary, while topical corticosteroid therapy remains the preferred treatment for lichen planus (LP) because of its economic and convenience benefits, it carries risks such as recurrence, corticosteroid dependence, and long-term side effects. PDT is a noninvasive topical treatment that offers a safe and effective alternative. Moreover, considering the potential of LP for malignant transformation, the unique antitumor and anti-inflammatory properties of ALA-PDT can help improve LP lesions and may also play a role in preventing LP-related carcinogenesis.

11.6 ALA-PDT for the Treatment of Epidermodysplasia Verruciformis, Xeroderma Pigmentosum and Other Genodermatoses

11.6.1 Overview of Genodermatosis Associated with Nonmelanoma Skin Cancer

Genodermatosis-associated nonmelanoma skin cancers, or keratinocyte carcinomas, are malignant skin cancers that originate from skin cells due to hereditary skin diseases and can result in patient mortality. Basal cell carcinoma (BCC) and cutaneous squamous cell carcinoma (cSCC) are the most common forms of these cancers. Additionally, precancerous conditions such as actinic keratosis (AK) and actinic cheilitis (AC) are prevalent. These diseases often occur more frequently within families and tend to have an earlier onset, often in childhood. Multiple lesions are typically located in sun-exposed areas, such as the face, neck, and limbs, and are prone to recurrence. In addition to skin cancer, genodermatoses can be associated with characteristic facial features, bone or limb deformities, hearing or vision impairments, visceral involvement, and other skin manifestations, such as pigmentation abnormalities, telangiectasia, and alopecia [147]. There are over 450 rare skin-related diseases classified into keratinization, pigmentary, metabolic, and autoimmune disorders and skin cancer-associated genodermatoses. Several genodermatoses manifest as skin cancer and can lead to death from skin cancers, including Gorlin syndrome, xeroderma pigmentosum, epidermodysplasia verruciformis, inherited epidermolysis bullosa, oculocutaneous albinism, dyskeratosis congenita, and Bazex-Dupré-Christol syndrome [148].

Genodermatosis-associated nonmelanoma skin cancers are rare diseases with a low incidence, but advancements in molecular diagnostic techniques have led to increased diagnoses and reports of these conditions, making what was once considered "rare" more prevalent. Current technologies allow for early molecular diagnosis of relevant genodermatoses through mutation screening of disease-causing genes. As a result, the demand for the diagnosis and treatment of secondary NMSC has increased. This surge in demand places a significant financial burden on patients' families and presents a substantial challenge to social care systems and prevention efforts.

11.6.2 Therapeutic Methods

Lesions associated with nonmelanoma skin cancers are characterized by early onset, frequent occurrence, and a tendency to recur. Clinical treatment requires a multidisciplinary approach involving dermatology, plastic surgery, ophthalmology, and sometimes dentistry and otolaryngology. Treatment methods can be divided into surgical options and nonsurgical options. Surgical treatment is highly destructive and often impractical due to the multiplicity of lesions. Nonsurgical treatments, such as imiquimod, 5-fluorouracil (5-FU), and cryotherapy, are typically reserved for early-stage lesions but have limited efficacy. With the advent of biologics, PD-1/PD-L1 and VEGFR antibodies have shown promise for treating multiple or advanced genodermatosis-associated nonmelanoma skin cancers. Hedgehog inhibitors are available for patients with multiple or aggressive BCC, but owing to their side effect profiles, limited response rates, and high treatment costs, they are not recommended as first-line therapies. Radiation and chemotherapy have been reported, but their use is limited by serious adverse reactions and limited efficacy [147, 149]. In conclusion, there is no universally recommended treatment for genodermatosis-associated nonmelanoma skin cancer, and effectively managing these conditions remains a significant clinical challenge.

11.6.3 Photodynamic Therapy

11.6.3.1 PDT for Gorlin Syndrome

Gorlin syndrome, also known as nevoid basal cell carcinoma syndrome, is a rare autosomal dominant disorder caused by mutations in the PTCH gene. It is characterized by congenital developmental abnormalities and increased susceptibility to BCCs. Early BCC lesions typically appear during adolescence or childhood and can occur in both sun-exposed and nonexposed areas, with common locations including the face, back, and chest. These lesions are often multiple [150]. A study summarized the clinical outcomes of 83 patients with Gorlin syndrome treated with MAL-PDT and concluded that MAL-PDT is an effective and safe treatment for BCC in this patient population. The recommended treatment protocol includes applying a 16% MAL solution to the skin lesions and keeping them away from light for 3 h, followed by exposure to 630 nm red light with a total dose of 37 J/cm^2. Two treatments should be performed at 1-week intervals, with reassessment at 3 months. If necessary, a second cycle of treatment can be administered [151]. In a study of seven patients, including two children treated with 16.8% MAL with a similar protocol, the overall clearance rates for superficial and nodular BCC were 78% and 79%, respectively, with excellent cosmetic results. Pediatric patients also demonstrated good tolerability of the treatment [152].

A study compared the efficacy of red and blue-light PDT for the treatment of BCC in three patients with a total of 141 lesions. Each patient underwent six PDT sessions, with half of their lesions receiving blue-light irradiation (417 nm, 10 J/cm^2) and the other half receiving red-light irradiation (630 nm, 75 J/cm^2). The treatments were administered at 2-week intervals, with light-avoidance incubation for 4 h with 20% ALA. The overall clearance rate for blue-light PDT was 98%, which was slightly higher than the 93% clearance rate for red-light PDT, although the difference was not statistically significant. Patients also reported less pain during blue-light PDT than during red-light PDT. The efficacy of the treatment was evaluated 6 months after the last session [153].

In 2017, a retrospective study compared the recurrence rates of wider local excision versus PDT combined with excision for multiple BCC lesions in patients with Gorlin syndrome. The first treatment group received two courses of ALA-PDT (20% ALA, 4 h of light-avoidance incubation, 635 nm red light, 62.5 mW/cm^2 irradiation for 20 min) after excision. The second group underwent wider local excision, with excision 0.5 cm away from the original incision. While there was no significant difference in recurrence rates, the ALA-PDT group demonstrated notable advantages in terms of economic burden, healing time, and aesthetic satisfaction [154]. In 2020, another case report described the use of microwave therapy followed by ALA-PDT to treat superficial BCC on the scalp in a patient with Gorlin syndrome. PDT was performed with 20% ALA, light-avoidance sealing for 4 h, 633 nm red light, and 40–60 mW/cm^2 irradiation for 30 min. No recurrence was observed 3 months after treatment [155].

11.6.3.2 PDT for Xeroderma Pigmentosum

Xeroderma pigmentosum (XP) is a rare autosomal recessive skin disorder, often with consanguineous parents, where the skin is highly sensitive to UV damage due to the absence of nucleic acid endonucleases, preventing the repair of UV-induced DNA damage. This results in an almost 100% likelihood of developing skin cancer, including BCC, cSCC, and melanoma [156]. XP is genetically heterogeneous and includes eight subtypes (XPA, XPB, XPC, XPD, XPE, XPF, XPG, XPH) and a variant, XPV, caused by mutations in specific genes, such as XPA, ERCC3 (XPB), XPC, ERCC2 (XPD), DDB2 (XPE), ERCC4 (XPF), ERCC5 (XPG), ERCC1, and POLH (XPV). The primary treatment approach for XP involves strict sun avoidance to reduce skin inflammation and delay cancer onset. Current therapeutic options include surgical excision, topical treatments such as 5-fluorouracil and imiquimod creams, and radiotherapy. Although PDT has been occasionally reported for XP, it is rarely used because of the need for strict light avoidance in the daily life of affected individuals [157].

In 1991, Wolf and Kerl reported the first case of XP with the XPC subtype treated via ALA-PDT in *The Lancet*. The patient, a 47-year-old woman with XP, had superficial cSCC on her dorsal hand. The treatment involved 40% ALA incubation for 4 h, followed by irradiation with a Lycra slide 250-W bulb filtered by a SCHOTT RG570 longwave-colored glass filter at an energy density of 90 J/cm^2. The patient experienced strong local reactions, including redness, swelling, and blisters lasting nearly 2 weeks. However, the lesion resolved completely after a single session with only local hyperpigmentation, and no recurrence was observed after 6 months [158]. The second patient involved a 16-year-old Hispanic female with XPC who had multiple AKs and NMSCs on her face. She underwent ALA-PDT on the entire face three times over a year, with 40 min of ALA incubation and 417–432 nm blue-light irradiation for 16 min at an energy density of 90 J/cm^2. The treatment showed no significant adverse effects and resulted in a favorable outcome [159]. More recently, a 12-year-old XP patient with multiple BCCs on the face and neck was treated with hematoporphyrin PDT. After 48 h of intravenous hematoporphyrin administration (3 mg/kg), the lesions were removed with a CO_2 laser combined with PDT. The irradiation used a wavelength of 630 nm, with an energy density of 100 mW/cm^2 for 1000 s. After 2 months, most lesions had disappeared, and dermoscopic examination revealed no abnormal tumor tissue in the treated area [160].

In addition to positive reports of PDT efficacy, there is also a case of ineffective PDT treatment. A child with a severe XP subtype (DeSanctis-Cacchione syndrome) developed invasive cSCC involving the conjunctiva and cornea. The patient was treated with hematoporphyrin PDT at a dosage of 1.5 mg/kg, 630-nm diode red light at a power density of 120 mW/cm^2, an energy density of 200 J/cm^2, and irradiation for 77 min. However, 3 months later, the tumor extent increased significantly, accompanied by severe visual impairment. This case highlights the potential risk of exacerbating ocular and periocular tumors in XP patients when hematoporphyrin PDT is used

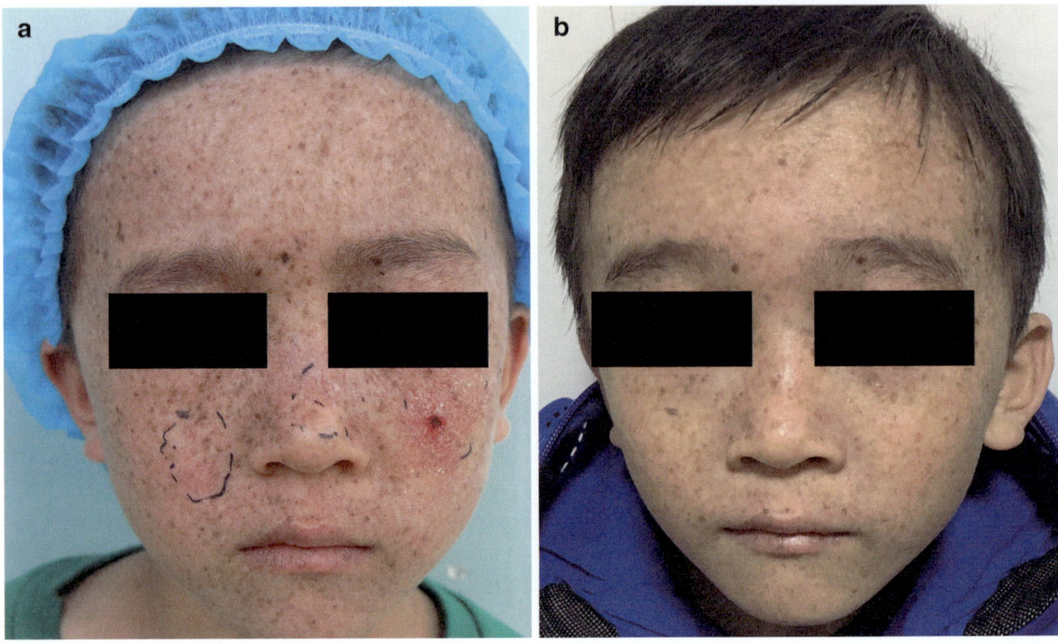

Fig. 11.24 Multiple NMSC on the face of a 7-year-old male child with XPC improved after three courses of ALA-PDT. (**a**) before treatment. (**b**) 6 months posttreatment

[161]. The authors' team also reported successful PDT treatment for early, multiple NMSCs on the faces of children with XP, confirming its efficacy in some cases (Fig. 11.24) [162]. However, due to the photosensitivity of XP, PDT remains an exploratory approach. Further clinical studies are needed to better evaluate the potential benefits and risks of PDT in this patient population.

11.6.3.3 PDT for Epidermodysplasia Verruciformis

Epidermodysplasia verruciformis (EV) is a rare autosomal recessive genodermatosis that increases susceptibility to skin cancer due to HPV infection, with lesions often appearing in sun-exposed areas. The first case of EV-associated nonmelanoma skin cancer (NMSC) treated with PDT was reported in 1999 [163] and involved a 65-year-old woman with multiple superficial BCCs on her arms and forehead. The patient was treated with 20% ALA in the dark for 6 h, followed by irradiation with a 580–740 nm incoherent light source. After one session, all the tumors were in complete clinical and histologic remission, but some recurrent lesions appeared after 1 year, suggesting that PDT could control disease progression but not fully eradicate lesions. A subsequent case involved a patient with eyelid Bowen's disease secondary to EV who was treated with 20% ALA and light avoidance for 4 h, followed by a 585-nm dye laser for three treatment courses [149]. The author's team also reported the successful use of ALA-PDT in two other EV patients. One of the patients was a 68-year-old woman with recurrent SCC after surgery on her left upper eyelid. The treatment involved 20% ALA light-avoidance incubation for 4 h, followed by six ALA-PDT sessions using a 635-nm semiconductor laser with a power density of 60 mw/cm^2 and an energy density of 100 J/cm^2. The team also used a holmium laser of 10 Hz, 0.5–0.8 J ablation, and a fiber diameter of 550 μm to treat thicker skin lesions and successfully removed SCC lesions. No recurrence was observed after 1 year (Fig. 11.25) [164]. The other patient was a 51-year-old male with multiple SCCs and AKs on his face and trunk who underwent 10% ALA treatment followed by 8 PDT sessions and achieved complete lesion clearance with no recurrence after 1 year (Fig. 11.26) [165].

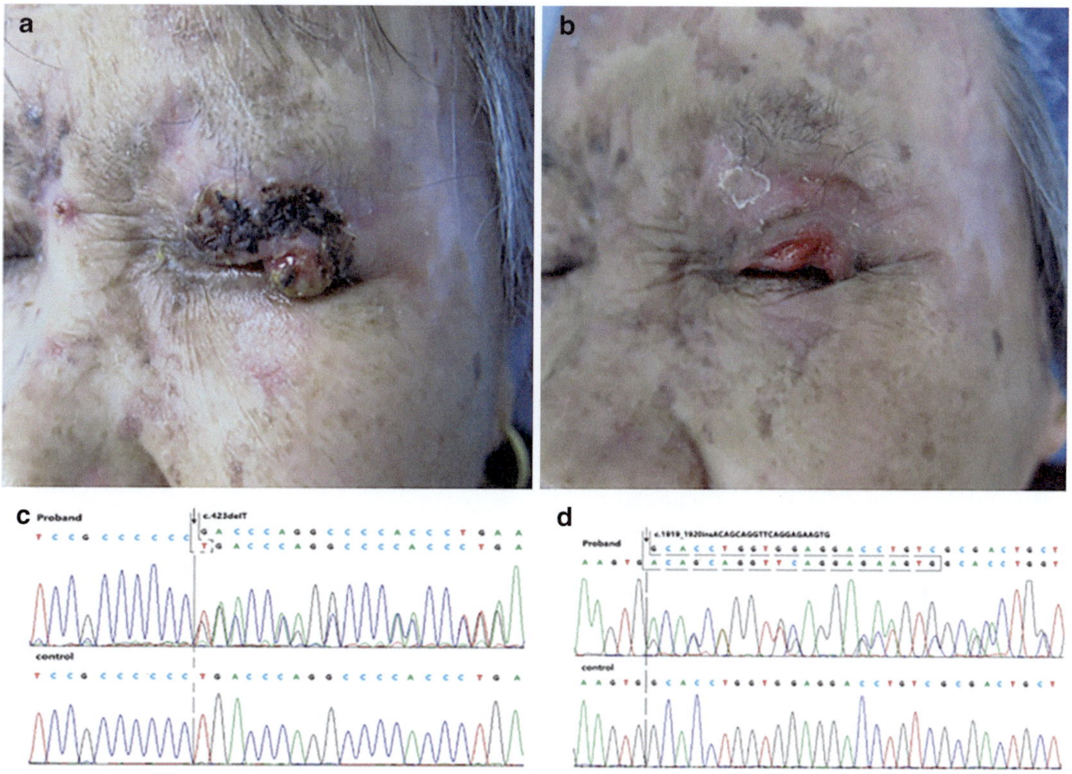

Fig. 11.25 SCC over the left upper eyelid of a 68-year-old female patient with EV, which was cleaned after 6 ALA-PDT sessions, in combination with a holmium laser: (**a**) before treatment. (**b**) After treatment. (**c**, **d**) The patient carries the compound heterozygous mutations c.423delT and c.1919_1920insACAGCAGGTTCAGGAGAAGTG in the TMC8 gene

11.6.3.4 PDT for Inherited Bullosa Epidermolysis

Inherited epidermolysis bullosa (EB) is a genetic disorder that is inherited in either an autosomal dominant or recessive manner and is caused by mutations in genes encoding structural proteins of the skin. Depending on the location of the blisters, they are classified as simplex EB (EBS), junctional EB (JEB), or dystrophic EB (DEB). EB increases the risk of localized skin cancers, particularly cSCC, which is a severe complication of DEB and the leading cause of death in affected individuals [166]. One study reported a 51-year-old female patient with DEB who developed Bowen's disease with scarring and deformity on the right ring finger. After one session of ALA-PDT, which involved the use of 20% ALA with light avoidance for 6 h and a 630-nm diode laser with a power density of 130 mW/cm^2, the lesions almost completely healed, with only mild erythema and no recurrence after 2 years. Compared with traditional surgery, this approach helps avoid the risk of scar contracture and finger dysfunction [167]. Another case involved a 22-year-old male DEB patient with a focal superficial BCC on the right forehead. After two sessions of MAL-PDT, some nodular lesions remained, leading to local surgical excision, which ultimately cured the BCC [168].

11.6.3.5 PDT for Oculocutaneous Albinism

Oculocutaneous albinism (OCA) is an autosomal recessive disorder characterized by the complete absence or reduction of melanin in the skin and adnexa due to tyrosinase deficiency. The clinical manifestations of OCA include white skin, white

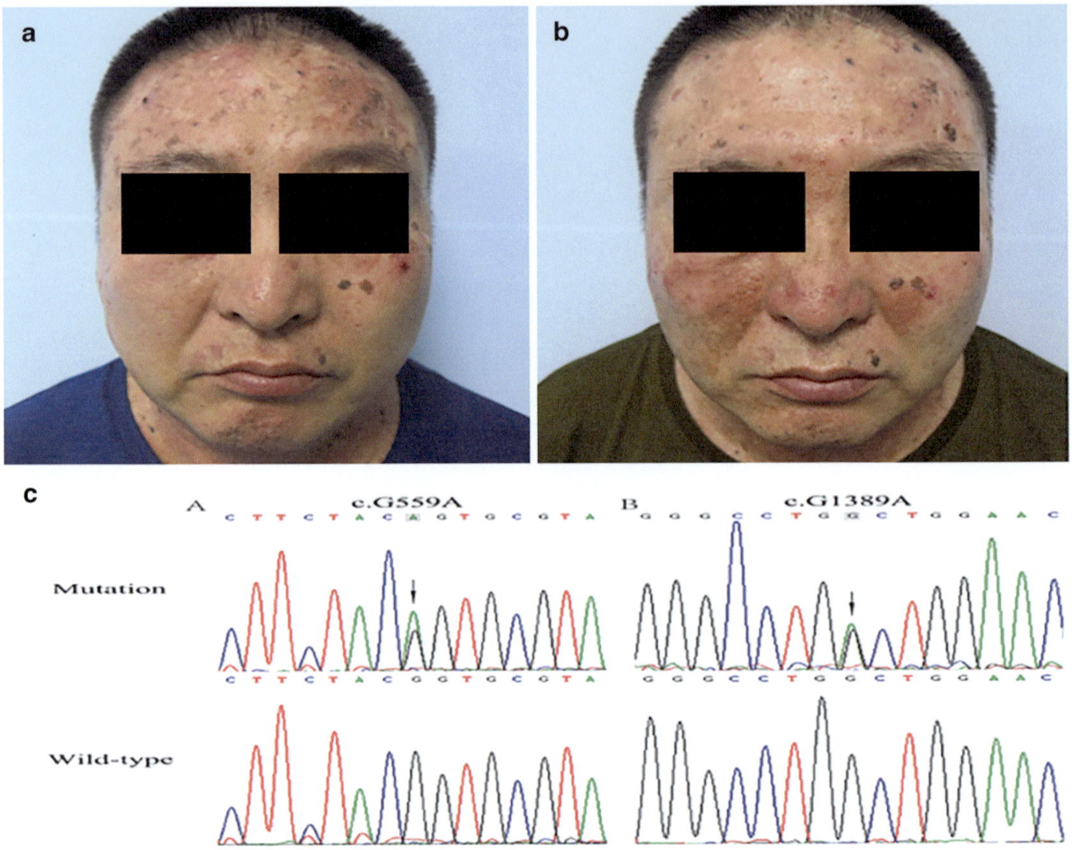

Fig. 11.26 A 51-year-old male EV patient with multiple SCCs and AKs on the face, with lesion clearance after 9 ALA-PDT sessions: (**a**) before treatment. (**b**) 1 month after treatment. (**c**) Patient carrying compound heterozygous mutations; c. G559A and c. C1389A in the TMC8 gene

or yellowish hair, congenital nystagmus, foveal hypoplasia, iris translucency, decreased retinal pigmentation, vision problems, and severe photophobia. Owing to the lack of melanin protection, individuals with OCA are highly susceptible to ultraviolet radiation and often develop AK and NMSCs before the age of 30 [169]. One study treated three female patients with 66 total facial AK lesions via DL-PDT over 24 weeks. The procedure involved curing AK lesions, applying SPF50 sunscreen, and then using 16% MAL, followed by outdoor treatment under shaded conditions in the early morning. After treatment at 4, 12, and 24 weeks, no pain or significant side effects occurred, and only one patient experienced mild erythema with itching. Clinical cure was achieved in 52 lesions at weeks 4 and 12, and 50 lesions were completely cured by week 24 [170]. The author's team also treated facial cSCC and multiple AKs in an 89-year-old OCA patient. cSCC was removed by debulking first, followed by 11 ALA-PDT sessions for the whole face; all lesions were cleaned after ALA-PDT, and no recurrence was observed after 1 year, although posttreatment erythema persisted (Fig. 11.27).

11.6.3.6 PDT for Other Genodermatoses Predisposing Patients to Skin Tumors

Bazex-Dupré-Christol is a sporadic X-linked dominant disorder that is clinically similar to Gorlin syndrome. It is typically associated with congenital hair reduction, follicular atrophy of the extremities, and a predisposition to BCCs. Oley syndrome, characterized by the triad of

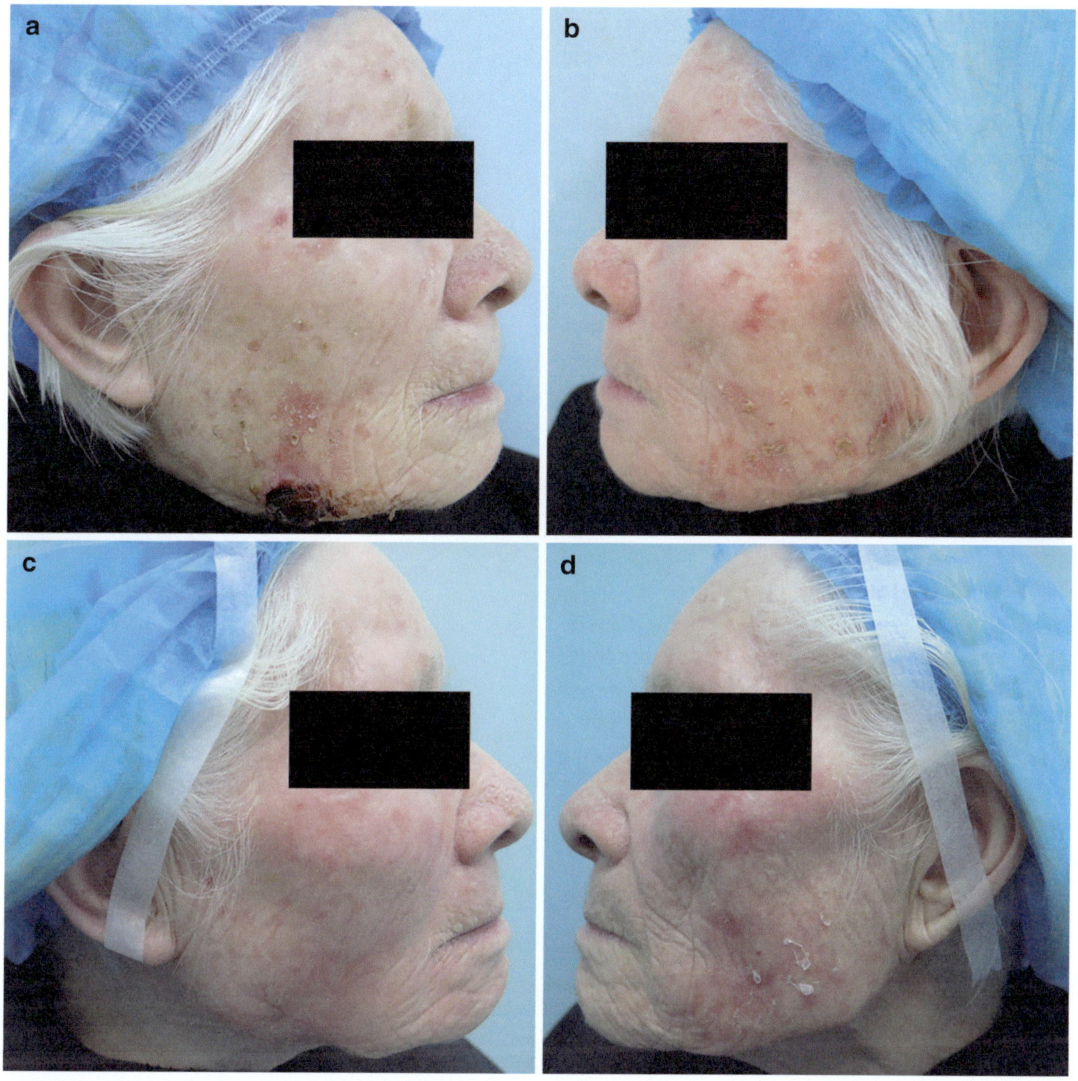

Fig. 11.27 Right mandibular cSCC and multiple AKs on the face of an 89-year-old female patient with OCA, which was cleared after surgical debulking combined with ALA-PDT. (**a**, **b**) Before treatment. (**c**, **d**) After treatment

BCC, hypotrichosis, and skin eruptions, is now recognized as a clinical variant of BDCS [171]. Because patients with BDCS are prone to developing multiple BCCs, nonsurgical treatments such as imiquimod, 5-fluorouracil, PDT, and cryotherapy may be theoretically considered for managing BCCs in these patients, in addition to traditional surgical approaches [147]. However, owing to the rarity of BDCS cases, no PDT treatments for this condition have been reported to date.

Dyskeratosis congenita (DC) is a genetic disorder caused by mutations in telomerase-related genes and was first described in 1906 as a hereditary skin disease. It typically presents with a characteristic mucocutaneous triad, including reticulated hyperpigmentation of the skin, nail deformities or atrophy, and leukoplakia of the oral mucosa. DC is often associated with decreased hematopoietic function [172]. Among them, oral leukoplakia (OLK), a common precancerous lesion in the oral cavity, can occur independently and presents as white lesions with epithelial hyperplasia and hyperkeratosis. While PDT is an established treatment for OML, no reports have yet linked PDT to DCs [173]. Other genodermatoses, such as Bloom syndrome, Rombo syndrome, Huriez syndrome, and Ferguson-Smith syndrome, also predispose individuals to skin tumors. Although PDT has not been reported in these conditions, it may offer a viable treatment option for skin tumors in patients who cannot tolerate surgery.

In summary, PDT offers several advantages, including preserving the original tissue structure, being minimally invasive, and inducing antitumor immunity, making it a promising therapeutic approach for genodermatosis-associated NMSCs. However, its application is limited by the need for strict light avoidance, particularly in conditions such as XP, EV, and OCA, leading to relatively few long-term studies on its use for these diseases. As PDT techniques continue to improve and more case reports demonstrate their effectiveness, PDT is increasingly being considered a viable clinical treatment option for genodermatosis-associated NMSC.

References

1. Lyu MY, Guo YS, Li S, et al. Hospital-based epidemiological and clinical characterisation of the malignant transformation of oral leukoplakia in a Chinese population. Int Dent J. 2017;67(4):252–9.
2. Wang T, Wang L, Yang H, et al. Development and validation of nomogram for prediction of malignant transformation in oral leukoplakia: a large-scale cohort study. J Oral Pathol Med. 2019;48(6):491–8.
3. Kasianandan A, Kannan K. Leukoplakia of the bladder: a case report and literature review. Int Urogynecol J. 2012;23(1):131–3.
4. Cheng LHH. Ubiquitin and malignant transformation of oral mucosa. Head Neck. 2001;23(11):972–8.
5. Pozhogina AG, Groshikov MI, Tsvetkova GM. Fluorescent histological and histochemical characteristics of leukoplakia of the oral mucosa and vermillion border. Stomatologiia. 1972;51(5):14–6.
6. Erira AT, Navarro AFR, Robayo DAG. Human papillomavirus, Epstein–Barr virus, and *Candida albicans* coinfection in oral leukoplakia with different degrees of dysplasia. Clin Exp Dent Res. 2021;7(5):914–23.
7. Greenslade R. Interventions for treating oral leukoplakia to prevent oral cancer. Nurs Stand. 2017;31(39):42.
8. Gomes CC, Fonseca-Silva T, Galv CF, et al. Inter- and intralesional molecular heterogeneity of oral leukoplakia. Oral Oncol. 2015;51(2):178–81.
9. Sperandio M, Brown AL, Lock C, et al. Predictive value of dysplasia grading and DNA ploidy in malignant transformation of oral potentially malignant disorders. Cancer Prev Res. 2013;6(8):822–31.
10. Rindum JL, Stenderup A, Holmstrup P. Identification of *Candida albicans* types related to healthy and pathological oral mucosa. J Oral Pathol Med. 1994;23(9):406–12.
11. Pentenero M, Sutera S, Lodi G, et al. Oral leukoplakia diagnosis and treatment in Europe and Australia: oral medicine practitioners' attitudes and practice. Oral Dis. 2022;29(8):3214–22.
12. Grant WE, Hopper C, Speight PM, et al. Photodynamic therapy of malignant and premalignant lesions in patients with 'field cancerization' of the oral cavity. J Laryngol Otol. 1993;107(12):1140–5.
13. Colin HFRCS, Path PMS, et al. Photodynamic therapy using 5-aminolevulinic acid for premalignant and malignant lesions of the oral cavity. Cancer. 1996;78(7):1374–83.
14. Tsai JC, Chiang CP, Chen HM, et al. Photodynamic therapy of oral dysplasia with topical 5-aminolevulinic acid and light-emitting diode array. Lasers Surg Med. 2010;34(1):18–24.
15. Chen HM, Yu CH, Tsai T, et al. Topical 5-aminolevulinic acid-mediated photodynamic therapy for oral verrucous hyperplasia, oral leukoplakia and oral erythroleukoplakia. Photodiagn Photodyn Ther. 2007;4(1):44–52.
16. Kawczyk-Krupka A, Waskowska J, Raczkowska-Siostrzonek A, et al. Comparison of cryotherapy and photodynamic therapy in treatment of oral leukoplakia. Photodiagn Photodyn Ther. 2012;9(2):148–55.
17. Selvam NP, Sadaksharam J, Singaravelu G, et al. Treatment of oral leukoplakia with photodynamic therapy: a pilot study. J Cancer Res Ther. 2015;11(2):464–7.
18. Chen Q, Dan H, Tang F, et al. Photodynamic therapy guidelines for the management of oral leucoplakia. Int J Oral Sci. 2019;11(2):14.
19. Zhang Y, Zhang L, Yang D, et al. Treatment of oral refractory large area mucosal leukoplakia with CO_2 laser combined with photodynamic therapy: case report. Photodiagn Photodyn Ther. 2017;20:193–5.
20. Fistarol SK, Itin PH. Diagnosis and treatment of lichen sclerosus: an update. Am J Clin Dermatol. 2013;14(1):27–47.
21. Lewis FM, Tatnall FM, Velangi SS, et al. British Association of Dermatologists guidelines for the management of lichen sclerosus, 2018. Br J Dermatol. 2018;178(4):839–53.

22. Shi L, Liu J, Zhang H, et al. Vulvar lichen sclerosus progressing to squamous cell carcinoma due to the poor compliance for the follow-up after ALA-PDT. Photodiagn Photodyn Ther. 2022;40:103171.
23. Gerkowicz A, Szczepanik-Kułak P, Krasowska D. Photodynamic therapy in the treatment of vulvar lichen Sclerosus: a systematic review of the literature. J Clin Med. 2021;10:23.
24. Hillemanns P, Untch M, Pröve F, et al. Photodynamic therapy of vulvar lichen sclerosus with 5-aminolevulinic acid. Obstet Gynecol. 1999;93(1):71–4.
25. Lan T, Zou Y, Hamblin MR, et al. 5-Aminolevulinic acid photodynamic therapy in refractory vulvar lichen sclerosus et atrophicus: series of ten cases. Photodiagn Photodyn Ther. 2017;21:234–8.
26. Mazdziarz A, Osuch B, Kowalska M, et al. Photodynamic therapy in the treatment of vulvar lichen sclerosus. Photodiagn Photodyn Ther. 2017;19:135–9.
27. Li Z, Wang Y, Wang J, et al. Evaluation of the efficacy of 5-aminolevulinic acid photodynamic therapy for the treatment of vulvar lichen sclerosus. Photodiagn Photodyn Ther. 2020;29:101596.
28. Prodromidou A, Chatziioannou E, Daskalakis G, et al. Photodynamic therapy for vulvar lichen sclerosus-a systematic review. J Low Genit Tract Dis. 2018;22(1):58–65.
29. Shi L, Miao F, Zhang LL, et al. Comparison of 5-Aminolevulinic acid photodynamic therapy and Clobetasol propionate in treatment of vulvar lichen Sclerosus. Acta Derm Venereol. 2016;96(5):684–8.
30. Neill SM, Lewis FM, Tatnall FM, et al. British Association of Dermatologists' guidelines for the management of lichen sclerosus 2010. Br J Dermatol. 2010;163(4):672–82.
31. Sen CK. Human wounds and its burden: an updated compendium of estimates. Adv Wound Care. 2019;8(2):39–48.
32. Morton LM, Phillips TJ. Wound healing and treating wounds: differential diagnosis and evaluation of chronic wounds. J Am Acad Dermatol. 2016;74(4):589–605.
33. Maida V, Ennis M, Kuziemsky C, et al. Symptoms associated with malignant wounds: a prospective case series. J Pain Symptom Manag. 2009;37(2):206–11.
34. Wilcox JR, Carter MJ, Covington S. Frequency of debridements and time to heal: a retrospective cohort study of 312,744 wounds. JAMA Dermatol. 2013;149(9):1050–8.
35. Peck B, Workeneh B, Kadikoy H, et al. Spectrum of sodium hypochlorite toxicity in man-also a concern for nephrologists. NDT Plus. 2011;4(4):231–5.
36. Opstrup MS, Johansen JD, Garvey LH. Chlorhexidine allergy: sources of exposure in the health-care setting. Br J Anesth. 2015;114(4):704–5.
37. Werner AH, Russell AD. Mupirocin, fusidic acid and bacitracin: activity, action and clinical uses of three topical antibiotics. Vet Dermatol. 1999;10(3):225–40.
38. Leaper D. Appropriate use of silver dressings in wounds: international consensus document. Int Wound J. 2012;9(5):461–4.
39. Goldman RJ. Hyperbaric oxygen therapy for wound healing and limb salvage: a systematic review. PM & R. 2009;1(5):471–89.
40. Khurram MF, Sarfraz Ali S, Yaseen M. Vacuum-assisted wound closure therapy in pediatric lower limb trauma. Int J Low Extrem Wounds. 2019;18(3):317–22.
41. Li X, Wang H, Wang X, et al. In vitro study of the inhibitory effect of photodynamic therapy with 5-aminolevulinic acid on planktonic *Staphylococcus epidermidis*. Chin J Dermatol. 2012;45(8):557–60.
42. Huang J, Guo M, Jin S, et al. Antibacterial photodynamic therapy mediated by 5-aminolevulinic acid on methicillin-resistant *Staphylococcus aureus*. Photodiagn Photodyn Ther. 2019;28:330–7.
43. Dai T, Tegos GP, Zhiyentayev T, et al. Photodynamic therapy for methicillin-resistant *Staphylococcus aureus* infection in a mouse skin abrasion model. Lasers Surg Med. 2010;42(1):38–44.
44. Hajim KI, Salih DS, Rassam YZ. Laser light combined with a photosensitizer may eliminate methicillin-resistant strains of *Staphylococcus aureus*. Lasers Med Sci. 2010;25(5):743–8.
45. Eming SA, Krieg T, Davidson JM. Inflammation in wound repair: molecular and cellular mechanisms. J Invest Dermatol. 2007;127(3):514–25.
46. Medzhitov R. Inflammation 2010: new adventures of an old flame. Cell. 2010;140(6):771–6.
47. Kundu JK, Surh YJ. Emerging avenues linking inflammation and cancer. Free Radic Biol Med. 2012;52(9):2013–37.
48. Chiu YJ, Huang TH, Chiu CS, et al. Analgesic and antiinflammatory activities of the aqueous extract from Plectranthus amboinicus (Lour.) Spreng. Both in vitro and in vivo. Evid Based Complement Alternat Med. 2012;2012:508137.
49. Choi JY, Park GT, Na EY, et al. Molecular changes following topical photodynamic therapy using methyl aminolaevulinate in mouse skin. J Dermatol Sci. 2010;58(3):198–203.
50. Nie S, Wang X, Wang H. NLRP3 Inflammasome mediated interleukin-1β production in cancer-associated fibroblast contributes to ALA-PDT for cutaneous squamous cell carcinoma. Cancer Manag Res. 2019;11:10257–67.
51. Wang P, Han J, Wei M, et al. Remodeling of dermal collagen in photoaged skin using low-dose 5-aminolevulinic acid photodynamic therapy occurs via the transforming growth factor-β pathway. J Biophotonics. 2018;11(6):e201700357.
52. Huang J, Wu S, Wu M, et al. Efficacy of the therapy of 5-aminolevulinic acid photodynamic therapy combined with human umbilical cord mesenchymal stem cells on methicillin-resistant *Staphylococcus aureus*-infected wound in a diabetic mouse model. Photodiagn Photodyn Ther. 2021;36:102480.

53. Huang J, Guo M, Wu M, et al. Effectiveness of a single treatment of photodynamic therapy using topical administration of 5-aminolevulinic acid on methicillin-resistant *Staphylococcus aureus*-infected wounds of diabetic mice. Photodiagn Photodyn Ther. 2020;30:101748.
54. Mai B, Gao Y, Li M, et al. Photodynamic antimicrobial chemotherapy for *Staphylococcus aureus* and multidrug-resistant bacterial burn infection in vitro and in vivo. Int J Nanomedicine. 2017;12:5915–31.
55. Wang C, Huang S, Zhu T, et al. Efficacy of photodynamic antimicrobial therapy for wound flora and wound healing of pressure sore with pathogen infection. Zhonghua Yi Xue Za Zhi. 2014;94(31):2455–9.
56. Karrer S, Bosserhoff AK, Weiderer P, et al. Influence of 5-aminolevulinic acid and red light on collagen metabolism of human dermal fibroblasts. J Invest Dermatol. 2003;120(2):325–31.
57. Nesi-Reis V, Lera-Nonose D, Oyama J, et al. Contribution of photodynamic therapy in wound healing: a systematic review. Photodiagn Photodyn Ther. 2018;21:294–305.
58. Morimoto K, Ozawa T, Awazu K, et al. Photodynamic therapy using systemic administration of 5-aminolevulinic acid and a 410-nm wavelength light-emitting diode for methicillin-resistant *Staphylococcus aureus*-infected ulcers in mice. PLoS One. 2014;9(8):e105173.
59. Schieber M, Chandel NS. ROS function in redox signaling and oxidative stress. Curr Biol. 2014;24(10):453–62.
60. Martin KR, Barrett JC. Reactive oxygen species as double-edged swords in cellular processes: low-dose cell signaling versus high-dose toxicity. Hum Exp Toxicol. 2002;21(2):71–5.
61. Sahu K, Sharma M, Dube A, et al. Topical antimicrobial photodynamic therapy improves angiogenesis in wounds of diabetic mice. Lasers Med Sci. 2015;30(7):1923–9.
62. Chiu WT, Tran TV, Pan SC, et al. Cystic fibrosis transmembrane conductance regulator: a possible new target for photodynamic therapy enhances wound healing. Adv Wound Care. 2019;8(10):476–86.
63. Dai T, Gupta A, Huang YY, et al. Blue light eliminates community-acquired methicillin-resistant *Staphylococcus aureus* in infected mouse skin abrasions. Photomed Laser Surg. 2013;31(11):531–8.
64. Miyamoto Y, Nishikiori D, Hagino F, et al. Effect of 630-NM pulsed laser irradiation on the proliferation of HeLa cells in Photofrin®-mediated photodynamic therapy. Laser Ther. 2011;20(2):135–8.
65. Li X, Wang H, Wang X. Photodynamic therapy of 5-aminolevulinic acid on *Staphylococcus epidermidis* biofilms. Chin J Dermatol. 2012;45(12):865–9.
66. Liu C, Zhou Y, Wang L, et al. Photodynamic inactivation of *Klebsiella pneumoniae* biofilms and planktonic cells by 5-aminolevulinic acid and 5-aminolevulinic acid methyl ester. Lasers Med Sci. 2016;31(3):557–65.
67. Liu C, Zhou Y, Wang L, et al. Mechanistic aspects of the photodynamic inactivation of vancomycin-resistant enterococci mediated by 5-aminolevulinic acid and 5-aminolevulinic acid methyl ester. Curr Microbiol. 2015;70(4):528–35.
68. Hsieh CM, Huang YH, Chen CP, et al. 5-Aminolevulinic acid induced photodynamic inactivation on *Staphylococcus aureus* and *Pseudomonas aeruginosa*. J Food Drug Anal. 2014;22(3):350–5.
69. Yang Z, Hu X, Zhou L, et al. Photodynamic therapy accelerates skin wound healing through promoting re-epithelialization. Burns Trauma. 2021;9:tkab008.
70. Lei X, Liu B, Huang Z, et al. A clinical study of photodynamic therapy for chronic skin ulcers in lower limbs infected with *Pseudomonas aeruginosa*. Arch Dermatol Res. 2015;307(1):49–55.
71. Li X, Kou H, Zhao C, et al. Efficacy and safety of ALA-PDT in treatment of diabetic foot ulcer with infection. Photodiagn Photodyn Ther. 2022;38:102822.
72. Grandi V, Bacci S, Corsi A, et al. ALA-PDT exerts beneficial effects on chronic venous ulcers by inducing changes in inflammatory microenvironment, especially through increased TGF-beta release: a pilot clinical and translational study. Photodiagn Photodyn Ther. 2018;21:252–6.
73. Light JG, Bomar L, McMichael A. Erosive pustular dermatosis in a patient with lichen planopilaris treated with aminolevulinic acid photodynamic therapy. Photodiagn Photodyn Ther. 2021;33:102207.
74. Shi J, Huang J, Yang D, et al. Successful application of ALA-PDT in rare cutaneous infection of mycobacterium parascrofulaceum. Photodiagn Photodyn Ther. 2023;43:103604.
75. Topaloglu N, Güney M, Yuksel S, et al. Antibacterial photodynamic therapy with 808 nm laser and indocyanine green on abrasion wound models. J Biomed Opt. 2015;20(2):28003.
76. Garcia VG, de Lima MA, Okamoto T, et al. Effect of photodynamic therapy on the healing of cutaneous third-degree-burn: histological study in rats. Lasers Med Sci. 2010;25(2):221–8.
77. Huang J, Fan Q, Shi L, et al. A novel chlorin derivative Shengtaibufen (STBF) mediated photodynamic therapy combined with iodophor for the treatment of chronic superficial leg wounds infected with methicillin-resistant *Staphylococcus aureus*: a retrospective clinical study. Photodiagn Photodyn Ther. 2024;48:104300.
78. Sahu K, Sharma M, Sharma P, et al. Effect of poly-L-lysine-chlorin P6-mediated antimicrobial photodynamic treatment on collagen restoration in bacterium-infected wounds. Photomed Laser Surg. 2014;32(1):23–9.
79. Vecchio D, Dai T, Huang L, et al. Antimicrobial photodynamic therapy with RLP068 kills methicillin-resistant *Staphylococcus aureus* and improves wound healing in a mouse model of infected skin abrasion PDT with RLP068/cl in infected mouse skin abrasion. J Biophotonics. 2013;6(9):733–42.

80. Nafee N, Youssef A, El-Gowelli H, et al. Antibiotic-free nanotherapeutics: hypericin nanoparticles thereof for improved in vitro and in vivo antimicrobial photodynamic therapy and wound healing. Int J Pharm. 2013;454(1):249–58.
81. Wang A, Li R. Differential diagnosis of cutaneous fungal diseases. Dermatol Venereal Dis. 2014;36(1):11–2.
82. Zhan P, Liu W. The changing face of dermatophytic infections worldwide. Mycopathologia. 2017;182(1–2):77–86.
83. Nenoff P, Krüger C, Ginter-Hanselmayer G, et al. Mycology - an update. Part 1: dermatomycoses: causative agents, epidemiology and pathogenesis. J German Soc Dermatol. 2014;12(3):188–209.
84. Wang X, Ding C, Xu Y, et al. Analysis on the pathogenic fungi in patients with superficial mycosis in the northeastern China during 10 years. Exp Ther Med. 2020;20(6):281.
85. Van Daele R, Spriet I, Wauters J, et al. Antifungal drugs: what brings the future? Med Mycol. 2019;57(Supplement_3):S328–43.
86. Zhang R. Guidelines for the diagnosis and treatment of tinea tinea and tinea pedis in China (Popular Science Edition 2022). Chin J Mycol. 2022;17(2):89–93.
87. Lv X. Chinese guidelines for the diagnosis and treatment of tinea corporis and tinea cruris (primary practice version 2022). Chin J Mycol. 2022;17(3):177–82.
88. Hudson A, Sturgeon A, Peiris A. Tinea versicolor. JAMA. 2018;320(13):1396.
89. Yu J, Zhu H. Guidelines for onychomycosis in China (2021 edition). Chin J Mycol. 2022;17(1):1–7.
90. Yu J, Zhu M. Chinese guidelines for diagnosis and treatment of tinea capitis (2018 revision). Chin J Mycol. 2019;14(1):4–6.
91. Li J, Huang J, Lu S, et al. Retrospective analysis of 254 subcutaneous tissue fungal infections (1990-2019). J Dermatol Venereol. 2020;27(4):223–6.
92. Sharma B, Sharma AK, Sharma U. Sporotrichosis: a comprehensive review on recent drug-based therapeutics and management. Curr Derm Rep. 2022;11(2):110–9.
93. Queiroz-Telles F, de Hoog S, Santos DW, et al. Chromoblastomycosis. Clin Microbiol Rev. 2017;30(1):233–76.
94. Yang Z, Liu C, Xiong H, et al. Photodynamic therapy, a promising treatment approach for cutaneous infectious granulomas. Photodiagn Photodyn Ther. 2022;39:102952.
95. Pfaller MA, Diekema DJ, Turnidge JD, et al. Twenty years of the SENTRY antifungal surveillance program: results for candida species from 1997-2016. Open Forum Infect Dis. 2019;6(Suppl 1):S79–94.
96. Zhu H, Wen H. Advances in terbinafine-resistant dermatophytes of lichen planus. Chin J Mycol. 2020;15(4):253.
97. Moan J, Peng Q. An outline of the hundred-year history of PDT. Anticancer Res. 2003;23(5):3591–600.
98. Hamblin MR. Antimicrobial photodynamic inactivation: a bright new technique to kill resistant microbes. Curr Opin Microbiol. 2016;33:67–73.
99. Ma W, Zhang M, Cui Z, et al. Aloe-emodin-mediated antimicrobial photodynamic therapy against dermatophytosis caused by Trichophyton rubrum. Microb Biotechnol. 2022;15(2):499–512.
100. Zhu Z, Tang Z, Phillips JA, et al. Regulation of singlet oxygen generation using single-walled carbon nanotubes. J Am Chem Soc. 2008;130(33):10856–7.
101. Calixto GMF, de Annunzio SR, Victorelli FD, et al. Chitosan-based drug delivery systems for optimization of photodynamic therapy: a review. AAPS PharmSciTech. 2019;20(7):253.
102. Scherer KM, Bisby RH, Botchway SW, et al. New approaches to photodynamic therapy from types I, II and III to type IV using one or more photons. Anticancer Agents Med Chem. 2017;17(2):171–89.
103. Kim WR, Bae SG, Oh TH. Photodynamic therapy of red and blue lights on Malassezia pachydermatis: an in vitro study. Pol J Vet Sci. 2018;21(1):185–91.
104. Shen JJ, Arendrup MC, Jemec GBE, et al. Photodynamic therapy: a treatment option for terbinafine resistant Trichophyton species. Photodiagn Photodyn Ther. 2021;33:102169.
105. Wan P, Guo W, Wang Y, et al. Photosensitizer-polypeptide conjugate for effective elimination of *Candida albicans* biofilm. Adv Healthc Mater. 2022;11(16):e2200268.
106. Trevisan E, Menegazzi R, Zabucchi G, et al. Effect of methylene blue photodynamic therapy on human neutrophil functional responses. J Photochem Photobiol B. 2019;199:111605.
107. Shi L, Wu Q, Yang J, et al. ALA-PDT successfully treated Majocchi's granuloma by directly killing Trichophyton tonsurans and recruiting T lymphocytes. Photodiagn Photodyn Ther. 2021;35:102328.
108. Sotiriou E, Koussidou T, Patsatsi A, et al. 5-Aminolevulinic acid-photodynamic treatment for dermatophytic tinea pedis of interdigital type: a small clinical study. J Eur Acad Dermatol Venereol. 2009;23(2):203–4.
109. Calzavara-Pinton PG, Venturini M, Capezzera R, et al. Photodynamic therapy of interdigital mycoses of the feet with topical application of 5-aminolevulinic acid. Photodermatol Photoimmunol Photomed. 2004;20(3):144–7.
110. Sotiriou E, Panagiotidou D, Ioannides D. 5-Aminolevulinic acid photodynamic therapy treatment for tinea cruris caused by Trichophyton rubrum: report of 10 cases. J Eur Acad Dermatol Venereol. 2009;23(3):341–2.
111. Shen JJ, Jemec GBE, Arendrup MC, et al. Photodynamic therapy treatment of superficial fungal infections: a systematic review. Photodiagn Photodyn Ther. 2020;31:101774.
112. Wu MF, Lv T, Wang HW. Successful photodynamic therapy of tinea capitis child with liver dysfunction caused by oral antifungal drugs: a case report. Photodiagn Photodyn Ther. 2020;30:101745.

113. Dai H, Gao Z, Chen J, et al. ALA-PDT combined with oral administration of terbinafine hydrochloride tablets in the treatment of kerion in a child. Chin J Mycol. 2020;15(4):236.
114. Bowornsathitchai N, Thammahong A, Shoosanglertwijit J, et al. Methylene blue-mediated photodynamic therapy may be superior to 5% amorolfine nail lacquer for nondermatophyte onychomycosis. Photodermatol Photoimmunol Photomed. 2021;37(3):183–91.
115. Navarro-Bielsa A, Gracia-Cazaña T, Robres P, et al. Combination of photodynamic therapy and oral antifungals for the treatment of onychomycosis. Pharmaceuticals. 2022;15(6):722.
116. Koren A, Salameh F, Sprecher E, et al. Laser-assisted photodynamic therapy or laser-assisted amorolfine lacquer delivery for treatment of toenail onychomycosis: an open-label comparative study. Acta Derm Venereol. 2018;98(4):467–8.
117. Sotiriou E, Koussidou-Eremonti T, Chaidemenos G, et al. Photodynamic therapy for distal and lateral subungual toenail onychomycosis caused by Trichophyton rubrum: preliminary results of a single-center open trial. Acta Derm Venereol. 2010;90(2):216–7.
118. Watanabe D, Kawamura C, Masuda Y, et al. Successful treatment of toenail onychomycosis with photodynamic therapy. Arch Dermatol. 2008;144(1):19–21.
119. Cai Q, Yang LJ, Chen J, et al. Successful sequential treatment with itraconazole and ALA-PDT for cutaneous granuloma by *Candida albicans*: a case report and literature review. Mycopathologia. 2018;183(5):829–34.
120. Alberdi E, Gómez C. Successful treatment of pityriasis versicolor by photodynamic therapy mediated by methylene blue. Photodermatol Photoimmunol Photomed. 2020;36(4):308–12.
121. García-Malinis AJ, Milagro Beamonte A, Torres Sopena L, et al. Cutaneous sporotrichosis treated with methylene blue-daylight photodynamic therapy. J Eur Acad Dermatol Venereol. 2018;32(3):e90–1.
122. Ko DY, Kim KH, Song KH. Comparative study of photodynamic therapy with topical methyl Aminolevulinate versus 5-aminolevulinic acid for facial actinic keratosis with long-term follow-up. Ann Dermatol. 2014;26(3):321–31.
123. Lee JW, Kim BJ, Kim MN. Photodynamic therapy: new treatment for recalcitrant Malassezia folliculitis. Lasers Surg Med. 2010;42(2):192–6.
124. Rosenthal I. Phthalocyanines as photodynamic sensitizers. Photochem Photobiol. 1991;53(6):859–70.
125. Morgado LF, Trávolo ARF, Muehlmann LA, et al. Photodynamic therapy treatment of onychomycosis with aluminum-phthalocyanine chloride nanoemulsions: a proof of concept clinical trial. J Photochem Photobiol B. 2017;173:266–70.
126. DeRossi SS, Ciarrocca KN. Lichen planus, lichenoid drug reactions, and lichenoid mucositis. Dent Clin N Am. 2005;49(1):77–89.
127. Li C, Tang X, Zheng X, et al. Global prevalence and incidence estimates of oral lichen planus: a systematic review and meta-analysis. JAMA Dermatol. 2020;156(2):172–81.
128. McCartan BE, Healy CM. The reported prevalence of oral lichen planus: a review and critique. J Oral Pathol Med. 2008;37(8):447–53.
129. Gonzalez-Moles MA, Warnakulasuriya S, Gonzalez-Ruiz I, et al. Worldwide prevalence of oral lichen planus: a systematic review and meta-analysis. Oral Dis. 2021;27(4):813–28.
130. Kirby B, Whitehurst C, Moore JV, et al. Treatment of lichen planus of the penis with photodynamic therapy. Br J Dermatol. 1999;141(4):765–6.
131. Wu MF, Wang B, Lv T, et al. Successful treatment of penile condyloma acuminata accompanied with lichen planus with photodynamic therapy. Photodiagn Photodyn Ther. 2018;24:142–4.
132. Maloth KN, Velpula N, Kodangal S, et al. Photodynamic therapy - a noninvasive treatment modality for precancerous lesions. J Lasers Med Sci. 2016;7(1):30–6.
133. Sulewska M, Duraj E, Sobaniec S, et al. A clinical evaluation of efficacy of photodynamic therapy in treatment of reticular oral lichen planus: a case series. Photodiagn Photodyn Ther. 2019;25:50–7.
134. He Y, Deng J, Zhao Y, et al. Efficacy evaluation of photodynamic therapy for oral lichen planus: a systematic review and meta-analysis. BMC Oral Health. 2020;20(1):302.
135. Aghahosseini F, Arbabi-Kalati F, Fashtami LA, et al. Methylene blue-mediated photodynamic therapy: a possible alternative treatment for oral lichen planus. Lasers Surg Med. 2006;38(1):33–8.
136. Aghahosseini F, Arbabi-Kalati F, Fashtami LA, et al. Treatment of oral lichen planus with photodynamic therapy mediated methylene blue: a case report. Med Oral Patol Oral Cir Bucal. 2006;11(2):126–9.
137. Sadaksharam J, Nayaki KP, Selvam NP. Treatment of oral lichen planus with methylene blue mediated photodynamic therapy–a clinical study. Photodermatol Photoimmunol Photomed. 2012;28(2):97–101.
138. Sobaniec S, Bernaczyk P, Pietruski J, et al. Clinical assessment of the efficacy of photodynamic therapy in the treatment of oral lichen planus. Lasers Med Sci. 2013;28(1):311–6.
139. Kvaal SI, Angell-Petersen E, Warloe T. Photodynamic treatment of oral lichen planus. Oral Surg Oral Med Oral Pathol Oral Radiol. 2013;115(1):62–70.
140. Jajarm HH, Falaki F, Sanatkhani M, et al. A comparative study of toluidine blue-mediated photodynamic therapy versus topical corticosteroids in the treatment of erosive-atrophic oral lichen planus: a randomized clinical controlled trial. Lasers Med Sci. 2015;30(5):1475–80.
141. Helgesen AL, Gjersvik P, Peng Q, et al. Biodistribution of protoporphyrin IX in female genital erosive lichen planus after topical application of hexaminolevulinate. Photodiagn Photodyn Ther. 2014;11(2):113–7.

142. Helgesen AL, Warloe T, Pripp AH, et al. Vulvovaginal photodynamic therapy vs. topical corticosteroids in genital erosive lichen planus: a randomized controlled trial. Br J Dermatol. 2015;173(5):1156–62.
143. Jurczyszyn K, Trzeciakowski W, Kozakiewicz M, et al. Fractal dimension and texture analysis of lesion autofluorescence in the evaluation of oral lichen planus treatment effectiveness. Materials. 2021;14(18):5448.
144. Mostafa D, Moussa E, Alnouaem M. Evaluation of photodynamic therapy in treatment of oral erosive lichen planus in comparison with topically applied corticosteroids. Photodiagn Photodyn Ther. 2017;19:56–66.
145. Saleh W, Tageldin S, Khashaba E, et al. Could photodynamic therapy be utilized as a treatment modality for oral lichen planus? Photodiagn Photodyn Ther. 2020;30:101677.
146. Mirza S, Rehman N, Alrahlah A, et al. Efficacy of photodynamic therapy or low level laser therapy against steroid therapy in the treatment of erosive-atrophic oral lichen planus. Photodiagn Photodyn Ther. 2018;21:404–8.
147. Schierbeck J, Vestergaard T, Bygum A. Skin cancer associated genodermatoses: a literature review. Acta Derm Venereol. 2019;99(4):360–9.
148. Babu NA, Rajesh E, Krupaa J, et al. Genodermatoses. J Pharm Bioallied Sci. 2015;7(Suppl 1):S203–6.
149. Sunohara M, Ozawa T, Morimoto K, et al. Dye laser photodynamic therapy for Bowen's disease in a patient with epidermodysplasia verruciformis. Osaka City Med J. 2012;58(2):77–82.
150. Bresler SC, Padwa BL, Granter SR. Nevoid basal cell carcinoma syndrome (Gorlin syndrome). Head Neck Pathol. 2016;10(2):119–24.
151. Basset-Seguin N, Bissonnette R, Girard C, et al. Consensus recommendations for the treatment of basal cell carcinomas in Gorlin syndrome with topical methylaminolaevulinate-photodynamic therapy. J Eur Acad Dermatol Venereol. 2014;28(5):626–32.
152. Girard C, Debu A, Bessis D, et al. Treatment of Gorlin syndrome (nevoid basal cell carcinoma syndrome) with methylaminolevulinate photodynamic therapy in seven patients, including two children: interest of tumescent anesthesia for pain control in children. J Eur Acad Dermatol Venereol. 2013;27(2):171–5.
153. Maytin EV, Kaw U, Ilyas M, et al. Blue light versus red light for photodynamic therapy of basal cell carcinoma in patients with Gorlin syndrome: a bilaterally controlled comparison study. Photodiagn Photodyn Ther. 2018;22:7–13.
154. Bu W, Zhang M, Zhang Q, et al. Preliminary results of comparative study for subsequent photodynamic therapy versus secondary excision after primary excision for treating basal cell carcinoma. Photodiagn Photodyn Ther. 2017;17:134–7.
155. Li C, Chen P, Li Z, et al. 5-aminolevulinic acid photodynamic therapy and excision surgery for nevoid basal cell carcinoma syndrome with multiple basal cell carcinomas and PTCH1 mutation. Photodiagn Photodyn Ther. 2020;32:101968.
156. Baykal C, Atci T, Yilmaz Z, et al. Skin tumors in xeroderma pigmentosum: evaluation of a large series and a literature review. J Cutan Pathol. 2021;48(7):884–95.
157. de Andrade FAG, Cavalcanti CEO, Isoldi FC, et al. Therapeutics of xeroderma pigmentosum: a PRISMA-compliant systematic review. Indian J Dermatol Venereol Leprol. 2021;87(2):176–89.
158. Wolf P, Kerl H. Photodynamic therapy in patient with xeroderma pigmentosum. Lancet. 1991;337(8757):1613–4.
159. Larson DM, Cunningham BB. Photodynamic therapy in a teenage girl with xeroderma pigmentosum type C. Pediatr Dermatol. 2012;29(3):373–4.
160. Cai H, Yang QQ, Ma C, et al. Photodynamic therapy in the treatment of xeroderma pigmentosum: a case report. Photodiagn Photodyn Ther. 2020;30:101761.
161. Procianoy F, Cruz AA, Baccega A, et al. Aggravation of eyelid and conjunctival malignancies following photodynamic therapy in DeSanctis-Cacchione syndrome. Ophthalmic Plast Reconstr Surg. 2006;22(6):498–9.
162. Zheng J, Liu W, Zhou Z, et al. Successful treatment of nonmelanoma skin cancer in three patients with Xeroderma Pigmentosum by modified ALA-PDT. Photodiagn Photodyn Ther. 2023;43:103694.
163. Karrer S, Szeimies RM, Abels C, et al. Epidermodysplasia verruciformis treated using topical 5-aminolaevulinic acid photodynamic therapy. Br J Dermatol. 1999;140(5):935–8.
164. Chen Q, Jiang L, Shi L, et al. Successful treatment of upper-left eyelid squamous cell carcinoma in an epidermodysplasia verruciformis patient by ALA-PDT/holmium laser combination therapy. Photodiagn Photodyn Ther. 2021;34:102277.
165. Zhao Z, Wu Y, Zhou Z, et al. ALA-PDT successfully treated multiple cSCC in situ and AK in a patient with epidermodysplasia verruciformis. Photodiagn Photodyn Ther. 2021;35:102395.
166. Mallipeddi R. Epidermolysis bullosa and cancer. Clin Exp Dermatol. 2002;27(8):616–23.
167. Souza CS, Felicio LB, Bentley MV, et al. Topical photodynamic therapy for Bowen's disease of the digit in epidermolysis bullosa. Br J Dermatol. 2005;153(3):672–4.
168. Lee MW, Varigos G, Foley P, et al. Photodynamic therapy for basal cell carcinoma in recessive dystrophic epidermolysis bullosa. ISRN Dermatol. 2011;2011:346754.
169. Marcon CR, Maia M. Albinism: epidemiology, genetics, cutaneous characterization, psychosocial factors. An Bras Dermatol. 2019;94(5):503–20.
170. Garcia Galvao LE, Tomaz R, de Sa Goncalves H. Daylight photodynamic therapy in the treatment of actinic keratosis in carriers of oculocutaneous albinism: report of three cases. Actas Dermosifiliogr. 2019;110(5):407–10.

171. Andreani V, Richard M, Folchetti G, et al. Congenital hypotrichosis and milia with spontaneous regression during adolescence or Oley syndrome: a variant of Bazex-dupre-Christol syndrome. Ann Dermatol Venereol. 2000;127(3):285–8.
172. Garofola C, Nassereddin A, Gross GP. Dyskeratosis congenita. In: StatPearls. Treasure Island: StatPearls Publishing; 2024.
173. Li Y, Wang B, Zheng S, et al. Photodynamic therapy in the treatment of oral leukoplakia: a systematic review. Photodiagn Photodyn Ther. 2019;25:17–22.

Neoadjuvant Use of PDT for Nonmelanoma Skin Cancers

12

Caihe Liao, Jia Yan, Peiru Wang, Bo Wang, and Xiuli Wang

12.1 Definition of Neoadjuvant PDT

Compared with conventional neoadjuvant therapy, which is limited to presurgical use, neoadjuvant PDT represents a comprehensive approach to photodynamic therapy, encompassing applications before surgery or laser treatments and in combination with postoperative therapies (Fig. 12.1). This advanced strategy for managing refractory NMSCs aims to reduce the tumor load, improve operability, and support definitive treatment [1, 2]. When used postoperatively, PDT targets residual tumors, reduces the risk of recurrence, and promotes wound healing.

PDT has emerged as a novel neoadjuvant therapy because of its ability to penetrate tumor tissue and induce cytotoxic effects through the generation of reactive oxygen species. ALA-PDT has been shown to trigger immunogenic cell death, recruit tertiary lymphoid structure-like intratumoral lymphoid aggregates, and enhance antitumor immunity [3, 4]. The density of tertiary lymphoid structures in cSCC correlates with increased histological differentiation, emphasizing the potential of neoadjuvant PDT as an emerging antitumor strategy [5]. By combining surgery, laser therapy, and systemic therapy, neoadjuvant PDT addresses the limitations of mono-PDT and is particularly suitable for advanced NMSCs with large, multiple, invasive tumors or those in cosmetically or functionally sensitive areas [6]. Furthermore, it offers a safe, minimally invasive option for elderly, frail patients or those unwilling to undergo invasive surgery.

C. Liao · J. Yan · P. Wang · X. Wang (✉)
Institute of Photomedicine, Shanghai Skin Disease Hospital, School of Medicine, Tongji University, Shanghai, China
e-mail: wangxiuli_1400023@tongji.edu.cn

B. Wang
Avera Medical Group Dermatology, Aberdeen, SD, USA

University of South Dakota, Vermillion, SD, USA
e-mail: makiwang@med.umich.edu

X. Wang, B. Wang (eds.), *Photodynamic Therapy in Dermatology*,
https://doi.org/10.1007/978-981-96-8915-6_12

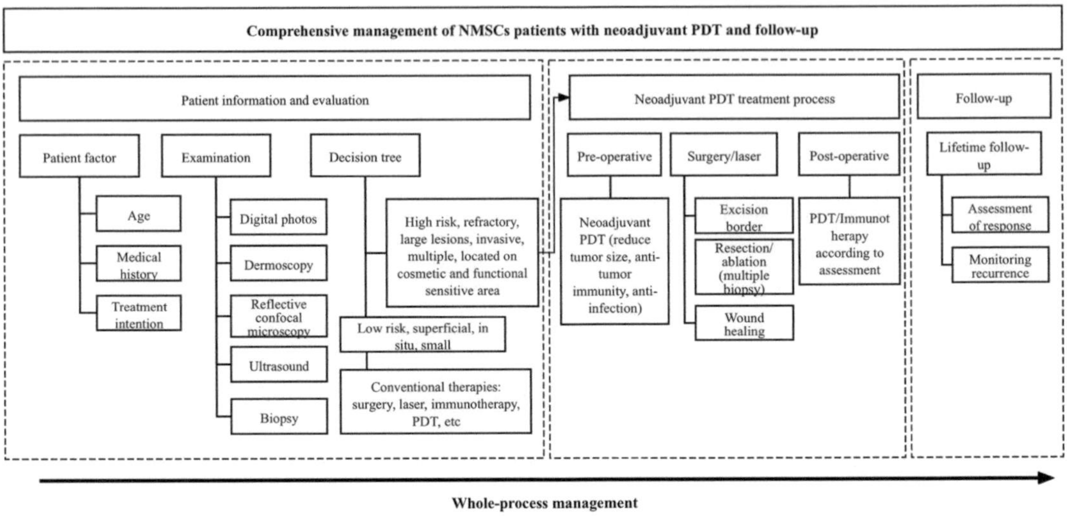

Fig. 12.1 Comprehensive management of NMSC patients receiving neoadjuvant PDT and follow-up. This information should be made available and discussed at multidisciplinary team (MDT) meetings

12.2 Therapeutic Process for Neoadjuvant PDT

12.2.1 Preoperative Treatment

Neoadjuvant PDT is employed to reduce the tumor size before surgery or ablative treatments, minimizing surgical defects and facilitating reconstruction. It is particularly advantageous for managing tumor erosion, ulceration, and local infection caused by rapid tumor growth and invasion. Compared with antibiotics, PDT provides broader antibacterial properties and serves as an effective antibiotic-free option for infection control in the perioperative period [7]. We recommend starting PDT 1 week prior to surgery. ALA at a 20% concentration is applied at a thin layer on the tumor surface and 0.5–1 cm peripherally, incubated for 0.5–1 h, and irradiated with 633-nm LED red light (150–200 J/cm^2, 28 mW/cm^2) without removing the ALA cream. Preoperative PDT is performed 1–3 times at 3–7-day intervals.

12.2.2 Surgery or Ablative Treatments

The increasing incidence of NMSCs in cosmetically and functionally sensitive areas, such as the scalp, face, or genital region, underscores the need for treatments that balance effective tumor clearance with functional and cosmetic preservation [8, 9].

Surgical excision is generally recommended for NMSCs to achieve a tumor-free margin [10]. While wider margins enhance safety, surgery can lead to pain, scarring, and potential functional impairment. Neoadjuvant PDT combined with surgical excision or ablative treatments such as electrodesiccation and curettage is an alternative approach [11, 12]. Surgical options include standard wide local excision, which removes all visible tumor borders with safety margins, and in situ excision, which involves narrow-margin resection along the tumor edge to preserve local tissue structure and function. The wound was left open for subsequent PDT treatment, followed by a postoperative pathological assessment of the lateral and deep margins.

12.2.3 Postoperative Treatments

In cases of positive or limited surgical margins, postoperative ALA-PDT is recommended. Leaving the excision site unsutured enhances ALA absorption and facilitates repeatable PDT treatments, improving treatment precision and making

PDT a more sustainable alternative to radiation and surgery. Neoadjuvant ALA-PDT begins the day after excision, and a 20% ALA solution is applied for 30 min before irradiation with 633-nm LED red light at 150–300 J/cm^2 and 28–60 mW/cm^2. PDT sessions are repeated every 1–2 weeks until complete wound healing is achieved.

ALA-PDT combined with immune checkpoint inhibitor programmed death-1 (PD-1) or programmed death-ligand 1 (PD-L1) monoclonal antibodies has synergistic antitumor effects, enhances the immunotherapy response, reduces the risk of recurrence or metastasis in high-risk NMSC patients, and improves outcomes in advanced cSCC patients [4, 13]. Additionally, epidermal growth factor receptor (EGFR) inhibitors have shown efficacy in advanced cSCC treatment [14], whereas Hedgehog pathway inhibitors are effective in advanced BCC [15]. The integration of ALA-PDT with immunotherapy or targeted therapy represents a promising approach for managing NMSCs.

12.3 Clinical Applications

12.3.1 Basal Cell Carcinoma

ALA-PDT is recommended for superficial BCC and thin nodules (thickness <2 mm), supported by a grade of recommendation A and a level of evidence I [8, 16]. Its efficacy is comparable to that of surgical treatment, with better cosmetic outcomes. Neoadjuvant PDT is recommended for BCC patients with a heavy tumor load or high recurrence risk. PDT has proven effective as a neoadjuvant therapy to reduce tumor burden and local morbidity in BCC treatment [17]. In a prospective study, 33 BCC patients who underwent neoadjuvant PDT achieved complete remission after an average of 1.8 ± 0.2 treatments, with no local recurrence at the 1-year follow-up [18]. Another study reported a 13.2–100% reduction in the lesion area, further supporting the efficacy of neoadjuvant PDT for facial BCC [6]. The author's group successfully treated a 91-year-old patient with locally advanced BCC via a combination of modified ALA-PDT, a Ho-YAG laser, and hematoporphyrin derivative photodynamic therapy (HpD-PDT), reducing the tumor thickness from 15 mm to 4 mm after six treatments [19]. Neoadjuvant PDT preserves hair follicles without cosmetic deformity, making it especially advantageous for hair-bearing areas, including the face and scalp [20]. Espiñeira Sicre et al. reported successful tumor volume reduction and elimination of peripheral lesions in a case of radiotherapy-induced recurrent multiple BCC using neoadjuvant PDT [21].

Recommended neoadjuvant therapies for BCC:

The general assessment confirms the diagnosis via ultrasound, dermoscopy, and biopsy, with additional tests tailored to the BCC location and potential risk of metastasis.

Preoperative ALA-PDT with 20% ALA cream was applied to the BCC lesions, which were subsequently incubated for 30 min. Red-light irradiation with an energy density of 200 J/cm^2 and a power density of 28 mW/cm^2 is recommended, which is repeated every 3 days for a total of two treatments. This approach is suitable for patients with erosion, ulceration, or concurrent infection of BCC. Although BCC grows slowly, it is invasive to surrounding tissues, especially in elderly patients with a long disease history and inadequate skin care. In this context, ALA-PDT serves as an ideal antibiotic-free, immunomodulatory treatment that controls infection and reduces the tumor load before surgery or ablative treatments.

Surgical or Ablative Treatments

Ultrasound or imaging methods provide details about the depth of BCC lesions.

- Curettage is recommended for BCC lesions with a depth of ≤2 mm, and a sterile curette with a 3–5 mm margin is used to scrape the lesions along the edges and base until clearance (Fig. 12.2).
- A carbon dioxide (CO_2) laser is recommended for BCC depths >2 mm and those in the dermis. A CO_2 laser was used to remove the BCC lesion, which included a 1-mm safety margin, and the burned tissue was wiped away with

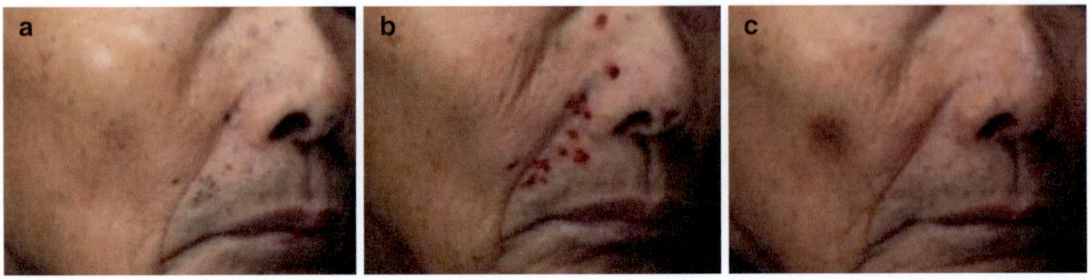

Fig. 12.2 Multiple BCC lesions before and after ALA-PDT combined with curettage. (**a**) There were more than 55 nodular BCC lesions on the face of a 75-year-old male patient before treatment. (**b**) Manifestation immediately after curettage. (**c**) After three sessions of ALA-PDT. No scar was observed in the treated area except for the case of dyspigmentation

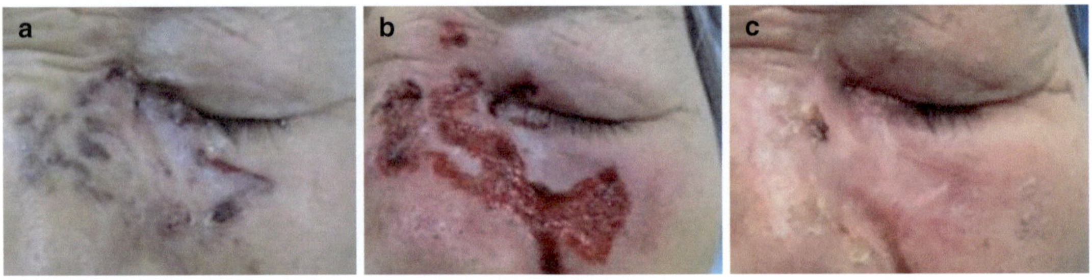

Fig. 12.3 Paranasal and inner canthus BCC lesions before and after ALA-PDT combined with carbon dioxide (CO_2) laser treatment. (**a**) 73-year-old female with a giant BCC (tumor size: 50 × 36 mm) before treatment, (**b**) manifestation immediately after CO_2 laser treatment, and (**c**) after four sessions of ALA-PDT treatments. The eye appearance and function were well preserved

saline gauze until the visible lesions were removed (Fig. 12.3).

- Narrow local excision for BCC is indicated for BCC that reaches subcutaneous soft tissue without breaching the deep fascia, with 2-mm surgical margins at the peripheral and deep margins. The wound was left open after hemostasis (Fig. 12.4).

Postoperative ALA-PDT Postoperative ALA-PDT treatment begins 24 h after surgery or ablative treatments. A 20% ALA solution was applied to the BCC wound, which was subsequently incubated for 30 min. Red-light irradiation with an energy density of 150–250 J/cm^2 and a power density of 28–60 mW/cm^2 was applied every 1–2 weeks until the wound was completely healed, and no BCC lesions were detected via dermoscopy or skin ultrasound. In cases of residual tumors, reneoadjuvant PDT combined with surgical treatment may be considered. For locally advanced or metastatic BCC, neoadjuvant PDT serves as a local palliative treatment, whereas Hedgehog pathway inhibitors are recommended as first-line treatments.

12.3.2 Invasive Cutaneous Squamous Cell Carcinoma

Wide local excision and Mohs micrographic surgery remain the first-line treatments for primary cSCC [10, 22]. However, the necessity of wider excision margins has been questioned. A retrospective study of 1000 high-risk cSCC patients compared narrow and wide clinical resection margins and revealed no significant difference in incomplete resection rates between wider (6–10 mm) and narrower (≤5 mm) margins (2.6% vs 3.0%, $P = 0.99$) or in recurrence or cSCC-

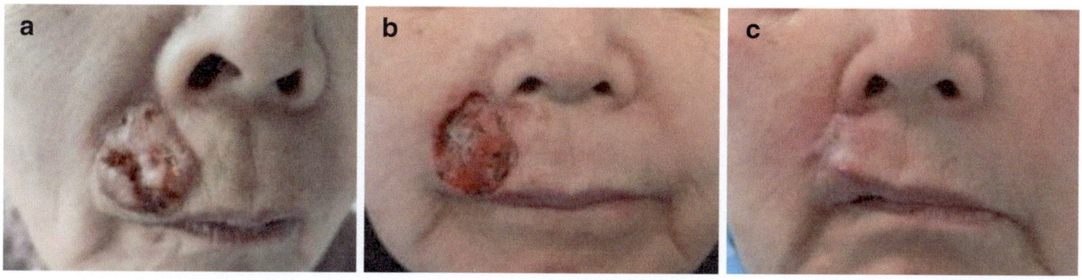

Fig. 12.4 BCC lesions at the right NLF before and after ALA-PDT combined with narrow margin surgery. (**a**) 78-year-old female with BCC (tumor size: 23 × 23 mm, tumor depth: 4.2 mm) before treatment and (**b**) manifestation immediately after a 2-mm narrow-margin excision. The defect was left open without reconstruction. (**c**) After three sessions of ALA-PDT, the wound healed, with mild scar contracture and lip traction changes

specific mortality rates [23]. These findings suggest that wider margins may have a limited impact on the prognosis of high-risk patients. Moreover, complete excision with wide margins can lead to functional impairment and poor cosmetic outcomes, particularly for lesions on the face, head, and genital areas.

PDT is a safe and effective therapy with good cosmetic outcomes and is recommended for treating actinic keratoses and squamous cell carcinoma in situ, with a Grade A recommendation and Level I evidence [8, 24]. Although PDT can be an alternative to surgery in certain cases, it is not suitable as a first-line treatment for invasive cSCC because of the limited penetration depth of the photosensitizer and light source. Neoadjuvant PDT addresses these limitations. Studies have shown that neoadjuvant ALA-PDT combined with surgery is effective for invasive cSCC [25], reducing tumor size before surgery, creating favorable conditions for surgical treatment, enhancing antitumor immunity, and improving complete remission rates. ALA-PDT can also be used for consolidation treatment after surgery to eliminate potential microlesions. A retrospective study by the author's group revealed that among 33 cSCC patients who were unable or unwilling to undergo surgery, 15.2% (5/33) achieved complete remission, and 72.7% (24/33) achieved partial remission after ALA-PDT combined with imiquimod [26].

The lips and eyelids are special sites for cSCC, and treatment can be challenging because of the risk of morphological and functional defects from surgery or radiation therapy. In such cases, neoadjuvant ALA-PDT offers an alternative treatment option that can achieve complete remission without functional or aesthetic sequelae [27]. A combination of superficial excision surgery and PDT is effective in treating lip cSCCs [28, 29]. For tumors in locations where surgical resection is limited, combining neoadjuvant PDT with holmium laser ablation has shown promising results for recurrent and invasive cSCC in the eyelid [30]. Huang et al. reported successful adjuvant PDT for a giant keratoacanthoma-like cSCC of the eyelid, removing residual malignant cells at the surgical margins [31]. This approach effectively eliminates the tumor while preserving normal tissue and reducing the risk of recurrence. Furthermore, PDT has a preventive effect on actinic keratosis and cSCC [32]. Randomized controlled trials have further demonstrated the potential of PDT in preventing the formation of new NMSCs in patients with regional cancer [33]. Thus, neoadjuvant PDT can not only effectively remove precancerous lesions and tumors but also reduce recurrence and prevent the development of new NMSCs.

Recommended neoadjuvant therapies for invasive cSCC:

General assessment: A biopsy and histological confirmation should be performed on suspected lesions. Once primary cSCC is diagnosed histologically, clinical evaluation should include patient demographics, tumor location, and diameter for staging. For patients with high-risk factors, imaging techniques such as ultrasound, computed tomography (CT), magnetic resonance imaging (MRI), or positron emission tomography-computed tomography (PET-CT) are recommended to assess local invasion and regional nodal metastasis. Staging systems help predict the risk of recurrence or metastasis. Several available staging systems include the UICC eighth edition (for cutaneous cSCC excluding eyelid, perianal, vulva, and penis), the American Joint Committee on Cancer eighth edition (for head and neck), the Brigham and Women's Hospital system, and the Breuninger staging system [34].

Preoperative ALA-PDT: Freshly prepared 20% ALA cream was applied to the cSCC lesions, and the lesions were protected from light for 0.5–1 h. The ALA cream was retained thinly on the surface of the lesions. Red-light irradiation with an energy density of 150–200 J/cm^2 and a power density of 28 mW/cm^2 is recommended. The treatment was repeated every 3–7 days, with the total number of treatments determined on the basis of the response to PDT. The goal of this approach is to reduce the tumor size, limit peripheral invasion, and eliminate infection.

Narrow local excision: This imaging techniques provide details about the depth of cSCC lesions and the presence of perivascular involvement. The tumor was resected with a 3-mm clinically narrow margin and evaluated through histological examination, including one point on the deep frontal margin and four points on the peripheral margins. The incision was kept open without suturing or reconstruction.

Postoperative ALA-PDT: Postoperative ALA-PDT treatment was initiated 24 h after surgery. A 20% ALA solution was applied and incubated for 30 min, followed by irradiation with 633-nm LED red light at a dose of 150–300 J/cm^2 and a power density of 28–60 mW/cm^2. PDT is repeated every 1–2 weeks until the incision is fully healed, with clinical response and noninvasive examinations (such as dermoscopy and skin ultrasound) used to assess progress (Fig. 12.5). A biopsy was conducted to confirm any suspicious lesions. For patients with locally advanced cSCC, immunotherapy or targeted therapy (such as PD-1 monoclonal antibodies or EGFR inhibitors) is recommended as part of combination therapy (Fig. 12.6). Additionally, neoadjuvant PDT may be employed as a palliative treatment for local tumor reduction in advanced metastatic cSCC when other treatments are not feasible or effective, thus improving patients' quality of life.

12.3.3 Extramammary Paget's Disease

Extramammary Paget's disease (EMPD) is a rare malignancy that typically affects the genital, perianal, and axillary areas of elderly individuals. Owing to its insidious nature and poorly defined borders, EMPD is often difficult to diagnose and prone to recurrence. Early diagnosis and appropriate therapy are critical for effective treatment. ALA-PDT is recommended as a palliative treatment for EMPD, particularly as a neoadjuvant therapy to reduce tumor size before surgery [35]. In a prospective trial, 13 patients with 19 EMPD lesions underwent surgery or neoadjuvant ALA-PDT, with lesion sizes reduced by more than 58% after 4 PDT sessions. The recurrence rate in the PDT group was 9.1%, whereas it was 25% in the surgery group [36]. Additionally, the average size of the surgical wound in the neoadjuvant PDT group was half that of the surgery-only group, leading to less structural damage and scarring. The author's group reported similar results, noting that the lesion size decreased after each treatment. A 71-year-old patient with recurrent postoperative EMPD in the right perineum was successfully treated with nine sessions of neoadjuvant PDT and four sessions of ultrasound-guided holmium laser treatments [37]. Another prospective study involving 11 patients with deep invasive EMPD treated with systemic HpD-PDT reported that 72.7% of patients achieved complete remission after 12–27 months, with recurrent patients treated with ALA-PDT, a holmium laser, or HpD-PDT [38]. PDT also serves as a palliative treatment for nonsurgical EMPD patients, reducing the tumor burden, improving quality of life, and prolonging survival [39]. A

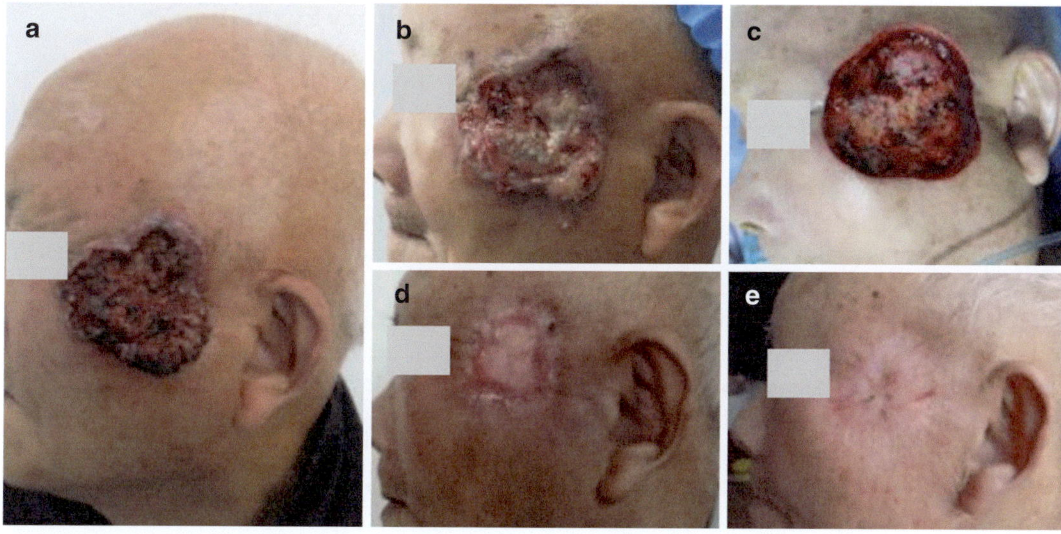

Fig. 12.5 Neoadjuvant ALA-PDT treatment in patients with very high-risk cSCC. (**a**) 92-year-old male with a giant cSCC (tumor size: 50 × 50 × 11.2 mm) at the left temple before treatment. (**b**) After two sessions of ALA-PDT treatments. (**c**) Manifestation immediately after a 3-mm narrow-margin excision. (**d**) The incision was healed after four sessions of ALA-PDT treatments. (**e**) The patient achieved a complete response at 20 months and achieved a good cosmetic outcome

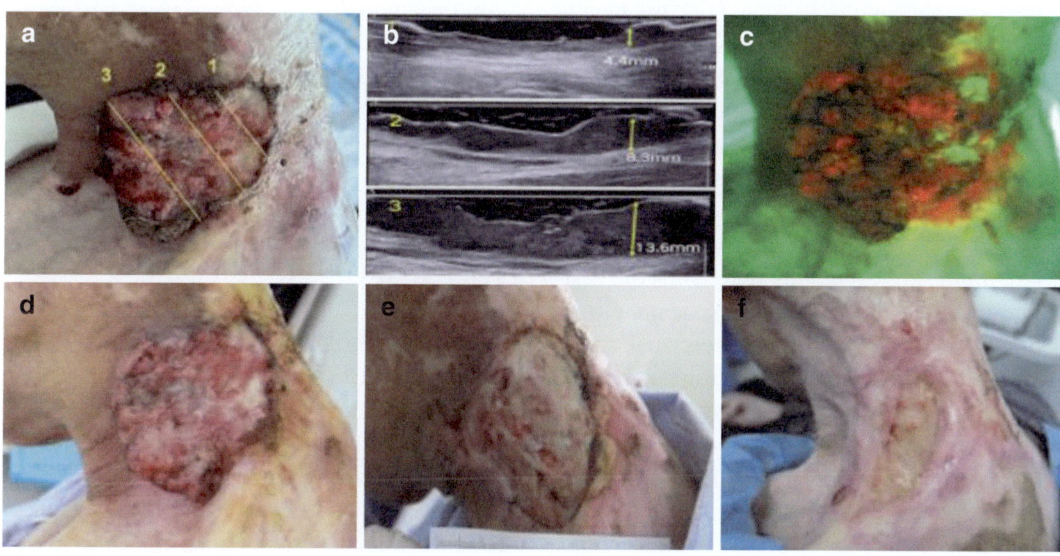

Fig. 12.6 Neoadjuvant ALA-PDT treatment in patients with a locally advanced cSCC with field cancer. (**a**) An 80-year-old male with cSCC in the left neck (tumor size: 55 × 44 mm) was diagnosed via an X-ray accident at work 55 years ago. (**b**) Skin ultrasound revealed that the thickness of the tumor was 4.4–13.6 mm. (**c**) After 30 min of incubation, the tumor and surrounding field cancerization showed red fluorescence. (**d**) After two sessions of ALA-PDT treatments before surgical excision. (**e**) Manifestation immediately after a 3-mm narrow-margin excision of cSCC. (**f**) After 11 sessions of ALA-PDT and 12 sessions of PD-1 immunotherapy (toripalimab, 240 mg, an interval of 3 weeks), the tumor with field cancerization improved

clinical trial involving 32 patients with EMPD treated with aminolevulinic acid methyl ester (M-ALA) PDT revealed that 9.4% achieved complete resolution, 78.1% achieved partial resolution, and 12.5% achieved stable disease after 3 PDT sessions. No patients experienced disease progression. Although PDT may not cure EMPD, it is a reliable strategy for managing the disease and its symptoms [40]. The selective enrichment of photosensitizers in tumor tissues also aids in fluorescence diagnosis, helping to delineate tumor boundaries and detect lesions beyond the clinical margins [41]. Treatment options should focus on tumor resection while preserving normal appearance and function. Neoadjuvant PDT combined with surgery or laser therapy is a promising approach to reduce recurrence and improve quality of life in patients with EMPD.

Recommended neoadjuvant therapies for EMPD:

- For superficial invasive EMPD (stage I, thickness <2 mm), multiple ALA-PDT treatments can achieve a complete response. Before PDT, plum blossom needle pretreatment was applied within 2 cm of the EMPD border. For thicker local areas, CO_2 laser or holmium laser ablation can be combined with pretreatment to increase the effectiveness of the treatment.
- For EMPD patients with deep invasion (≥2 mm), surgical treatment remains the first-line approach. However, for large and multiple tumors located in the genital/perianal areas, neoadjuvant ALA-PDT is strongly recommended. This treatment aims to reduce tumor size and the extent of surgical resection, leading to a lower recurrence rate than simple surgical resection.
- For advanced invasive or metastatic EMPD, ALA-PDT serves as a palliative treatment to alleviate the tumor burden and improve patients' quality of life. In cases of EMPD with deep infiltration or involvement of special locations, HpD-PDT can be used if necessary.

12.4 Efficacy Evaluation

12.4.1 Testing Methods

There are various methods used to assess the efficacy of neoadjuvant PDT, including both objective and subjective evaluations. Noninvasive examinations are preferred, with invasive methods reserved for necessary cases:

- Clinical examination: The treated site was inspected, a total body skin exam was performed, and regional lymph nodes were identified.
- Noninvasive diagnostic methods: Dermatoscopy, reflectance confocal microscopy, and high-frequency ultrasound are recommended for evaluating the treated area. Imaging techniques such as CT and MRI are recommended for assessing the risk of local invasion or distant metastasis.
- Invasive diagnostic methods**:** Skin biopsy and sentinel lymph node biopsy were performed when necessary.
- Tools such as the Skin Cancer Index and the Skin Cancer Quality of Life Assessment Tool can be employed to evaluate a patient's quality of life.

12.4.2 Assessment

The Response Evaluation Criteria in Solid Tumors, version 1.1 (RECIST 1.1), is strongly recommended for assessing treatment efficacy. A complete response refers to complete resection of the tumor, a partial response refers to tumor reduction >70%, a progressive response refers to tumor enlargement >20%, and a stable response refers to the degree of tumor change between PR and PD. Evaluations are performed before and after treatment, with a focus on reducing recurrence and complications while incorporating patient perspectives. Feedback and statements from patients offer valuable insights to optimize overall treatment management [42].

12.5 Adverse Reactions

12.5.1 Pain

The modified PDT is the preferred treatment to minimize patient pain (visual analog scale score $\leq$3 points) during treatment. However, for tumors complicated by infection, located on the head or face, or in elderly patients, significant pain may still occur. Symptomatic treatments such as cold air cooling, ice packs, or local infiltration anesthesia are recommended to alleviate discomfort.

12.5.2 Acute Cutaneous Reactions

Acute local adverse reactions typically arise at the start of PDT treatment and last 1–3 days; these reactions are characterized by the infiltration of inflammatory cells, primarily neutrophils. Common symptoms include erythema, pain, burning, itching, edema, and blisters, especially in open incisions. Mild to moderate reactions generally resolve without specific treatment but require proper wound care and infection prevention. Severe reactions may necessitate the use of topical or systemic steroids to suppress inflammation.

12.5.3 Wound Healing

Local adverse reactions during the recovery period typically occur 4 days after ALA-PDT and may include exudation, crusting, and dyspigmentation. These reactions usually resolve with topical care and symptomatic management. While red light promotes wound healing, large nasal defects pose a greater risk of scar formation, potentially impacting facial appearance and functionality. Thus, for such cases, healing with secondary intention is not advised; instead, repair with a flap is recommended to address the wound defect effectively.

12.6 Patient Management

Post-ALA-PDT follow-up should occur monthly for the first 3 months and then every 3–6 months for 2 years, with prompt reexamination for any abnormalities. High-risk groups require more frequent follow-up and lifelong monitoring. EMPD, which has a higher recurrence rate than other NMSCs do, necessitates more frequent follow-up. Noninvasive diagnostic methods, such as dermatoscopy, reflectance confocal microscopy, and skin ultrasound, are recommended, with skin biopsy with histopathology performed as needed. Patient education is crucial, as it emphasizes NMSC recognition, protection, self-examination, the importance of early treatment, and adherence to follow-up schedules. This approach improves prevention, early detection, prognosis, and management of NMSCs.

In conclusion, neoadjuvant PDT shows promise as a treatment for NMSCs, especially when surgery is not the preferred option. However, further randomized controlled trials are essential to comprehensively evaluate its safety and efficacy in managing NMSCs.

References

1. Frei E. Clinical cancer research: an embattled species. Cancer. 1982;50(10):1979–92. https://doi.org/10.1002/1097-0142(19821115)50:10<1979::aid-cncr2820501002>3.0.co;2-d.
2. Frei E. What's in a name–neoadjuvant. J Natl Cancer Inst. 1988;80(14):1088–9. https://doi.org/10.1093/jnci/80.14.1088.
3. Ji J, Zhang Y, Chen WR, Wang X. DC vaccine generated by ALA-PDT-induced immunogenic apoptotic cells for skin squamous cell carcinoma. Onco Targets Ther. 2016;5(6):e1072674. https://doi.org/10.1080/2162402X.2015.1072674.
4. Zeng Q, Yang J, Ji J, Wang P, Zhang L, Yan G, et al. PD-L1 blockade potentiates the antitumor effects of ALA-PDT and optimizes the tumor microenvironment in cutaneous squamous cell carcinoma. Onco Targets Ther. 2022;11(1):2061396. https://doi.org/10.1080/2162402X.2022.2061396.

5. Wu YH, Wu F, Yan GR, Zeng QY, Jia N, Zheng Z, et al. Features and clinical significance of tertiary lymphoid structure in cutaneous squamous cell carcinoma. J Eur Acad Dermatol Venereol. 2022;36(11):2043–50. https://doi.org/10.1111/jdv.18464.
6. Jeremic G, Moore CC, Brandt MG, Doyle PC. Neoadjuvant use of photodynamic therapy in basal cell and squamous cell carcinomas of the face. ISRN Dermatol. 2011;2011:809409. https://doi.org/10.5402/2011/809409.
7. de Oliveira AB, Ferrisse TM, Fontana CR, Basso FG, Brighenti FL. Photodynamic therapy for treating infected skin wounds: a systematic review and meta-analysis from randomized clinical trials. Photodiagn Photodyn Ther. 2022;40:103118. https://doi.org/10.1016/j.pdpdt.2022.103118.
8. Shi L, Wang H, Chen K, Yan J, Yu B, Wang S, et al. Chinese guidelines on the clinical application of 5-aminolevulinic acid-based photodynamic therapy in dermatology (2021 edition). Photodiagn Photodyn Ther. 2021;35:102340. https://doi.org/10.1016/j.pdpdt.2021.102340.
9. Maeda T, Yoshino K. Management of elderly patients with advanced cutaneous squamous cell carcinoma. Jpn J Clin Oncol. 2022;52(3):214–20. https://doi.org/10.1093/jjco/hyab213.
10. Stratigos AJ, Garbe C, Dessinioti C, Lebbe C, van Akkooi A, Bataille V, et al. European consensus-based interdisciplinary guideline for invasive cutaneous squamous cell carcinoma: part 2. Treatment-update 2023. Eur J Cancer. 2023;193:113252. https://doi.org/10.1016/j.ejca.2023.113252.
11. Yu N, Luo X, Wei T, Zhang Q, Yu J, Wu L, et al. Dermabrasion combined with photodynamic therapy: a new option for the treatment of nonmelanoma skin cancer. Lasers Med Sci. 2022;37(2):1255–63. https://doi.org/10.1007/s10103-021-03381-3.
12. Yu N, Wu L, Su J, Chen M, Lu L, Huang K, et al. Photodynamic therapy combined with surgery versus Mohs micrographic surgery for the treatment of difficult-to-treat basal cell carcinoma: a retrospective clinical study. J Dermatolog Treat. 2023;34(1):2200871. https://doi.org/10.1080/09546634.2023.2200871.
13. Newman JG, Hall MA, Kurley SJ, Cook RW, Farberg AS, Geiger JL, et al. Adjuvant therapy for high-risk cutaneous squamous cell carcinoma: 10-year review. Head Neck. 2021;43(9):2822–43. https://doi.org/10.1002/hed.26767.
14. Savoia P, Cremona O, Fava P. New perspectives in the pharmacological treatment of non-melanoma skin cancer. Curr Drug Targets. 2016;17(3):353–74. https://doi.org/10.2174/138945011666615080612371 7.
15. Peris K, Fargnoli MC, Kaufmann R, Arenberger P, Bastholt L, Seguin NB, et al. European consensus-based interdisciplinary guideline for diagnosis and treatment of basal cell carcinoma-update 2023. Eur J Cancer. 2023;192:113254. https://doi.org/10.1016/j.ejca.2023.113254.
16. Cosgarea R, Susan M, Crisan M, Senila S. Photodynamic therapy using topical 5-aminolaevulinic acid vs. surgery for basal cell carcinoma. J Eur Acad Dermatol Venereol. 2013;27(8):980–4. https://doi.org/10.1111/j.1468-3083.2012.04619.x.
17. Zelin E, Zalaudek I, Agozzino M, Dianzani C, Dri A, Di Meo N, et al. Neoadjuvant therapy for nonmelanoma skin cancer: updated therapeutic approaches for basal, squamous, and merkel cell carcinoma. Curr Treat Options in Oncol. 2021;22(4):35. https://doi.org/10.1007/s11864-021-00826-3.
18. Jeremic G, Brandt MG, Jordan K, Doyle PC, Yu E, Moore CC. Using photodynamic therapy as a neoadjuvant treatment in the surgical excision of nonmelanotic skin cancers: prospective study. J Otolaryngol Head Neck Surg. 2011;40(Suppl 1):82–9.
19. Liao C, Shi L, Wang D, Wang X. Bimodal photodynamic therapy for treatment of a 91-year-old patient with locally advanced cutaneous basal cell carcinoma and postoperative scar management. Photodiagn Photodyn Ther. 2021;36:102553. https://doi.org/10.1016/j.pdpdt.2021.102553.
20. Liao C, Zhang G, Wang P, Sun X, Wang X. Combination curettage and modified ALA-PDT for multiple basal cell carcinomas of the face and head. Photodiagn Photodyn Ther. 2021;35:102393. https://doi.org/10.1016/j.pdpdt.2021.102393.
21. Espineira Sicre J, Garcia Sirvent L, Ruiz Sanchez J, Garcia Fernandez L, Soro Martinez P, Miralles Botella J, et al. Neoadjuvant photodynamic therapy as a therapeutic alternative in multiple basal cell carcinoma induced by radiotherapy. Photodiagn Photodyn Ther. 2023;44:103820. https://doi.org/10.1016/j.pdpdt.2023.103820.
22. Schmults CD, Blitzblau R, Aasi SZ, Alam M, Andersen JS, Baumann BC, et al. NCCN guidelines(R) insights: squamous cell skin cancer, version 1.2022. J Natl Compr Cancer Netw. 2021;19(12):1382–94. https://doi.org/10.6004/jnccn.2021.0059.
23. Baba N, Kato H, Nakamura M, Matsushita S, Aoki M, Fujimoto N, et al. Narrower clinical margin in high or very high-risk squamous cell carcinoma: a retrospective, multicenter study of 1,000 patients. J Dtsch Dermatol Ges. 2022;20(8):1088–99. https://doi.org/10.1111/ddg.14810.
24. Sharma A, Birnie AJ, Bordea C, Cheung ST, Mann J, Morton CA, et al. British Association of Dermatologists guidelines for the management of people with cutaneous squamous cell carcinoma in situ (Bowen disease) 2022. Br J Dermatol. 2023;188(2):186–94. https://doi.org/10.1093/bjd/ljac042.
25. Lu YG, Wang YY, Yang YD, Zhang XC, Gao Y, Yang Y, et al. Efficacy of topical ALA-PDT combined with excision in the treatment of skin malignant tumor. Photodiagn Photodyn Ther. 2014;11(2):122–6. https://doi.org/10.1016/j.pdpdt.2014.02.006.
26. Zhang GL, Keyal U, Shi L, Wang PR, Zhang LL, Bhatta AK, et al. Photodynamic therapy as an alternative treatment in patients with invasive cutaneous

SCC where surgery is not feasible: single center experience. Photodiagn Photodyn Ther. 2020;32:101980. https://doi.org/10.1016/j.pdpdt.2020.101980.
27. Wang P, Zhang G, Zhang L, Zhou Z, Shi L, Zeng Q, et al. 5-Aminolevulinic acid photodynamic therapy for early-stage lip squamous cell carcinoma. Photodiagn Photodyn Ther. 2021;35:102321. https://doi.org/10.1016/j.pdpdt.2021.102321.
28. Wang Y, Yang Y, Yang Y, Lu Y. Surgery combined with topical photodynamic therapy for the treatment of squamous cell carcinoma of the lip. Photodiagn Photodyn Ther. 2016;14:170–2. https://doi.org/10.1016/j.pdpdt.2016.04.008.
29. Yan J, Wang P, Li L, Zhang L, Zhang G, Tang Y, et al. Surgery sequential with 5-Aminolevulinic acid photodynamic therapy for lip squamous cell carcinoma: two cases reports. Photodiagn Photodyn Ther. 2020;32:102043. https://doi.org/10.1016/j.pdpdt.2020.102043.
30. Chen Q, Jiang L, Shi L, Li C, Wu Y, Yang J, et al. Successful treatment of upper-left eyelid squamous cell carcinoma in an epidermodysplasia verruciformis patient by ALA-PDT/holmium laser combination therapy. Photodiagn Photodyn Ther. 2021;34:102277. https://doi.org/10.1016/j.pdpdt.2021.102277.
31. Huang J, Liu Y, Wu M, Wang X, Wang H. Successful treatment of a giant keratoacanthoma-like squamous cell carcinoma in the eyebrow using surgery combined with photodynamic therapy: a case report. Photodiagn Photodyn Ther. 2021;35:102474. https://doi.org/10.1016/j.pdpdt.2021.102474.
32. Liew YCC, De Souza NNA, Sultana RG, Oh CC. Photodynamic therapy for the prevention and treatment of actinic keratosis/squamous cell carcinoma in solid organ transplant recipients: a systematic review and meta-analysis. J Eur Acad Dermatol Venereol. 2020;34(2):251–9. https://doi.org/10.1111/jdv.15852.
33. Apalla Z, Sotiriou E, Chovarda E, Lefaki I, Devliotou-Panagiotidou D, Ioannides D. Skin cancer: preventive photodynamic therapy in patients with face and scalp cancerization. A randomized placebo-controlled study. Br J Dermatol. 2010;162(1):171–5. https://doi.org/10.1111/j.1365-2133.2009.09492.x.
34. Stratigos AJ, Garbe C, Dessinioti C, Lebbe C, van Akkooi A, Bataille V, et al. European consensus-based interdisciplinary guideline for invasive cutaneous squamous cell carcinoma. Part 1: diagnostics and prevention-update 2023. Eur J Cancer. 2023;193:113251. https://doi.org/10.1016/j.ejca.2023.113251.
35. Kibbi N, Owen JL, Worley B, Wang JX, Harikumar V, Downing MB, et al. Evidence-based clinical practice guidelines for extramammary Paget disease. JAMA Oncol. 2022;8(4):618–28. https://doi.org/10.1001/jamaoncol.2021.7148.
36. Wang HW, Lv T, Zhang LL, Lai YX, Tang L, Tang YC, et al. A prospective pilot study to evaluate combined topical photodynamic therapy and surgery for extramammary Paget's disease. Lasers Surg Med. 2013;45(5):296–301. https://doi.org/10.1002/lsm.22142.
37. Li C, Guo L, Wang P, Shi L, Sun X, Hu C, et al. ALA-PDT combined with holmium laser therapy of postoperative recurrent extramammary Paget's disease. Photodiagn Photodyn Ther. 2019;27:92–4. https://doi.org/10.1016/j.pdpdt.2019.05.011.
38. Wang D, Wang P, Li C, Zhou Z, Zhang L, Zhang G, et al. Efficacy and safety of HpD-PDT for extramammary Paget's disease refractory to conventional therapy: a prospective, open-label and single arm pilot study. Photodiagn Photodyn Ther. 2022;37:102670. https://doi.org/10.1016/j.pdpdt.2021.102670.
39. Shen S, Zhang G, Wang P, Zhang Y, Keyal U, Ji J, et al. ALA-PDT as palliative care in a patient with secondary perineum EMPD. Photodiagn Photodyn Ther. 2018;22:166–8. https://doi.org/10.1016/j.pdpdt.2018.04.002.
40. Fontanelli R, Papadia A, Martinelli F, Lorusso D, Grijuela B, Merola M, et al. Photodynamic therapy with M-ALA as non surgical treatment option in patients with primary extramammary Paget's disease. Gynecol Oncol. 2013;130(1):90–4. https://doi.org/10.1016/j.ygyno.2013.04.008.
41. Li X, Zhao C, Kou H, Zhu F, Yang Y, Lu Y. PDD-guided tumor excision combined with photodynamic therapy in patients with extramammary Paget's disease. Photodiagn Photodyn Ther. 2022;38:102841. https://doi.org/10.1016/j.pdpdt.2022.102841.
42. Yan J, Wang B, Zhang G, Liao C, Zhao Z, Wang P, et al. Neoadjuvant photodynamic therapy: an updated therapeutic approach for non-melanoma skin cancers. Curr Treat Options in Oncol. 2024;25(6):813–26. https://doi.org/10.1007/s11864-024-01209-0.

HMME-PDT for the Treatment of Superficial Vascular Skin Diseases

13

Yunfeng Zhang, Dixin Wang, Bo Wang, and Xiuli Wang

13.1 HMME-PDT in the Treatment of Port Wine Stain

13.1.1 Introduction

The incidence of vascular diseases, including vascular tumors and malformations, is 2% among newborns, with the frequency increasing with age. The head and neck region is most commonly affected, accounting for approximately 60% of cases, followed by the trunk and limbs. These conditions primarily manifest in skin, subcutaneous, and mucosal tissues, although they can also involve internal organs [1, 2].

13.1.1.1 Clinical Features

Port wine stains (PWS) are congenital microvascular malformations and the most common type of capillary malformation, with an incidence of 0.3–0.5% among newborns. PWS typically do not resolve on its own and tend to thicken with age. Clinically, they are classified into three types: the pink type, characterized by a flat lesion that fades completely under finger pressure and ranges from light pink to red; the violaceous type, which also has a flat lesion but varies from light violaceous to deep violaceous, fading incompletely under fingertip pressure; and the hypertrophic type, presenting as thickened or nodular hyperplastic skin lesions with incomplete to no fading under finger pressure [3]. Skin lesions in exposed areas can significantly affect a patient's physical and mental well-being, underscoring the importance of early intervention [4].

13.1.1.2 Histopathology

Histopathological examination of PWS typically reveals a normal epidermis, with dilated capillaries and venules in the papillary and reticular dermis. The vessel walls consist of a single layer of endothelial cells, with diameters ranging from 10 μm to 300 μm and depths between 100 μm and 1000 μm. In pink PWS, mild vascular dilation in the superficial dermal layer is prominent, with increased capillary dilation as patient's age. Violaceous PWS shows further dilation of dermal blood vessels extending into the superficial dermis and subcutaneous tissues without endothelial cell proliferation. The hypertrophic type may display various features, including vascular dilation in the dermis, enlarged sebaceous glands, hair follicle enlargement, and accumulation of sebaceous secretions. Extensive dilation of dermal blood vessels can form a honeycomb pattern with

Y. Zhang · D. Wang · X. Wang (✉)
Institute of Photomedicine, Shanghai Skin Disease Hospital, School of Medicine, Tongji University, Shanghai, China
e-mail: wangxiuli_1400023@tongji.edu.cn

B. Wang
Avera Medical Group Dermatology, Aberdeen, SD, USA

University of South Dakota, Vermillion, SD, USA
e-mail: makiwang@med.umich.edu

X. Wang, B. Wang (eds.), *Photodynamic Therapy in Dermatology*,
https://doi.org/10.1007/978-981-96-8915-6_13

minimal interstitial tissue. Sometimes there is less vascular dilation, diffuse tissue collagenization, a loose interstitium, focal lymphocytic infiltration, and lymphedema-like changes [5].

13.1.2 Treatment Methods for Port Wine Stains

Traditional treatment methods for port wine stains (PWS) include radiation, liquid nitrogen cryotherapy, electrocautery, chemical exfoliation, superficial X-ray, traditional Chinese medicine, and surgical excision with skin grafting. However, these largely nonselective and destructive treatments often result in adverse reactions, such as scar formation and pigment changes, and are rarely used in clinical practice [6]. The authors' group previously utilized chicken combs as animal models to investigate the effects of ALA-PDT on microvascular malformations, observing changes in overall morphology, histology, and blood vessel numbers before and after treatment. The results indicated that ALA-PDT did not damage dermal capillaries in the chicken combs and had no therapeutic effect on microvascular malformations, suggesting that local ALA-PDT is not suitable for treating PWS [7].

13.1.2.1 Pulsed Dye Laser

In 1983, Anderson and Parrish introduced the theory of selective photothermal decomposition, which led to the development of pulsed dye lasers (PDLs) and significantly advanced the treatment of PWS by improving both their effectiveness and safety. PDL, which typically uses 585-nm or 595-nm lasers, remains the "gold standard" for PWS treatment. However, as clinical use has progressed, several limitations have emerged. PDL is most effective for skin lesions with diameters ranging from 50 μm to 150 μm, and factors such as patient's age, lesion area, depth, and classification can influence clinical outcomes. These factors may also contribute to potential adverse reactions, including pigmentation changes and scarring [8, 9].

13.1.2.2 Other Laser Treatments

With the rapid advancement of optomedical technology, various new treatment devices, such as intense pulsed light (IPL), variable pulse width doubling lasers (Nd:YAG 532 nm), and Alexandrite lasers, have been introduced and applied to treat different types of PWS with some therapeutic effects. However, the cure rates with these lasers remain suboptimal, as only 12–85% of patients experience less than 50% improvement, and there is a tendency for recurrence after treatment [10].

Several factors limit the effectiveness of treatment for PWS, including the competitive absorption of laser energy by melanin in the epidermis, rapid dispersion of heat energy due to small superficial blood vessels, difficulty in achieving sufficient thermal coagulation, and partial vascular damage followed by reperfusion and regeneration. These issues contribute to poor clinical outcomes and recurrence. As a result, many PWS patients still lack comprehensive and ideal treatment, making PWS management a significant clinical challenge [11].

13.1.2.3 HMME-PDT

Photosensitizers for HMME-PDT Currently, the photosensitizers used for PWS treatment include mixtures of hematoporphyrin derivatives (such as HpD and PSD-007) and monomeric photosensitizers such as hematoporphyrin monomethyl ether (HMME). The former contains complex components, some of which are slowly excreted in the skin, leading to high phototoxicity and prolonged light avoidance. HMME, a novel monomeric porphyrin photosensitizer developed in China, offers advantages such as a single chemical composition, good tissue selectivity, strong photosensitization, high photodynamic efficacy, low toxicity, rapid in vivo clearance, and high safety. Its absorption peak is in the green light band, and pharmacokinetic studies have shown that HMME is enriched primarily in the liver after intravenous administration, with absorption peaks at 395 nm, 497 nm and 531 nm (Fig. 13.1) [12]. This allows minimal absorption by the epidermis compared with the blue–purple band, ensuring adequate light penetration to

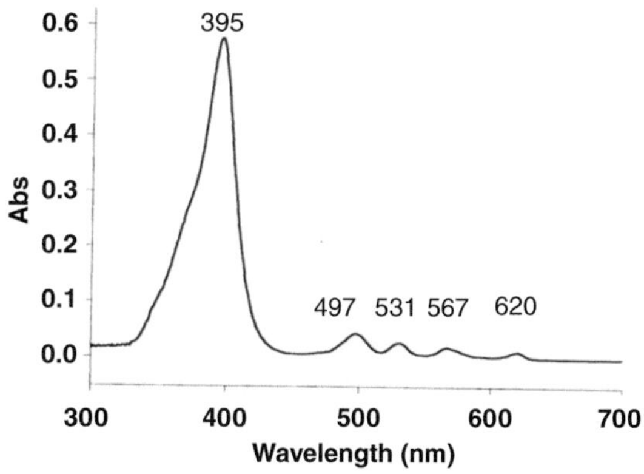

Fig. 13.1 Absorption spectrum of HMME. In the ultraviolet and visible light range, HMME exhibited absorption peaks at 395, 497, and 531 nm

target blood vessels while protecting deeper dermal layers. Studies have shown fewer adverse reactions, shorter light avoidance periods, and reduced intervals between treatments, making HMME an ideal approach for treating PWS. In 2005, HMME was approved by the National SFDA as a photosensitizer for PDT in PWS treatment, completing phase I, II, and III clinical trials by 2009. It received SFDA certification in 2012 and CFDA production approval in 2016 (drug product name: Fumeda, national drug approval number H20163349), although its current approved indication is PWS treatment, despite potential applications for tumor diagnosis and treatment [12].

Light Sources of HMME-PDT Coherent light sources, such as lasers, and incoherent light sources, such as intense pulsed light (IPL) and light-emitting diodes (LEDs), are commonly used for treatment. Continuous lasers, such as 532-nm semiconductor lasers or dynamic pulsed light (DPL), are preferred because of their high efficiency in exciting photosensitive drugs. High-frequency pulsed light and 630-nm semiconductor lasers can also be utilized, with the latter offering deeper penetration but increasing the risk of scar formation after dermal penetration. Studies by Gu Ying's team showed that continuous 532-nm laser PDT was more effective than pulsed 532-nm laser PDT in treating PWS with the same wavelength [13]. Recently, 532-nm LED machines have replaced earlier light sources because of their small size, face mask design, continuous treatment, stable energy, long lifespan, and low cost, making them the preferred light source for HMME-PDT treatment of PWS in clinical practice [14].

Mechanism of HMME-PDT The mechanism of HMME-PDT in treating PWS involves the photosensitizer reaching a concentration peak in the blood immediately after intravenous injection, where it is rapidly absorbed by vascular endothelial cells, while minimal absorption occurs in epidermal cells. This results in a significant concentration difference between vascular endothelial cells and epidermal cells. A specific wavelength of laser light, which penetrates the surface and is selectively absorbed by endothelial cells, is then applied. This causes the photosensitizer to generate reactive oxygen species, such as singlet oxygen, which selectively disrupts the dilated capillary network in the affected area. Importantly, the normal epidermis remains undamaged due to the lack of photosensitizers, and the deeper dermal tissue beneath the abnormal capillary network is protected by shallow laser penetration, preventing effective stimulation of the deeper layers [15, 16].

Clinical Applications of HMME-PDT In 1991, Gu Ying's team first applied PDT to treat PWS in China, achieving significant clinical efficacy, particularly for large and deep skin lesions [17]. Sun Peihong et al. evaluated the safety and tolerability of a single intravenous constant velocity injection of HMME in healthy Chinese subjects, as well as single-dose pharmacokinetic trials during phase I clinical testing, laying the foundation for the medication regimen in phase II trials. The results showed that HMME is safe and well tolerated at doses ranging from 2.5 mg/kg to 10 mg/kg. Following intravenous injection, HMME is rapidly cleared from the blood with a short half-life, demonstrating high safety, a brief light avoidance period, ease of care, and shorter intervals between treatments. These characteristics improve both patient compliance and the efficiency of clinical use [12].

In a 2011 prospective clinical trial investigating the optimal protocol, 5 mg/kg HMME was used as a photosensitizer, followed by 532-nm frequency-doubling Nd:YAG laser treatment for PWS. To balance efficacy and safety, a treatment protocol involving 10 min after intravenous HMME injection followed by 20 min of laser irradiation is recommended [18]. In 2016, Zhao et al. conducted a randomized, double-blind, placebo-controlled phase III clinical trial with an optimized regimen of 5 mg/kg HMME and 532-nm light source irradiation for 20 min in 440 adolescent and adult patients (aged 14–65) at eight clinical centers across China. The results demonstrated that the HMME-PDT is an effective and safe treatment for PWS, with high satisfaction among both doctors and patients [19]. In 2018, Gan Liqiang et al. treated 82 children aged 1–14 years with PWS via the HMME-PDT. Patients received 5 mg/kg HMME intravenously, followed by skin lesion irradiation with 532-nm LED green light at a power density of 80–85 mW/cm^2 for 20–25 min. After two rounds of treatment, all 82 patients showed varying degrees of improvement, suggesting that HMME-PDT is a safe and effective method for treating PWS in children [20]. Additionally, combining PDT with laser therapy may complement each other and improve therapeutic outcomes [21]. However, the authors acknowledged the challenges of achieving complete fairness in comparing these methods owing to differing operational approaches and variable factors, highlighting the need for further research with larger sample sizes and more in-depth comparative analyses.

Moreover, it is important to emphasize the need for noninvasive, efficient, and accurate efficacy evaluation methods in clinical practice, as current methods rely primarily on subjective naked-eye observation. While pathological biopsy remains the gold standard, its invasive nature makes routine implementation difficult. Consequently, noninvasive diagnostic techniques offer significant advantages and potential for broader application in the evaluation of PWS treatment efficacy.

The authors' group has attempted and explored the application of HMME-PDT for PWS (Figs. 13.2 and 13.3) and noninvasive diagnostic techniques in PWS detection, such as the VISIA-CRTM skin analysis system, dermatoscopy, laser speckle contrast imaging (LSCI), and ultrahigh frequency skin ultrasound (HFUS), to observe the morphology, quantity, depth, and blood flow perfusion changes in blood vessels [22]. The VISIA-CR™ skin analyzer can collect images according to standards and accurately analyze the resolution of erythema through the erythema index (Fig. 13.4). Dermatoscopy can assist in the clinical classification of PWS and detect the degree of vascular damage in the skin lesion area after treatment, guiding the adjustment of the treatment dose and the selection of the final treatment endpoint, which is highly important for effi-

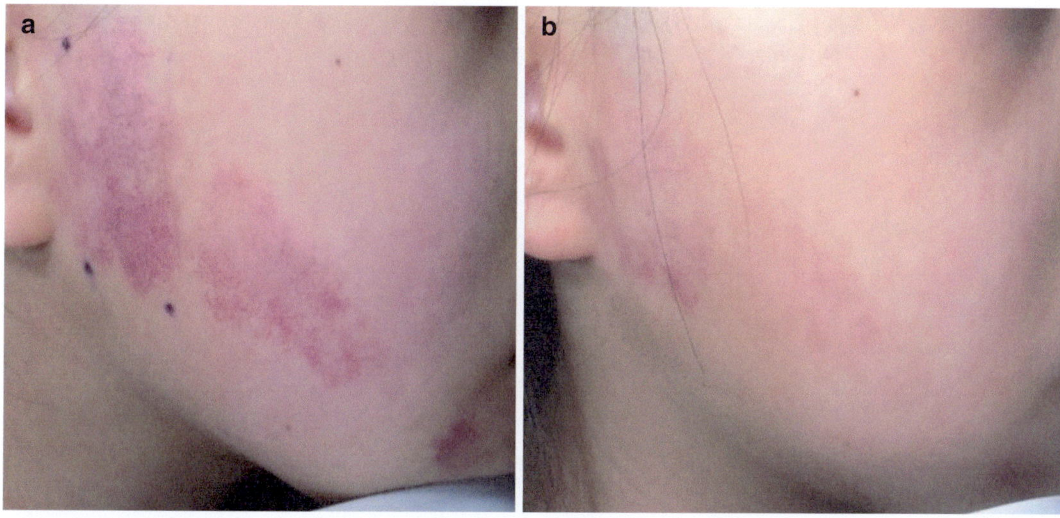

Fig. 13.2 HMME-PDT treatment for pediatric PWS. (**a**) irregular patchy erythematous lesions on the right cheek before treatment. (**b**) a significant reduction in erythematous lesions on the right cheek 1 month after two treatments

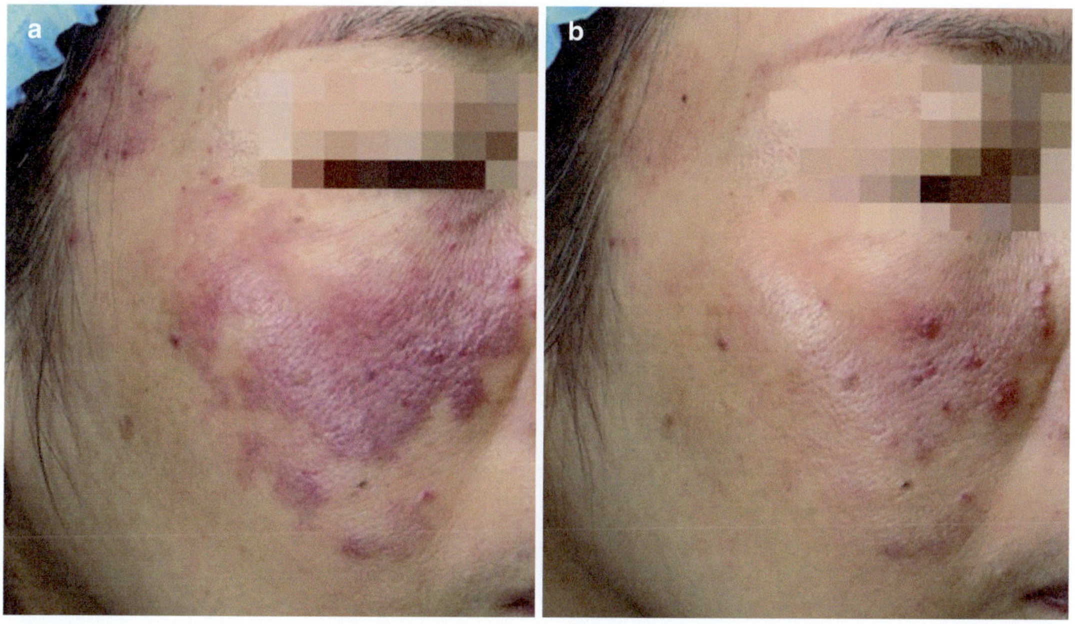

Fig. 13.3 HMME-PDT treatment for adult PWS. (**a**) Before treatment, irregular patchy violaceous lesions with localized nodular hyperplasia were visible on the right cheek. (**b**) One month after two treatments, a significant reduction in erythematous lesions on the right cheek was observed, with some residual nodules

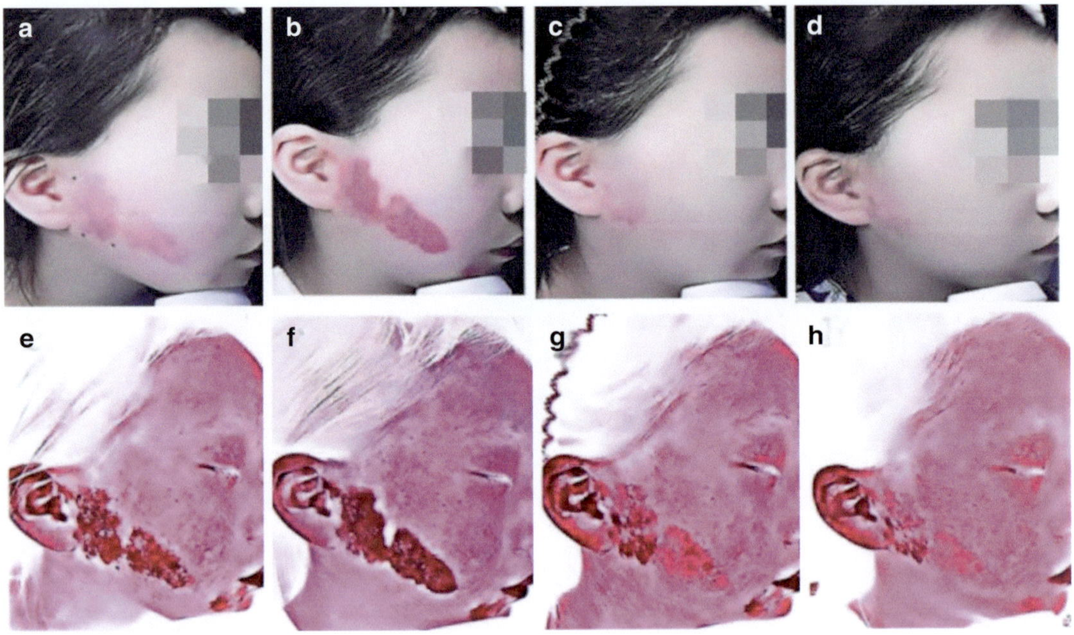

Fig. 13.4 Application of the VISIA-CRTM skin analysis system in HMME-PDT for PWS. (**a**–**d**) Standard images display changes in lesion color before and after HMME-PDT treatment. (**e**–**h**) RBX-red images reveal heightened and densely distributed blood vessels in the lesion area that gradually fade after treatment

cacy evaluation (Fig. 13.5). HFUS and LSCI aid in evaluating therapeutic effects by detecting changes in skin thickness and blood flow perfusion before and after treatment. In addition, the authors' group has successfully built the latest photoacoustic imaging system, which combines optical and ultrasound imaging, provides higher spatial resolution and deeper tissue imaging, allowing for the detection of various tissue components, such as collagen, fat, blood vessels, hemoglobin, and melanin. A new quantitative evaluation biomarker, the PWS level, which is based on average photoacoustic signal intensity, has been proposed to assess lesion severity and treatment improvement. Compared with conventional noninvasive diagnostics, this method offers a more quantitative and accurate approach and can assist in PWS classification and the evaluation of therapeutic outcomes [23]. Research published in authoritative dermatology journals shows the potential of noninvasive technologies for assessing the efficacy of HMME-PDT for PWS, although further exploration and refinement are still needed (see Chap. 16 for details).

Treatment Steps of HMME-PDT First, ensure that only the target skin area is exposed to the treatment, protecting the surrounding normal skin. The distance from the skin lesion varies depending on the treatment device. For example, with a 532-nm LED device, the treatment spot is typically 10 × 10 cm (with slight variations depending on the device). The treatment head should be positioned approximately 10 cm from the lesion, perpendicular to the skin. For larger areas, treatment should be conducted in stages, typically starting from the sides and then at the center. Second, the dosage of HMME was calculated on the basis of body weight (5 mg/kg), and a fresh 50-mL solution was prepared with physiological saline. A larger vein, such as the antecubital vein, is selected for intravenous injection. After the vein was successfully punctured, the channel was rinsed with saline before the photosensitizer was slowly administered at 2.5 mL/min over a 20-min infusion via an injection pump. After the injection, the channel was rinsed with saline to ensure that the drug fully entered the bloodstream. During this process, direct exposure to strong

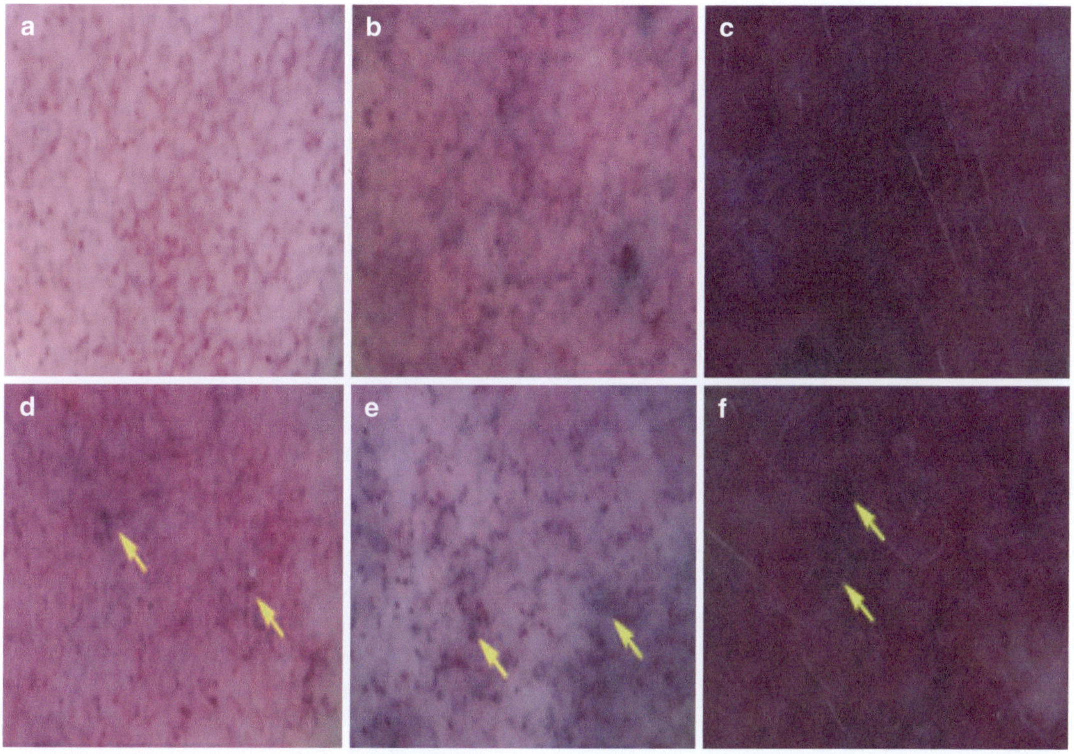

Fig. 13.5 Application of dermatoscopy in HMME-PDT diagnosis and treatment of PWS. (**a**) The pink type shows irregular dot-like and linear vessels on a bright red background. (**b**) Violaceous type presents as densely distributed globular and thick linear vessels on a dark red background. (**c**) Hypertrophic type is characterized by cluster-like vessels on a dark red background. (**d–f**) After HMME-PDT treatment, signs of vascular rupture (yellow arrows) are observed in the lesion area

light is avoided. Third, illumination begins 10 min after the intravenous infusion starts, with the treatment parameters adjusted on the machine. The illumination power is typically set between 80 mW/cm^2 and 100 mW/cm^2, with the illumination energy ranging from 96 J/cm^2 to 115 J/cm^2.

Precautions of HMME-PDT HMME-PDT are suitable for treating all types of PWS, particularly large lesions over 5 cm in diameter, as well as cases in which previous treatments failed. However, it is important to exclude patients with certain conditions. Contraindications include allergic reactions, scar-prone skin, and photosensitive diseases such as porphyria, photosensitivity, or porphyrin allergy. Patients allergic to any component of HMME drugs, those who are pregnant, who are breastfeeding, or who are trying to conceive during the treatment period should also be excluded.

During HMME-PDT treatment, several precautions are crucial. Local drug leakage during administration should be avoided; if leakage occurs, the infusion should be stopped immediately, a cold compress should be applied, and the affected area should be completely shaded from light until the swelling resolves. Protect perilesional normal skin by covering it with a light-blocking cloth before illumination to avoid unnecessary exposure. To prevent scarring, local reactions should be monitored closely during treatment to avoid blisters caused by excessive light energy. The treatment endpoint is determined by the reaction type of the erythema area (detailed below), which serves as a key indicator of photosensitive damage to the abnormal vascular network, aiding in determining the optimal irradiation time and ensuring a safe and effective outcome.

After treatment, a cold compress was applied immediately after light exposure and intermittently for 3 days to reduce swelling. For redness, swelling, and erosion, topical antibiotic ointment was used. If a scab forms, avoid forced removal and potential scar formation. Additionally, patients should avoid direct sunlight for 2 weeks posttreatment to ensure optimal healing and prevent complications.

Common erythema reactions immediately after HMME-PDT include the following: (1) Fading type, where the treatment area becomes lighter or even clears, (2) dark purple with black spots characterized by a noticeable dark purple color and small black spots in the treatment area, (3) obvious dark purple type, where the treatment area shows a distinct dark purple color, and and (4) slightly dark type, where the area appears slightly darker. The relationships between these erythema reaction types and lesion classification, treatment frequency, and treatment efficacy remain unclear and warrant further investigation.

Adverse Reactions and Management of HMME-PDT Adverse reactions to HMME-PDT for PWS are categorized into systemic and local reactions. Systemic reactions may include abnormal hepatobiliary function (elevated transaminases and bilirubin), gastrointestinal disturbances (nausea, vomiting), cardiovascular issues (sinus arrhythmias, conduction disorders, nonspecific ECG abnormalities), respiratory symptoms (shortness of breath), ocular conditions (conjunctivitis, dry eye), hematologic abnormalities (elevated white blood cells), neurological effects (dizziness), and urinary abnormalities (hematuria, proteinuria). No serious adverse events were reported. Local reactions primarily involve pain, burning, itching, swelling, blisters, purpura, and scabbing. Most reactions are mild to moderate, transient, and self-resolving without special treatment. For further details, refer to Chap. 15, Sect. 15.3.

Recommended Protocols There are some recommended protocols including key treatment parameters for HMME-PDT in the treatment of port wine stains, which can be seen in Table 13.1.

- Appropriate patient age: Unlimited.
- Appropriate lesion sites: There are no special restrictions on PWS lesion sites, but precautions should be taken when treating special sites, such as the eyes, mouth, nose, and ears.
- Appropriate lesion types: HMME-PDT is suitable for all types of PWS, especially for large lesions (diameter > 5 cm) or patients who have failed previous treatment.
- Treatment interval: Every 2 months.
- Frequency: Depending on lesion size and therapeutic effect.
- Efficacy evaluation: Depending on the clinical observation. Noninvasive diagnostic techniques such as dermatoscopy and skin ultrasound can also be used to assist in the evaluation of clinical efficacy.
- Endpoint assessment: Based on the treatment response in the erythema area.

13.1.3 Conclusions

HMME-PDT offers a promising new treatment option for PWS, providing hope for patients. However, its treatment protocols and light source selection require further refinement and optimi-

Table 13.1 Recommended protocols for HMME-PDT in the treatment of port wine strains

	HMME				Dose of light	
Pretreatment	HMME formulation	HMME concentration	Medication time	Light source	Power density	Energy density
Expose skin lesions Protect surrounding normal skin	Solution	5 mg/mL	10 min	532 nm laser/ LED light	80–100 mW/ cm^2	96–115 J/ cm^2

zation. Additionally, exploring the potential benefits of combining HMME-PDT with other therapeutic methods could help enhance its overall efficacy.

13.2 HMME-PDT for the Treatment of Other Vascular Skin Diseases

13.2.1 Arteriovenous Malformations and Venous Malformations

Arteriovenous malformations (AVMs) and venous malformations (VMs) account for two-thirds of systemic vascular malformations [24]. They have traditionally been treated through surgical resection, endovascular therapy, or a combination of AVMs and surgical resection, sclerotherapy, laser therapy, or combination therapy for VMs [24]. While research on AVMs and VMs has been limited, the advancement and application of PDT in treating PWS highlight its potential applicability for these vascular malformation lesions as well [25].

In 2009, Waseem Jerjes et al. utilized optical fiber-mediated interstitial photodynamic therapy (iPDT) to treat 23 patients with various head and facial vascular abnormalities, including VMs, hemangiomas, lymphoid malformations, neurofibromas, rhabdomyosarcoma, basal cell carcinoma, and squamous cell carcinoma. Using timopofen as a photosensitizer at a concentration of 0.15 mg/kg, patients received intravenous injections followed by semiconductor laser irradiation via fiber optics at a wavelength of 652 nm and an energy density of 20 J/cm^2, guided by ultrasound imaging 96 h later. Each patient underwent 1–10 treatments on the basis of their condition, and a significant decrease in lesion size (50–80%) was observed in patients with VMs, hemangiomas, lymphoid malformations, and neurofibromas after 6 weeks, demonstrating satisfactory efficacy [26]. In 2011, Waseem Jerjes et al. used iPDT to treat 43 patients with head and neck vascular abnormalities, including hemangiomas, VMs, lymphatic malformations, and AVMs, with tetrahydroxychlorophenol used as a photosensitizer under similar conditions. Imaging showed significant efficacy in 34.9% and moderate efficacy in 25.6% of patients after 6 weeks, with lymphatic malformations responding best, followed by AVMs [27]. The team highlighted the advantages of ultrasound-guided PDT in accurately targeting tissues, protecting vital organs, and minimizing adverse reactions.

13.2.2 Infantile Hemangioma

Infantile hemangioma (IH) is the most common vascular and soft tissue tumor in infants and young children and is more common in the head and neck. IH exhibits unique growth cycles, including a proliferation period (0–1 year old), a regression period (1–5 years old), and a regression completion period (5–10 years old). Traditional treatment methods for IH include drug therapy (propranolol, etc.), laser therapy, vascular embolization, sclerotherapy injection, and surgical intervention [28]. Pulse dye lasers (PDLs) are currently the primary method for treating superficial IHs. While there have been few reports on the use of PDT for treating IHs in the past, recent studies have shown promising clinical efficacy, indicating its potential as a viable treatment option.

Waseem Jerjes et al. demonstrated the efficacy of iPDT in treating head and facial vascular abnormalities, including deep IH patients, highlighting the potential of PDT in managing these conditions [26]. In another study, Jaehoon Choi et al. transplanted IH specimens into nude mice and applied PDT treatment 6–10 weeks post-transplantation via photoporphyrin as a photosensitizer (1 mg/mL, 5 mg/kg via tail vein injection). After 24 h, 630-nm semiconductor excitation light delivered through optical fibers (100 J/cm^2 energy density, 150 mW/cm^2 power density) significantly reduced the graft volume within 24 h of irradiation, primarily through endothelial cell apoptosis, establishing a mechanism for early-stage destruction of hemangioma [29].

13.2.3 Kaposi's Sarcoma

Kaposi's sarcoma (KS), also known as multiple idiopathic hemorrhagic sarcoma, is a rare malignant tumor characterized by spindle cell proliferation and angiomatous structures that affect the skin, blood vessels, and potentially internal organs. It presents as purple nodular skin lesions and can progress from localized skin involvement to widespread lesions in the skin, oral cavity, lymph nodes, and internal organs [30]. Traditional treatments for KS include surgery, physical therapy, cytotoxic drug injections, sclerosing agents, interferon therapy, chemotherapy, antiangiogenic medications, retinoic acid, and radiotherapy, all of which have certain adverse effects [31]. PDT offers a promising approach for treating KS by targeting tumor cells and human herpesvirus-8 (HHV-8), which is implicated in KS pathogenesis. PDT not only kills HHV-8-infected cells but also activates local immune responses, increasing the number of CD8+ T cells, whose cytotoxic activity helps eliminate HHV-8-infected cells, thereby providing therapeutic benefits for KS [32].

Min Young Park et al. treated a case of classic Kaposi's sarcoma in a 70-year-old male patient via PDT. The patient, who tested negative for HIV, had a purple–red skin lesion on his left foot, with cytological staining showing positive results for human herpesvirus-8 (HHV-8) and CD31. A 20% ALA solution was prepared as the photosensitizer and injected into each lesion at a dose of 0.3 mL/cm^2. The lesions were irradiated with red light at an energy density of 100 J/cm^2 and a power density of 100 mW/cm^2. Treatment was performed every 2 weeks, for a total of two sessions. The lesions were significantly reduced with minimal pigmentation, and no recurrence was noted after a 6-month follow-up [30]. In another case, Tardivo et al. used PDT to treat AIDS-related Kaposi's sarcoma in a patient who had not responded to several rounds of chemotherapy. Methylene blue and toluidine blue were used as photosensitizers at a concentration of 2% and were injected into the skin lesions until they turned dark blue. The lesions were irradiated with light at a wavelength of 600–750 nm, with an energy density of 18 J/cm^2 and a power density of 100 mW/cm^2. After weekly treatment for 4 months, followed by biweekly treatment for another 6 months, the skin lesions significantly improved [33].

13.2.4 Vascular Sarcoma

Angiosarcoma (AS), also known as malignant angioendothelioma, is a rare and highly malignant skin soft tissue tumor that originates from endothelial cells in blood vessels or lymphatic vessels. Its clinical manifestations lack distinct characteristics, and it can be classified into nodular, ulcerative, and diffuse types. Some lesions resemble pedunculated hemangiomas, whereas others are large, diffuse, and infiltrative skin lesions that may present as skin-colored, grayish-black, or purplish-blue nodules or plaques with a soft texture. These lesions can lead to ulcers and bleeding [34]. Traditional treatment primarily involves surgery, often combined with radiotherapy and chemotherapy; however, complete removal is challenging, and the recurrence rate remains high [35].

In 2007, Thong et al. conducted PDT on a 64-year-old male patient with head and neck angiosarcoma and distant metastasis. The photosensitizer Fotolon was intravenously injected at doses ranging from 2.0 mg/kg to 5.7 mg/kg for 10–20 min. After 3 h, the patient was irradiated with 665-nm wavelength light at a power density of 80–150 mW/cm^2 and an energy density of 65–200 J/cm^2. The patient received approximately four treatments, with mild pain during the sessions and no complications. After 10 months, new skin lesions appeared on both upper limbs. PDT was applied again to the right upper limb, and interestingly, untreated tumors in the same area improved after 2 months, whereas lesions in the left upper limb spontaneously improved after 4 months. Pathological examination of the left upper limb revealed infiltration of CD8+ and CD4+ T lymphocytes, indicating the immune effect of PDT in treating angiosarcoma, which plays a crucial role in preventing recurrence [36]. In 2017, Yang Gao treated an 81-year-old male patient with epithelioid angiosarcoma located in the left medial corner of the eye. The patient underwent surgical resection followed by ALA-PDT, which involved the use of 10% ALA cream and laser irradiation at a wavelength of 635 nm, a power density of 200 mW/cm^2, and an energy density of 120 J/cm^2. The PDT was repeated three times over 3 weeks. One year later, the patient experienced no recurrence or significant adverse reactions and was satisfied with the outcome [32]. For facial angiosarcoma, which is challenging to resect fully and prone to recurrence, combining surgical resection with PDT is a promising treatment option [37].

13.2.5 Conclusions

In summary, PDT is an effective treatment for skin vascular diseases, offering advantages such as repeatability, noninvasiveness, high selectivity, and fewer side effects. It is emerging as a promising option for treating vascular malformations and hemangiomas. Compared with traditional therapies, PDT has superior selectivity, making it particularly suitable for large-area PWS. Its benefits, including reduced treatment frequency and low recurrence rates, have contributed to its growing preference in PWS management. However, further clinical observations are needed to optimize treatment protocols, particularly the selection of treatment parameters such as the light source, photosensitizer, and irradiation dose. Additionally, research into new PSs and light sources is essential for continued advancements in this field.

There is limited research on the use of PDT for treating IH, AVMs, and VMs. However, clinical studies indicate that PDT can be an effective treatment option for these conditions, particularly when traditional therapies such as medication or surgery are not suitable or have proven ineffective. iPDT offers innovative solutions for deep vascular lesions, presenting a potential alternative. Nonetheless, extensive clinical research is needed to establish a solid theoretical foundation and refine treatment strategies for IH, AVMs, and VMs, including the optimization of photosensitizers, light sources, and treatment methods. For Kaposi's sarcoma, PDT has shown promising results, although pretreatment, such as CO_2 laser use to enhance photosensitizer penetration in thicker lesions, should be considered. While the clinical outcomes are encouraging, the lack of standardized and individualized treatment parameters, including the photosensitizer concentration, irradiation dose, and number of treatment cycles, requires further investigation to improve clinical decision-making.

References

1. Arumugam Venkatachalam Sargurunathan E, Gowda Venkatesha RR, et al. Port-wine stains and intraoral hemangiomas: a case series. Cureus. 2024;16(6):e63532.
2. Urban MJ, Williams EF. Vascular lesions. Facial Plast Surg Clin North Am. 2024;32(1):13–25.
3. Updyke KM, Khachemoune A. Port-wine stains: a focused review on their management. J Drugs Dermatol. 2017;16(11):1145–51.
4. Jiang F, Shao J, Chen L, et al. Influence of port-wine stains on quality of life of children and their parents. Acta Derm Venereol. 2021;101(8):adv00516.
5. Yu W, Zhu J, Gu Y, et al. Port-wine stains on the neck respond better to a pulsed dye laser than lesions on the face: an intrapatient comparison study with histopathology. J Am Acad Dermatol. 2019;80(3):779–81.
6. Goldberg DJ. Treatment of port wine stains. J Cosmet Laser Ther. 2010;12(1):1.
7. Wei ML, Zhang HY, Wang PR, et al. A study on the effects of 532 nm continuous laser combined with photodynamic therapy versus 595 nm pulsed dye laser on a chicken comb model of vascular malformation. Photon Lasers Med. 2016;5(3):15.
8. Gao K, Huang Z, Yuan KH, et al. Side-by-side comparison of photodynamic therapy and pulsed-dye laser treatment of port-wine stain birthmarks. Br J Dermatol. 2013;168(5):1040–6.
9. Wlotzke U, Hohenleutner U, Abd-El-Raheem TA, et al. Side-effects and complications of flashlamp-pumped pulsed dye laser therapy of port-wine stains. A prospective study. Br J Dermatol. 1996;134(3):475–80.
10. Wang B, Mei X, Wang Y, et al. Adjuncts to pulsed dye laser for treatment of port wine stains: a literature review. J Cosmet Laser Ther. 2021;23(7–8):209–17.
11. Faurschou A, Olesen AB, Leonardi-Bee J, et al. Lasers or light sources for treating port-wine stains. Cochrane Database Syst Rev. 2011;11:Cd007152.
12. Sun PH, Zhao X, Zhou Y, et al. Tolerance and pharmacokinetics of single-dose intravenous hemoporfin in healthy volunteers. Acta Pharmacol Sin. 2011;32(12):1549–54.

13. Yuzhi W, Zheng H, Kaihua Y. Clinical comparative study of KTP laser and novel LED light source for photodynamic therapy of fresh red nevus. J Pract Med. 2015;31(24):4.
14. Ying G, Fanguang L, Kai W, et al. Clinical analysis of 1216 cases of red wine stains treated with photodynamic therapy. Chin J Laser Med. 2001;10(2):86–9.
15. Mei Y, Xiao X, Fan L, et al. In vitro photodynamic therapy of endothelial cells using hematoporphyrin monomethyl ether (Hemoporfin): relevance to treatment of port wine stains. Photodiagn Photodyn Ther. 2019;27:268–75.
16. Zhang Q, Li ZH, Li YY, et al. Hypericin-photodynamic therapy induces human umbilical vein endothelial cell apoptosis. Sci Rep. 2015;5:18398.
17. Ying G, Junheng L, Yiping J, et al. Mechanism exploration of photodynamic therapy for selective treatment of port wine stains. Chin J Laser Med. 1992;1(3):5.
18. Zhao Y, Zhou Z, Zhou G, et al. Efficacy and safety of hemoporfin in photodynamic therapy for port-wine stain: a multicenter and open-labeled phase IIa study. Photodermatol Photoimmunol Photomed. 2011;27(1):17–23.
19. Zhao Y, Tu P, Zhou G, et al. Hemoporfin photodynamic therapy for port-wine stain: a randomized controlled trial. PLoS One. 2016;11(5):e0156219.
20. Li-Qiang G, Hua W, Si-Li N, et al. A clinical study of HMME-PDT therapy in Chinese pediatric patients with port-wine stain. Photodiagn Photodyn Ther. 2018;23:102–5.
21. Kelly KM, Kimel S, Smith T, et al. Combined photodynamic and photothermal induced injury enhances damage to in vivo model blood vessels[J]. Lasers Surg Med. 2004;34(5):407–13.
22. Wen L, Zhang Y, Zhang L, et al. Application of different noninvasive diagnostic techniques used in HMME-PDT in the treatment of port wine stains. Photodiagn Photodyn Ther. 2019;25:369–75.
23. Zhang H, Zhang G, Zhang Y, et al. Quantitatively assessing port-wine stains using a photoacoustic imaging method: a pilot study. J Am Acad Dermatol. 2021;85(6):1613–6.
24. AlShamekh S. Arteriovenous malformations. Dermatol Clin. 2022;40(4):445–8.
25. Patel AM, Chou EL, Findeiss L, et al. The horizon for treating cutaneous vascular lesions. Semin Cutan Med Surg. 2012;31(2):98–104.
26. Jerjes W, Upile T, Vincent A, et al. Management of deep-seated malformations with photodynamic therapy: a new guiding imaging modality. Lasers Med Sci. 2009;24(5):769–75.
27. Jerjes W, Upile T, Hamdoon Z, et al. Interstitial PDT for vascular anomalies. Lasers Surg Med. 2011;43(5):357–65.
28. Höger PH, Hamm H. Infantile hemangioma: clinical manifestation, treatment, and differential diagnoses. Dermatologie. 2023;74(5):331–9.
29. Choi J, Kim WJ, Park SW, et al. Photodynamic therapy suppresses tumor growth in an in vivo model of human hemangioma. Arch Dermatol Res. 2014;306(1):81–91.
30. Park MY, Kim YC. Classic Kaposi sarcoma treated with intralesional 5-aminolevulinic acid injection photodynamic therapy. Arch Dermatol. 2009;145(10):1200–2.
31. Schneider JW, Dittmer DP. Diagnosis and treatment of kaposi sarcoma. Am J Clin Dermatol. 2017;18(4):529–39.
32. Iftode N, Rădulescu MA, Aramă ȘS, et al. Update on Kaposi sarcoma-associated herpesvirus (KSHV or HHV8) - review. Rom J Intern Med. 2020;58(4):199–208.
33. Tardivo JP, Del Giglio A, Paschoal LH, et al. New photodynamic therapy protocol to treat AIDS-related Kaposi's sarcoma. Photomed Laser Surg. 2006;24(4):528–31.
34. Young RJ, Brown NJ, Reed MW, et al. Angiosarcoma. Lancet Oncol. 2010;11(10):983–91.
35. Sturm EC, Marasco IS, Katz SC. Multidisciplinary management of angiosarcoma - a review. J Surg Res. 2021;257:213–20.
36. Thong PS, Ong KW, Goh NS, et al. Photodynamic-therapy-activated immune response against distant untreated tumors in recurrent angiosarcoma. Lancet Oncol. 2007;8(10):950–2.
37. Gao Y, Wang WS, Wang HL, et al. Treatment of epithelioid angiosarcoma with topical ALA-PDT in the course of surgery. Photodiagn Photodyn Ther. 2017;19:153–5.

14 Application of Photosensitizer-Mediated Fluorescence Diagnosis

Peiru Wang, Chunxiao Li, Hongwei Wang, Bo Wang, and Xiuli Wang

14.1 Introduction

Photosensitizer-mediated fluorescence diagnosis, also known as photodynamic diagnosis (PDD), is part of fluorescence diagnosis, alongside autofluorescence detection, which uses intrinsic tissue fluorescence to assess variations. PDD is a noninvasive method that employs fluorescence emitted by photosensitizers during de-excitation for disease diagnosis. After the administration of photosensitizers systemically or locally, specific light wavelengths illuminate the tissue, exciting the photosensitizer and causing the targeted tissues to emit diagnostic fluorescence signals [1, 2]. This emerging technology offers ease of operation, high sensitivity, and real-time monitoring, making it a promising diagnostic tool for certain skin diseases.

14.1.1 Development History

The development of PDD began in the early twentieth century. In 1924, Lam first reported the fluorescent localization effect of porphyrins in malignant tumors, which was initially misinterpreted as an infection-induced phenomenon [3]. In 1942, Auler and Figge reported that hematoporphyrin (Hp) preferentially accumulated in tumors when it was injected into rats [4, 5]. In 1948, *H. pylori* was reported to accumulate in tumor, embryonic, and wound tissues, suggesting the use of photosensitizer fluorescence for tumor diagnosis [6]. In 1951, Manganiello reported that porphyrin compounds could also accumulate in wounds, lymph nodes, and placenta [7]. In 1953, Peck reported that metal porphyrin compounds were localized in tumors and noted that Hp did not accumulate at lower doses (<120 mg/person) [8]. In 1955, Rassmussen-Taxdal reported orange–red fluorescence in the tumor tissues of 8 out of 11 patients injected with 500–1000 mg of Hp, aiding in diagnosis and surgical guidance [9]. These findings indicate that porphyrins easily accumulate at tumor sites and emit fluorescence, which is beneficial for tumor diagnosis and

P. Wang · C. Li · X. Wang
Institute of Photomedicine, Shanghai Skin Disease Hospital, School of Medicine, Tongji University, Shanghai, China
e-mail: wangxiuli_1400023@tongji.edu.cn

H. Wang (✉)
Department of Dermatology, Huadong Hospital, Fudan University, Shanghai, People's Republic of China

B. Wang
Avera Medical Group Dermatology, Aberdeen, SD, USA

University of South Dakota, Vermillion, SD, USA
e-mail: makiwang@med.umich.edu

X. Wang, B. Wang (eds.), *Photodynamic Therapy in Dermatology*,
https://doi.org/10.1007/978-981-96-8915-6_14

"visual" guidance for tumor resection. A breakthrough came in 1959 when Lipson from the Mayo Clinic demonstrated that hematoporphyrin derivatives had superior tumor fluorescence localization characteristics, with clinical studies reporting diagnostic accuracies of over 80% in bronchial and esophageal cancers. This marked the introduction of the concept of "fluorescence endoscopy diagnosis" [10]. In 1968, Gregorie documented PDD in 226 tumor patients, achieving a positive concordance rate of 76.3% for malignant tumors on the basis of characteristic orange–red fluorescence in 132 of 173 cases [11].

In 1990, Kennedy first proposed the use of ALA-induced protoporphyrin IX (PpIX) fluorescence imaging for diagnosing oral mucosal cancer and precancerous lesions [12]. PDD has since been applied in the diagnosis of various skin diseases, treatment evaluation, and posttreatment follow-up. In 1996, Professors Shizheng Xu and Xiuli Wang pioneered ALA-PDT for treating skin tumors in China, and in 1997, Professor Wang began exploring ALA-PDT for treating condyloma acuminatum, conducting fluorescence kinetic studies and officially introducing ALA-PDD in China. In 2004, the authors' group internationally reported the effectiveness and safety of ALA-PDT for condyloma acuminatum [13]. A 2007 study on ALA conversion to PpIX in the treatment of condyloma acuminatum revealed significant fluorescence in the epidermis but not in the dermis, confirming that ALA-PDT primarily affects epidermal tissue without causing scarring [14]. In 2005, the authors' team used ALA-PDT to treat follicular sebaceous gland-related diseases, particularly severe acne, marking a breakthrough in the treatment of refractory conditions [15, 16]. This result drew clinical attention, as previous fluorescence kinetic studies had shown fluorescence only in the epidermis, with no fluorescence in the dermis where the nodular and cystic lesions in patients with moderate-to-severe acne involve mainly pathological changes. It was speculated that ALA might accumulate in the hair follicle sebaceous gland via the pilosebaceous duct. In 2011, this team conducted PDD research on acne patients via fluorescence microscopy for the first time, confirming that ALA accumulates in the hair follicle sebaceous gland via the pilosebaceous duct, making the hair follicle sebaceous gland the direct target of ALA-PDT for the treatment of severe acne [17]. The authors' group also applied ALA-PDD to fungal infections such as tinea cruris and tinea corporis, providing evidence supporting the use of ALA-PDT in the treatment of fungal infections. In 2019, they extended their research to apply HpD-PDD in HpD-PDT for the treatment of skin tumors [18].

14.1.2 Mechanism of Action

In PDD, photosensitizers are administered to tumor or proliferating tissues and incubated for a specific duration, allowing fluorescent substances to accumulate within tumors or hyperactive cells. When the lesions are illuminated with light of an appropriate wavelength, the fluorescent substances absorb the energy of the excitation light, transitioning to an unstable excited state. They then release energy through physical deexcitation, emit fluorescence, and return to a stable ground state (Fig. 14.1). The fluorescence emitted from tumors or hyperactive cells indicates the presence of skin lesions, aiding their identification through PDD.

The choice of photosensitizer is critical in PDD and directly influences diagnostic efficacy. The most commonly used locally applied photosensitizers are ALA and 5-aminolevulinic acid methyl ester (MAL), both precursors in porphyrin synthesis that promote PpIX production within cells. Studies have shown that ALA provides better tissue distribution homogeneity and is rapidly metabolized due to its small molecular size, minimizing accumulation, irritation, and toxicity, making it ideal for skin or mucosal applications. The brick-red fluorescence induced by PpIX is easily visible under Wood's lamp [4], a filtered ultraviolet lamp emitting 320–400 nm light that is commonly used for diagnosing skin pigmentary abnormalities and infections. This emission wavelength aligns with the excitation wavelengths of PpIX and HpD, allowing clear observation of fluorescence. Systemic photosen-

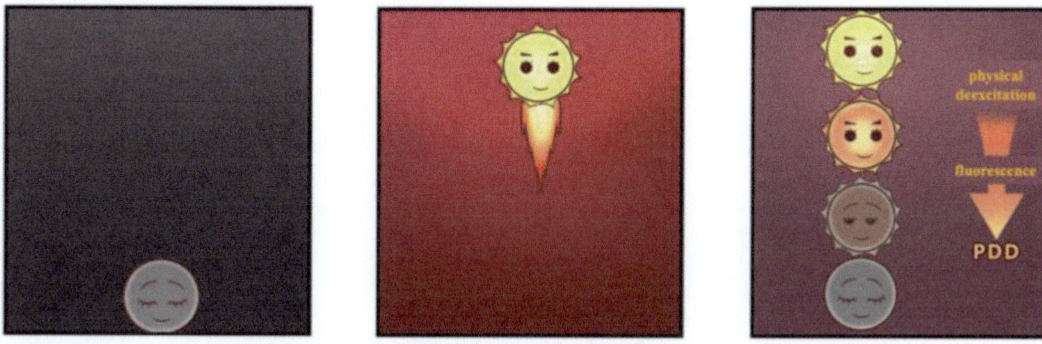

Fig. 14.1 The mechanism of PDD

sitizers such as HpD and HMME further broaden the scope of PDD.

14.2 The Application of PDD in Skin Diseases

In the field of dermatology, PDD is primarily used for the diagnosis and treatment of nonmelanoma skin cancers, HPV-related diseases, follicular/sebaceous gland-related disorders, and other skin conditions.

14.2.1 Application of the PDD in Skin Cancers

PDD is primarily employed for the diagnosis of nonmelanoma skin cancers, assessment of drug penetration and accumulation, determination of the margins of skin lesions prior to treatment, evaluation of treatment efficacy, and monitoring of patient prognosis.

14.2.1.1 Diagnosis of Nonmelanoma Skin Cancers

PDD is an effective tool for the diagnosis of nonmelanoma skin cancers, including actinic keratosis (AK) and its subclinical lesions, basal cell carcinoma (BCC), cutaneous squamous cell carcinoma (cSCC), Bowen's disease (BD), and extramammary Paget's disease (EMPD). During ALA-PDD, skin cancer lesions exhibit distinct brick-red fluorescence, which contrasts sharply with the nonfluorescent appearance of normal skin. This fluorescence contrast highlights clear lesion margins, aiding in the diagnosis. When combined with clinical findings, PDD enhances the accuracy of diagnosing skin tumors, showing high consistency with pathological examinations [19].

14.2.1.2 Evaluation of Drug Penetration and Accumulation

PDD enables the assessment of photosensitizer application in nonmelanoma skin tumors and precancers by comparing fluorescence intensity across varying conditions. Drug permeation was determined by evaluating fluorescence at different skin depths and time points after topical administration. In a study by the authors' group, PDD demonstrated that ALA penetration in AK lesions was greater following plum-blossom needling pretreatment than following CO_2 fractional laser pretreatment. The PpIX fluorescence within the skin lesions was stronger at 2 and 3 h after plum-blossom needling pretreatment, indicating greater diffusion of ALA in the superficial dermis. Plum-blossom needling pretreatment has proven cost-effective, making it more suitable for clinical application (Fig. 14.2) [20]. Another study on ALA-PDT for Bowen's disease revealed improved lesion clearance with plum-blossom needling pretreatment, as confirmed by enhanced ALA penetration through the PDD [21]. Additionally, in systemic PDT,

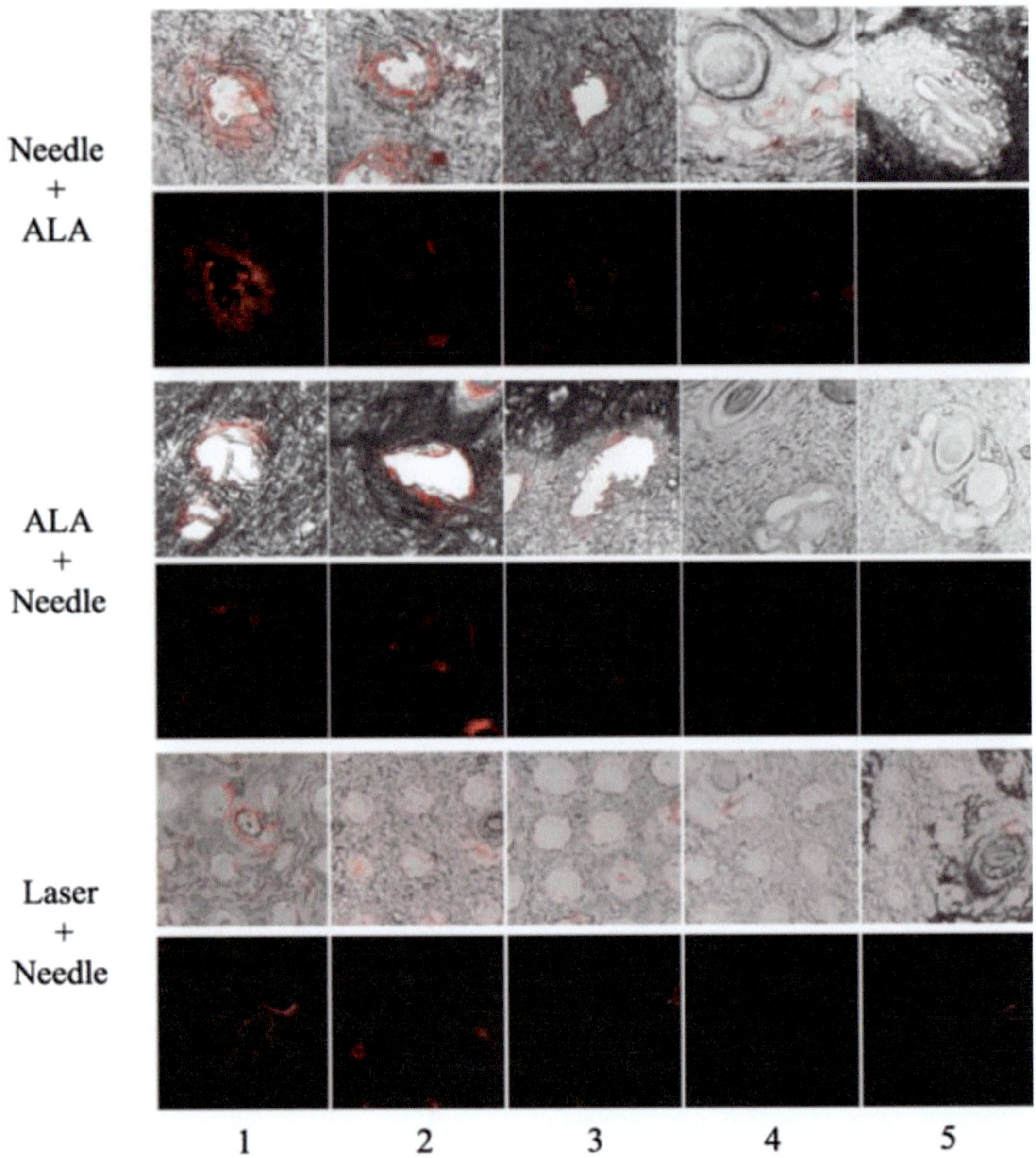

Fig. 14.2 PDD demonstrates the enhancement of ALA penetration by plum-blossom needling pretreatment during PDT for actinic keratosis (AK). Skin tissue sections and fluorescence images at five different depths before and after plum blossoming or CO_2 ablative fractional laser pretreatment following 180 min of ALA occlusion (Plum-Blossom Needling + ALA group, ALA + Plum-Blossom Needling group, Laser + Plum-Blossom Needling group). (1) 120 μm (±12 μm); (2) 500 μm (±48 μm); (3) 1000 μm (±48 μm); (4) 1500 μm (±48 μm); (5) 1800 μm (±48 μm)

fluorescence detection at various time points in lesions and surrounding areas aids in evaluating drug accumulation, optimizing treatment timing, and assessing drug metabolism post-PDT to ensure safety and guide postoperative light protection [18].

14.2.1.3 Definition of Lesion Margins

Determining Cancer Margins before Mohs Surgery

PDD has potential as a preoperative tool for Mohs micrographic surgery by measuring tumor size and accurately identifying lesion margins, helping to minimize surgical layers, reduce operating time, and improve efficiency [22]. For non-pigmented BCC, PDD-guided margin determination prior to Mohs surgery has demonstrated promising results in reducing surgical incision size. This precise localization enhances clearance rates, supports better wound healing, and decreases postoperative recurrence, making PDD a valuable adjunct in preoperative planning for skin lesion surgeries [23].

Defining Margins of Skin Lesions in PDT Treatment

In systemic PDT for nonmelanoma skin cancers, photosensitizers such as HpD accumulate within cancer tissues at 48–72 h after intravenous administration. By treating an area 1–2 cm beyond the visible lesion boundaries, PDT can target residual lesions and reduce the risk of recurrence (Fig. 14.3). Furthermore, PDD-enabled fluorescence diagnosis enhances the detection of occult, multiple, or residual lesions often missed by visual or conventional diagnostic methods. For example, the authors' group applied HpD-PDD to identify recurrent EMPD (Fig. 14.4), where brick-red fluorescence in Fig. 14.4f revealed a suspicious lesion undetected clinically or noninvasively. A subsequent biopsy

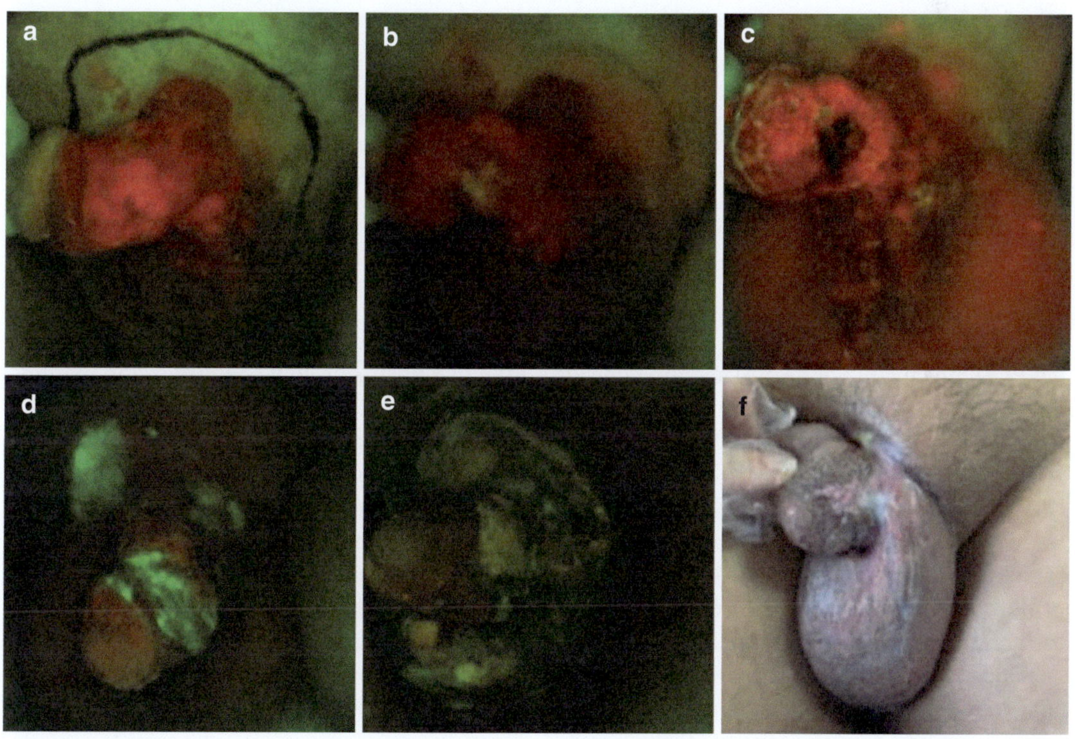

Fig. 14.3 PDD detection of the accumulation of the photosensitizer HpD in local skin lesions during HpD-PDT treatment. (**a–e**) Fluorescence images of the lesion under Wood's lamp at various time points after intravenous injection of HpD (5 mg/kg) in an EMPD patient: immediately after the first light treatment with HpD-PDT (the area 1–2 cm outside the skin lesion is demarcated with a black marker pen for photodynamic therapy), 48 h after HpD injection, 72 h after injection, 1 week after injection, and 4 weeks after injection. (**f**) Clinical photograph taken 3 months after HpD-PDT treatment in an EMPD patient showing complete clearance of the skin lesion

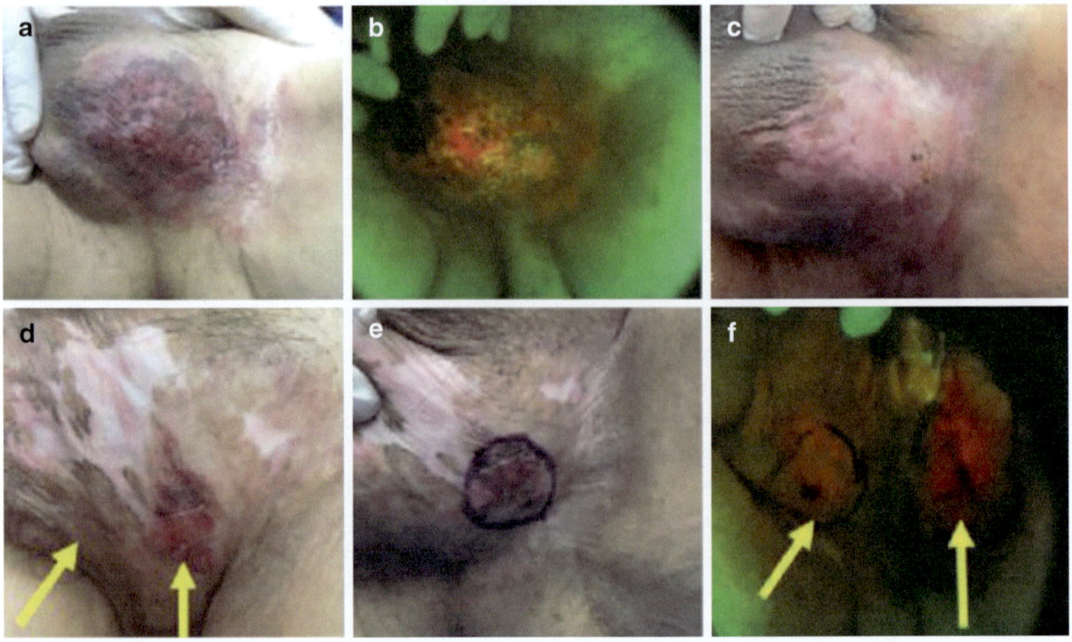

Fig. 14.4 PDD detection of recurrent skin lesions after EMPD treatment, revealing hidden lesions. (**a**) Clinical photo of a scrotal EMPD lesion, (**b**) fluorescence image 48 h after intravenous injection of HpD during HpD-PDT, indicating local drug accumulation, (**c**) follow-up visit 4 months after clearance of the skin lesion post-HpD-PDT, (**d**) suspected recurrent lesion found during a follow-up visit 11 months after HpD-PDT, (**e**) biopsy marking of the local skin lesion in the patient, and (**f**) HpD-PDD fluorescence diagnosis revealing a suspicious skin lesion that was not detected by the naked eye or noninvasive diagnosis, further biopsy indicating the presence of cancer cells

confirmed tumor cells at the site, demonstrating that PDD effectively improves detection rates for hidden and multiple nonmelanoma skin cancers [24].

14.2.1.4 Efficacy Evaluation and Follow-Up

The development of PDD is intrinsically linked to PDT, as the photosensitizer used in PDD also targets tumor cells during PDT, allowing both techniques to be effectively combined [25]. PDD can assess lesion size in nonmelanoma skin tumors, enabling dynamic efficacy evaluation by comparing lesion size before and after treatment. A pioneering study by the authors' group combined local PDT with surgery for EMPD, utilizing PDD to delineate lesion margins, guide treatment, and assess efficacy. Pretreatment with ALA-PDD clearly visualized lesion areas, and after two ALA-PDT sessions, fluorescence imaging revealed decreased fluorescence, indicating effective treatment. PDD defines lesion margins, guides surgical margins, and identifies residual lesions postexcision, with fluorescence highlighting tumor margins for photodynamic combination therapy [26]. Compared with Mohs surgery alone, combining surgery with ALA-PDT reduced recurrence rates to 5.9% while minimizing recovery challenges associated with excessive excision [27]. Additionally, PDD facilitates long-term follow-up by noninvasively assessing lesion recurrence at multiple time points [28].

14.2.2 Application of PDD in HPV-Related Diseases

The authors' group conducted a study on 60 patients with urethral condyloma acuminatum, using PpIX fluorescence intensity localization and quantitative analysis. After skin lesions were incubated with various ALA concentrations for various durations, the PpIX fluorescence intensity significantly increased at 2 h, peaking between 3 and 5 h, with 10% ALA resulting in notably greater fluorescence than that of the controls [29, 30]. PDD detected previously undetectable HPV subclinical infection lesions missed by the acetic acid test (Fig. 14.5), introducing a novel "field clearance" approach that expands ALA application up to 2 cm beyond lesion edges. Compared with conventional "spot clearance" CO_2 laser methods, this strategy effectively eradicates subclinical and latent HPV infections, reducing recurrence. Although ALA-PDD has diagnostic value for subclinical and latent HPV lesions, its high cost and testing requirements limit its clinical use as a replacement for the acetic acid test, which, despite low specificity and high false-positive rates, remains a common rapid screening tool. In practice, PDD evaluations of lesions and adjacent tissues before ALA-PDT treatment aid in diagnosing warts, subclinical lesions, and latent infections while assessing ALA incubation adequacy, ensuring readiness for PDT. Early diagnosis and treatment significantly lower recurrence rates and reduce medical costs. Additionally, ALA-PDD aids in early diagnosis, recurrence prevention, and subclinical infection detection in condyloma acuminatum while serving as a diagnostic tool for cervical intraepithelial neoplasia. Research findings indicate a positive correlation between the severity of cervical intraepithelial neoplasia and fluorescence intensity, enabling PDD to guide the development of clinical parameters and treatment regimens for PDT [31, 32]. Additionally, PDD has been successfully applied in assisting in the diagnosis of Bowenoid papulosis, vulvar lichen sclerosus, and oral lichen planus [30, 33, 34].

14.2.3 Application of PDD in Hair Follicle and Sebaceous Gland-Related Diseases

In 2004, the authors' group pioneered the use of ALA-PDT for acne treatment in China, demonstrating its effectiveness and optimizing treatment parameters. They identified a 3–5% ALA concentration with a 1–3 h application time as optimal for treating severe acne with ALA-PDT [16]. This study was the first to reveal the accumulation of brick-red PpIX fluorescence derived from ALA absorption, specifically within hair follicles and sebaceous gland units, confirming that these compounds are primary targets for ALA-PDT in severe acne treatment [17]. Additionally, PDD has been applied to other hair follicle- and sebaceous gland-related diseases, such as folliculitis decalvans, pyoderma, and rosacea. Clinically, PDD helps define treatment areas, determine appropriate treatment parameters, and evaluate therapeutic outcomes.

14.2.4 Research and Application of PDD in Other Skin Diseases

PDD is increasingly being explored for various skin diseases, broadening its clinical applications. This includes conditions such as papulosquamous dermatosis and fungal infections. For example, the authors' team studied PDD in 104 lesions of 30 psoriasis patients and analyzed blue light ALA-PDD fluorescence intensity and PASI scores before and after narrowband ultraviolet therapy. Certain psoriasis lesions presented pinpoint red PpIX fluorescence, with higher PASI scores than nonfluorescent lesions did. These findings suggest that fluorescence intensity is positively correlated with disease severity and progression, offering valuable insights into psoriasis management (Fig. 14.6) [35].

The authors' group was the first to apply PDD to infectious skin diseases such as tinea cruris. Typically, tinea cruris does not fluoresce under Wood's lamp, but after topical ALA application, noticeable brick-red fluorescence appears, indicating the conversion of ALA into PpIX and suggesting PDT as a treatment option. Further studies confirmed the effectiveness of ALA-PDT for tinea cruris, although its use is limited by the need for multiple treatments and considerations of cost and convenience compared with antifungal medications. Despite this, ALA-PDT remains

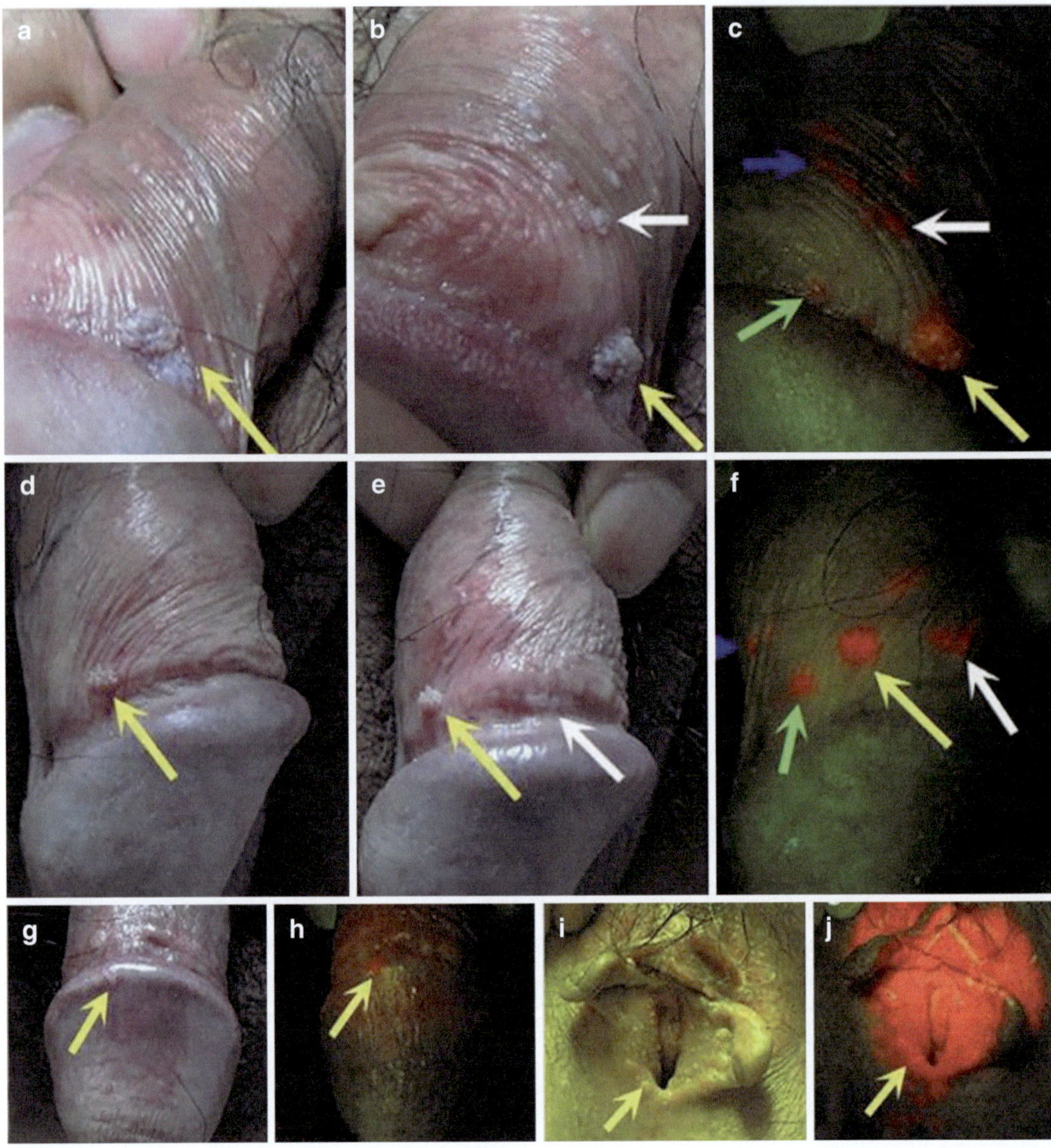

Fig. 14.5 Application of the PDD in patients with condyloma acuminatum. Patient 1 (**a**) clinical image of a male patient with condyloma acuminatum for 5 months, with yellow arrows indicating active lesions (HPV+), (**b**) acetic acid whitening test of the skin lesion, with white arrows indicating subclinical lesions (HPV+), (**c**) ALA fluorescence examination clearly showing clinical, subclinical, and latently infected skin lesions, with green arrows indicating latent infection 1 cm from the edge of the clinical lesion (HPV+), and blue arrows indicating latent infection 2 cm from the edge of the clinical lesion (HPV+), Patient 2 (**d**) clinical image of a male patient with condyloma acuminatum for 2 months, with yellow arrows indicating the lesions (HPV+), (**e**) acetic acid whitening test of the skin lesion, with white arrows indicating subclinical lesions (HPV+), (**f**) ALA fluorescence examination clearly showing clinical, subclinical, and latently infected skin lesions, with green arrows indicating latent infection 0.5 cm from the edge of the clinical lesion (HPV+), and blue arrows indicating latent infection 1.5 cm from the edge of the clinical lesion (HPV+), Patient 3 (**g**) a male patient with condyloma acuminatum for 2 months, accompanied by balanitis, (**h**) PDD showing nonspecific red fluorescence (0.5–2 cm from the edge of the lesion, HPV−, yellow arrows indicating the lesion), Patient 4 (**i**) a female patient with condyloma acuminatum for 5 months, accompanied by candidal vaginitis, and (**j**) PDD image showing nonspecific red fluorescence (0.5–1 cm HPV+, 1–2 cm HPV−, yellow arrows indicating the lesion)

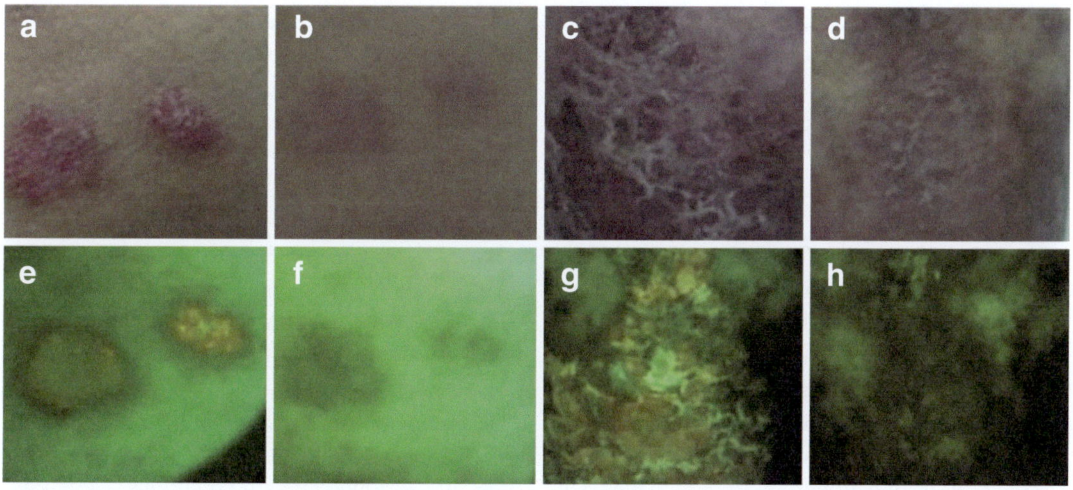

Fig. 14.6 PDD was used to detect PpIX accumulation in lesions at different stages of psoriasis, indicating the severity and progression of psoriasis. (**a**) Images of active psoriasis lesions at the right thigh, (**b**) images of the recovery stage of the same lesions, (**c**) images of active psoriasis lesions in the left popliteal fossa and on the curved side of the leg, (**d**) images of the recovery stage of the same lesions, and (**e–h**) corresponding to the fluorescence images of psoriasis lesions in (**a–d**) with Wood's lamp irradiation

a promising alternative or adjunct therapy when antifungal drugs are unavailable or restricted. Additionally, PDD has been used to visualize the extent of Majocchi granulomas before treatment and to guide clinical interventions [36]. In vascular conditions such as port wine staining, PDD is employed prior to hematoporphyrin treatment to visualize skin lesions, and the light dosage is adjusted on the basis of fluorescence quenching after treatment [37, 38].

In basic research, photosensitizer-mediated photodynamic diagnosis and therapy are applied to various animal models of tumors, inflammatory conditions, and vascular diseases. These studies often compare different drug concentrations, doses, administration routes, timings, and corresponding treatment regimens to assess the photosensitivity of the photosensitizer. By analyzing and comparing these factors, researchers can determine the optimal parameters for photodynamic therapy in different animal models, providing a foundation for further exploration of its efficacy and underlying mechanisms.

14.3 Procedure and Precautions for PDD

Local PDD for skin diseases requires the selection of different concentrations of ALA cream on the basis of the specific disease type. The cream is applied topically to the skin lesions and their margins, after which the area is covered with a light-proof material and incubated for several hours. Following incubation, the lesion area is illuminated with ultraviolet light from an LED source, typically Wood's lamp, in a darkroom. Distinct brick-red fluorescence indicates positive demarcation of the skin lesion and its boundaries, whereas the absence of fluorescence suggests a negative result. For skin cancers, histopathological confirmation is essential, and in cases of HPV-related diseases, adjunctive acetic acid testing is recommended for further diagnosis.

Precautions during the procedure:

- It is recommended that an ALA concentration of 2–3% be used for PDD. Higher concentrations should be avoided, as they may cause unclear boundaries between the lesion and background, leading to false positives and interference with accurate detection and diagnosis.

- The application time of ALA for PDD should be shorter than that for PDT, ideally between 1 and 3 h. This prevents excessive absorption by normal tissues, ensuring clear delineation of the lesion and minimizing the risk of false positives.
- Mucosal sites have a greater capacity for nonspecific ALA absorption. Therefore, when performing PDD on mucosal areas and adjacent regions, it is important to reduce the ALA concentration and shorten the application time to achieve maximum contrast in fluorescence intensity between pathological and normal tissues, thereby minimizing background interference and reducing the likelihood of false positives.
- A light source at approximately 405 nm was used for fluorescence excitation. A Wood's lamp is a commonly selected light source for PDD. The lesion and surrounding areas were observed in a darkroom setting to enhance fluorescence visibility.
- During photography, the use of special yellow filters can help reduce interference from the blue light emitted by Wood's lamp, ensuring clearer imaging of the lesion's fluorescence.

PDD is a noninvasive diagnostic technique with significant clinical value for nonmelanoma skin cancers, HPV-related diseases, follicular sebaceous gland disorders, and various inflammatory, infectious, and vascular conditions. It is primarily used for visualizing drug accumulation, locating potential infections or subclinical skin lesions, detecting recurrent or multifocal lesions, and assessing fluorescence intensity to adjust photosensitizer concentrations during treatment. PDD also helps in selecting optimal treatment time points, guiding light parameters, and exploring the targets of PDT therapy for skin diseases. It enables the evaluation of treatment efficacy by observing changes in fluorescence intensity before and after PDT, aiding in delineating treatment boundaries, maximizing PDT effects, and reducing disease recurrence. Additionally, PDD serves as an adjunct detection tool for follow-up and recurrence monitoring. The key advantages of clinical PDD applications include its speed and convenience, especially for early diagnosis, treatment processes, and follow-up of mobile and recurrent lesions; its safety, noninvasiveness, and painlessness; and its ability to provide dynamic observation and semiquantitative detection for objective analysis. However, the specificity of PDD needs further improvement, particularly for mucosal skin lesions. The accuracy of PDD is influenced by factors such as the photosensitizer, excitation wavelength, light intensity, lesion type, and surrounding skin conditions. More controlled studies are needed to provide evidence-based support for clinical applications. As PDD continues to develop and improve, including parameter optimization, the development of new photosensitizers, and the introduction of more sensitive detection methods, this technology will play an increasingly valuable role in clinical examinations, auxiliary diagnoses, and treatment efficacy evaluations in dermatology.

References

1. Andrade CT, Vollet-Filho JD, Salvio AG, Bagnato VS, Kurachi C. Identification of skin lesions through aminolaevulinic acid-mediated photodynamic detection. Photodiagn Photodyn Ther. 2014;11(3):409–15. https://doi.org/10.1016/j.pdpdt.2014.05.006.
2. Osman E, Alnaib Z, Kumar N. Photodynamic diagnosis in upper urinary tract urothelial carcinoma: a systematic review. Arab J Urol. 2017;15(2):100–9. https://doi.org/10.1016/j.aju.2017.01.003.
3. Lam S, Macaulay C, Leriche JC, Ikeda N, Palcic B. Early localization of bronchogenic carcinoma. Diagn Ther Endosc. 1994;1(2):75–8. https://doi.org/10.1155/DTE.1.75.
4. Auler H, Banzer G. Untersuchungen über die Rolle der Porphyrine bei geschwulstkranken Menschen und Tieren. Z Krebsforsch. 1942;53(2):65–8. https://doi.org/10.1007/bf01792783.
5. Figge FH. Near-ultraviolet rays and fluorescence phenomena as aids to discovery and diagnosis in medicine. Univ Md Med Bull. 1942;26:165–8.
6. Figge FH, Weiland GS, Manganiello LOJ. Cancer detection and therapy. Affinity of neoplastic, embryonic, and traumatized tissues for porphyrins and metalloporphyrins. Proc Soc Exp Biol Med. 1948;68(3):640–1.

7. Manganiello L, Figge FJ. Cancer detection and therapy. II Methods of preparation and biological effects of metallo-porphyrins. Bull Sch Med Univ Md. 1951;36(1):3–7.
8. Peck GC, Mack HP, Figge FJ. Cancer detection and therapy. III. Affinity of lymphatic tissues for hematoporphyrin. Bull Sch Med Univ Md. 1953;38(3):124–7.
9. Rassmussen-Taxdal DS, Ward GE, Figge FHJ. Fluorescence of human lymphatic and cancer tissues following high doses of intravenous hematoporphyrin. Cancer. 1955;8(1):78–81. https://doi.org/10.1002/1097-0142(1955)8:1<78::Aid-cncr2820080109>3.0.Co;2-l.
10. Lipson RL, Baldes EJ, Olsen AM. Hematoporphyrin derivative: a new aid for endoscopic detection of malignant disease. J Thorac Cardiovasc Surg. 1961;42(5):623–9. https://doi.org/10.1016/s0022-5223(19)32560-7.
11. Gregorie HB Jr, Horger EO, Ward JL, Green JF, Richards T, Robertson HC Jr, Stevenson TB. Hematoporphyrin-derivative fluorescence in malignant neoplasms. Ann Surg. 1968;167(6):820–8. https://doi.org/10.1097/00000658-196806000-00002.
12. Moan J, Peng Q. An outline of the hundred-year history of PDT. Anticancer Res. 2003;23(5):3591–600.
13. Wang X, Wang H, Wang HS, Xu S, Liao K, Hillemanns PJB. Topical 5-aminolaevulinic acid-photodynamic therapy for the treatment of urethral condylomata acuminata. Br J Dermatol. 2004;151(4):880–5.
14. Wang XL, Wang HW, Huang Z, Stepp H, Baumgartner R, Dannecker C, et al. Study of protoporphyrin IX (PpIX) pharmacokinetics after topical application of 5-aminolevulinic acid in urethral condylomata acuminata. Photochem Photobiol. 2007;83(5):1069–73.
15. Zhang L, Wang X, Wang H, SU, L., & Guo, M. Topical aminolevulinic acid-photodynamic therapy in acne. Chin J Dermatol. 2009;42(2):78–80.
16. Wang XL, Wang HW, Zhang LL, Guo MX, Huang Z. Topical ALA PDT for the treatment of severe acne vulgaris. Photodiagn Photodyn Ther. 2010;7(1):33–8. https://doi.org/10.1016/j.pdpdt.2010.01.003.
17. Ding HL, Wang XL, Wang HW, Huang Z. Successful treatment of refractory facial acne using repeat short-cycle ALA-PDT: case study. Photodiagn Photodyn Ther. 2011;8(4):343–6. https://doi.org/10.1016/j.pdpdt.2011.07.003.
18. Li C, Wang P, Wang D, Shi L, Zhou Z, Zhang L, et al. Fluorescence kinetics study of twice laser irradiation based HpD-PDT for nonmelanoma skin cancer. Lasers Surg Med. 2022. https://doi.org/10.1002/lsm.23538.
19. Neuß S, Gambichler T, Bechara FG, Wöhl S, Lehmann P. Preoperative assessment of basal cell carcinoma using conventional fluorescence diagnosis. Arch Dermatol Res. 2009;301(4):289–94. https://doi.org/10.1007/s00403-008-0911-9.
20. Chen J, Zhang Y, Wang P, Wang B, Zhang G, Wang X. Plum-blossom needling promoted PpIX fluorescence intensity from 5-aminolevulinic acid in porcine skin model and patients with actnic keratosis. Photodiagn Photodyn Ther. 2016;15:182–90. https://doi.org/10.1016/j.pdpdt.2016.06.012.
21. Wu Y, Wang P, Zhang L, Wang B, Wang X. Enhancement of photodynamic therapy for Bowen's disease using plum-blossom needling to augment drug delivery. Dermatologic Surg. 2018;44(12):1516–24. https://doi.org/10.1097/DSS.0000000000001608.
22. de Leeuw J, van der Beek N, Neugebauer WD, Bjerring P, Neumann HA. Fluorescence detection and diagnosis of nonmelanoma skin cancer at an early stage. Lasers Surg Med. 2009;41(2):96–103. https://doi.org/10.1002/lsm.20739.
23. Jeon SY, Kim KH, Song KH. Efficacy of fluorescence diagnosis-guided Mohs micrographic surgery for pigmented vs nonpigmented basal cell carcinoma. Acta Derm Venereol. 2014;94(5):568–73. https://doi.org/10.2340/00015555-1783.
24. Wozniak Z, Trzeciakowski W, Chlebicka I, Ziolkowski P. Photodynamic diagnosis and photodynamic therapy in basal cell carcinoma using a novel laser light source. Photodiagn Photodyn Ther. 2020;31:101883. https://doi.org/10.1016/j.pdpdt.2020.101883.
25. Casas A. Clinical uses of 5-aminolaevulinic acid in photodynamic treatment and photodetection of cancer: a review. Cancer Lett. 2020;490:165–73. https://doi.org/10.1016/j.canlet.2020.06.008.
26. Wang HW, Lv T, Zhang LL, Lai YX, Tang L, Tang YC, et al. A prospective pilot study to evaluate combined topical photodynamic therapy and surgery for extramammary Paget's disease. Lasers Surg Med. 2013;45(5):296–301. https://doi.org/10.1002/lsm.22142.
27. Bayan CY, Khanna T, Rotemberg V, Samie FH, Zeitouni NC. A review of noninvasive imaging in extramammary Paget's disease. J Eur Acad Dermatol Venereol. 2018;32(11):1862–73. https://doi.org/10.1111/jdv.15072.
28. Kleinpenning MM, Wolberink EW, Smits T, Blokx WAM, Van De Kerkhof PCM, Van Erp PEJ, Gerritsen RMJP. Fluorescence diagnosis in actinic keratosis and squamous cell carcinoma. Photodermatol Photoimmunol Photomed. 2010;26(6):297–302. https://doi.org/10.1111/j.1600-0781.2010.00546.x.
29. Wang HW, Wang XL, Zhang LL, Guo MX, Huang Z. Aminolevulinic acid (ALA)-assisted photodynamic diagnosis of subclinical and latent HPV infection of external genital region. Photodiagn Photodyn Ther. 2008;5(4):251–5. https://doi.org/10.1016/j.pdpdt.2008.11.004.
30. Wang X, Wang H, Zhang L, Guo M, Su L, Tao J. 5-aminolevulinic acid-mediated photodynamic diagnosis for condylomata acuminata. Chin J Dermatol. 2008;29(3):149–59.
31. Andikyan V, Kronschnabl M, Hillemanns M, Wang X, Stepp H, Hillemanns P. Fluorescence diagnosis with 5-ALA thermogel of cervical intraepithelial neoplasia. Gynakol Geburtshilfliche Rundsch. 2004;44(1):31–7. https://doi.org/10.1159/000074315.
32. Hillemanns P, Wang X, Hertel H, Andikyan V, Hillemanns M, Stepp H, Soergel P. Pharmacokinetics

and selectivity of porphyrin synthesis after topical application of hexaminolevulinate in patients with cervical intraepithelial neoplasia. Am J Obstet Gynecol. 2008;198(3):301–7. https://doi.org/10.1016/j.ajog.2007.07.045.
33. Cao Y, Zhang G, Wang P, Li C, Wang X. Treatment of hyperkeratotic vulvar lichen sclerosus with combination of holmium laser therapy and ALA-PDT: case report. Photodiagn Photodyn Ther. 2020;31:101762. https://doi.org/10.1016/j.pdpdt.2020.101762.
34. Fan Z-X, Zhang L-L, Wang H-W, Wang P-R, Huang Z, Wang X-L. Treatment of cutaneous lichen planus with ALA-mediated topical photodynamic therapy. J Innov Opt Health Sci. 2015;8(1):15400040. https://doi.org/10.1142/s1793545815400040.
35. Wang B, Xu Y-T, Zhang L, Zheng J, Sroka R, Wang H-W, et al. Protoporphyrin IX fluorescence as potential indicator of psoriasis severity and progression. Photodiagn Photodyn Ther. 2017;19:304–7.
36. Cai Q, Yang L-J, Chen J, Yang H, Gao Z-Q, Wang X-LJM. Successful sequential treatment with itraconazole and ALA-PDT for cutaneous granuloma by Candida albicans: a case report and literature review. Mycopathologia. 2018;183(5):829–34.
37. Lai Y, Zhang H, Wei M, Ji J, Shi L, Wang P, et al. Can red-light 5-aminolevulinic photodynamic therapy cure port wine stains on comb animal model? Photodiagn Photodyn Ther. 2018;22:253–62. https://doi.org/10.1016/j.pdpdt.2018.04.017.
38. Lei TC, Glazner GF, Duffy M, Scherrer L, Pendyala S, Li B, et al. Optical properties of hematoporphyrin monomethyl ether (HMME), a PDT photosensitizer. Photodiagn Photodyn Ther. 2012;9(3):232–42. https://doi.org/10.1016/j.pdpdt.2012.01.003.

Management of Adverse Reactions to Photodynamic Therapy

15

Yutong Yang, Dixin Wang, Bo Wang, and Xiuli Wang

15.1 Adverse Reactions to ALA-PDT and Relevant Treatment Measures

It has been 29 years since ALA-PDT was first introduced in dermatology in China in 1996. Over this period, it has been widely adopted in more than 3000 hospitals across the country, with its safety and efficacy consistently recognized. Following 29 years of clinical practice and groundbreaking basic research, the authors' group systematically reviewed the adverse reactions associated with ALA-PDT in dermatological treatments, categorizing them into those occurring during treatment and those occurring after treatment.

Y. Yang · D. Wang · X. Wang
Institute of Photomedicine, Shanghai Skin Disease Hospital, School of Medicine, Tongji University, Shanghai, China
e-mail: wangxiuli_1400023@tongji.edu.cn

B. Wang (✉)
Avera Medical Group Dermatology, Aberdeen, SD, USA

University of South Dakota, Vermillion, SD, USA
e-mail: makiwang@med.umich.edu

15.1.1 Adverse Reactions during Treatment

The primary adverse reaction during treatment is pain, which typically peaks a few minutes after irradiation begins, subsides or diminishes once the irradiation ends, and usually returns to normal within 1–3 days posttreatment. Pain significantly impacts both the patient's treatment experience and the overall clinical outcome.

Pain during ALA-PDT treatment is thought to result from the generation of reactive oxygen species during irradiation, activation of TRPV1 channels, and epigenetic factors, although the precise mechanism remains unclear. Pain intensity and sensitivity vary on the basis of factors such as disease type, lesion location and size, light dose, and individual differences [1–14]. Clinically, pain can also be mitigated through daylight ALA-PDT or newer painless ALA-PDT techniques [15, 16]. Effective pain management is crucial in ALA-PDT for skin diseases, with a numeric pain rating (NPRS, 0–10) recommended during irradiation to guide treatment adjustments on the basis of pain grading, as outlined in Table 15.1.

X. Wang, B. Wang (eds.), *Photodynamic Therapy in Dermatology*,
https://doi.org/10.1007/978-981-96-8915-6_15

Table 15.1 Pain grading and management protocol for ALA-PDT

Pain grading	Management protocol
Mild (1 ≤ NPRS ≤ 3)	The patient was advised to relax, while local cooling measures, including cold air and cold spray, were applied. Additionally, lidocaine aerosol was used to alleviate pain
Moderate (3 < NPRS ≤ 6)	Based on mild pain treatment, local infiltration anesthesia, nerve block anesthesia, and two-step intermittent illumination to reduce the illumination power density
Severe (6 < NPRS ≤ 10)	Monitor patient's vital signs, and recommend oral tramadol and morphine, topical fentanyl patch, terminate treatment if necessary, and use general anesthesia in special cases

NPRS numeric pain rating scale

15.1.2 Adverse Reactions After Treatment

The authors' group conducted a retrospective study analyzing adverse reactions in 439 patients treated with ALA-PDT for various skin conditions from January to December 2019. These included appendage diseases, skin tumors, precancerous lesions, HPV-related diseases, and other refractory skin conditions, such as actinic cheilitis, Majocchi granulomas, lichen sclerosus et atrophicus, leukoplakia, xeroderma pigmentosum, sporotrichosis, and follicular hamartoma. The recorded adverse reactions included pain during treatment (98.8%), erythema (92.4%), edema (35.0%), exudation (23.0%), dyspigmentation (27.3%), fever (2.4%), and hypopigmentation (1.9%) [17]. In a 2022 prospective study focusing on moderate to severe acne treated with ALA-PDT, 40 patients were recruited, 35 of whom met the inclusion criteria. Adverse reactions were recorded as follows: pain posttreatment (91.4%), a burning sensation (91.4%), dry skin (91.4%), itching (85.7%), erythema (94.3%), pustules (82.9%), crusting (65.7%), oozing (48.6%), dyspigmentation (42.7%), edema (20%), and blistering (11.4%) [3].

The findings from these two studies can be categorized into the acute phase, recovery phase, and other systemic or local adverse reactions on the basis of the timing of their occurrence. Acute-phase reactions typically appear within 1–3 days following ALA-PDT and include erythema, edema, itching, a burning sensation, posttreatment pain, dry skin, blisters, and pustules. Recovery phase reactions generally manifest 4 days or later post-ALA-PDT and predominantly include exudation, crusting, and dyspigmentation, as illustrated in Figs. 15.1 and 15.2.

15.1.2.1 Adverse Reactions in the Acute Phase

Mechanism Acute adverse reactions to ALA-PDT typically occur at the start of treatment and persist for 1–3 days; these adverse reactions are characterized by the infiltration of inflammatory cells, predominantly neutrophils. These reactions, including erythema, pain, a burning sensation, dry skin, itching, edema, pustules, and blisters, reflect the inflammatory effects and systemic immune responses induced by ALA-PDT. The mechanisms underlying these reactions involve four key aspects: (1) The release of damage-associated molecular patterns (DAMPs) from target cells or stromal cells due to damage after PDT. (2) Early vascular changes, including increased vascular permeability, vascular occlusion, and the release of various vasoactive substances and proinflammatory mediators. (3) Activation of the alternative pathway leads to chemokine release. (4) Induction of signal transduction cascades and transcription factors leads to the release of cytokines, matrix metalloproteinases, and adhesion molecules [18].

Influencing Factors The severity of acute adverse reactions to ALA-PDT is influenced by several factors, including the type and concentration of photosensitizer, the type of light source, the power density and dose of light, and the content of reactive oxygen species. Other factors, such as the type of disease being treated, the number of treatments, and patient characteristics, such as age and sex, also play a role. Notably, phototoxicity during PDT treatment is most strongly correlated with the inflammatory response observed after treatment [19].

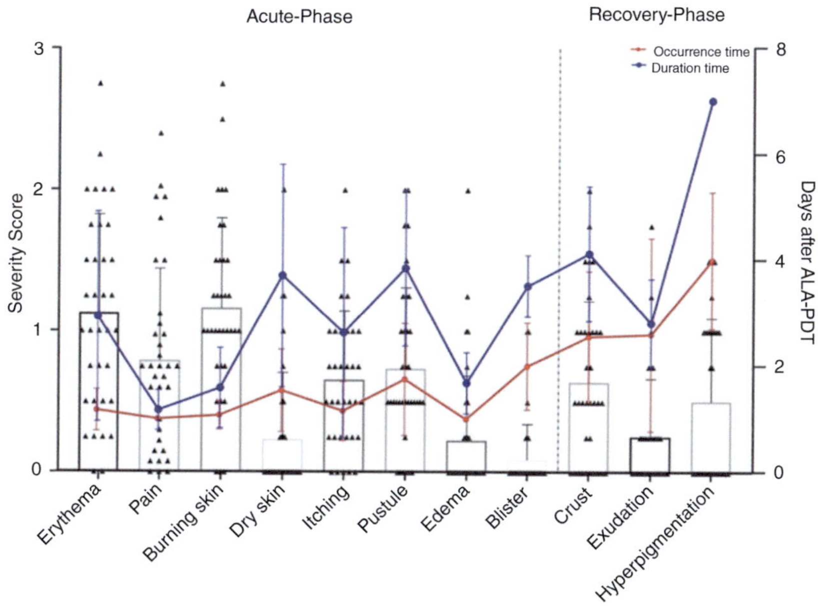

Fig. 15.1 Severity, occurrence time, and duration of adverse reactions after ALA-PDT (Reproduced from [2])

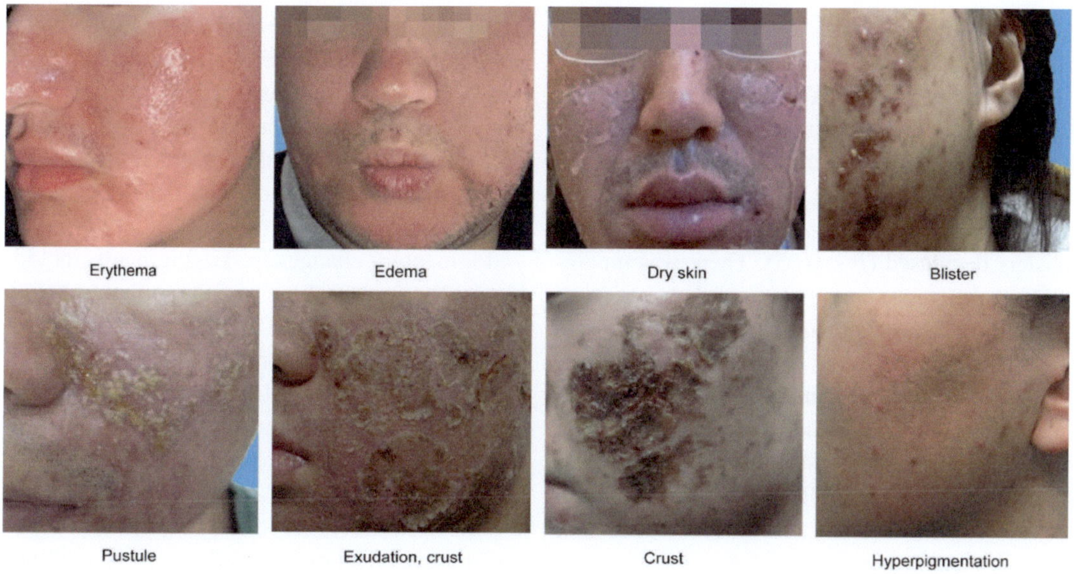

Fig. 15.2 Clinical manifestations of local adverse reactions after ALA-PDT (Reproduced from [2])

There were no significant differences in the severity distributions of erythema, pain, burning sensations, itching, or pustules after ALA-PDT. However, the severity of dry skin is primarily mild to moderate and significantly lower than that of erythema, pain, burning sensations, and pustules ($P < 0.05$) [3]. As patient age increases, the severity of acute-phase adverse reactions generally decreases, except for pruritus, as shown in Fig. 15.3. The heightened severity of pruritus in elderly patients may be attributed to changes in the barrier function of the stratum corneum, an

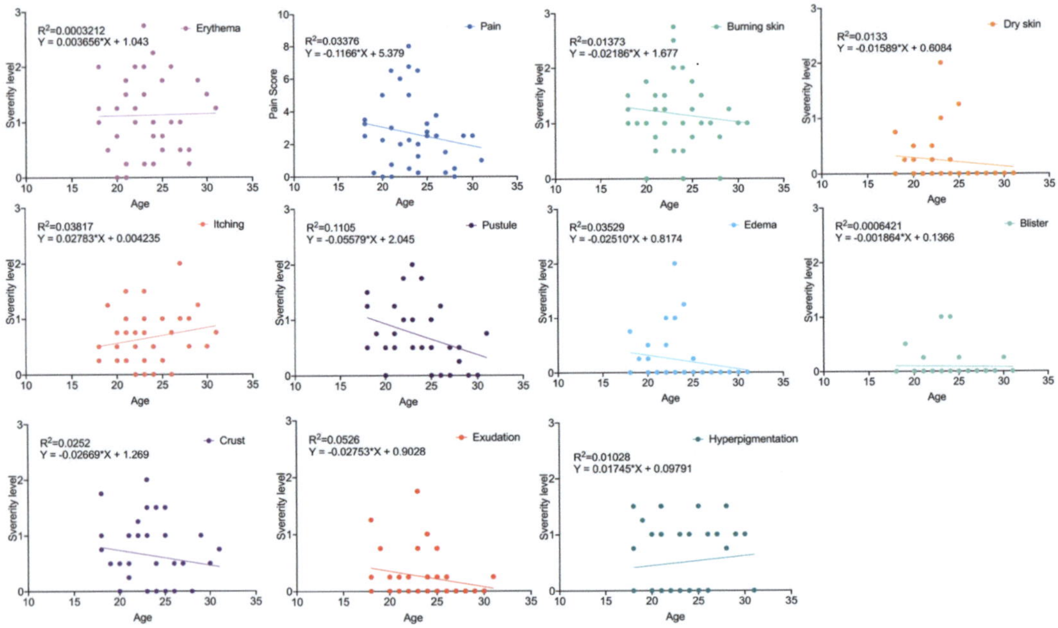

Fig. 15.3 Association between adverse reactions after ALA-PDT and patient age (reproduced from [2])

alkaline shift in skin pH, and reduced activity of sebaceous and sweat glands [20, 21].

Throughout the ALA-PDT course, the incidence of erythema, dry skin, and pustules remained stable after each treatment, whereas the incidence of burning sensation and edema increased and the incidence of pain, itching, and blisters decreased ($P < 0.05$). There was no significant difference in the severity distribution of pain, erythema, dry skin, or edema between the treatments. However, as the course progresses, the severity of itching and pustules significantly decreases ($P < 0.05$), and while the severity of blisters tends to decrease, it is not statistically significant. Conversely, the severity of the burning sensation tended to increase with the number of ALA-PDT sessions (Fig. 15.4).

15.1.2.2 Adverse Reactions During the Recovery Phase

Exudation and crusting following ALA-PDT treatment typically occur 2–5 days after treatment and last 2–4 days, whereas crusting also appears during this period, lasting 3–6 days. Both reactions are generally mild to moderate in severity and are influenced by factors such as patient age, number of treatments, treatment parameters, and disease type. Younger patients are more prone to exudation and crusting (Fig. 15.3). However, as the number of ALA-PDT treatments increased, the incidence and severity of these reactions gradually decreased (Fig. 15.4).

Pigmentary changes in skin pigments, including hyperpigmentation and hypopigmentation, can occur after ALA-PDT, with hyperpigmentation being more common [20, 21].

In a study of ALA-PDT for skin diseases, the incidence of hyperpigmentation was 27.5%. Specifically, for skin appendage diseases, the incidence was greater at 42.5%, likely due to the inflammatory response around the lesion and increased pigment production by melanocytes [17, 20–22]. The occurrence of hyperpigmentation is influenced by factors such as Fitzpatrick skin type, treatment dose, and disease type [7, 18, 19]. Moseley's study of 762 patients revealed that individuals with skin types I–III had a rare incidence of pigment changes of only 1% [23]. Changes such as melasma and freckles have also been reported following PDT treatment [24].

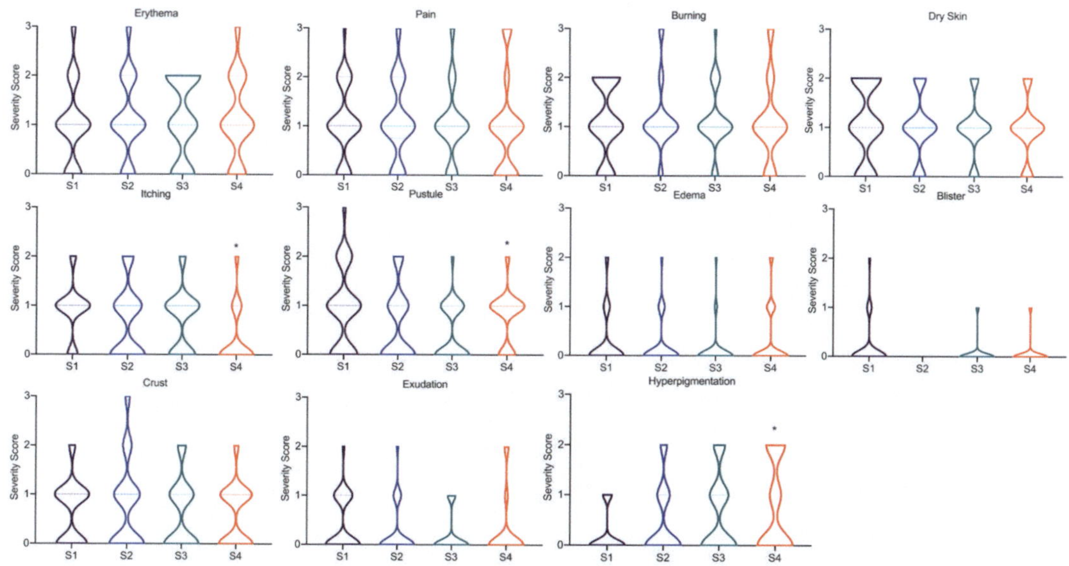

Fig. 15.4 Relationships between adverse reactions and the number of treatments after ALA-PDT (reproduced from [2])

Hyperpigmentation after ALA-PDT treatment typically resolves on its own within 3–6 months and generally does not require special treatment. To promote resolution, oral vitamin C or its derivatives, iontophoresis with vitamin C derivatives, and intense pulsed light (IPL) therapy can be used. It is crucial to avoid exposure to light for 48 h following ALA-PDT treatment, as this can help alleviate or reduce the occurrence of hyperpigmentation.

The incidence of hypopigmentation following ALA-PDT treatment was 1.9%, with a higher prevalence in female patients and a positive correlation with patient age. In a group of patients, hypopigmentation occurred in areas such as the scalp, forehead, corners of the eyes, or both cheeks in four patients with actinic keratoses (Fig. 15.5), on the forearm and upper arm in two patients with Bowen disease, and on the back of the nose in three patients with cutaneous squamous cell carcinoma (cSCC). Hypopigmentation was most commonly observed in exposed areas (66%), and patients undergoing ALA-PDT in these regions should be informed of the potential risk of hypopigmentation.

Hypopigmentation following ALA-PDT is thought to result from inflammatory damage to target lesions [23]. Treatment induces the generation of reactive oxygen species (ROS) and inflammatory cytokines, which activate the innate immune response and subsequently promote the adaptive T-cell response. These T-cell subsets produce soluble factors such as TNF-α and IFN-γ, which contribute to the development of hypopigmentation [25]. Older patients are more prone to hypopigmentation, likely due to delayed responses associated with aging, such as slower T-cell penetration into the treated area, delayed epithelial regeneration, or reduced melanocyte activity [26]. Most cases of hypopigmentation resolve spontaneously and do not require specific treatment, but severe cases may be managed with autologous melanocyte transplantation [24].

15.1.2.3 Management of Adverse Reactions

After ALA-PDT treatment, it is important to keep the treated area clean to prevent secondary infection. Topical moisturizers are recommended for individuals with dry skin, whereas for mild erythema, edema, itching, and burning, topical ice can be applied for cooling. If erythema persists, residual ALA should be removed by cleaning the area. Severe itching can be treated with

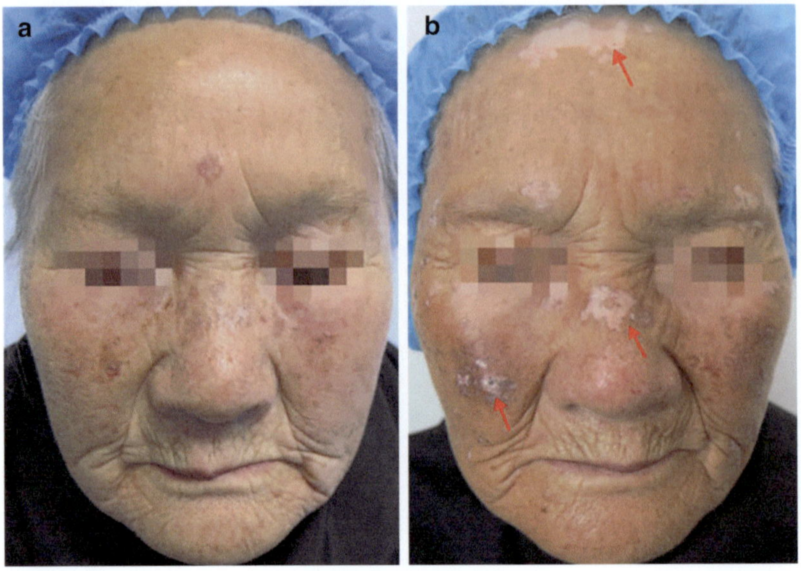

Fig. 15.5 Hypopigmentation occurred 6 months after ALA-PDT treatment for actinic keratosis (*red arrow*)

oral antihistamines, and pain may be alleviated with oral painkillers such as tramadol. For exudation, blisters, erosion, and ulcers, wound protection should be enhanced, and symptomatic treatment, such as topical antibiotics, may be necessary. When scabs are present and another ALA-PDT treatment is needed, the scabs should be removed before treatment. Sun exposure should be avoided for patients with pigment changes, and symptomatic treatments should be applied as needed.

15.1.2.4 Other Adverse Reactions

In addition to pain and local adverse reactions, ALA-PDT can also induce other rare complications, such as herpes simplex, bullous pemphigoid, pemphigus, and fever.

Herpes simplex mechanism induced after ALA-PDT treatment is unknown and may be related to local short-term immunosuppression induced by PDT treatment [27], and the initiation of antiviral therapy is recommended.

Currently, there is only one reported case of bullous pemphigoid after MAL-PDT for Bowen disease, which occurred 3 months after treatment, as described by Rakvit et al. [28]. However, no cases of bullous pemphigoid associated with ALA-PDT have been reported to date.

Pemphigus The authors reported a case involving an elderly patient with facial BCC who developed pemphigus vulgaris 2 weeks after the third ALA-PDT treatment. The patient presented with blisters on the face, trunk, and extremities following treatment [29].

Fever The authors reported that the incidence of fever after ALA-PDT treatment was 2.4%, with most patients experiencing fever on the day of treatment. The axillary body temperature ranged between 38.0 °C and 39.0 °C, peaking the day after treatment and gradually returning to normal. Physical cooling treatment may be necessary if required [29]. Fever, a common symptom of infection and inflammatory conditions, is primarily mediated by prostaglandin E2 (PGE2), which binds to the prostaglandin E3 (EP3) receptor in the preoptic hypothalamus [30]. After ALA-PDT, the inflammatory cytokines IL-1, IL-6, and TNF-α are significantly upregulated within 24 h, which may contribute to fever [31]. The subsequent increase in PGE2 synthesis can bind to receptors in the hypothalamus, triggering fever as part of the immune response. This fever response is considered normal and may help promote the immune response and aid in lesion clearance.

Other rare adverse reactions, such as urticaria, hypertension, psoriasis, and transient amnesia, can also occur after ALA-PDT treatment [32, 33], and attention should be given during follow-up.

In summary, the common adverse reactions of ALA-PDT include pain, erythema, edema, exudation, and pigmentation, as well as less common reactions such as herpes simplex, bullous pemphigoid, pemphigus, and fever. Clinically, it is important to fully understand these potential adverse reactions, provide patients with timely and appropriate symptomatic treatment, and adjust the treatment parameters of ALA-PDT as needed. For effective clinical recording and management evaluation of these adverse reactions, Table 15.2 can be consulted.

15.2 Adverse Reactions of Hematoporphyrin Derivative Photodynamic Therapy (HpD-PDT) and Related Treatments

Hematoporphyrin derivative photodynamic therapy (HpD-PDT) has been successfully applied in the treatment of various nonmelanotic skin cancers, such as squamous cell carcinoma (SCC), basal cell carcinoma (BCC), and extramammary Paget's disease (EMPD), as well as conditions such as port wine stain (PWS). It has shown significant therapeutic efficacy [34, 35]. However, owing to the systemic intravenous application of photosensitizers, their metabolism in the body takes a considerable amount of time. As a result, some adverse reactions, such as pain, skin ulceration, infection, scar formation, photosensitivity, and phototoxic reactions, may occur and are often more pronounced than those associated with topical 5-aminolevulinic acid (ALA)-PDT. To ensure optimal clinical efficacy and improve patient compliance, it is essential to manage these adverse reactions effectively. Various strategies have been explored to improve PDT outcomes and reduce side effects, including adjusting the incubation concentration, duration, light spectrum, and light source properties [36]. On the basis of a review of the literature and clinical practice, the mechanisms and treatment strategies for these adverse reactions are further discussed.

15.2.1 Topical Adverse Reactions

15.2.1.1 Pain

Photodynamic pain refers to the discomfort caused by PDT, which can be categorized into intra-PDT pain and post-PDT pain. This type of pain significantly hinders the success of PDT. The severity of photodynamic pain is influenced by factors such as the light source and the presence of protoporphyrin IX (PpIX), and it typically manifests as burning, electrical sensations and tingling. Intra-PDT pain typically occurs within the first few seconds of light exposure and is significantly alleviated as soon as light therapy is stopped. On the other hand, post-PDT pain may last longer, usually subsiding within 8 days after treatment [37].

The pain induced by PDT may be related to various generation mechanisms, such as reactive oxygen species production, transient receptor potential (TRP) channel activation, and the inflammatory response. The essence of pain management should be focused on patient experience, aiming to minimize pain while maintaining the therapeutic efficacy of PDT. A balance should be sought between the treatment's effectiveness and the management of pain, with the approach tailored to the intensity of pain and the individual physical condition of the patient. For mild pain, cooling methods such as electric fans, air coolers, and cold sprays can be effective. Moderate pain can be managed with oral analgesics, local infiltration anesthesia, nerve-blocking anesthesia, stepwise light therapy, or fentanyl patches. In cases of severe pain, nerve-blocking anesthesia or even intravenous systemic anesthesia may be needed. If these treatments fail to alleviate pain effectively, the pain management strategy can be escalated as needed to minimize discomfort while preserving the curative effect.

Table 15.2 Evaluation form for the management of adverse reactions to ALA-PDT

Name	Age	Gender	Diagnosis	Treatment parameters		Number of treatments	
		None	Mild	Moderate	Severe	Time of occurrence	Time of resolution
Adverse effects in acute phase							
Erythema							
Pain							
Burning							
Pruritus							
Pustules							
Dry skin							
Edema							
Blisters							
Others							
Adverse reactions in recovery phase							
Exudation							
Crust							
Hyperpigmentation							
Hypopigmentation							
Others							
Other adverse reactions							
Fever							
Psoriasis							
Dermatitis							
Pemphigoid							
Transient amnesia							
Others							
Suggestion							
Types of skin diseases		Tumors and precancerous lesions HPV-related skin diseases Diseases of the skin appendages Other:			Painful erythema, pigment problems Pain, erythema, edema, oozing Pain, erythema, pigmentation Pain, erythema, edema, oozing		
Gender		Woman			Edema, hypopigmentation, fever		
Age		The younger you are Older you get			Pain, burning, dry skin, edema, pustules, blisters, crusting, oozing, fever Itching, pigment problems		
ALA-PDT treatment		Progress of the course of treatment			Itching, itching, pigmentation		

15.2.1.2 Scar Formation

Most scars after PDT are hypertrophic. When HpDs damage subcutaneous tissue and cause deep ulcers, excessive production of collagen is triggered, leading to hypertrophic scars and secondary pain. Factors such as overprocessing, improper management of scabs, blisters, and infections during PDT can contribute to this. Overprocessing may result from excessive drug and/or light doses, as well as uneven light distribution, especially on irregularly shaped lesions. These conditions cause certain areas to receive higher light doses, increasing the likelihood of hypertrophic scarring.

While ALA-PDT or solar photodynamic therapy typically does not cause scarring [37–39], HpD-PDT, which uses a systemic photosensitizer that targets deeper skin lesions, has a longer action time and may affect the basal layer, increasing the likelihood of scarring. A previous study reported a patient with port wine stain who developed superficial vein involvement on the back of the hand after PDT, with continuous swelling at the infusion site leading to scar formation and pigmentation after 1 month. Although the exact cause is unclear, photosensitizer extravasation may have played a role in this rare complication [24]. The authors' group reported that HpD-PDT for EMPD caused varying degrees of scar formation, but it did not affect skin structure or function [40]. Additionally, for locally advanced BCC, the authors' group combined ALA-PDT and HpD-PDT to treat a 91-year-old patient with BCC on the scalp, resulting in pain and hypertrophic scarring. Local corticosteroids and a 980 nm laser, along with a 595-nm pulsed dye laser, were used to improve the scar within 3 months [41] (Fig. 15.6).

To prevent accidental injection or leakage of photosensitizers into surrounding tissues, strict protective measures must be implemented. Thicker scabs should be allowed to heal fully to avoid external damage and forced stripping. Injections of glucocorticoids or laser treatments can be used to address scarring. For infants and children, additional safety precautions are necessary to minimize the risk of scarring from overtreatment, as their skin is more prone to phototoxicity, and posttreatment care can be more challenging.

15.2.1.3 Skin Photosensitivity and Phototoxicity

Previous studies have shown no significant changes in the central nervous system, cardiovascular system, or respiratory system following HpD injection in animals. The median acute lethal dose (LD50) was 218.2 mg/kg in adult rats and 279.1 mg/kg in adult mice. Acute toxicity tests in young mice revealed major adverse reactions, such as tachypnea, slow motility, crusting of the ear tips, tail edema, and ulceration. The minimum toxic dose (MTD) in young mice was 215 mg/kg. Acute and long-term toxicity tests on HpD revealed that overdose symptoms were similar to those of porphyria and occurred only in dogs and rats at doses 10–20 times greater (5 mg/kg intravenously). Histopathological examinations revealed that the liver, kidneys, and red blood cells were the primary organs or systems involved. The severity of the toxic reaction was dose dependent, with recovery observed after 2 weeks of drug withdrawal. The phototoxicity to mouse skin caused by ultraviolet (UV) light is far less severe than that caused by HpD [42].

Photosensitive reactions and phototoxic reactions are common adverse effects of PDT, typically manifesting as erythema, edema, pustules, erosion, exudation, and pruritus. Previous studies have shown that pruritus and edema, as manifestations of photosensitive dermatitis, are second only to pain in terms of frequency during PDT [37]. It was found that photosensitive dermatitis is the most common acute adverse effect, with an incidence ranging from 20.0% to 35.0%. The symptoms of photosensitive dermatitis are generally mild and resolve within 1–14 days after onset [43].

The mechanism of photosensitive and phototoxic reactions induced by PDT may involve (1) the release of damage-associated molecular patterns (DAMPs) by tumor or stromal cells following treatment, (2) early vascular changes, such as increased vascular permeability, vessel occlusion, and the release of various vasoactive substances and proinflammatory mediators, (3)

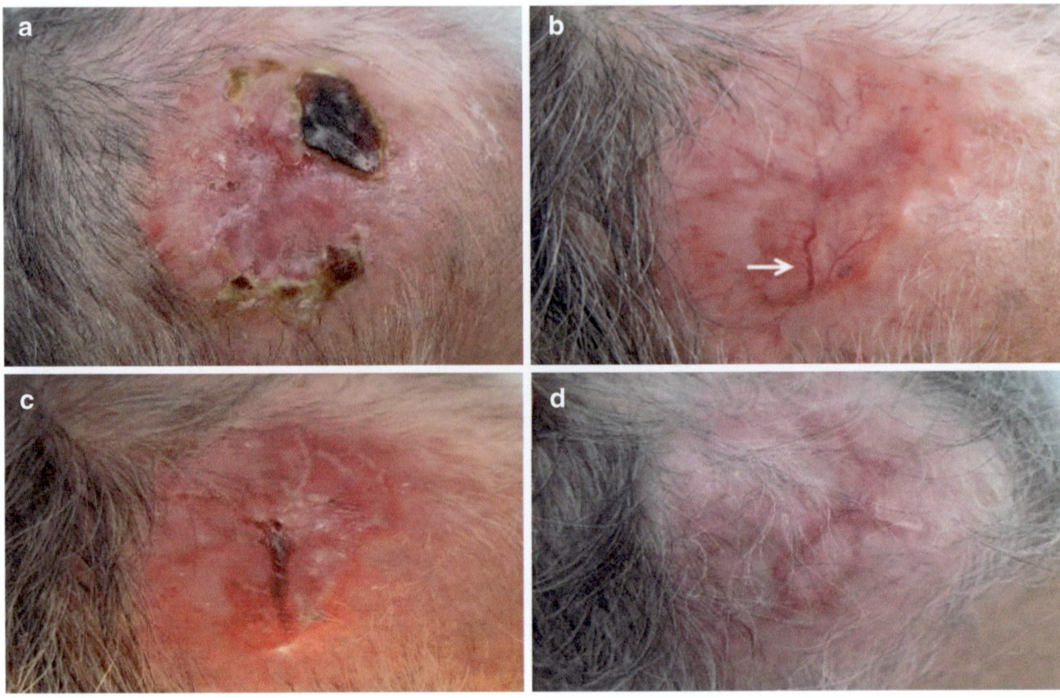

Fig. 15.6 Scars after HDD-PDT treatment of BCC. (**a**) Scar formation and scabbing were observed 6 weeks after treatment. (**b**) Neovascularization was observed in the scar (arrow). (**c**) Vessel occlusion was observed immediately after 980-nm laser treatment. (**d**) Scars significantly improved after 6 months of follow-up

activation of the bypass pathway leading to chemokine release, and (4) induction of signal transduction cascades and transcription factors, resulting in the release of cytokines, matrix metalloproteinases, and adhesion molecules [44].

Influencing Factors of the Photosensitive/Phototoxic Reactions PDT-related acute inflammation affected by the photosensitizer type and concentration, light source type, light power density and dosage, reactive oxygen species concentration, and disease type, with phototoxicity being most closely linked to the inflammatory response following PDT [45].

Clinical Manifestations of Photosensitive/Phototoxic Reactions Phototoxicity, which commonly manifests as erythema and edema, is a frequent side effect of PDT. A review of 2031 patients treated with PDT over 5 years reported erythema and edema in 89% of the patients. Erythema typically peaks 1–2 h postirradiation and resolves within 1–2 weeks, although rare cases may persist beyond 3 months. Histamine release following ALA-PDT peaks at 30 min postirradiation [46].

In a clinical study on PDT for AK patients, erythema occurred in all patients, with 90.9% also developing edema and 59.1% developing pustules. Erythema appeared immediately after irradiation and gradually resolved within 4 days. Edema emerged the day after treatment, peaking and beginning to subside 4 days later. Pustules typically form on the fourth day posttreatment; scratching should be avoided to prevent infection and scarring [37]. All patients with port wine stain developed edema after hematoporphyrin monomethyl ether (HMME) treatment, which was caused mainly by capillary destruction and increased vascular permeability after PDT. Edema usually appears after a short period of treatment and peaks after 2 days, lasting for 3–5 days [24].

Compared with topical ALA, the systemic photosensitizer HpD results in significantly prolonged skin allergic reaction times, typically lasting

8–12 weeks [47]. Programmed light avoidance is the primary strategy for preventing phototoxicity and photosensitivity. Upon treatment initiation, a light intensity below 100 lux is permissible. For the first 24 h post-HpD infusion, patients must remain in a dark ward (≥18 m^2) with their curtains closed and bulb power ≤40 W. For the following 7 days, patients should stay in rooms with bulb power ≤60 W in spaces of similar size. Outdoor activities are restricted to presunrise and postsunset hours for 7–30 days, starting with 30 min and increasing by 20 min daily, with caps and long sleeves needed. Between 30 and 90 days posttreatment, outdoor activities in direct sunlight (10:00 AM to 4:00 PM) should be avoided, and protective clothing should be worn. After 3 months, outdoor activities may resume if there is no pigmentation. In cases of pigmentation, the previous light avoidance protocol should continue until recovery. Fundus examinations are contraindicated for 3 months posttreatment.

Pruritus and pigmentation during PDT can largely be prevented by avoiding light exposure in a dark room for 1 month. A photosensitizer patch test is advisable before treatment. If a photosensitive reaction occurs, antiallergic drugs can effectively alleviate symptoms, and preadministration of beta carotene may help prevent or mitigate such reactions. Mild-to-moderate acute inflammation usually does not require additional treatment but requires proper care at the treatment site to avoid infection. Because severe inflammation affects daily life, steroids can control the inflammatory response [43]. Studies report varying incidences of hives post-PDT, with rates as high as 34% in one study and as low as 0.9–3.8% in others [48]. While cetirizine has been shown to double the median minimum itch dose without affecting phototoxic or erythema dose responses, prophylactic antihistamines are not routinely recommended according to relevant reviews [49].

15.2.2 Systemic Adverse Reactions

15.2.2.1 Infection

The risk of infection from PDT is relatively low, likely due to the antimicrobial activity of PDT itself, with an estimated incidence of less than 1%. Reported infections associated with PDT, including infections caused by *Staphylococcus aureus*, herpes simplex virus (HSV), and genital warts, typically occur after ALA-PDT. Infections following HpD-PDT are often attributed to lesion exposure, emphasizing the importance of proper lesion care, especially in sensitive or hard-to-manage locations, for effective infection prevention and control.

PDT often causes erosion and crusting, making it challenging to differentiate HSV. Pain, including burning sensations, vesicles, and pustules, typically peaks within 24 h after treatment. If symptoms arise after 24 h, reassessment for HSV is recommended. While the exact mechanism of PDT-induced HSV is unclear, it may involve local short-term immunosuppression [27]. Conventional antiviral therapy is effective upon diagnosis. Notably, HSV recurrence after PDT is rare, and prophylactic antiviral therapy is not currently advised.

Reports of systemic infections caused by HPD-PDT are rare, possibly due to the lower clinical use of systemic photosensitizers than of topical photosensitizers. The authors' group conducted HPD-PDT on 11 patients with EMPD, among whom one developed a urinary tract infection successfully treated with antibiotics [40]. Larger multicenter studies are needed to validate these findings, given the small sample size and single-center nature of the research.

The occurrence of skin infection after photodynamic therapy (PDT) is often linked to topical care. Before PDT, the treatment area should be thoroughly cleansed, and light therapy should avoid the menstrual period in female patients. Posttreatment, as skin lesion necrosis develops, lesions must be kept dry and clean, disinfected with Aner iodine, and covered with sterile dressings, which should be changed twice daily. During the later stages of edema, minimal exudation can be managed by gently drying with sterile cotton balls. Patients should limit physical activity, wear loose cotton clothing, avoid scratching, and seek medical support if radiation-induced redness, swelling, or exudation occurs. The scab period, which occurs 2–4 weeks after treatment, requires the area to be kept dry. If yellow exudate appears under the scab with surrounding redness, oral antibiotics should be taken, the scab should be removed, and surgical dressing should be applied. For pustules over the scab, puncture and drainage in a sterile setting, removal of pus, and application of antibiotic ointment are recommended. Subscab infection necessitates timely anti-infective treatment if thick scabs are present (Fig. 15.7).

15.2.2.2 Stress Response to Pain

Pain-related stress responses may lead to gastrointestinal and cardiovascular issues, including gastric ulcers or perforations, atrial fibrillation, and hypertension. Additionally, stress-induced pain can result in depression, claustrophobia, and loss of appetite, whereas lesional fluid loss may decrease albumin levels, affecting wound healing and increasing the risk of infection. To manage these stress responses, measures should include thorough preoperative assessments, the use of gastric mucosa protective medications when necessary, such as ECG monitoring during light exposure, and psychological counseling. Effective analgesia is essential for mitigating these adverse reactions.

15.2.2.3 Abnormal Hepatic and Renal Function and the Hematological System

Previous studies have shown that when HpD is administered to rats, the liver intake of HpD is 1.5 times greater than that of the digestive tract. During HpD treatment, abnormal hepatic function levels, such as ALT, γ-GT, AKP, total bile acids, and total bilirubin, may occur within 24 h to 7 days after administration. Additionally, HpD-PDT may be associated with a reduction in certain peripheral blood cell counts, warranting further investigation. HpD should be used with caution in patients with abnormal hepatic or renal function or decreased peripheral blood cell counts, and close follow-up monitoring after treatment is essential.

Pain, infection, scarring, and photosensitivity/phototoxicity are the main adverse events during HpD-PDT. An optimal balance between treatment efficacy and preventing adverse reactions can be achieved only when the mechanisms of these adverse effects and their relevant therapies are fully understood. This comprehensive understanding is crucial for improving adverse reaction management and advancing the development of PDT.

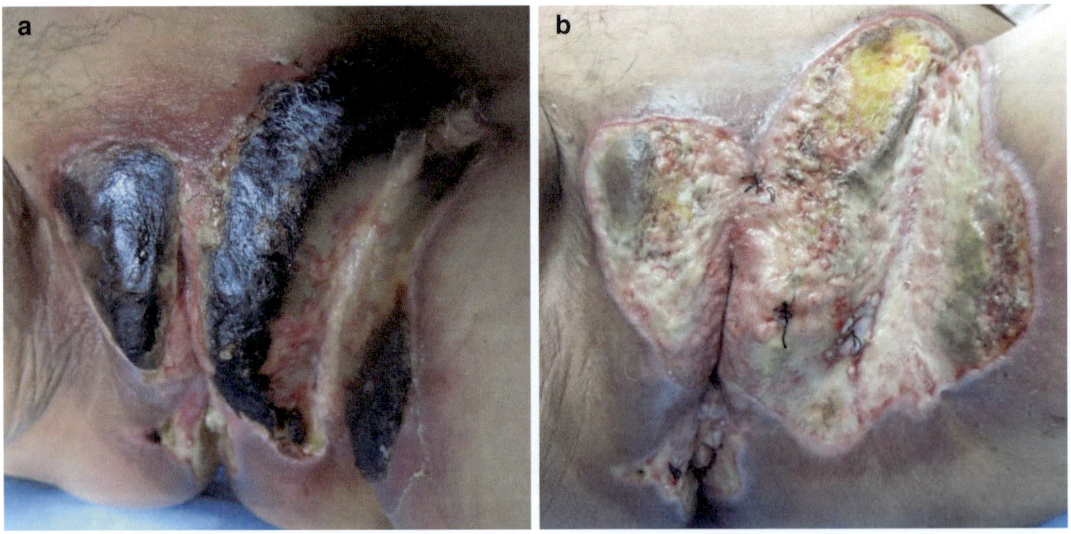

Fig. 15.7 Two to four weeks after HpD-PDT is the scab period. (**a**) A thick black scab was visible over the wound, and yellow granulation was visible below the local area. (**b**) After the debridement treatment, the wound was dry and new granulation tissue was visible at the base

15.3 Adverse Reactions of HMME-PDT and Treatment Measures

In 2016, hematoporphyrin monomethyl ether (HMME) was introduced as a photosensitizer for use in the venous system, with port wine stains (PWS) being its primary indication for treatment. The adverse reactions associated with HMME-PDT include both systemic and local reactions.

15.3.1 Systemic Adverse Reactions

Early pharmacological toxicological studies by Professor Xu Deyu and colleagues demonstrated that intravenous injection of 20 mg/kg HMME into S180 sarcoma mice did not significantly affect the central nervous system, cardiovascular system, or respiratory system. The acute toxicity was low, with no allergic, hemolytic, or vascular irritant effects observed, and no mutagenic effects were found. The extent of damage to the main target organs, including the liver, kidneys, and red blood cell system, was directly proportional to the drug dose. Additionally, teratogenic sensitivity period toxicity tests in rats revealed no adverse effects, such as bone marrow deformities or visceral organ malformations, in the groups treated with the test drug [50].

In 2011, Peihong Sun et al. conducted a pharmacokinetic study involving 36 healthy adults aged 18–45 years and reported that after a single intravenous dose of 7.5 mg/kg or 10 mg/kg HMME, gastrointestinal adverse reactions such as nausea (8.3%), gastric discomfort (5.6%), abdominal pain (5.6%), and vomiting (2.8%) were observed. Additionally, elevated alanine aminotransferase (ALT) levels were noted in three subjects on the fourth or seventh day post-administration, and one subject in the 5 mg/kg group presented elevated alkaline phosphatase (ALP) levels. However, all the levels returned to normal by day 14 without further treatment, and no other systemic adverse reactions occurred [51]. In a subsequent multicenter phase IIa clinical study involving 40 patients with PWS, mild-to-moderate somnolence, dizziness, and mood depression were reported in two patients, with all symptoms resolving spontaneously within 1–3 days [43]. In a phase III clinical study involving 440 PWS patients, systemic adverse reactions included elevated total bilirubin (TBil), sinus arrhythmias, conduction disorders, nonspecific ECG abnormalities, shortness of breath, conjunctivitis, dry eye, leukocytosis, hematuria, proteinuria, fatigue, increased sweating, and pulpitis [52]. The authors' group treated an 18-year-old male patient with midfacial PWS using a 5 mg/kg intravenous dose of HMME and noted immediate nasal congestion and chest tightness after irradiation, leading to treatment interruption. The symptoms were relieved after oxygen and a 5 mg intramuscular injection of dexamethasone, and the follow-up treatment proceeded without recurrence of symptoms. In 2018, Gan Liqiang et al. reported the treatment of 82 pediatric patients with PWS via HMME-PDT, with no significant systemic adverse reactions observed [53].

15.3.2 Topical Adverse Reactions

The local adverse reactions associated with HMME-PDT primarily include erythema, edema, and varying degrees of pain immediately after irradiation. Other possible adverse reactions include burning, itching, blisters, purpura, and crusting [54]. In the phase III clinical study of HMME-PDT, nearly all patients (approximately 99.5%) experienced topical adverse reactions, with the majority of these reactions being mild to moderate in severity.

15.3.2.1 Pain

Pain is the most significant adverse effect of HMME-PDT [55]. The mechanisms and influencing factors contributing to pain are similar to those discussed in the previous sections. In the phase III clinical study, 99.3% of patients experienced pain, with 80.1% reporting mild-to-moderate pain. The majority (98.5%) of pain occurred 5–10 min after the start of treatment, with the duration of pain varying. Notably, 42.1% of patients experienced relief on the same day, while the longest duration of pain was 19 days.

Pain levels vary among individuals, with some patients discontinuing or abandoning treatment due to severe pain.

On the basis of the authors' group's analgesic experience in PDT treatment, the following methods are recommended for HMME-PDT treatment.

Cold Air Analgesia It is a simple and effective method with definite therapeutic benefits for managing pain in HMME-PDT treatments. This technique may work by modulating pain signaling pathways, such as promoting vasoconstriction, reducing the production of ROS and inflammatory factors in vascular endothelial cells, and stimulating myelinated Aδ fibers. These fibers can activate pain inhibition pathways, increase pain thresholds, reduce capsaicin receptor activation, and decrease the transmission of nociceptive sensations [55–58]. In clinical practice, commonly used cooling devices include 4 °C air coolers and electric fans. The authors' group reported that using a cold fan during HMME-PDT resulted in a 4–5 °C reduction in the skin surface temperature and a corresponding reduction in pain, with a decrease in the pain score (VAS) of 2–4 points. However, it is important to assess whether cold air treatment might impact the therapeutic efficacy of HMME-PDT for PWS. In their studies, the authors reported no significant difference in efficacy between treatment groups with or without air coolers, although further confirmation through larger-scale clinical trials is necessary. As a result, air coolers are routinely used in clinical HMME-PDT treatments, whereas electric fans are often recommended for use after treatment or at home for continued relief.

Intermittent Illumination It can be useful for patients who experience significant or even unbearable pain despite cold air treatment. In such cases, light exposure can be paused until the pain is slightly alleviated, allowing the treatment to continue. However, the pause time should be short, as prolonged interruption can cause a decrease in the blood concentration of HMME, which may reduce the effectiveness of treatment [50]. While intermittent light exposure can help reduce pain, it is not the first choice because of the limited 50-min time window for HMME-PDT treatment. Prolonged exposure increases the risk of drug penetration beyond the blood vessels, potentially affecting the treatment's efficacy and, more critically, increasing the risk of scarring.

There have been no reports on the specific effectiveness of analgesic drugs for HMME-PDT treatment of PWS. The authors' group has attempted various medications for pain relief, including oral analgesics such as the nonsteroidal anti-inflammatory drug ibuprofen, the centrally acting analgesic dihydrocodeine, and intramuscular injections of morphine. However, the results from these attempts have been unsatisfactory, indicating that more research is needed to identify effective pharmacological pain management options for patients undergoing HMME-PDT for PWS.

For children who experience unsatisfactory pain relief with cold air analgesia, severe fear of pain, and difficulty cooperating with treatment, HMME-PDT can be performed under general anesthesia. However, this approach requires careful evaluation and implementation by a qualified anesthesiologist to ensure the child's safety during the procedure.

15.3.2.2 Burning Sensation and Itching

The data from the phase III clinical study indicated that burning sensations and itching were common side effects during HMME-PDT treatment. A total of 85.6% of patients reported experiencing a burning sensation during irradiation, with most cases being mild to moderate in intensity. These sensations typically do not require special treatment and are alleviated by the completion of irradiation. Pruritus, or itching, was reported by 64.7% of patients; it is also predominantly mild to moderate and can occur during or after treatment.

Cold air is commonly used to alleviate the burning sensation associated with HMME-PDT. In most cases, itching does not require special treatment; however, if pruritus is significant, it can be managed with topical corticosteroids or oral antihistamines to relieve discomfort.

15.3.2.3 Edema

Almost all treated patients experienced immediate swelling, which peaked at 24 h and gradually subsided between 72 and 96 h. Cold compresses can help reduce the degree of swelling. For patients with head and facial lesions, positioning the patient in a high occipital position is recommended to avoid laryngeal edema.

15.3.2.4 Blisters

Treatment with HMME-PDT should aim to avoid blisters. In phase III clinical studies, the incidence of blisters was 10%, with a median remission time of 3 days (1–24 days). Small blisters (<1–2 mm) typically resolve on their own without special treatment. For larger blisters, it is recommended that the patient visit the hospital for blister treatment, including daily wet compresses with normal saline or boric acid solution. Scratching should be avoided to reduce the risk of infection and scarring [24].

15.3.2.5 Purpura

Mild purpura occurred in 11.5% of the patients, with 27.1% of the cases appearing on the same day as the treatment. The median onset time was 1 day (0–3 days), and the median remission time was 4 days (2–15 days). Purpura is a manifestation of local vascular rupture following HMME-PDT treatment and typically does not require special treatment.

15.3.2.6 Crust

Crust formation is a relatively late and long-lasting treatment response. In phase III clinical trials, most patients who developed crusts had thin crusts. For thin crusts, topical antibiotics such as mupirocin ointment can be applied to prevent infection and promote crust shedding. For thick crusts, it is recommended that patients visit the hospital for appropriate symptomatic treatment when convenient to avoid the risk of scarring.

15.3.2.7 Photosensitivity Reaction

In phase I clinical trials, the half-lives of intravenous HMME injection in humans at 2.5 mg/kg, 5 mg/kg, and 7.5 mg/kg doses were 1.26 h, 1.31 h, and 1.70 h, respectively. The peak plasma concentration (Cmax) was observed 20 min after intravenous administration, after which it decreased rapidly. No HpD was detected in most plasma samples after 6 h, and no obvious skin photosensitivity reaction occurred after 52 h of administration and irradiation with a daylight simulator. However, if the nonlesional parts of the body are exposed to strong light within a few hours after administration, severe photosensitivity reactions may occur. These reactions may include skin burns, photophobia, dizziness, acute urticaria, and shortness of breath, which require immediate treatment. Therefore, patient education before clinical PDT treatment, including the preparation of sunscreen products such as sunglasses, long sleeves, and hats on the day of treatment, is crucial. After treatment, patients must avoid sunlight for 2 weeks and continue to protect themselves from the sun to prevent photosensitivity reactions.

15.3.2.8 Pigmentary Changes

Hyperpigmentation or hypopigmentation can occur 1–2 months after treatment, with incidences of 22.9% and 1.9%, respectively. Most patients recover spontaneously within 3–6 months. Mild hyperpigmentation or hypopigmentation typically does not require treatment.

15.3.2.9 Scarring

The incidence of scarring in phase III clinical studies was only 0.5%, with all cases being mild atrophic scars. Scarring may be associated with excessive light doses or inadequate posttreatment care, especially in young children (Fig. 15.8). To prevent scarring, frictional irritation should be avoided in the treated area, as it can lead to skin breakdown, infection, ulcers, and scarring. Once a scar forms, it should be treated as usual for scarring.

In summary, HMME-PDT treatment for PWS has relatively few adverse effects and is generally

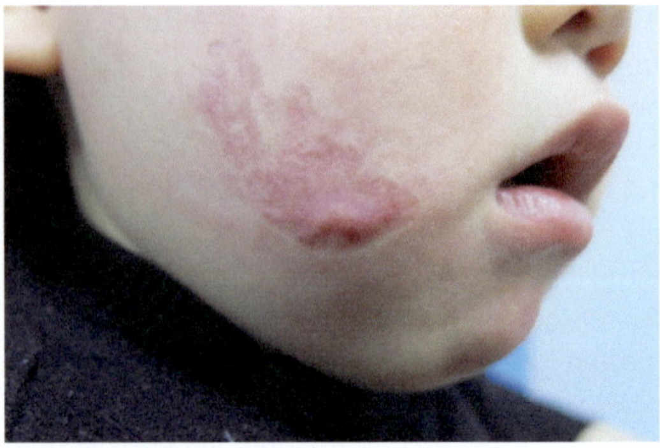

Fig. 15.8 Scarring of a child with PWS after HMME-PDT treatment due to improper topical care

considered safe. However, as the use of HMME-PDT for PWS becomes more widespread, further studies are needed to confirm and better understand its long-term safety profile.

References

1. Ko DY, Kim KH, Song KH. Comparative study of photodynamic therapy with topical methyl aminolevulinate versus 5-aminolevulinic acid for facial actinic keratosis with long-term follow-up. Ann Dermatol. 2014;26(3):321–31. https://doi.org/10.5021/ad.2014.26.3.321.
2. Shi L, Yang J, Zhang L, Zhang Y, Yan G, Zhang H, et al. A prospective study of adverse reactions of ALA-PDT for acne vulgaris. Photodiagnosis Photodyn Ther. 2022;38:102752. https://doi.org/10.1016/j.pdpdt.2022.102752.
3. Wiegell SR, Wulf HC. Photodynamic therapy of acne vulgaris using 5-aminolevulinic acid versus methyl aminolevulinate. J Am Acad Dermatol. 2006;54(4):647–51. https://doi.org/10.1016/j.jaad.2005.12.033.
4. Kuijpers DI, Thissen MR, Thissen CA, Neumann MH. Similar effectiveness of methyl aminolevulinate and 5-aminolevulinate in topical photodynamic therapy for nodular basal cell carcinoma. J Drugs Dermatol. 2006;5(7):642–5.
5. Fritsch C, Homey B, Stahl W, Lehmann P, Ruzicka T, Sies H. Preferential relative porphyrin enrichment in solar keratoses upon topical application of delta-aminolevulinic acid methylester. Photochem Photobiol. 1998;68(2):218–21.
6. Fritsch C, Stege H, Saalmann G, Goerz G, Ruzicka T, Krutmann J. Green light is effective and less painful than red light in photodynamic therapy of facial solar keratoses. Photodermatol Photoimmunol Photomed. 1997;13(5–6):181–5.
7. Radakovic-Fijan S, Blecha-Thalhammer U, Schleyer V, Szeimies RM, Zwingers T, Honigsmann H, et al. Topical aminolaevulinic acid-based photodynamic therapy as a treatment option for psoriasis? Results of a randomized, observer-blinded study. Br J Dermatol. 2005;152(2):279–83. https://doi.org/10.1111/j.1365-2133.2004.06363.x.
8. Schleyer V, Radakovic-Fijan S, Karrer S, Zwingers T, Tanew A, Landthaler M, et al. Disappointing results and low tolerability of photodynamic therapy with topical 5-aminolaevulinic acid in psoriasis. A randomized, double-blind phase I/II study. J Eur Acad Dermatol Venereol. 2006;20(7):823–8. https://doi.org/10.1111/j.1468-3083.2006.01651.x.
9. Barge J, Glanzmann T, Zellweger M, Salomon D, van den Bergh H, Wagnieres G. Correlations between photoactivable porphyrins' fluorescence, erythema and the pain induced by PDT on normal skin using ALA-derivatives. Photodiagn Photodyn Ther. 2013;10(4):683–93. https://doi.org/10.1016/j.pdpdt.2013.08.005.
10. Mandadi S, Tominaga T, Numazaki M, Murayama N, Saito N, Armati PJ, et al. Increased sensitivity of desensitized TRPV1 by PMA occurs through PKCepsilon-mediated phosphorylation at S800. Pain. 2006;123(1–2):106–16. https://doi.org/10.1016/j.pain.2006.02.016.
11. Stender IM, Na R, Fogh H, Gluud C, Wulf HC. Photodynamic therapy with 5-aminolaevulinic acid or placebo for recalcitrant foot and hand warts: randomized double-blind trial. Lancet. 2000;355(9208):963–6. https://doi.org/10.1016/S0140-6736(00)90013-8.
12. Alexiades-Armenakas M. Laser-mediated photodynamic therapy. Clin Dermatol. 2006;24(1):16–25. https://doi.org/10.1016/j.clindermatol.2005.10.027.
13. Babilas P, Knobler R, Hummel S, Gottschaller C, Maisch T, Koller M, et al. Variable pulsed light is less painful than light-emitting diodes for topical photodynamic therapy of actinic keratosis: a prospective randomized controlled trial. Br J Dermatol. 2007;157(1):111–7. https://doi.org/10.1111/j.1365-2133.2007.07959.x.
14. Voets T, Droogmans G, Wissenbach U, Janssens A, Flockerzi V, Nilius B. The principle of temperature-dependent gating in cold- and heat-sensitive TRP channels. Nature. 2004;430(7001):748–54. https://doi.org/10.1038/nature02732.
15. Rabindranathnambi A, Jeevankumar B. Dapsone in hidradenitis suppurativa: a systematic review. Dermatol Ther. 2022. https://doi.org/10.1007/s13555-021-00674-x.
16. Zhang Y, Zhang H, Zhang L. Modified 5-aminolevulinic acid photodynamic therapy to reduce pain in the treatment of moderate to severe acne vulgaris: a prospective, randomized split-face study. J Am Acad Dermatol. 2020;84(1):218–20. https://doi.org/10.1016/j.jaad.2020.04.146.

17. Shi L, Yang J, Zhang L, Zhang Y, Yan G, Zhang H, et al. Adverse reactions of ALA-PDT for the treatment of cutaneous diseases: a retrospective study. Photodiagn Photodyn Ther. 2022;38:102783. https://doi.org/10.1016/j.pdpdt.2022.102783.
18. Hongcharu W, Taylor CR, Chang Y, Aghassi D, Suthamjariya K, Anderson RR. Topical ALA-photodynamic therapy for the treatment of acne vulgaris. J Invest Dermatol. 2000;115(2):183–92. https://doi.org/10.1046/j.1523-1747.2000.00046.x.
19. Itoh Y, Ninomiya Y, Tajima S, Ishibashi A. Photodynamic therapy of acne vulgaris with topical delta-aminolaevulinic acid and incoherent light in Japanese patients. Br J Dermatol. 2001;144(3):575–9.
20. Chung BY, Um JY, Kim JC. Pathophysiology and treatment of pruritus in elderly. Int J Mol Sci. 2020;22(1):174. https://doi.org/10.3390/ijms22010174.
21. Choi EH. Gender, age, and ethnicity as factors that can influence skin pH. Curr Probl Dermatol. 2018;54:48–53. https://doi.org/10.1159/000489517.
22. Monfrecola G, Procaccini EM, D'Onofrio D, Roberti G, Liuzzi R, Staibano S, et al. Hyperpigmentation induced by topical 5-aminolaevulinic acid plus visible light. J Photochem Photobiol B. 2002;68(2–3):147–55.
23. Moseley H, Ibbotson S, Woods J, Brancaleon L, Lesar A, Goodman C, et al. Clinical and research applications of photodynamic therapy in dermatology: experience of the Scottish PDT Centre. Lasers Surg Med. 2006;38(5):403–16. https://doi.org/10.1002/lsm.20369.
24. Yuan KH, Gao JH, Huang Z. Adverse effects associated with photodynamic therapy (PDT) of port-wine stain (PWS) birthmarks. Photodiagn Photodyn Ther. 2012;9(4):332–6. https://doi.org/10.1016/j.pdpdt.2012.03.007.
25. Boniface K, Seneschal J, Picardo M, Taieb A. Vitiligo: focus on clinical aspects, immunopathogenesis, and therapy. Clin Rev Allergy Immunol. 2018;54(1):52–67. https://doi.org/10.1007/s12016-017-8622-7.
26. Guo S, Dipietro LA. Factors affecting wound healing. J Dent Res. 2010;89(3):219–29. https://doi.org/10.1177/0022034509359125.
27. Nobbe S, Trueb RM, French LE, Hofbauer GF. Herpes simplex virus reactivation as a complication of photodynamic therapy. Photodermatol Photoimmunol Photomed. 2011;27(1):51–2. https://doi.org/10.1111/j.1600-0781.2010.00552.x.
28. Rakvit P, Kerr AC, Ibbotson SH. Localized bullous pemphigoid induced by photodynamic therapy. Photodermatol Photoimmunol Photomed. 2011;27(5):251–3. https://doi.org/10.1111/j.1600-0781.2011.00609.x.
29. Zhou Q, Wang P, Zhang L, Wang B, Shi L, Keyal U, et al. Pemphigus vulgaris induced by 5-aminolaevulinic acid-based photodynamic therapy. Photodiagn Photodyn Ther. 2017;19:156–8. https://doi.org/10.1016/j.pdpdt.2017.05.014.
30. Blomqvist A, Engblom D. Neural mechanisms of inflammation-induced fever. Neuroscientist. 2018;24(4):381–99. https://doi.org/10.1177/1073858418760481.
31. Zhang L, Yang J, Liu X, Xu D, Shi L, Liu J, et al. 5-Aminolaevulinic acid photodynamic therapy amplifies intense inflammatory response in the treatment of acne vulgaris via CXCL8. Exp Dermatol. 2021;30(7):923–31. https://doi.org/10.1111/exd.14357.
32. Reinholz M, Heppt MV, Hoffmann FS. Transient memory impairment and transient global amnesia induced by photodynamic therapy. Br J Dermatol. 2015;173(5):1258–62. https://doi.org/10.1111/bjd.13985.
33. Shi L, Zhou C, Li C. Ulceration occurring after ALA-PDT combined with plum-blossom needle percussion for the treatment of pretibial Bowen's disease: a case report. Photodiagn Photodyn Ther. 2020;32:101958. https://doi.org/10.1016/j.pdpdt.2020.101958.
34. Wang Y, Lin Y, Zhang H-G, Zhu J. A photodynamic therapy combined with topical 5-aminolevulinic acid and systemic hematoporphyrin derivative is more efficient but less phototoxic for cancer. J Cancer Res Clin Oncol. 2016;142(4):813–21. https://doi.org/10.1007/s00432-015-2066-3.
35. Huang Z. Photodynamic therapy in China: over 25 years of unique clinical experience part two-clinical experience. Photodiagn Photodyn Ther. 2006;3(2):71–84. https://doi.org/10.1016/j.pdpdt.2006.03.001.
36. Yin R, Hao F, Deng J, Yang XC, Yan H. Investigation of optimal aminolaevulinic acid concentration applied in topical aminolaevulinic acid-photodynamic therapy for treatment of moderate to severe acne: a pilot study in Chinese subjects. Br J Dermatol. 2010;163(5):1064–71. https://doi.org/10.1111/j.1365-2133.2010.09860.x.
37. Gholam P, Kroehl V, Enk AH. Dermatology life quality index and side effects after topical photodynamic therapy of actinic keratosis. Dermatology. 2013;226(3):253–9. https://doi.org/10.1159/000349992.
38. Dai S, He S, Huang X, Chen P, Li Q, Guo J, et al. Safety and effectiveness of 5-aminolevulinic acid photodynamic therapy combined with fractional microplasma radio-frequency treatment for verrucous epidermal nevus: a retrospective study with long-term follow-up. J Dermatol. 2021;48(8):1229–35. https://doi.org/10.1111/1346-8138.15923.
39. Yoon J, Kim YC. Daylight photodynamic therapy with ablative carbon dioxide fractional laser for treating actinic keratosis in Asians: a case series. Photodiagn Photodyn Ther. 2020;31:101905. https://doi.org/10.1016/j.pdpdt.2020.101905.
40. Wang D, Wang P, Li C, Zhou Z, Zhang L, Zhang G, et al. Efficacy and safety of HpD-PDT for Extramammary Paget's disease refractory to conventional therapy: a prospective, open-label and single arm pilot study.

Photodiagn Photodyn Ther. 2022;37:102670. https://doi.org/10.1016/j.pdpdt.2021.102670.
41. Liao C, Shi L, Wang D, Wang X. Bimodal photodynamic therapy for treatment of a 91-year-old patient with locally advanced cutaneous basal cell carcinoma and postoperative scar management. Photodiagn Photodyn Ther. 2021;36:102553. https://doi.org/10.1016/j.pdpdt.2021.102553.
42. Pu Y, Chen W, Yu Z. Research progress of Hemoporfin–part one: preclinical study. Photodiagn Photodyn Ther. 2012;9(2):180–5. https://doi.org/10.1016/j.pdpdt.2011.09.004.
43. Zhao Y, Zhou Z, Zhou G, Tu P, Zheng Q, Tao J, et al. Efficacy and safety of hemoporfin in photodynamic therapy for port-wine stain: a multicenter and open-labeled phase IIa study. Photodermatol Photoimmunol Photomed. 2011;27(1):17–23. https://doi.org/10.1111/j.1600-0781.2010.00555.x.
44. Firczuk M, Nowis D, Gołąb J. PDT-induced inflammatory and host responses. Photochem Photobiol Sci. 2011;10(5):653–63. https://doi.org/10.1039/c0pp00308e.
45. Lerche CM, Fabricius S, Philipsen PA, Wulf HC. Correlation between treatment time, photobleaching, inflammation and pain after photodynamic therapy with methyl aminolevulinate on tape-stripped skin in healthy volunteers. Photochem Photobiol Sci. 2015;14(5):875–82. https://doi.org/10.1039/c5pp00069f.
46. Lehmann P. Side effects of topical photodynamic therapy. Z Dermatol. 2007;58(7):597–603.
47. Maier A, Tomaselli F, Matzi V, Rehak P, Pinter H, Smolle-Jüttner FM. Photosensitization with hematoporphyrin derivative compared to 5-aminolaevulinic acid for photodynamic therapy of esophageal carcinoma. Ann Thorac Surg. 2001;72(4):1136–40.
48. Ibbotson SH. Adverse effects of topical photodynamic therapy. Photodermatol Photoimmunol Photomed. 2011;27(3):116–30. https://doi.org/10.1111/j.1600-0781.2010.00560.x.
49. Ozog DM, Rkein AM, Fabi SG, Gold MH, Goldman MP, Lowe NJ, et al. Photodynamic therapy: a clinical consensus guide. Dermatologic Surg. 2016;42(7):804–27. https://doi.org/10.1097/DSS.0000000000000800.
50. Xu DY, Chen WH, Zhang H, Shen NC. Studies on a new drug for photodynamic therapy, hematoporphyrin monomethyl ether (HMME). Chin J Laser Med. 1993;1:3–7.
51. Sun PH, Zhao X, Zhou Y, Liang Y, Zhang HL, Cui YM, et al. Tolerance and pharmacokinetics of single-dose intravenous hemoporfin in healthy volunteers. Acta Pharmacol Sin. 2011;32(12):1549–54. https://doi.org/10.1038/aps.2011.132.
52. Zhao Y, Tu P, Zhou G, Zhou Z, Lin X, Yang H, et al. Hemoporfin photodynamic therapy for port-wine stain: a randomized controlled trial. PLoS One. 2016;11(5):e0156219. https://doi.org/10.1371/journal.pone.0156219.
53. Li-Qiang G, Hua W, Si-Li N, Chun-Hua T. A clinical study of HMME-PDT therapy in Chinese pediatric patients with port-wine stain. Photodiagn Photodyn Ther. 2018;23:102–5. https://doi.org/10.1016/j.pdpdt.2018.06.006.
54. Wen L, Zhang Y, Zhang L, Liu X, Wang P, Shen S, et al. Application of different noninvasive diagnostic techniques used in HMME-PDT in the treatment of port wine stains. Photodiagn Photodyn Ther. 2019;25:369–75. https://doi.org/10.1016/j.pdpdt.2019.01.008.
55. Wang B, Shi L, Zhang YF, Zhou Q, Zheng J, Szeimies RM, et al. Gain with no pain? Pain management in dermatological photodynamic therapy. Br J Dermatol. 2017;177(3):656–65. https://doi.org/10.1111/bjd.15344.
56. Warren CB, Karai LJ, Vidimos A, Maytin EV. Pain associated with aminolevulinic acid-photodynamic therapy of skin disease. J Am Acad Dermatol. 2009;61(6):1033–43. https://doi.org/10.1016/j.jaad.2009.03.048.
57. Tyrrell J, Campbell SM, Curnow A. The effect of air cooling pain relief on protoporphyrin IX photobleaching and clinical efficacy during dermatological photodynamic therapy. J Photochem Photobiol B. 2011;103(1):1–7. https://doi.org/10.1016/j.jphotobiol.2010.12.011.
58. Corti L. Nonpharmaceutical approaches to pain management. Top Companion Anim Med. 2014;29(1):24–8. https://doi.org/10.1053/j.tcam.2014.04.001.

16 Application of Noninvasive Diagnostic Techniques in Photodynamic Therapy

Xiaojing Liu, Peiru Wang, Long Wen, Bo Wang, and Xiuli Wang

16.1 Overview of Noninvasive Skin Diagnosis

The diagnosis of skin diseases has traditionally relied on the accurate assessment of skin lesion manifestations and affected tissues. This information is primarily obtained through naked-eye observation and histopathological examination. Direct clinical observation, while useful, is limited to visualizing only the surface of the skin lesions and cannot penetrate the epidermis, and it is also subject to subjective variations on the basis of the observer's expertise. Histopathology, often considered the "gold standard," provides more detailed diagnostic information; however, it is invasive, and its timeliness, operability, and accessibility are limited. Additionally, dermatopathologists are still relatively rare in many regions, further restricting their application.

In recent years, various new skin imaging diagnostic technologies have emerged, offering noninvasive, in vivo, real-time, and dynamic capabilities (Fig. 16.1). These technologies have significantly increased the accuracy and efficiency of skin disease diagnosis, making them indispensable tools in clinical dermatology. Commonly used noninvasive diagnostic methods include Wood's lamp, dermoscopy, high-frequency ultrasound (HFUS), reflectance confocal microscopy (RCM), photodynamic fluorescence diagnosis (PDD), VISIA-CR™ skin analysis, laser speckle contrast imaging (LSCI), optical coherence tomography (OCT), and photoacoustic imaging (PAI). These advancements allow for more comprehensive and accessible skin assessments, providing critical support in the diagnosis and management of various skin conditions [1, 2].

16.1.1 Wood's Lamp

The Wood's lamp has been an established diagnostic tool in dermatology for nearly a century [3], but its clinical use has been limited in recent decades. Since the 1970s, the frequency of studies and actual clinical applications involving the Wood's lamp have significantly decreased, and the device has almost fallen out of favor. However, in 2014, the authors' team published the world's first textbook on the application of Wood's lamp in dermatology in China, titled *"Practical Atlas of Wood's Light in Dermatology."* This textbook, which is based on initial clinical applications of

X. Liu · P. Wang (✉) · L. Wen · X. Wang
Institute of Photomedicine, Shanghai Skin Disease Hospital, School of Medicine, Tongji University, Shanghai, China
e-mail: wangpeiru@tongji.edu.cn

B. Wang
Avera Medical Group Dermatology, Aberdeen, SD, USA

University of South Dakota, Vermillion, SD, USA
e-mail: makiwang@med.umich.edu

X. Wang, B. Wang (eds.), *Photodynamic Therapy in Dermatology*,
https://doi.org/10.1007/978-981-96-8915-6_16

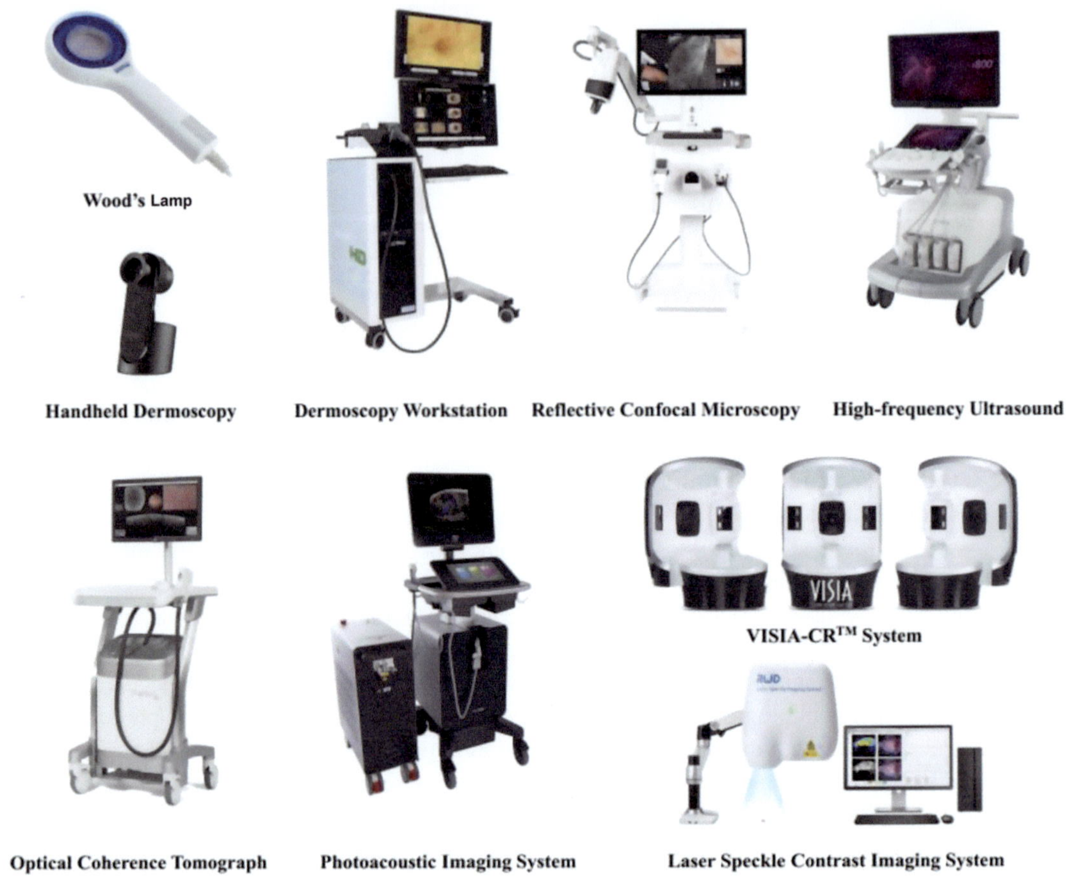

Fig. 16.1 Noninvasive diagnostic techniques in PDT

Wood's lamp in photodynamic therapy (PDT) and subsequent specialized clinical research, garnered worldwide attention among dermatologists in China [4]. It reignited interest in Wood's lamp and spurred its renewed application and popularization in clinical dermatology, bringing the technology back into prominence after it had been on the verge of being forgotten.

The Wood's lamp uses a high-pressure mercury lamp as its light source, emitting light with a wavelength range of 320–400 nm, peaking at 365 nm. The emitted ultraviolet (UV) light is filtered through a barium silicate filter containing 9% nickel oxide, known as Wood's filter. When this UV light is directed onto the skin, it is scattered or reflected by the epidermis. Melanin in the epidermis and dermis, as well as collagen in the dermis, absorbs light and emits nonspecific fluorescence, which primarily appears as blue or white light. In dermatology, Wood's lamp is primarily used for the clinical diagnosis and differential diagnosis of pigmentation disorders, infectious skin diseases, and certain metabolic skin conditions. It helps outline skin lesions, assess treatment efficacy, and conduct follow-up evaluations, particularly for skin with increased pigmentation. For cosmetic laser treatments, it is useful for evaluating the number and extent of pigmentation spots, allowing for monitoring of treatment results [5]. Additionally, Wood's lamp is valuable in PDD for skin tumors and precancerous lesions. PDD is a noninvasive diagnostic technique that uses the fluorescence produced by a photosensitizer when irradiated by a Wood's lamp. This fluorescence aids in the diagnosis of certain superficial skin tumors and assists in pre-

and posttreatment evaluations without causing harm. In 1996, Xu and the author's group pioneered the use of ALA-PDT for treating skin tumors in Chinese dermatology, but the significance of PDD research was highlighted by Wang's study on the fluorescence dynamics of urethral condyloma acuminata in 1997. Since then, Wang's team has expanded PDD applications to various dermatological conditions, including genital warts, skin tumors, moderate-to-severe acne, and treatments such as HMME-PDT and HpD-PDT [6–11]. PDD works via the selective absorption of photosensitizers by target tissues such as tumor cells or actively proliferating cells. This selective absorption enables the monitoring of photosensitizer distribution, differentiating between target tissues and normal tissues. This technique can help outline tumor margins, guide surgical practices for margin dissection, and optimize photodynamic therapy strategies for better treatment efficacy [5, 12].

16.1.2 Dermoscopy

Dermoscopy is a widely utilized noninvasive diagnostic technology that employs either polarized or nonpolarized light to filter out excess reflected light from the skin's surface. This allows for the magnification of skin lesions, enabling the observation of the deeper epidermis and superficial dermis, areas that are typically not visible to the naked eye. The technique is highly valued for its simplicity, cost-effectiveness, and high diagnostic specificity. It has become an essential tool for dermatologists, particularly in European and American countries [13]. Initially, dermoscopy was used primarily for diagnosing and differentiating pigmented skin conditions such as nevi and malignant melanoma. However, as technology has advanced and its clinical applications have expanded, dermoscopy has found significant use in diagnosing a wide range of common skin diseases. Additionally, it plays an important role in disease monitoring and treatment evaluation, making it a versatile tool in dermatological practice.

16.1.3 High-Frequency Ultrasound

High-frequency ultrasound (HFUS) is an advanced extension of traditional ultrasound technology that has gained significant traction in dermatology since the late 1970s. HFUS works by emitting ultrasound signals through high-frequency equipment, which are then reflected by the target tissue. These reflected signals are used to create a two-dimensional ultrasound image based on the strength, weakness, or spot density of the reflections [14]. HFUS devices operating at frequencies between 20 MHz and 75 MHz provide high resolution, making them particularly well suited for the shallow penetration depth required to examine skin tissues. It allows for detailed observation of both skin and subcutaneous tissues, offering structural insights into skin layers and some functional information about superficial organs [15]. Additionally, HFUS is valued for its simplicity, low cost, and excellent potential in skin disease diagnosis, particularly for skin cancers, increasing its application prospects in clinical dermatology.

16.1.4 Reflection Confocal Microscopy

Reflection confocal microscopy (RCM) uses an 830-nm diode laser as a point light source to emit monochromatic and coherent light, which passes through a beam splitter, scanning and focusing optical lenses, and a skin contact device. The reflected light from the focal plane is captured by a detector for imaging. By adjusting the focus plane, RCM enables real-time, dynamic, noninvasive, and continuous scanning of skin lesions, producing high-resolution images at 0.5–1 μm at the cellular level, a process known as "optical sectioning" [16]. Recently, RCM has seen rapid application growth in diagnosing pigmented and inflammatory skin diseases, with expert consensus emerging on its manifestations in these conditions [17, 18].

16.1.5 VISIA-CR™ Skin Analysis System

The VISIA-CR™ skin analysis system captures images under 6500 K standard white light, UV light, and polarized light sources. Its red area imaging mode utilizes Canfield-based RBX technology, which clearly distinguishes the special chromophore characteristics of the superficial skin and allows for quantitative analysis. The rhodopsin imaging mode accurately displays the fluorescence distribution of the skin's natural fluorescent substances and exogenous photosensitizers under UV light [19].

16.1.6 Laser Speckle Contrast Imaging

Laser speckle contrast imaging (LSCI) is a noncontact near-infrared imaging system that operates on the principle that irregular intensity patterns are formed when coherent light is reflected from a rough surface or backscattered from within a medium containing scattering matter. This creates randomly distributed spots, which can be used to measure superficial blood microcirculation in the skin [20]. LSCI can assess microcirculatory parameters such as skin blood vessel diameter, blood vessel density, blood flow velocity, and blood perfusion in the detection area. It offers advantages such as noncontact, noninvasive operation, fast imaging, and high temporal and spatial resolution.

16.1.7 Optical Coherence Tomography

Optical coherence tomography (OCT) is an imaging technology that uses low-coherence interference gating to resolve depth-direction information of biological tissues or materials [21]. It enables *in vivo* tomographic micron-level imaging, with a current resolution of less than 7.5 μm, and some high-resolution OCT systems can even reach 1 μm [22]. This capability allows OCT to clearly present the hierarchical structure of the skin. In recent years, OCT has developed rapidly, especially in biological tissue detection and imaging, making it a promising new tomographic technology.

16.1.8 Photoacoustic Imaging

Photoacoustic imaging (PAI) is an emerging noninvasive, nonionizing biomedical imaging technology that offers high sensitivity, satisfactory imaging depth, and good spatial resolution. With an imaging depth of 3–5 cm and a resolution of 100 μm, PAI is suitable for molecular imaging, providing information on the distribution, content, and microstructure size of biological macromolecules within tissues. It combines both structural and functional imaging [23–25]. However, its application in dermatology is still limited, with only a few studies conducted in this field [26, 27].

16.2 Application of Noninvasive Diagnosis in PDT

In recent years, as medical needs have increased, noninvasive diagnostic technologies have gained increasing attention from both doctors and patients. During PDT, these technologies have progressively shown advantages and promising application prospects, enhancing diagnosis, monitoring, and treatment strategies.

16.2.1 Application of Noninvasive Diagnosis in PDT for Skin Cancers

16.2.1.1 Basal Cell Carcinoma

Basal cell carcinoma (BCC) is more common in elderly individuals and typically occurs on sun-exposed areas such as the head, face, neck, and back of the hands. The incidence of BCC is closely related to sun exposure. While BCC generally grows slowly, in its final stages, it can become more aggressive, progressing to necrosis and potentially infiltrating deeper soft tissue and bone [28].

Dermoscopy features: BCC is categorized into five types: pigmented, nodular-ulcerative, superficial, morphea-like, and nonpigmented, with each type displaying distinct characteristics under dermoscopy [29, 30]: (1) Pigmented BCC, typical diagnostic patterns include one negative criterion (absence of a pigment network) and six positive features: large blue-gray ovoid nests, blue-gray globules, leaf-like structures, spoke-wheel structures, ulceration, and arborizing blood vessels. Diagnosis is possible with one negative criterion and at least one positive feature. (2) Superficial BCCs exhibit leaf-like structures, short arborizing capillaries, bright white or red structureless areas, and superficial erosion. (3) Nodular-ulcerative BCC is characterized by arborizing vessels and ulceration. (4) Mophoraform BCC presents a bright white background, pink-white structureless areas, arborizing blood vessels, and a star-like pattern with radial blood vessels and white stripes extending from the lesion to normal skin. (5) Nonpigmented BCCs display dilation of small or branched capillaries, superficial erosion, and bright white structureless areas. Dermoscopy is highly accurate for diagnosing BCC, with a diagnostic accuracy ranging from 95% to 99%, and it is widely used for the diagnosis, classification, and differential diagnosis of BCC.

HFUS features: HFUS features primarily indicate that the lesions are located in the epidermis and/or dermis with clear boundaries. These lesions exhibit punctate strong echoes and anechoic areas inside [31]. Guo et al. suggested that HFUS could differentiate between noninvasive and invasive BCC, with infiltrative BCC penetrating the dermis and exhibiting a crawling growth. HFUS helps define the scope and depth of BCC lesions, and when combined with color Doppler ultrasound, it can also reveal blood flow signals, providing additional diagnostic information.

RCM features: The RCM characteristics of BCC are closely associated with the histopathological subtype. Key features include parakeratosis in the stratum corneum, bright dendritic structures in the basal layer, and elongated mononuclear cells in the dermis with polarized nuclei aligned in the same direction. These cells form nodular, spoke-like, cord-like, or palisade-like patterns, often accompanied by prominent inflammatory infiltrates [32]. RCM also aids in diagnosing specific BCC subtypes [33]. For example, superficial BCC appears with cord-like protrusions connected to the epidermis (Fig. 16.2b); nodular BCC presents larger tumor nests with bright tumor islands, peripheral collagen bundles, and dilated blood vessels (Fig. 16.2f). Additionally, low-refractive cleft-like dark spaces can be observed (Fig. 16.2j). Thus, RCM significantly enhances the clinicians' ability to detect suspected BCC and differentiate its subtypes before surgical intervention.

OCT features of BCC typically present as low-reflective ovoid structures, sometimes with a bright center. Key characteristics include a dark halo surrounding the tumor, thinning of the epidermis, compression of collagen, and disruption of the epidermal-dermal junction [35]. OCT can also assist in distinguishing between BCC subtypes. For nodular BCC, the most characteristic manifestation is the presence of oval structures, often with dark areas or cysts (Fig. 16.2g). Superficial BCC typically shows a dark border separating the tumor from the dermis, with a bulge or cone extending from the epidermis to the dermis (Fig. 16.2c). In infiltrative BCC, a "grapelike" appearance with elongated structures in the dermis is observed (Fig. 16.2c, k) [34]. These distinctive OCT features can increase the diagnostic accuracy for BCC.

In the application of noninvasive diagnosis in PDT treatment before PDT, noninvasive diagnostic technologies play a crucial role in assisting in the diagnosis, classification, and determination of PDT parameters for BCC. Currently, Chinese guidelines recommend ALA-PDT for superficial and nodular BCC with depths less than 2 mm [36]. HFUS can accurately display the structure and invasive depth of skin lesions, aiding in both surgery planning and PDT parameter determination. RCM help detect atypical cells in skin lesions that may not be visible to the naked eye, whereas the combination of RCM and OCT can assist in BCC subtype classification. The characteristic patterns of the BCC subtypes identified through

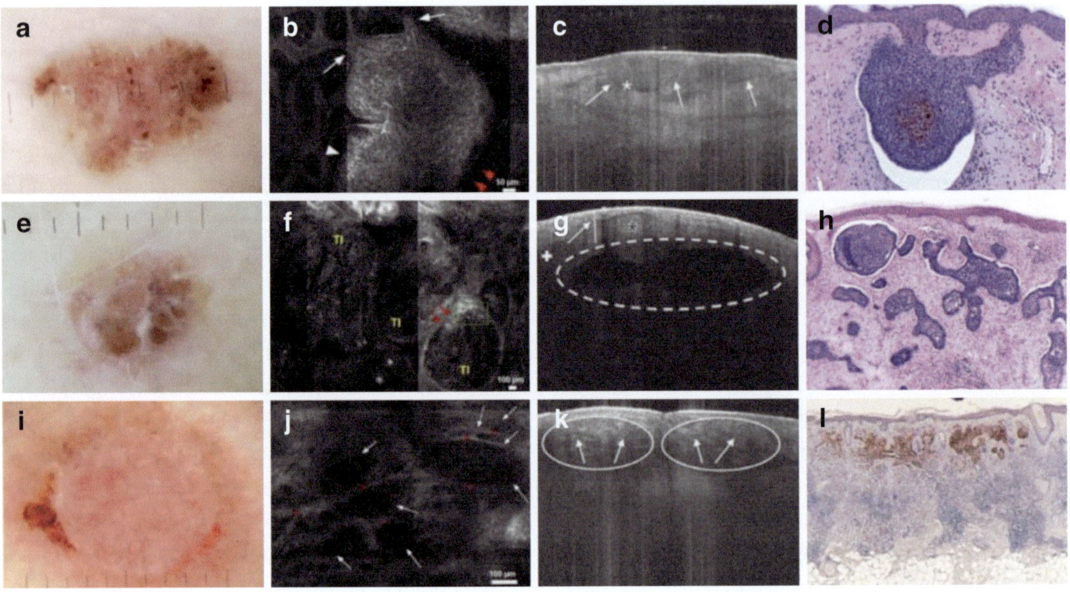

Fig. 16.2 Application of noninvasive diagnosis in the diagnosis of BCC [33, 34]· (**a–d**) Dermoscopy, RCM, OCT, and histopathological manifestations of superficial BCC (**a–d**), nodular BCC (**e–h**), and infiltrative BCC (**i–l**)

these noninvasive technologies can guide the formulation of PDT parameters and provide a basis for evaluating their efficacy during treatment.

PDD helps further define the BCC margin status, assess protoporphyrin IX transformation, and determine the PDT incubation time and illumination area. After PDT, noninvasive diagnostic technologies also offer advantages in evaluating and following up on BCC. Dermoscopy and RCM are effective for assessing the efficacy of PDT in superficial BCC, with dermoscopy showing reduced or absent blue-gray oval nests, globules, and arborizing blood vessels, along with flattened ulcerations, whereas RCM reveals blurred or absent tumor cells arranged in nodules, spokes, cords, or palisades [37]. During follow-up, certain features detected by these methods, such as blue-gray nests, globules, arborizing vessels under dermoscopy, and abnormal cells under RCM, may indicate recurrence. Owing to the deep location and extensive nature of nodular BCC, dermoscopy and RCM may not capture the full lesion, whereas HFUS effectively monitors thickness changes in skin lesions, aiding in determining tumor regression. Thus, noninvasive diagnostic technologies in PDT follow-up provide real-time, multipoint, and repeatable monitoring of skin lesion changes, guiding subsequent treatment and helping prevent recurrence (Fig. 16.3).

16.2.1.2 Actinic Keratosis

Actinic keratosis (AK) is a precancerous skin lesion commonly found in middle-aged and elderly individuals, primarily due to ultraviolet exposure. According to the 2021 expert consensus on the clinical diagnosis and treatment of AK in China, AK carries the risk of malignant transformation or progression to other nonmelanoma skin cancers (NMSCs), necessitating the management and/or treatment of all patients. Early detection and diagnosis are crucial for effective prevention and treatment. The gold standard for diagnosing AK is histopathology, which involves alternating parakeratosis and hyperkeratosis of the stratum corneum, atypical keratinocytes with large, dark-stained nuclei, and mildly disordered cell arrangement in a bud-like hyperplasia pattern in the epidermis, alongside solar elastosis and lymphocyte infiltration in the dermis. As AK primarily affects the epidermis, it can be easily detected via noninvasive diagnostic techniques such as dermoscopy and RCM.

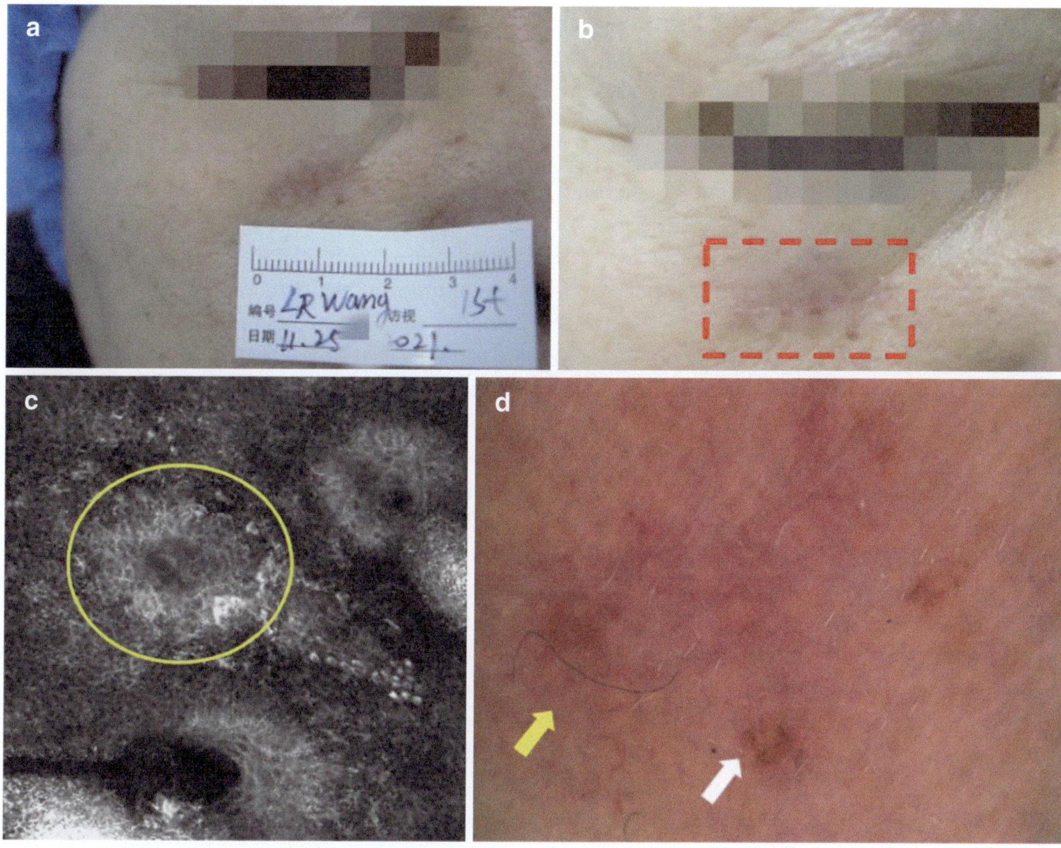

Fig. 16.3 Dermoscopy and RCM for evaluating residual BCC and indicating the continuation of photodynamic therapy. (**a**, **b**) Clinical images of BCC lesions after surgical resection. (**c**) RCM image showed that the epidermal cells were arranged in a disordered manner and that the tumor cells were arranged in a spoke-wheel shape. Bright tumor islands and highly refractive dendritic cells could be observed. (**d**) Dermoscopy revealed a red background with a central pink structureless area, surrounded by blue-gray globules at the periphery. Linear and small arbo- rizing blood vessels were noted at the edge of the skin lesion. Dermoscopy and RCM indicated residual BCC and further photodynamic therapy was considered

Dermoscopy features: Dermoscopy features of AK skin lesions are divided into three grades: Grade 1 shows a red pseudonetwork pattern, where hair follicle openings without pigment are visible against a red background, with discrete white scales on the surface and dot-like or linear blood vessels around the follicles. Grade 2 exhibited a strawberry-like pattern, with yellow-white, keratotic, enlarged follicular openings surrounded by a white halo and dot-like and irregular linear blood vessels. Grade 3 is characterized by obvious hyperkeratosis, yellow-white structureless areas, and enlarged follicular openings filled with keratotic plugs, with the surface covered by yellow-white scales and crust [38–40]. Dermoscopy is especially valuable for early screening of AK lesions.

RCM features: The main manifestations of AK skin lesions under RCM include: (1) hyperkeratosis or parakeratosis of the stratum corneum; (2) the arrangement of keratinocytes in the stratum spinosum is disordered, and the normal honeycomb structure is lost; and (3) keratinocytes are pleomorphic. Atypical keratinocytes with different sizes and shapes of nuclei are surrounded by highly reflective structures and blurred cell boundaries, which appear as target-shaped cells. (4) Medium-refractive substances around dermal collagen bundles. (5) Dilated blood vessels penetrate into the dermal papilla, and perivascular inflammatory infiltrates can be observed [41]. Disordered arrangement of the stratum spinosum and atypical keratinocytes are the key indications for RCM in diagnosing AK [42].

ALA-PDT is widely used to treat AK, particularly lesions on the head or face or those involving multiple or large areas [43]. The concept of "field cancerization" in AK has further highlighted the benefits of the "surface clearance" capabilities of PDT [44]. Noninvasive diagnostic tools such as Wood's lamp, dermoscopy, and RCM are integral to the entire ALA-PDT treatment and follow-up process, offering real-time, accurate, and noninvasive diagnostic support.

Before PDT treatment, dermoscopy and RCM can assist in diagnosis and differential diagnosis, such as detecting suspicious lesions, and help determine the target site for PDT [45]. The combined use of these methods allows comprehensive screening of AK lesions on the face, highlighting key or suspicious areas to guide treatment. During PDT, PDD helps mark the margins of the lesion, facilitating the treatment of "field cancerization." After PDT, dermoscopy can be used to monitor features such as basal pseudonetworks and yellow keratotic plugs, whereas RCM can be used to assess keratinocyte arrangement and morphology (Figs. 16.4 and 16.5). Changes in these features help evaluate treatment efficacy and guide decisions on continuing or terminating therapy. During follow-up, these tools enable real-time, noninvasive monitoring for potential AK recurrence, often detecting early signs before they are visible to the naked eye.

16.2.1.3 Cutaneous Squamous Cell Carcinoma

ALA-PDT is suitable for treating superficial and small cSCC, particularly in patients ineligible for surgery. Noninvasive diagnostic techniques such as dermoscopy and HFUS assist in the early diagnosis of cSCC, although the identification of invasive cSCC remains challenging [46–48].

Dermoscopic features: Dermatically, cSCC can present different characteristics depending on its subtype. Well-differentiated cSCC shows (1) yellow-white keratin in the center; (2) hairpin-like, irregular linear, and coiled vessels at the periphery; and (3) a pearl-like structure. If it is derived from the AK, the dermoscopic features of the AK can also be identified. Moderately differentiated cSCC commonly presents with peripheral loop-like blood vessels, diffuse yellow to light brown structureless areas, large erosions or ulcerations, and pearl-like structures. Poorly differentiated cSCC presents a polymorphous vascular pattern (>50% of the lesion), including numerous small linear irregular, hairpin, and coiled vessels on an erythematous background, occasionally with a peripheral white structureless area [40, 49].

HFUS features: cSCC under HFUS may present a hypoechoic irregular structure involving the dermis or the whole thickness of the skin. Owing to hyperkeratosis, the cSCC structure shows thick linear strong echoes with poorly defined irregular boundaries and a tendency to invade deep layers with enriched blood flow signals [50].

For application in PDT for cSCC, dermoscopy reveals characteristic patterns such as linear, hairpin, and polymorphous blood vessels, including coiled vessels, whereas HFUS accurately displays the depth and extent of tumor invasion. These diagnostic insights can be used to guide PDT treatment. HFUS can also identify tumor invasion into subcutaneous tissues, providing valuable information on tumor aggressiveness and prognosis. After effective PDT treatment, dermoscopy reveals the disappearance or reduction of cSCC-related features such as polymorphous vessels and pearl-like structures, whereas HFUS reveals reduced flow signals in the tumor area. The persistence or reappearance of these features posttreatment may indicate cSCC recurrence.

16.2.1.4 Other Skin Cancers

Extramammary Paget disease (EMPD) is a rare intraepithelial or invasive adenocarcinoma that occurs in anogenital skin. Dermoscopy features, though not fully elucidated, include the following [45]: (1) white-pink area; (2) irregularly distributed punctate, linear and glomerular blood vessels; (3) light gray to blue-gray punctate

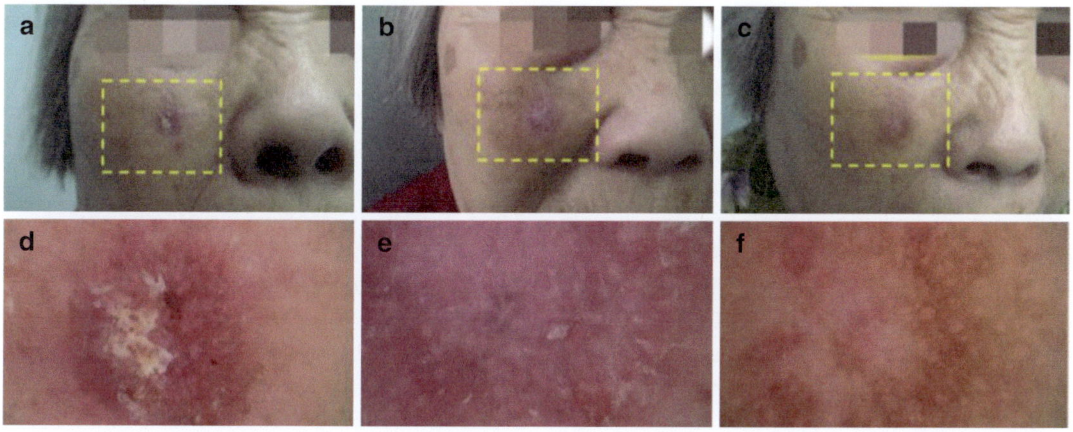

Fig. 16.4 The application of dermoscopy in the PDT of AK. (**a**, **d**) Before treatment, yellow scales, keratotic plugs, rosette signs, and pseudonetworks were obvious, exceeding the visible range of the naked eye. (**b**, **e**) After one session of ALA-PDT, a few scales could be observed, and the erythema subsided, while keratotic plugs and rosette signs remained, indicating the need to continue PDT. (**c**, **f**) After 3 sessions of ALA-PDT, there were no scales, and the erythema had basically subsided. Follicular keratotic plugs were not obvious, and the rosette sign disappeared, indicating the end point of PDT

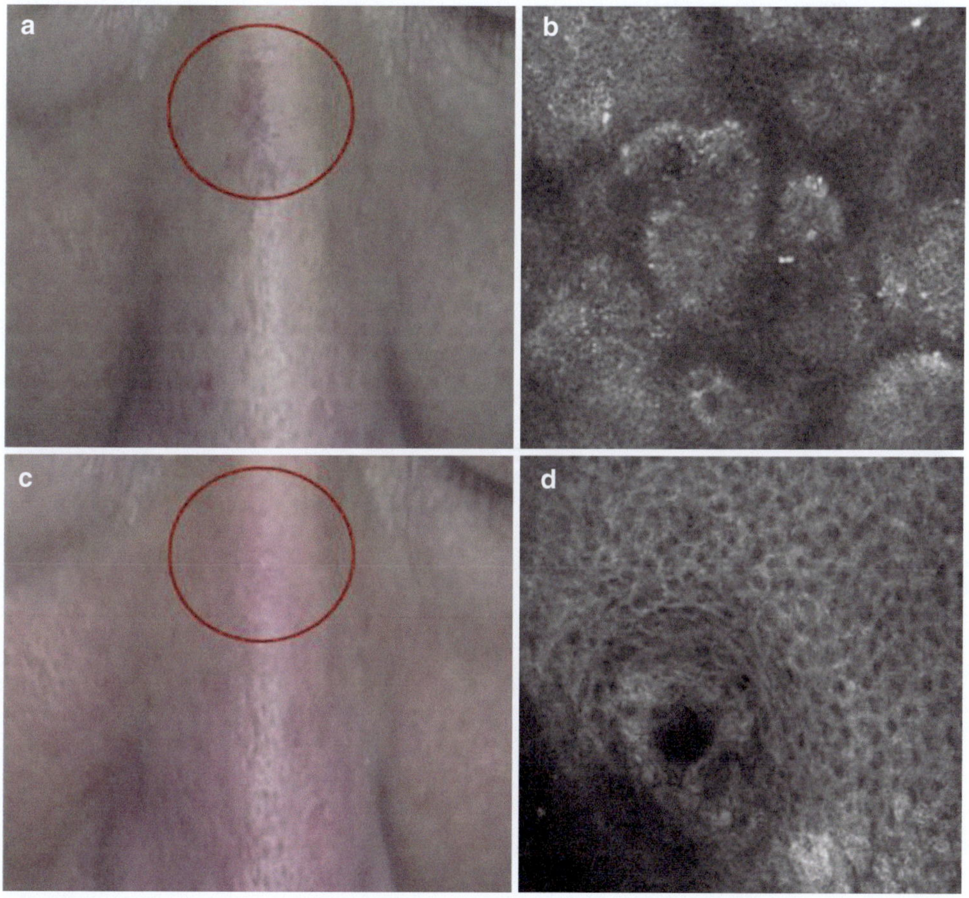

Fig. 16.5 Application of RCM in ALA-PDT of AK. (**a**, **b**) RCM before treatment revealed that the keratinocytes in the lesion area were arranged in a disordered manner, and a target-shaped distribution of atypical keratinocytes could be observed. (**c**, **d**) After three sessions of ALA-PDT, the arrangement of keratinocytes returned to normal

pigmentation (pepper powder-like); (4) shiny white streaks; (5) surface scales; and (6) ulceration. RCM reveals a disordered keratinocyte arrangement, Paget cells in the epidermis as large hypo-reflective cells with bright nuclei, dark glandular tumor nests in the basal layer and dermoepidermal junction, dilated tortuous vessels, inflammatory infiltrates [51], and highly reflective dendritic cells [52, 53]. HFUS distinguishes diffuse and tumor types of EMPD with features such as thickened skin, poorly defined margins, uneven echoes, and varying internal blood flow [54]. Although dermoscopy, RCM, and HFUS face limitations due to EMPD's extensive involvement and genital location, they are valuable for noninvasive, real-time, repeatable assessment. Before hematoporphyrin derivative photodynamic therapy (HpD-PDT) for EMPD, PDD aids in treatment planning and lesion identification, whereas HFUS can be used to evaluate invasion depth. Post-PDT, regular follow-up with dermoscopy, RCM, and HFUS helps monitor for recurrence and guide further management [10] (Fig. 16.6).

16.2.2 Application of Noninvasive Diagnosis in HMME-PDT for Port Wine Stain

Noninvasive diagnostic technology is increasingly applied in PDT treatment for various diseases. HMME-PDT is effective for treating PWS, where traditional efficacy evaluation relies largely on visual assessment, often capturing only the "tip of the iceberg." Recently, noninvasive or minimally invasive methods have demonstrated significant advantages in evaluating the clinical efficacy of PWS, offering more accurate, comprehensive, and objective assessments [55].

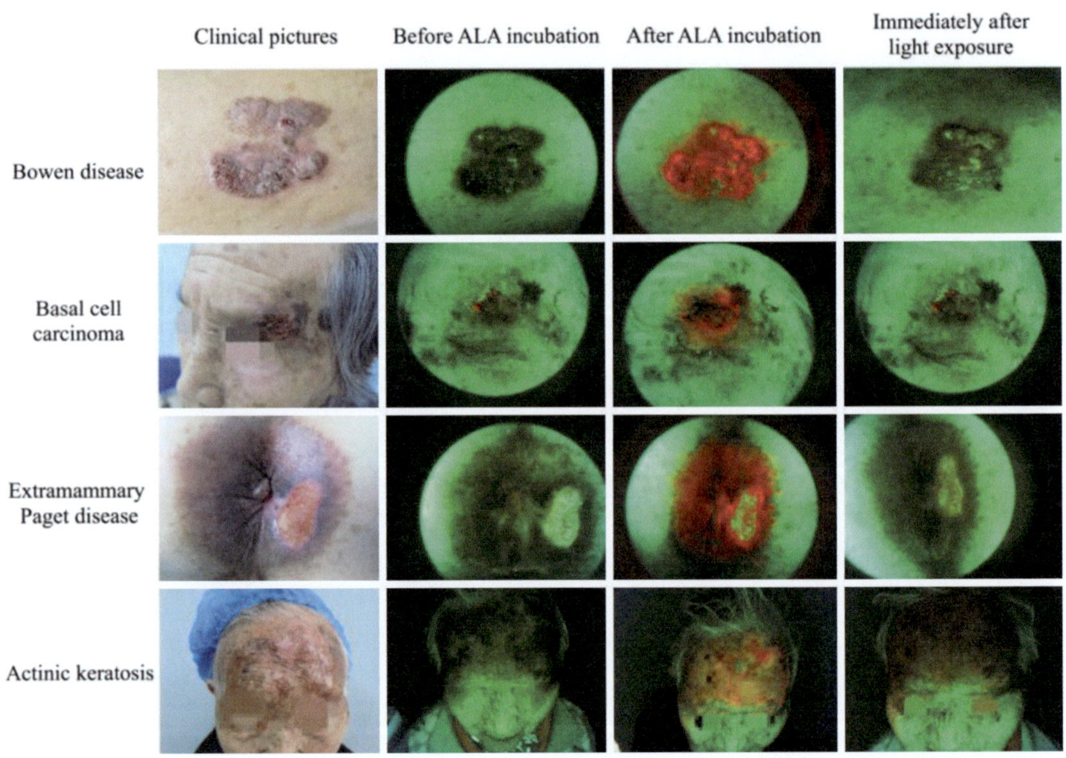

Fig. 16.6 PDD is used in the diagnosis and treatment of NMSC and AK lesions. There was no fluorescence in the skin lesions under Wood's light before ALA incubation. After incubation, PpIX fluorescence was enriched in the tumor lesions, and the true margin was slightly larger than the clinically determined margin. After illumination, the fluorescence-enriched area is significantly reduced

Among noninvasive techniques, the VISIA-CR™ skin analysis system, dermoscopy, HFUS, and LSCI are widely used for evaluating PWS lesions before and after HMME-PDT because of their ability to reflect vascular features, blood perfusion, and lesion thickness [2]. Research by the authors' group revealed that the VISIA-CR™ system captures standard images and accurately analyzes erythema regression through RBX red imaging (see Fig. 13.4 in Chap. 13). Dermoscopy aids in the clinical classification of PWS and the assessment of vascular injury in lesion areas post-PDT, guiding treatment dose adjustments and determining end points, which are critical for evaluating efficacy (see Fig. 13.5 in Chap. 13). HFUS and LSCI detect skin and lesion thickness pre- and post-treatment, whereas LSCI also measures blood perfusion, supporting therapeutic effect evaluation (Figs. 16.7 and 16.8). Together, these techniques complement one another, offering insights into lesion depth, resolution, and dynamic changes during HMME-PDT for PWS.

Tao et al. identified two main dermoscopic patterns for PWS: Type 1, a superficial pattern of red globules and dots corresponding to dilated capillaries in the dermal papilla, and Type 2, a deep pattern of red annular structures linked to a dilated vascular plexus in the deep dermis. During HMME-PDT for PWS, Type 1 lesions show a good response and are easier to clear, whereas Type 2 lesions are more resistant and less effective to treat [56]. Further research revealed that dotted and bulbous blood vessels, short rod-shaped vessels, and curved vessels respond well to HMME-PDT, whereas pale halos and arborizing vessels show a partial response. Lesions with mixed blood vessels, gray-white homogeneous structures, and reticular patterns respond poorly [57]. Therefore, dermoscopy aids in evaluating vessel patterns, supporting pre- and post-HMME-PDT assessments and monitoring treatment efficacy in PWS.

Liu et al. utilized 15 MHz HFUS to assess the thickness and density of lesions in 45 PWS patients and reported that after HMME-PDT, the skin thickness decreased while the density increased. Notably, lesion thickness changed most significantly in the treatment-responsive groups. These findings suggest that the therapeutic efficacy of HMME-PDT is closely associated with the thickness and density of PWS lesions [58].

In addition to HMME-PDT, noninvasive skin diagnostic technologies have been used for other therapies for PWS. Lu et al. focused on RCM to observe the diameter, depth, density, and blood flow of blood vessels in PWS lesions before and after pulsed dye laser treatment and reported that blood flow, vessel diameter, and depth were key factors contributing to laser resistance, whereas vessel density was not [59]. Marta Fusano et al. identified three RCM patterns in refractory PWS lesions: (1) linear blood vessels in the superficial dermis with smaller diameters and higher blood flow velocity; (2) dilated vessels with high blood flow velocity in the neural plexus below the dermal papilla; and (3) aneurysmal vasodilation in the deep dermis with slower blood flow than the other types [60]. While RCM has not been widely used for diagnostic evaluation in HMME-PDT treatment, these studies highlight its potential for pretreatment efficacy prediction and parameter optimization.

OCT can also be used to assess the PWS, although traditional OCT is limited by its insufficient resolution for imaging skin blood vessels. Gu's team developed a functional mode of OCT, optical coherence tomography angiography (OCTA), by combining it with complex algorithms, which allows for the extraction of quantitative information within 800 μm from the skin surface, such as blood vessel density, diameter, and depth. Using this technology, the team characterized the vascular morphology of PWS lesions and quantified the depth of dilated blood vessels on the basis of OCTA images. Their results revealed that blood vessels in PWS lesions had larger diameters and greater density than those in contralateral normal skin, with PWS lesions having a blood vessel diameter of 73 μm ± 14 μm, ranging from 10 μm to 150 μm, compared with 28 μm ± 2 μm in normal skin, ranging from 10 μm to 60 μm. Among the different types of PWS lesions, the thickened type has larger blood vessel diameters and higher density

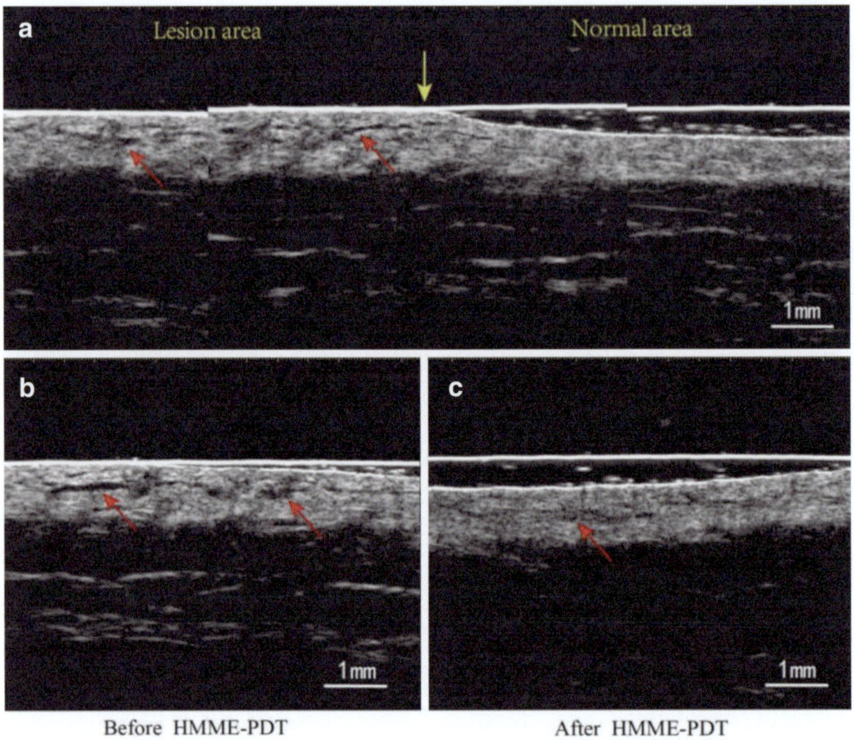

Fig. 16.7 HFUS for PWS patients with HMME-PDT. (**a**) HFUS revealed greater thickness in lesional skin than in normal nonlesional skin, the dermis was loosely arranged, and a linear hypoechoic signal was observed. (**b**, **c**) After HMME-PDT, the thickened dermis became thinner The linear hypoechoic signal was significantly reduced to normal. (Red arrows: abnormal dermal blood vessels; yellow arrows: boundaries between lesional and normal skin)

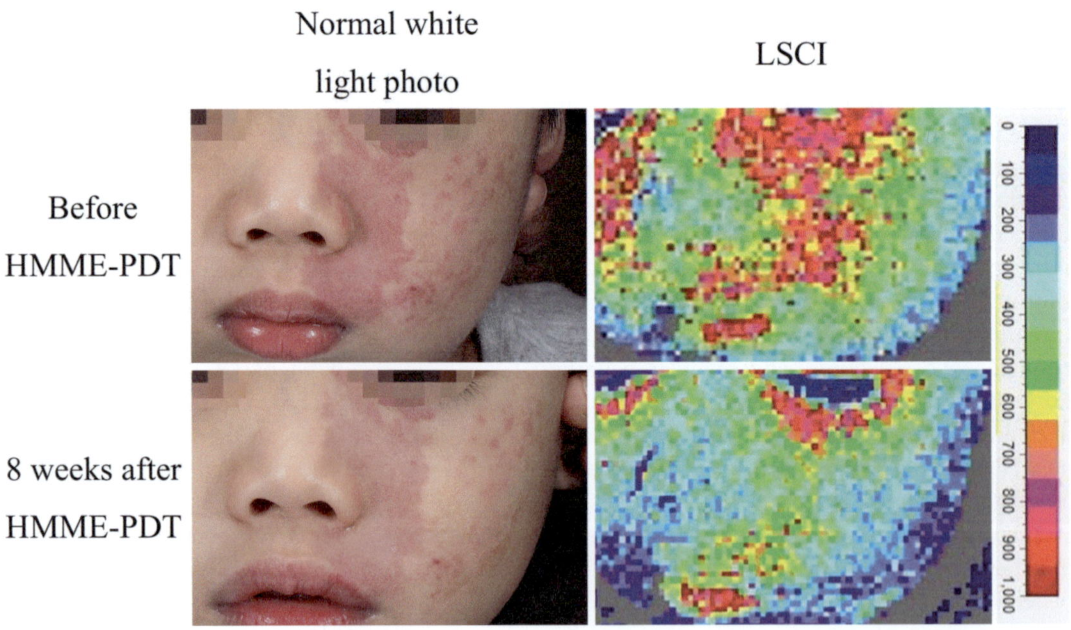

Fig. 16.8 LSCI for PWS patients with HMME-PDT. Compared with before treatment (**a**, **c**), the erythema in the treatment area subsided (**b**), and LSCI revealed that the blood perfusion signal was significantly reduced (**d**) in 8 weeks after treatment

than the purple-red type does [61]. Therefore, OCTA provides three-dimensional visualization of the in vivo structure and vasculature of PWS lesions, offers superior capabilities for accurately and comprehensively assessing skin lesions, and holds promise for full evaluation of the HMME-PDT of PWS.

In recent years, photoacoustic imaging (PAI), an emerging noninvasive diagnostic technology, has been explored in dermatology. As PAI combines structural and functional imaging, the authors' team applied it for the clinical evaluation of PWS and the efficacy evaluation of HMME-PDT for the first time [62] (Fig. 16.9). Through PAI of the PWS lesion area, we introduced a quantitative biomarker for PWS evaluation, the PWS level (PWS level = average PAI signal intensity in the PWS lesion area/average PAI signal intensity in the normal skin area). This approach is more quantitative and accurate than conventional noninvasive techniques and aids in the classification of PWS. Furthermore, comparing the level of PWS before and after treatment can be used to quantify improvements in skin lesions. In our comparison, the PWS of patients younger than 18 years ($n = 25$) was significantly lower than that of patients older than 18 years ($n = 10$). Additionally, the level of PWS in patients with purple–red-type PWS ($n = 20$) was significantly greater than that in those with red-type PWS ($n = 13$). Therefore, PAI may serve as an innovative and practical tool in the diagnosis and treatment of vascular-related skin diseases.

16.2.3 Application of Noninvasive Diagnosis in Other Diseases

As PDT treatment has become increasingly widespread in dermatology, the application of noninvasive diagnostic technologies in PDT has also expanded. For example, dermoscopy combined with RCM can be used to evaluate and monitor the efficacy of PDT for the treatment of rosacea. Dermoscopy can clearly show improvements in erythema and dilated blood vessels, whereas RCM can provide direct visualization of reduced inflammation and decreased Demodex in hair follicles (Fig. 16.10). These techniques are also valuable for clinical efficacy evaluation and disease follow-up in PDT treatment for conditions such as acne, genital warts, and other skin disorders.

Noninvasive skin diagnostic technologies offer the advantages of being noninvasive, real-time, multifocal, and repeatable, playing a crucial role in the diagnosis, PDT treatment, and follow-up of skin diseases. These technologies have significant clinical value throughout the entire PDT process, including disease diagnosis, monitoring of activity, parameter selection, treatment strategy adjustment, and recurrence monitoring.

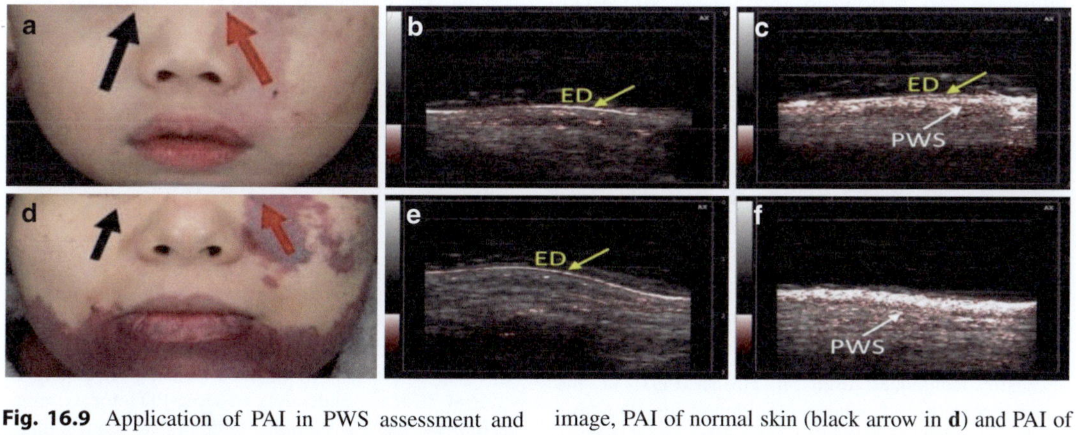

Fig. 16.9 Application of PAI in PWS assessment and HMME-PDT. (**a**–**c**) Gross image, PAI of normal skin (black arrow in figure **a**) and PAI of a PSW lesion (red arrow in figure **a**) in a red-type PWS child; (**d**–**f**) gross image, PAI of normal skin (black arrow in **d**) and PAI of the skin lesion (red arrow in **d**) in an adult patient with purple-red PWS

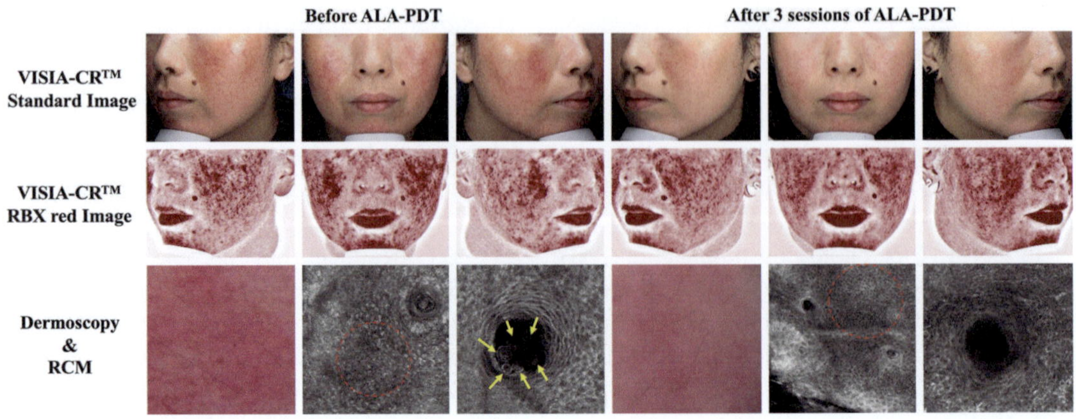

Fig. 16.10 Application of noninvasive diagnostic technology in the ALA-PDT of rosacea. The VISIA-CR™ system clearly showed the regression of erythema, which is more obvious on RBX imaging. Dermoscopy revealed that dilated capillaries were reduced and subsided after treatment. RCM revealed a decrease in lesional inflammation and Demodex colonization in hair follicles

Before PDT, noninvasive diagnostics assist in diagnosis with high consistency, repeatability, and precise positioning, aiding in determining the treatment area and assessing the stage and differentiation of NMSCs. During treatment, they help define lesion margins and track lesion changes after each session, facilitating treatment response evaluation and determining treatment endpoints. During follow-up, they allow for dynamic monitoring of lesion changes, disease outcomes, and recurrence. In conclusion, the optimal selection and combination of noninvasive skin diagnostic technologies provide comprehensive, three-dimensional support for diagnosis and follow-up throughout the PDT treatment process.

References

1. Schneider SL, Kohli I, Hamzavi IH, Rossi AM, Ozog DM. Emerging imaging technologies in dermatology: part I: basic principles. J Am Acad Dermatol. 2019;80(4):1114–20. https://doi.org/10.1016/j.jaad.2018.11.042.
2. Wen L, Zhang Y, Zhang L, Liu X, Wang P, Shen S, et al. Application of different noninvasive diagnostic techniques used in HMME-PDT in the treatment of port wine stains. Photodiagn Photodyn Ther. 2019;25:369–75. https://doi.org/10.1016/j.pdpdt.2019.01.008.
3. Klatte JL, van der Beek N, Kemperman PM. 100 years of wood's lamp revised. J Eur Acad Dermatol Venereol. 2015;29(5):842–7. https://doi.org/10.1111/jdv.12860.
4. Hong-wei W, Xiu-li W. Wood lamp dermatology practical technique diagram. Shanghai: Shanghai Scientific and Technical Publishers; 2014.
5. Ting LV, Bo W, Hongwei W. Application of wood lamp in pigmented and infectious skin diseases. Chin Med Abstr. 2018;35(2):210–5.
6. Wu Y, Wang P, Zhang L, Wang B, Wang X. Enhancement of photodynamic therapy for Bowen's disease using plum-blossom needling to augment drug delivery. Dermatol Surg. 2018;44(12):1516–24. https://doi.org/10.1097/dss.0000000000001608.
7. Chen J, Zhang Y, Wang P, Wang B, Zhang G, Wang X. Plum-blossom needling promoted PpIX fluorescence intensity from 5-aminolevulinic acid in porcine skin model and patients with actnic keratosis. Photodiagn Photodyn Ther. 2016;15:182–90. https://doi.org/10.1016/j.pdpdt.2016.06.012.
8. Ding HL, Wang XL, Wang HW, Huang Z. Successful treatment of refractory facial acne using repeat short-cycle ALA-PDT: case study. Photodiagn Photodyn Ther. 2011;8(4):343–6. https://doi.org/10.1016/j.pdpdt.2011.07.003.
9. Wang HW, Wang XL, Zhang LL, Guo MX, Huang Z. Aminolevulinic acid (ALA)-assisted photodynamic diagnosis of subclinical and latent HPV infection of external genital region. Photodiagn Photodyn Ther. 2008;5(4):251–5. https://doi.org/10.1016/j.pdpdt.2008.11.004.
10. Wang D, Wang P, Li C, Zhou Z, Zhang L, Zhang G, et al. Efficacy and safety of HpD-PDT for extramammary Paget's disease refractory to conventional therapy: a prospective, open-label and single arm pilot

study. Photodiagn Photodyn Ther. 2022;37:102670. https://doi.org/10.1016/j.pdpdt.2021.102670.
11. Xiu-li W, Hongwei W, Ling-lin Z, Ming-xia GUO, Lina SU, Ji-ning TAO. Application of 5-amino-ketovalerate photodynamics in diagnosis of condyloma acuminatum. Chin J Dermatol. 2008;41(5):296–300. https://doi.org/10.3321/j.issn:0412-4030.2008.05.006.
12. Gunaydin G, Gedik ME, Ayan S. Photodynamic therapy for the treatment and diagnosis of cancer-a review of the current clinical status. Front Chem. 2021;9:686303. https://doi.org/10.3389/fchem.2021.686303.
13. Yélamos O, Braun RP, Liopyris K, Wolner ZJ, Kerl K, Gerami P, et al. Dermoscopy and dermatopathology correlates of cutaneous neoplasms. J Am Acad Dermatol. 2019;80(2):341–63. https://doi.org/10.1016/j.jaad.2018.07.073.
14. Levy J, Barrett DL, Harris N, Jeong JJ, Yang X, Chen SC. High-frequency ultrasound in clinical dermatology: a review. Ultrasound J. 2021;13(1):24. https://doi.org/10.1186/s13089-021-00222-w.
15. Menglong R, Hang L, Man L. Expert consensus on high-frequency skin ultrasound diagnosis of common skin diseases. Chin Med Front J. 2019;11(8):23–8. https://doi.org/10.12037/yxqy.2019.08-04.
16. Csuka EA, Ward SC, Ekelem C, Csuka DA, Ardigò M, Mesinkovska NA. Reflectance confocal microscopy, optical coherence tomography, and multiphoton microscopy in inflammatory skin disease diagnosis. Lasers Surg Med. 2021;53(6):776–97. https://doi.org/10.1002/lsm.23386.
17. Yan L, Huaxu L. Expert consensus on diagnostic features of reflective confocal microscopy for pigmented dermatosis. Chin Med Front J. 2019;11(8):29–33. https://doi.org/10.12037/yxqy.2019.08-05.
18. Liuqing C, Qian J. Expert consensus on diagnostic features of reflective confocal microscopy for inflammatory skin diseases. Chin Med Front J. 2019;11(8):34–40. https://doi.org/10.12037/yxqy.2019.08-06.
19. Goldsberry A, Hanke CW, Hanke KE. VISIA system: a possible tool in the cosmetic practice. J Drugs Dermatol. 2014;13(11):1312–4.
20. Shen D, Wei J, Chen L, Shen X, Wang L. In addition to photothermal effects, low-level CO(2) laser irradiation can potentiate skin microcirculation through photobiomodulation mechanisms. Photobiomodul Photomed Laser Surg. 2019;37(3):151–8. https://doi.org/10.1089/photob.2018.4570.
21. Levine A, Wang K, Markowitz O. Optical coherence tomography in the diagnosis of skin cancer. Dermatol Clin. 2017;35(4):465–88. https://doi.org/10.1016/j.det.2017.06.008.
22. Münter M, Vom Endt M, Pieper M, Casper M, Ahrens M, Kohlfaerber T, et al. Dynamic contrast in scanning microscopic OCT. Opt Lett. 2020;45(17):4766–9. https://doi.org/10.1364/ol.396134.
23. Olsovsky C, Hinsdale T, Cuenca R, Cheng YL, Wright JM, Rees TD, et al. Handheld tunable focus confocal microscope utilizing a double-clad fiber coupler for in vivo imaging of oral epithelium. J Biomed Opt. 2017;22(5):56008. https://doi.org/10.1117/1.Jbo.22.5.056008.
24. Li R, Phillips E, Wang P, Goergen CJ, Cheng JX. Label-free in vivo imaging of peripheral nerve by multispectral photoacoustic tomography. J Biophotonics. 2016;9(1–2):124–8. https://doi.org/10.1002/jbio.201500004.
25. Huang S, Qin Y, Chen Y, Pan J, Xu C, Wu D, et al. Interstitial assessment of aggressive prostate cancer by physio-chemical photoacoustics: an ex vivo study with intact human prostates. Med Phys. 2018. https://doi.org/10.1002/mp.13061.
26. Chu Z, Long W, Peiru W, Xiu-li W. Progress in the application of photoacoustic imaging in skin tumors. Chin J Dermatol. 2021;54(3):256–9. https://doi.org/10.35541/cjd.20190884.
27. Long WEN, Pei-ru W, Xiu-li W. Research progress of photoacoustic technology in skin diseases. Chin J Laser Med. 2019;28(2):107–11. https://doi.org/10.13480/j.issn1003-9430.2019.0107.
28. Kuflik AS, Janniger CK. Basal cell carcinoma. Am Fam Physician. 1993;48(7):1273–6.
29. Wozniak-Rito A, Zalaudek I, Rudnicka L. Dermoscopy of basal cell carcinoma. Clin Exp Dermatol. 2018;43(3):241–7. https://doi.org/10.1111/ced.13387.
30. Dermatology Imaging Group of Dermatology and Venereology Committee of Chinese Association of Integrated Traditional and Western Medicine. Expert consensus on dermoscopic features of basal cell carcinoma in China. Chin J Dermatol. 2019;52(6):371–7. https://doi.org/10.3760/cma.j.issn.0412-4030.2019.06.001.
31. Wang SQ, Liu J, Zhu QL, Zhao CY, Qu T, Li F, et al. High-frequency ultrasound features of basal cell carcinoma and its association with histological recurrence risk. Chin Med J. 2019;132(17):2021–6. https://doi.org/10.1097/cm9.0000000000000369.
32. Rubinstein G, Garfinkel J, Jain M. Live, remote control of an in vivo reflectance confocal microscope for diagnosis of basal cell carcinoma at the bedside of a patient 2500 miles away: a novel tele-reflectance confocal microscope approach. J Am Acad Dermatol. 2019;81(2):e41–2. https://doi.org/10.1016/j.jaad.2019.02.016.
33. Lupu M, Popa IM, Voiculescu VM, Boda D, Caruntu C, Zurac S, et al. A retrospective study of the diagnostic accuracy of in vivo reflectance confocal microscopy for basal cell carcinoma diagnosis and subtyping. J Clin Med. 2019;8(4):449. https://doi.org/10.3390/jcm8040449.
34. Holmes J, von Braunmühl T, Berking C, Sattler E, Ulrich M, Reinhold U, et al. Optical coherence tomography of basal cell carcinoma: influence of location, subtype, observer variability and image quality on diagnostic performance. Br J Dermatol. 2018;178(5):1102–10. https://doi.org/10.1111/bjd.16154.

35. Meekings A, Utz S, Ulrich M, Bienenfeld A, Nandanan N, Fisher J, et al. Differentiation of basal cell carcinoma subtypes in multi-beam swept source optical coherence tomography (MSS-OCT). J Drugs Dermatol. 2016;15(5):545–50.
36. Branch Light Medical Treatment Equipment Group. Clinical application guide of photodynamic therapy for dermatology (2021 edition). Chin J Dermatol. 2021;54(1):1–9. https://doi.org/10.35541/cjd.20200731.
37. Venturini M, Sala R, Gonzàlez S, Calzavara-Pinton PG. Reflectance confocal microscopy allows in vivo real-time noninvasive assessment of the outcome of methyl aminolaevulinate photodynamic therapy of basal cell carcinoma. Br J Dermatol. 2013;168(1):99–105. https://doi.org/10.1111/bjd.12052.
38. Gutzmer R, Wiegand S, Kölbl O, Wermker K, Heppt M, Berking C. Actinic keratosis and cutaneous squamous cell carcinoma. Dtsch Arztebl Int. 2019;116(37):616–26. https://doi.org/10.3238/arztebl.2019.0616.
39. Labadie JG, Compres E, Sunshine JC, Alam M, Gerami P, Harikumar V, et al. Actinic keratosis color and its associations: a retrospective photographic, dermoscopic, and histologic evaluation. Dermatol Surg. 2022;48(1):57–60. https://doi.org/10.1097/dss.0000000000003281.
40. Dermatological Department of China Council for the Promotion of Health Care International Exchange Branch Skin Image Group Chinese Medicine Skin Disease. Expert consensus on dermoscopic features of squamous cell tumors. Chin J Dermatol. 2018;51(2):87–91. https://doi.org/10.3760/cma.j.issn.0412-4030.2018.02.001.
41. Arisi M, Zane C, Polonioli M, Tomasi C, Moggio E, Cozzi C, et al. Effects of MAL-PDT, ingenol mebutate and diclofenac plus hyaluronate gel monitored by high-frequency ultrasound and digital dermoscopy in actinic keratosis - a randomized trial. J Eur Acad Dermatol Venereol. 2020;34(6):1225–32. https://doi.org/10.1111/jdv.16123.
42. Prow TW, Tan JM, Pellacani G. Reflectance confocal microscopy: hallmarks of keratinocyte cancer and its precursors. Curr Probl Dermatol. 2015;46:85–94. https://doi.org/10.1159/000366541.
43. Chinese Medicine Skin Disease Rehabilitation Skin Venereology Professional Committee of the Chinese Medical Association Branch of Photodynamic Therapy Research Center. Expert consensus on the clinical diagnosis and treatment of photolinear keratosis in China. Chin J Dermatol. 2021;54(12):1048–56. https://doi.org/10.35541/cjd.20210561.
44. Willenbrink TJ, Ruiz ES, Cornejo CM, Schmults CD, Arron ST, Jambusaria-Pahlajani A. Field cancerization: definition, epidemiology, risk factors, and outcomes. J Am Acad Dermatol. 2020;83(3):709–17. https://doi.org/10.1016/j.jaad.2020.03.126.
45. Xiaoqin Y, Chan H, Long W, Yuting X, Keyal U, Guolong Z, et al. Dermoscopic monitoring for treatment and follow-up of actinic keratosis with 5-aminolaevulinic acid photodynamic therapy. Technol Cancer Res Treat. 2018;17:1533033818820091. https://doi.org/10.1177/1533033818820091.
46. Fania L, Didona D, Di Pietro FR, Verkhovskaia S, Morese R, Paolino G, et al. Cutaneous squamous cell carcinoma: from pathophysiology to novel therapeutic approaches. Biomedicine. 2021;9(2):171. https://doi.org/10.3390/biomedicines9020171.
47. Keyal U, Bhatta AK, Zhang G, Wang XL. Present and future perspectives of photodynamic therapy for cutaneous squamous cell carcinoma. J Am Acad Dermatol. 2019;80(3):765–73. https://doi.org/10.1016/j.jaad.2018.10.042.
48. Venereology Branch Skin Cancer Research Center of Chinese Medical Association Dermatologists Branch. Expert consensus on skin squamous cell carcinoma. Chin J Dermatol. 2021;54(8):653–64. https://doi.org/10.35541/cjd.20201140.
49. Hu C, Liu X, Wang P, Guo L, Li C, Xu M, et al. Dermoscopy and ultrosound monitoring actinic keratosis with cutaneous squamous cell carcinoma: a case report and literature review. Photodiagn Photodyn Ther. 2022;37:102709. https://doi.org/10.1016/j.pdpdt.2021.102709.
50. Chen ZT, Yan JN, Zhu AQ, Wang LF, Wang Q, Li L, et al. High-frequency ultrasound for differentiation between high-risk basal cell carcinoma and cutaneous squamous cell carcinoma. Skin Res Technol. 2022;28(3):410–8. https://doi.org/10.1111/srt.13121.
51. Ishizuki S, Nakamura Y. Extramammary Paget's disease: diagnosis, pathogenesis, and treatment with focus on recent developments. Curr Oncol. 2021;28(4):2969–86. https://doi.org/10.3390/curroncol28040260.
52. Pan ZY, Liang J, Zhang QA, Lin JR, Zheng ZZ. In vivo reflectance confocal microscopy of extramammary Paget disease: diagnostic evaluation and surgical management. J Am Acad Dermatol. 2012;66(2):47–53. https://doi.org/10.1016/j.jaad.2010.09.722.
53. Yélamos O, Hibler BP, Cordova M, Hollmann TJ, Kose K, Marchetti MA, et al. Handheld reflectance confocal microscopy for the detection of recurrent extramammary Paget disease. JAMA Dermatol. 2017;153(7):689–93. https://doi.org/10.1001/jamadermatol.2017.0619.
54. Lei Z, Panpan Y, Liya Z, Yangcan D. Characteristic analysis of high frequency color Doppler ultrasound in Paget disease outside breast. Chin J Dermatol. 2021;54(7):625–8. https://doi.org/10.35541/cjd.20200425.
55. Li DC, Nong X, Hu ZY, Fang TW, Zhao TT, Sun SH, et al. Efficacy and related factors analysis in HMME-PDT in the treatment of port wine stains. Photodiagn Photodyn Ther. 2020;29:101649. https://doi.org/10.1016/j.pdpdt.2020.101649.
56. Li Y, Wang X, Liu Y, Tao J. Dermoscopy predicts outcome in hemoporfin-mediated photodynamic therapy of port-wine stains: a prospective observational study.

J Am Acad Dermatol. 2020;83(6):1765–7. https://doi.org/10.1016/j.jaad.2020.03.063.
57. Wang X, Suo H, Gao Y, Du H, Fu Y, Sha S, et al. Correlation between the hemoporfin-mediated photodynamic treatment response and the dermoscopy vascular pattern in patients with a port-wine stain: a prospective study. J Eur Acad Dermatol Venereol. 2020;34(12):2795–801. https://doi.org/10.1111/jdv.16596.
58. Khalaf AT, Sun Y, Wang F, Sheng M, Li Y, Liu X. Photodynamic therapy using HMME for port-wine stains: clinical effectiveness and sonographic appearance. Biomed Res Int. 2020;2020:6030581. https://doi.org/10.1155/2020/6030581.
59. Fu Z, Huang J, Xiang Y, Huang J, Tang Z, Chen J, et al. Characterization of laser-resistant port wine stain blood vessels using in vivo reflectance confocal microscopy. Lasers Surg Med. 2019;51(10):841–9. https://doi.org/10.1002/lsm.23134.
60. Fusano M, Bencini PL. Capillaroscopy and reflectance confocal microscopy characterization of refractory port-wine stains. Lasers Med Sci. 2021;36(2):407–12. https://doi.org/10.1007/s10103-020-03084-1.
61. Liu Y, Chen D, Xu J, Tan Y, Wang Y, Zhao H, et al. Quantitative assessment of vascular features in port wine stains through optical coherence tomography angiography. Photodiagn Photodyn Ther. 2021;36:102607. https://doi.org/10.1016/j.pdpdt.2021.102607.
62. Zhang H, Zhang G, Zhang Y, Wen L, Zhang M, Pan J, et al. Quantitatively assessing port-wine stains using a photoacoustic imaging method: a pilot study. J Am Acad Dermatol. 2021;85(6):1613–6. https://doi.org/10.1016/j.jaad.2020.12.024.

Future Prospects of Photodynamic Therapy in Dermatology

17

Peiru Wang, Bo Wang, and Xiuli Wang

Photodynamic therapy (PDT) and photodynamic fluorescence diagnosis (PDD) have widespread applications across various medical fields, including dermatology, gynecology, dentistry, ophthalmology, otolaryngology, gastroenterology, pulmonology, and neurology. Among these, ALA-PDT is the most widely used and well-established method in dermatology. This book provides a comprehensive review of the development of PDT, covering key topics such as the development of skin disease-specific photosensitizers, light sources, the mechanisms of PDT, and solutions to PDT-related pain management. The clinical section is divided into ten chapters, primarily focusing on ALA-PDT treatments for skin cancers, HPV-related diseases, follicular and sebaceous gland disorders, hemangiomas, skin aging, and other refractory conditions. It also introduces HMME-PDT for treating vascular malformations and HpD-PDT for treating invasive skin squamous cell carcinoma and extramammary Paget's disease.

The application of PDT in dermatology has expanded to over 3000 hospitals in China, benefiting hundreds of thousands of patients. However, the clinical adoption of PDT varies across countries and regions, with some areas not fully recognizing its potential. Many clinicians still adhere to traditional diagnostic and treatment approaches, limiting their understanding of recent developments in PDT. In tumor treatment, both the depth and clinical efficacy of PDT need further enhancement. Additional research on the mechanisms, as well as improvements in photosensitizers and light sources, is essential for advancing clinical applications. The adoption of PDT as a new adjunctive therapy concept will also help expand its clinical use. For refractory skin conditions, the advantages of PDT, such as being minimally invasive, repeatable, almost no drug resistant, and causing fewer side effects, should be fully utilized, with ongoing refinement of targeted PDT strategies. The pain issue that once limited use of PDT has been addressed with the introduction of modified painless ALA-PDT, though further research on PDT-related pain could significantly improve future applications. For common dermatological diseases, such as hair follicle and sebaceous gland disorders or antiaging treatments, PDT is increasingly moving toward home use, allowing more individuals to benefit. Addressing the ongoing challenges

P. Wang · X. Wang (✉)
Institute of Photomedicine, Shanghai Skin Disease Hospital, School of Medicine, Tongji University, Shanghai, China
e-mail: wangpeiru@tongji.edu.cn; wangxiuli_1400023@tongji.edu.cn

B. Wang
Avera Medical Group Dermatology, Aberdeen, SD, USA

University of South Dakota, Vermillion, SD, USA
e-mail: makiwang@med.umich.edu

X. Wang, B. Wang (eds.), *Photodynamic Therapy in Dermatology*,
https://doi.org/10.1007/978-981-96-8915-6_17

and bottlenecks in PDT will be key areas of focus for future research.

17.1 Improving the Efficiency of Photodynamic Therapy

PDT has been successfully applied to treat various malignant cancers, but some cancers remain resistant to PDT, requiring improvements in the efficacy and management of adverse reactions. A common limitation is the photosensitizer precursor ALA, which has limited penetration and light depth, reducing the clinical effectiveness of PDT. Future research should focus on the following areas: (1) New photosensitizers that can be targeted and uniformly delivered to the treatment area, enhance the oxygen effect, improve permeability, and distribute the photosensitizer more uniformly to improve therapeutic outcomes have been developed. Additionally, dual-reactive photosensitizers that combine PDT and photothermal therapy could enhance antitumor efficacy, particularly for cancers such as malignant melanoma that are resistant to traditional PDT. The main challenge for new nanoloaded PSs remains their compatibility and safety for clinical use, although nanoliposomes such as BF-200 and verteporfin, which have already been used in clinical practice, offer promising examples. (2) New light sources or excitation sources are needed to address the depth limitations of current light sources in PDT. This includes intratissue irradiation, longer wavelength light sources, and new excitation methods based on upconversion materials. Nonlaser excitation sources, such as ultrasound and X-rays, could also be explored for their ability to induce antitumor effects similar to those of PDT. Although their excitation efficiency is currently lower than that of lasers, improving photosensitizers could make these alternatives more viable for clinical use. (3) The development of PDT adjuvants is crucial to improving their efficacy. Previous studies, such as those by Xiuli Wang's team, have shown that immune adjuvants such as imiquimod and PD-1 antibodies can enhance the antitumor effects of PDT. PDT can trigger tumor antigen release, recruit immune cells, and promote antitumor immunity through mechanisms such as apoptosis, pyroptosis, and ferroptosis. Further research into the immune mechanisms of PDT and the development of immune adjuvants could significantly improve the effectiveness of tumor PDT treatment.

17.2 The Concept of Neoadjuvant PDT in Cancer

An increasing number of studies have highlighted that the mechanism of PDT treatment extends beyond the synergistic effects of photosensitizers, light, and oxygen in targeted tissues. PDT also has other promising effects, including antitumor immune responses and the promotion of tissue repair, which deserve further attention. PDT is a local, targeted therapy that is not prone to drug resistance, and it can activate local antitumor immunity, improve the tumor microenvironment, and potentially uncover additional mechanisms still to be explored. In clinical practice, PDT plays a vital role throughout the entire process of skin tumor treatment, including reversing skin photoaging; treating precancerous lesions and superficial cancers; assisting in the treatment of thicker, deeper cancers when combined with surgery or laser therapy; and providing palliative care for advanced cancers to improve patient quality of life. Drawing on 26 years of clinical application and foundational research by the authors' team, PDT can be performed before or after tumor surgery and combined with laser therapy to reduce the tumor burden and activate antitumor immune effects. This innovative concept, called tumor neoadjuvant PDT treatment, represents a new approach in tumor therapy. Recently, Xiuli Wang's research team successfully applied tumor adjuvant immunotherapy, such as PD-1 antibody-assisted PDT for cSCC and extramammary Paget's disease, with the aim of overcoming tumor immune suppression, enhancing the antitumor immune effect of PDT, reshaping the tumor microenvironment, and improving treatment efficiency. The advantages of PDT—good targeting, repeatable treatment, nonresistance, and the potential to overcome tumor resistance mechanisms—position it as a promising new adjuvant in cancer treatment. It is expected to become a key therapeutic tool for various types of cancers in clinical practice, further enriching the landscape of tumor therapy.

17.3 PDT Clinical Transformation and the Expansion of PDT Indications

Since the initial application of ALA-PDT in skin cancers and Professor Xiuli Wang's pioneering use in treating urethral genital warts in 1997, Wang's research team has consistently expanded the indications for ALA-PDT in China. These include treatments for moderate to severe acne, folliculitis decalvans, and other follicular and sebaceous gland disorders. PDT has also shown good therapeutic effects for common yet clinically challenging skin conditions such as rosacea, hidradenitis suppurativa, seborrhea, lichen sclerosus, and fungal and mycobacterial infections. PDT has significant advantages in treating infectious diseases, as it eliminates the risk of drug resistance. For patients with granulomatous or drug-resistant bacterial infections, where traditional treatments often fail, PDT has promising development potential. Additionally, PDT can damage bacterial biofilms, although research is still ongoing to increase the permeability of photosensitizers. This area needs further development to transition from basic research to clinical applications. For diseases that are difficult to treat with conventional methods (those that have poor efficacy, high recurrence rates, or high risks of complications), PDT presents a valuable new treatment option.

17.4 Painless Photodynamic Promotion and Improvement

Since the inception of PDT treatment, pain has remained a major obstacle, reducing patient compliance and limiting its clinical application. Xiuli Wang's research team reported that PDT-related pain is positively correlated with light power density and pioneered a new type of painless ALA-PDT. This innovation has been successfully applied to treat acne, genital warts, and actinic keratosis, forming a new comfort-focused PDT treatment. Previous studies have demonstrated that a two-step illumination approach can alleviate pain and that, compared with traditional red-light PDT, PDT with sunlight or intense pulsed light results in milder discomfort. However, painless PDT protocols have yet to be effectively implemented in the treatment of Heimpofen and Xipofen PDT, which requires further exploration, particularly for systemic photosensitizers. Moving forward, the development of a painless PDT protocol will improve the patient experience and expand the accessibility of PDT for a wider range of patients.

17.5 Home PDT Treatment

Owing to the proven efficacy of ALA-PDT in treating common skin diseases and promoting skin rejuvenation, coupled with the development of smart PDT devices, the trend toward home use of PDT treatment is inevitable. The creation of a household PDT treatment system that complements hospital-based treatments is promising. This includes advancements in photosensitizers and dosage forms, as well as supporting light sources, household air conditioners, and other medical devices tailored for home PDT use. Innovations such as microneedle patch PSs can help enhance public and home accessibility to PDT treatments, making them more convenient and affordable for a wider population.

As more researchers continue to explore and advance PDT applications, the technology is becoming increasingly refined, with new indications and breakthroughs overcoming previous treatment bottlenecks. Additionally, increasing public awareness of PDT is contributing to its widespread acceptance, propelling treatment to new heights. We believe that "photodynamic therapy in dermatology" will play a pivotal role in achieving this goal, offering innovative solutions and improving patient outcomes in the field of dermatology.

MIX
Papier aus verantwortungsvollen Quellen
Paper from responsible sources
FSC® C105338

If you have any concerns about our products,
you can contact us on
ProductSafety@springernature.com

In case Publisher is established outside the EU,
the EU authorized representative is:
Springer Nature Customer Service Center GmbH
Europaplatz 3, 69115 Heidelberg, Germany

Printed by Libri Plureos GmbH
in Hamburg, Germany